NURSING THEORIES

The Base for Professional Nursing Practice

FIFTH EDITION

Julia B. George, R.N., Ph.D.
Department of Nursing
California State University, Fullerton
Fullerton, CA

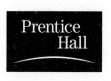

Prentice
Hall

Upper Saddle River, New Jersey 07458

Library of Congress Cataloging-in-Publication Data

Nursing theories : the base for professional nursing practice / [edited by] Julia B.
George — 5th ed.
    p. ; cm.
  Includes bibliographical references and index.
  ISBN 0-8385-7110-7
    1. Nursing—Philosophy. I. George, Julia B.
    [DNLM: 1. Nursing Theory. WY 86 N9755 2002]
  RT84.5 .N89 2002
  610.73'01—dc21   2001036930

Publisher: Julie Levin Alexander
Executive Editor: Maura Connor
Editorial Assistant: Beth Ann Romph/Sladjana Repic
Marketing Manager: Nicole Benson
Director of Manufacturing and Production: Bruce Johnson
Managing Editor: Patrick Walsh
Production Editor: Lisa Garboski
Production Liaison: Cathy O'Connell
Manufacturing Buyer: Pat Brown
Cover Design: Joe Sengotta
Composition: UG / GGS Information Services, Inc.
Printing and Binding: RR Donnelley and Sons, Harrisonburg
Design Director: Cheryl Asherman
Senior Design Coordinator: Maria Guglielmo Walsh

Pearson Education LTD.
Pearson Education Australia PTY, Limited
Pearson Education Singapore, Pte. Ltd
Pearson Education North Asia Ltd.
Pearson Education Canada, Ltd.
Pearson Educación de Mexico, S.A. de C.V.
Pearson Education — Japan
Pearson Education Malaysia, Pte. Ltd

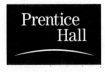

10 9 8 7 6 5 4 3 2 1
ISBN 0-8385-7110-7

CONTRIBUTORS

Janice V. R. Belcher, R.N., Ph.D.
Associate Professor
Wright State University
Dayton, Ohio

Agnes M. Bennett, R.N., M.S.
Assistant Professor, Retired
Department of Nursing
Miami University
Oxford, Ohio

Susan Stanwyck Bowman, R.N.,
  Ph.D.
Professor Emeritus, Nursing
Humboldt State University
Arcata, California

Suzanne M. Falco, R.N., Ph.D.
Associate Professor
School of Nursing
The University of Wisconsin,
  Milwaukee
Milwaukee, Wisconsin

Lois J. Brittain Fish, R.N., M.S.N.
Supportive Home Services Specialist,
  Retired
Riverside School and R. T. Industries,
  Inc.
Troy, Ohio

Peggy Coldwell Foster, R.N., M.S.N.
Perinatal Clinical Nurse Specialist
Maternity Home Care Coordinator
Mercy Hospital Anderson
Cincinnati, Ohio

Noreen Cavan Frisch, R.N., Ph.D.
Professor and Chair
Department of Nursing
Cleveland State University
Cleveland, Ohio

Chiyoko Yamamoto Furukawa, R.N.,
  Ph.D.
Professor, Emerita
College of Nursing
University of New Mexico
Albuquerque, New Mexico

Julia Gallagher Galbreath, R.N., C.S.,
  M.S.
Associate Professor
Edison State Community College
Piqua, Ohio

Julia B. George, R.N., Ph.D.
Professor Emeritus, Nursing
California State University, Fullerton
Fullerton, California

Maryanne Garon, R.N., D.N.Sc.
Faculty
Department of Nursing
California State University, Fullerton
Fullerton, California

Janet S. Hickman, R.N., Ed.D.
Professor, Graduate Program
  Coordinator
Department of Nursing
West Chester University
West Chester, Pennsylvania

Joan Swartz Howe, R.N., M.S.
Assistant Professor in Nursing
Lima Technical College
Lima, Ohio

Brenda Johnson, R.N., Ph.D.
Assistant Professor
Department of Nursing
Southeast Missouri State University
Cape Girardeau, Missouri

Jane H. Kelley, R.N., Ph.D.
Professor
School of Nursing
University of Mississippi Medical
    Center
Jackson, Mississippi

Marie L. Lobo, R.N., Ph.D., F.A.A.N.
Associate Professor
Graduate Program
College of Nursing
Medical University of South Carolina
Charleston, South Carolina

**Charlotte Paul, R.N., Ph.D.,
    F.N.S.**
Professor (retired)
Edinboro University of Pennsylvania
Edinboro, Pennsylvania

Susan G. Praeger, R.N., Ed.D.
Professor of Nursing
Wright State University
Dayton, Ohio

**Joan S. Reeves, R.N., Dr.P.H.,
    C.T.N.**
Assistant Professor
Department of Nursing
University of New Hampshire
Durham, New Hampshire

CONTENTS

PREFACE

A unique knowledge base, and the means to communicate it, are requisite for a profession. Nursing continues to be deeply involved in developing its own unique knowledge base and in educating students about it. In identifying this base, various concepts, models, and theories specific to nursing have been recognized, defined, and developed. Although these concepts, models, and theories have been published in a variety of journals and in books by individual theorists, there is a need for them to be gathered in one volume and applied to nursing practice to help the individual student and practitioner of nursing in making optimum use of theory in practice.

OVERVIEW

Nursing Theories, 5th Edition is designed to consider the ideas of twenty-five nursing theorists and relate the work of each to the clinical practice of nursing. As appropriate, this application to practice may be within the framework of the nursing process or within the framework of the particular theory or model under discussion. It must be recognized that the book serves as a secondary source in relation to the statements and purposes of the individuals whose writings are discussed. It is intended as a tool for the thoughtful and considered application of nursing concepts and theories to nursing practice, and through four editions this book has served students in nursing programs and nurses in this country and around the world. This fifth edition is intended to continue this service.

There are essentially four areas of focus. First, Chapters 1 and 2 present the place of concepts and theories in nursing and discuss the use of theory in nursing practice. These chapters provide a common base for the next twenty-two chapters and should be read first. In previous editions, Chapter 2 focused solely on the nursing process. In recognition of the number of theories that are based in qualitative relations and require qualitative research methods, and thus may be less than compatible with the nursing process, this chapter has been expanded to include other methods of guiding clinical practice.

Next, Chapters 3 through 23 present the major components of the work of Florence Nightingale, Hildegard E. Peplau, Virginia Henderson, Lydia E. Hall, Dorothea E. Orem, Dorothy E. Johnson, Myra Estrin Levine, Imogene M. King, Martha E. Rogers, Sister Callista Roy, Betty Neuman, Josephine G. Paterson and Loretta T. Zderad, Jean Watson, Rosemarie Rizzo Parse, Helen Erickson, Evelyn M. Tomlin, and Mary Ann P. Swain, Madeleine M. Leininger, Margaret Newman, and Anne Boykin and Savina Schoenhofer. Each chapter presents one theorist (or group of theorists) and is a secondary source in relation to the contents of the theory. Each chapter is also a primary source in relation to the chapter author(s)'s work about the application of the theory to practice.

Although an effort has been made to present the information chronologically, these chapters may be read in any order. Each chapter gives the historical setting of the nurse theorist(s) and the specific components identified as meaningful to nursing. This material is drawn from the work of each theorist or group of theorists. The components are then interpreted and discussed by the chapter authors in relation to the use of the theory in clinical practice and to at least the four basic concepts in nursing's metaparadigm: (1) the human or individual, (2) health, (3) society/environment, and (4) nursing. In addition, the work of each theorist is discussed in relation to the theory critique questions included in Chapter 1. This discussion is not to be considered a comprehensive critique of the work but rather an effort to give one view of the strengths and weaknesses of the work, and to stimulate the reader's thought processes about the characteristics of a theory and those of the particular work. The terms *theory*, *model*, *conceptual framework*, and *conceptual model* are not used consistently in the nursing literature. Thus the work being presented may be strongly supported in the responses to the critique questions and still not be generally accepted as a theory. Where there was significant literature, either research, practice, or theoretical, about the work discussed in the chapter, an annotated bibliography appears at the end of the chapter.

Chapter 24 is an aid to the reader for using several or all of these theories in nursing practice in a given situation. This chapter gives some examples of application of the components as a guide and stimulus to the reader's use of theory for professional nursing practice. Chapter 24 will be most meaningful if it is read after becoming familiar with the contents of Chapters 1 through 23. A glossary is also provided for quick reference to some common terms and to terms specific to the work of particular theories.

In reflection of changes in health care practice settings, Chapter 25 presents three models for nursing practice with other disciplines. Each of these models is discussed in relation to their compatibility with the nursing theories discussed in this book. The intent of this chapter is to provide nurses with a framework for interacting with other disciplines to serve the best interests of those being served.

Some of the theorists, as appropriate to their times, used *she* to refer to the nurse, and *he* to refer to the recipient of care. In some chapters, it would have been awkward to change the theorist's use of such words. In these situations, we have indicated that the use is that of the original author. In like manner, we have tried to reflect the original author's use of the terms *patient* and *client*.

NEW TEACHING AND LEARNING RESOURCES

For the first time, both students and instructors can benefit from additional supplements accompanying this textbook. Readers of this textbook can go to the free Companion Website at *www.prenhall.com/george* to access the interactive, chapter-specific modules. Each module consists of a variety of critical thinking and other exercises, links to other online resources regarding nursing theory, and objectives.

Faculty adopting this textbook have free access to the online Syllabus Manager™ feature of the Companion Website, *www.prenhall.com/george*. It offers a whole host of features that facilitate the students' use of the Companion Website, and allows faculty to post syllabi, course information, and assignments online for their students. Finally, online course management companions for *Nursing Theories, 5th Edition* are available for schools using Blackboard, Course Compass, or WebCT course management systems. The online course management solutions feature interactive modules and an electronic test bank for teaching this course content through distance learning. For more information or a demonstration of Syllabus Manager™ or Prentice Hall's online course companions, please contact your Prentice Hall Sales Representative.

ACKNOWLEDGMENTS

A special "thank you" is due the staff at Prentice Hall Health for their help and encouragement during the process of developing the fifth edition of this book. They have been patient, understanding, and supportive during the many changes that have occurred, both within the publishing industry and within the lives of the various contributors to this book, during the development of the manuscript for the book.

Suggestions and comments from users of this text are requested and welcomed.

Julia B. George

REVIEWERS

Patricia Dardano, D.N.Sc.
Regis College
Weston, MA

Alice Gaudine, R.N., Ph.D.
Memorial University of Newfoundland
St. John's, NF
Canada

Mira Lessick, Ph.D., R.N.
Rush University
Chicago, IL

Patsy L. Ruchala, D.N.Sc., R.N.
St. Louis University
St. Louis, MO

Helen J. Streubert, B.S.N., M.S.N., Ed.D.
College of Misericordia
Dallas, PA

CHAPTER 1

AN INTRODUCTION TO NURSING THEORY

Janet S. Hickman

The purpose of this chapter is to provide the learner with the tools necessary to understand the nursing theories presented in this book. These tools include learning the language and definitions of theoretical thinking, acquiring a perspective of the historical development of nursing theories, and learning methods to analyze and evaluate nursing theories. Understanding nursing theory is the prerequisite to choosing and using a theory to guide one's nursing practice.

Nursing theories have developed from the choices and assumptions about the nature of what a particular theorist believes about nursing, what the basis of nursing knowledge is, and what nurses do or how they practice in the real world. Each theory carries with it a worldview, a way of seeing nursing and human events that highlights certain aspects of reality, and possibly shades or ignores aspects in other areas (Ray, 1998). Each theorist was influenced by her own values, the historical context of the discipline of nursing, and a knowledge base rooted in the world of nursing science.

A FEW WORDS ABOUT NURSING SCIENCE . . .

What nursing science is, and what it is not, is a topic of significant debate in the current nursing literature. This is especially true now at the dawn of a new century, after a decade of cost containment, nursing staff reductions, and managed care. Despite a nurse/client-unfriendly health care delivery situation in the United States, thinking about nursing science has achieved some areas of consensus on an international level. The Spring 1997 issue of *Nursing Science Quarterly* presented an international dialogue on the question: "What is nursing science?" In the following responses, note the patterns of agreement of thinking from the different respondents.

Dr. John Daly—Australia

Nursing science is an identifiable, discrete body of knowledge comprising paradigms, frameworks, and theories. . . . This structure is vested in nursing's totality and simultaneity paradigms. These competing paradigms posit mutually exclusive perspectives on the human-universe inter-relationship, health, and the central phenomenon of nursing. . . . Nursing science is in development; it will continue to evolve (p. 10).

Dr. Gail J. Mitchell—Canada

Nursing science represents clusters of precisely selected beliefs and values that are crafted into distinct theoretical structures. Theoretical structures exist for the purpose of giving direction and meaning to practice and research activities. . . . Nursing theories can be learned through committed study, but to understand a theory's contribution to humankind, it must be experienced as a way of being with others. It is within the nurse-person process or the researcher-participant process, that theory can be judged as meaningful, or not (p. 10).

Tuulikki Toikkanen—Finland

In nursing science we are dwelling in questions emerging from human life which are illuminating meanings in relation to the human-universe process (p. 11).

Dr. Brian Millar—Great Britain

. . . nursing science is that body of knowledge developed from questions raised by nurses and investigated by them, concerning the relationship of the human-health-environment (p. 11).

Dr. Renzo Zanotti—Italy

. . . The goal of nursing science is to test new interpretations and to explore different explanations, under general laws, about phenomena referring to caring, well-being, and autonomy of persons as harmonious entities. . . (p. 11).

Dr. Teruko Takahashi—Japan

Nursing science is a unique human science which focuses on phenomena related to human health. . . . Unlike natural sciences such as medicine, nursing science focuses on the quality of life for each person. Therefore, nursing science does not investigate health phenomena based on causality. Health as lived experience is investigated from the point of view of healthcare consumers. . . (p. 11).

Dr. Ania M. L. Willman—Sweden

Nursing as a science has both a practical and a theoretical aspect. The aim to foster human health is the practical aspect. This is an ethical aim because health is viewed as something good. To reach this goal research is a necessity, and this is the theoretical aspect of nursing science which concerns nursing and health (p. 12).

Dr. Elizabeth Ann Manhart Barrett—United States of America

Nursing science is the substantive, abstract knowledge describing nursing's unique phenomenon of concern, the integral nature of unitary human beings and their environments. The creation of this knowledge occurs through synthesis as well as qualitative and quantitative modes of inquiry. . . . Nursing science-based practice is the imaginative and creative use of nursing knowledge to promote the health and well-being of all people (p. 12).

Dr. William K. Cody—United States of America

The discipline of nursing requires knowledge and methods other than nursing science, *but nursing science is the essence of nursing as a scholarly discipline*; without it, there would be no *nursing*, only care. . . . As a *science,* nursing's *richness* is manifest in the availability of cutting-edge philosophies and theories to provide guidance for practice, . . . and a growing body of literature describing nursing theory-based practice. . . (pp. 12–13).

THE LANGUAGE OF THEORETICAL THINKING

The previous section of this chapter presented state-of-the-art thinking about the definition of nursing science from international experts. Clearly it has been a long journey from Nightingale's *Notes on Nursing* (1859/1992) to the state of nursing science in the twenty-first century. This chapter will provide you with the tools to examine the theories that were developed by nurses during this more than 140-year journey. As you proceed through this textbook, the commentary in the previous section will take on new and different meanings to you. You are about to begin a new journey that will take you into the realm of theoretical thinking in nursing as it evolved in the context of nursing history. This journey will provide you with an appreciation of the implications of nursing theory for professional nursing practice, nursing science, and nursing research.

Concepts

The first unit to consider in the language of theoretical thinking is the *concept.* A concept is an idea, thought, or notion conceived in the mind. Concepts may be empirical or abstract, depending on their ability to be observed in the real world. Concepts are said to be *empirical* when they can be observed or experienced through the senses. A stethoscope is an example of an empirical concept; it can be seen and touched. *Abstract* concepts are those that are not observable, such as caring, hope, and infinity. All concepts become abstractions in the absence of the object. For example, once you have become familiar with a stethoscope, you are able to see the concept of a stethoscope in your mind without having one physically present. Abstractions such as caring, hope, or infinity are more difficult to picture, as one has never had the opportunity to observe these concepts in reality.

To understand the presentations of nursing theories in this book, it will be of critical importance to look at the definitions of the concepts provided. Some of the theories will use concepts with which you are familiar, but they may be used in unfamiliar ways; others will introduce new concepts, some with new or unfamiliar labels.

The term *metaparadigm* is defined as the core content of a discipline, stated in the most global or abstract of terms. Kim (1989) states that the functions of a metaparadigm are to summarize the intellectual and social missions of a discipline and place a boundary on the subject matter of that discipline.

Until recently, there was general agreement in the literature that the metaparadigm of the discipline of nursing consisted of four major concepts: person, health, environment, and nursing. Each of these four concepts was presented as an abstraction. Specific definitions of each of the four concepts will differ depending on the author. For the purposes of this text, the following general definitions will be used. *Person* may represent an individual, a family, a community, or all of mankind. In this context, *person* is the focus of nursing practice. *Health* represents a state of wellbeing mutually decided on by the client and the nurse. *Environment* may represent the immediate person's physical surroundings, the community, or the universe and all that it contains. *Nursing* is the practice of the science and art of the discipline.

Current literature suggests that a four-concept metaparadigm for the discipline of nursing is too restrictive. Meleis (1997) maintains that the domain of nursing knowledge encompasses seven concepts: nursing client, transitions, interaction, nursing process, environment, nursing therapeutics, and health. Parse (1995a) states that the major phenomena of concern to nursing include self-care, adaptation, interpersonal relations, goal attainment, caring, energy fields, human becoming, and others. To these, Cody (1996) adds the concerns of nursing's unique traditions of respect for human dignity and the uniqueness of each client—dimensions of the discipline that he believes find no expression in a metaparadigm limited to four concepts and their definitions. Malinski (1995) suggests dropping the entire idea of a metaparadigm of nursing as she considers it to be no longer warranted and states that the development of metaparadigms is an evolving process. She indicates that as nursing is now more diverse than homogeneous, any attempt to provide a simple definition of the scope of the discipline will be so broad as to be meaningless.

Despite the scholarly controversies regarding metaparadigms and their current status (or lack of status) in nursing science, it is important to consider their impact on theory development in nursing. In analyzing the theories in this book, the reader will be able to identify the presence (or absence) of global or metaparadigm concepts upon which the different theories are based (or not based). For purposes of consistency, each chapter will discuss the theorists definitions or viewpoints on the original four concept metaparadigm of person, health, environment, and nursing, as well as consider other concepts in each theory.

Theories

Concepts are the elements used to generate theories. Chinn and Kramer (1999) define a theory as "a creative and rigorous structuring of ideas that project a tentative, purposeful, and systematic view of phenomena" (p. 51). They state that the word *creative* underscores the role of human imagination and vision in theory development, but caution that the creative processes are also rigorous, systematic, and disciplined. In their view, theories are *tentative*, and therefore open to revision as new evidence emerges. Their definition of theory requires that there be a purpose for the theory. Simply stated, a theory suggests a direction in how to view facts and events.

Theories cannot be equated with scientific laws, which predict the results of given experiments 100 percent of the time. Laws compose the basis of most of the natural sciences. As nursing is a human science, the rigor and objectivity of the laboratory are both inappropriate and impossible to duplicate. In the future, the predictability of nursing theories will become more reliable as the research base from which theories develop and from which they are tested grows.

Meleis (1997) defines nursing theory as ". . . a conceptualization of some aspect of reality (invented or discovered) that pertains to nursing. The concept is articulated for the purpose of describing, explaining, predicting, or prescribing nursing care" (p. 16). This definition adds the importance of communicating nursing theory and the purpose of prescription of nursing care.

Theories are composed of concepts (and their definitions) and propositions that explain the relationships between the concepts. For example, Nightingale *proposed* a beneficial relationship between fresh air and health. Theories are based on stated assumptions that are presented as givens. Theoretical assumptions may be taken as "truth" because they cannot be empirically tested, such as in a value statement or ethic. Theories may be presented as models that provide a diagram or map of the theory's content.

Barnum (1994) states that a complete nursing theory is one that contains context, content, and process. Context is the environment in which the nursing act takes place; content is the subject of the theory; and process is the method the nurse uses in applying the theory. The nurse acts on, with, or through the content elements of the theory.

Although some texts differentiate between "theories" and "conceptual models" of nursing, the majority of authors believe that this is an artificial distinction. Meleis (1997) goes so far as to say, "These differences are tentative at best and hair-splitting, unclear, and confusing at worst" (pp. 14–15). For the purposes of this text, the existing nursing conceptualizations presented *are* theories.

Levels of Theory

The level of a theory refers to the scope, or range, of phenomena to which the theory applies. The level of abstraction of the concepts in the theory is closely tied to its scope. Chinn and Kramer (1999) state that theory may be characterized as *micro, macro, molecular, midrange, molar, atomistic,* and *holistic*. Micro, molecular, and atomistic suggest relatively narrow-range phenomena, whereas macro, holistic, and molar imply that the theory covers a broad scope. Midrange theories deal with a portion of nursing's total concern but not with the totality of the discipline. Chinn and Kramer provide the example of pain alleviation as a midrange theory, and the explanation of the physiology of the phenomena known as pain as a possible micro theory. Both of these deal with a portion of a person. Macro theories deal with persons as a whole. These labels are arbitrary and may differ in different disciplines.

Grand theory is also a term used in the literature. It means theory that covers broad areas of concern within a discipline. In the same vein, a *school of thought* has been defined by Parse (1998) as a theoretical point of view held by a community of scholars. It is a tradition, including specific assumptions and principles, a specified focus of inquiry, and congruent approaches to research and practice. *Metatheory* is a term used to label theory about the theoretical process and theory development.

Another way of looking at levels of theory is to look at what it is that the theory does. For Dickoff and James (1968), theory develops on four levels: factor-isolating, factor-relating, situation-relating, and situation-producing. Level 1, factor-isolating, is descriptive in nature. It involves naming or classifying facts/events. Level 2, factor-relating, requires correlating or associating factors in such a way that they meaningfully depict a larger situation. Level 3, situation-relating, explains and predicts how situations are related. Level 4, situation-producing, requires sufficient knowledge about how and why situations are related, so that when the theory is used as a guide, valued situations can be produced. When using this method, one speaks of the relative power of the theory, with Level 4 being the most powerful, because it controls (or does more than describe, explain, or predict).

Worldviews

A worldview is one's philosophical frame of reference in looking at one's world. The worldview of the philosophy of science is that of logical empiricism. This worldview requires that all truths must be confirmed by sensory experiences. Logical empiricism requires objectivity and is relatively value free. Objectivity requires study of the smallest parts of phenomena by using the scientific method. In this worldview, the whole is equal to the sum of its parts. In the literature, this worldview is also called the *received view*. It is from this view of nursing science that the nursing process was created.

One of the worldviews that opposes logical empiricism is that of the human science or the *perceived view*. A human science worldview focuses on human beings as wholes and their lived experiences within a given context.

Parse (1987) posits two worldviews of nursing related to the received and the perceived views. The description of the totality paradigm reflects the received view, while her description of the simultaneity paradigm reflects the perceived view. A basic difference in these paradigms is the perception of person. The totality paradigm looks at the bio-psycho-social-spiritual aspects of person, whereas the simultaneity paradigm views person as an irreducible whole in constant interrelationship with the universe. Theorists of the totality paradigm tend to define health as a state of well-being as measured against norms, while simultaneity theorists view health as something the client determines individually.

Cody (1995) affirms Parse's position on paradigms: "Basic assumptions that Parse made about the totality and simultaneity paradigms ten years ago hold true today. There really are only two sets of essential beliefs about human beings and health in nursing" (p. 146).

CYCLICAL NATURE OF THEORY, RESEARCH, AND PRACTICE

It is important to understand that theory, research, and practice impact each other in circular ways. Middle-range theories can be tested in clinical practice by clinical research. The research process may validate the theory, cause it to be modified, or invalidate it. The more research that is conducted about a specific theory, the more useful the theory is to practice. Practice is based on the theories of the discipline that are validated through research (see Fig. 1–1). Research findings are published in periodical literature and books, are presented at conferences, and are available through abstracts, such as Dissertation Abstracts International.

Research may be based on the received or perceived worldview. Received view research is *quantitative*, where statistical data represent empirical facts and events. The methodology of the research is based on the scientific method. Perceived view research is *qualitative* in nature, based on the thoughts, feelings, and beliefs of the research subjects. A number of methodologies have been proposed to conduct qualitative research.

Polit and Hungler (1995) state that *quantitative* research tends to emphasize deductive reasoning, the rules of logic, and the measurable attributes of human experience. They state that quantitative research methods *generally* focus on a small number of concepts, begin with hunches as to how the concepts are related, use formal instruments and structured processes to collect data (under conditions of control),

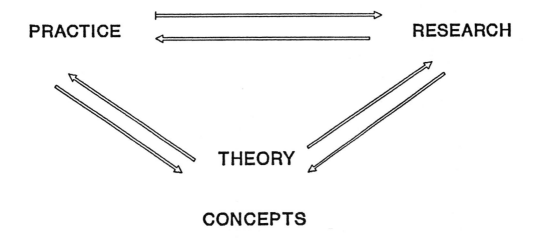

Figure 1–1. Cyclical nature of theory, research, and practice.

emphasize objectivity in both data collection and analysis, and analyze numerical data using statistical procedures.

Qualitative research is described by Polit and Hungler (1995) as emphasizing the dynamic, holistic, and individual aspects of the human experience and attempting to capture those aspects in their entirety, within the context of those experiencing them. They state that research using qualitative methods *generally* focuses on attempts to understand the entirety of some phenomenon rather than focusing on specific concepts; relies on the subject's interpretation of events rather than hunches of the researcher; collects data without formal, structured instruments; does not attempt to control the context of the research, but rather attempts to capture it in its entirety; capitalizes on the subjectivity of the data as a means for understanding and interpreting human experiences; and analyzes narrative data in an organized, but intuitive fashion.

According to Haase and Meyers (1988), quantitative and qualitative approaches differ in the following ways:

1. Quantitative methods assume a singular reality; qualitative methods assume multiple interrelated realities.
2. Quantitative methods assume that objective reality is the appropriate domain; qualitative methods assume that subjective experiences are also legitimate.
3. Quantitative methods are reductionistic; qualitative methods take an ecological view in which they attempt to gain a full understanding of the reality.
4. Quantitative methods reveal the whole through its parts; qualitative methods assume that the whole is greater than its parts.
5. Quantitative methods assume that discrepancies are to be accounted for or eliminated; qualitative methods recognize that discrepancies may be existentially real.

Table 1–1 provides a comparison of quantitative and qualitative research methods.

TABLE 1–1. COMPARISON OF RESEARCH METHODS*

Quantitative	Qualitative
Objective	Subjectivity value
One reality	Multiple realities
Reduction, control, prediction	Discovery, description, and understanding
Measurable	Interpretative
Mechanistic	Organismic
Parts equal the whole	Whole is greater than the parts
Report statistical analyses	Report rich narrative
Researcher separate	Researcher part of the research process
Subjects	Participants
Context free	Context dependent

*Streubert and Carpenter (1995, p. 12)

HISTORICAL PERSPECTIVE

The history of theory development and theoretical thinking in nursing began with the writings of Florence Nightingale and continues to the present. This section highlights significant events in this history.

Florence Nightingale

Nightingale's (1859/1992) *Notes on nursing* presents the first nursing theory that focuses on the manipulation of the environment for the benefit of the patient. Although Nightingale did not present her work as a "nursing theory," it has directed nursing practice for over 140 years.

The Columbia School—The 1950s

In the 1950s the need to prepare nurses at the graduate level for administrative and faculty positions was recognized. Columbia University's Teachers College developed graduate education programs to meet these functional needs. The first theoretical conceptualizations of nursing science came from graduates of these programs. These include Peplau (1952, 1988), Henderson (1955), Hall (1959), and Abdellah (Abdellah, Beland, Martin, & Metheney, 1960).

Theorists of the Columbia School operated from a biomedical model that focused primarily on what nurses do, that is, their functional roles. They considered patient problems and needs to be the practice focus. Independent of the Columbia theorists, Johnson (at the University of California, Los Angeles) suggested that nursing knowledge is based on a theory of nursing diagnosis that is different from medical diagnosis (Meleis, 1997).

The Yale School—The 1960s

In the 1960s the focus of theoretical thinking in nursing moved from a problem/need and functional role focus to the relationship between the nurse and the patient. The Yale School's theoretical position was influenced by the Columbia Teacher's College graduates who became faculty members there (Henderson (1960, 1966), Orlando (1961/1990), and Wiedenbach (1964, 1969)).

Theorists of the Yale School view nursing as a process rather than an end in itself. Their theories look at how nurses do what they do and how the patient perceives his or her situation. Theorists of this school include Orlando and Wiedenbach. Independent of the Yale School, Levine (1967) presented her four conservation principles of nursing.

In 1967 Yale faculty—Dickoff, James, and Wiedenbach (two philosophers and a nurse, respectively)—presented a definition of nursing theory and goals for theory development in nursing. Their paper was published in *Nursing Research* a year later and has become a classic document in the history of theoretical thinking in nursing (Dickoff, James, & Wiedenbach, 1968).

It is important to note that it was during the 1960s that federal monies were made available for doctoral study for nurse educators. The resulting doctorally prepared individuals became the next wave of nurse theorists.

The 1970s

The 1970s was the decade in which many nursing theories were first presented. Most of these theories have been revised since their original presentations. Table 1–2 lists the theoretical publications of this decade.

The 1980s

In the 1980s, many nursing theories were revised based on the research findings that expanded them. In addition, the works of Dorothy Johnson; Rosemarie Rizzo Parse; Madeleine Leininger; and Erickson, Tomlin, and Swain were added to the body of theoretical thought in nursing. The theoretical publications of the 1980s are presented in Table 1–3.

The 1990s

In the 1990s, research studies that tested and expanded nursing theory were numerous. *Nursing Science Quarterly* (edited by Rosemarie Rizzo Parse and published by Chestnut House 1988–1998, Sage, 1999–) is devoted exclusively to the presentation of nursing theory-based research findings and theoretical topics.

Rogers published "Nursing: Science of Unitary, Irreducible, Human Beings: Update 1990," (in *Visions of Rogers' science-based nursing*, edited by Barrett), which is the latest refinement of her theory. Barrett's (1990) text contains 24 additional chapters about Rogers' theory and its implications for practice, research, education, and the future.

In 1992 Parse changed the language of her theory from Man-Living-Health to the theory of Human Becoming. She explained that the reason for the change is that contemporary dictionary definitions of "man" tend to be gender-based, as opposed

TABLE 1–2. NURSING THEORIES OF THE 1970s

Theorist	Year	Title
M. Rogers	1970	*An introduction to the theoretical basis of nursing*
I. King	1971	*Toward a theory for nursing: General concepts of human behavior*
D. Orem	1971	*Nursing: Concepts of practice*
M. Levine	1973	*Introduction to clinical nursing*
B. Neuman	1972	A model for teaching total person approach to patient problems (with R. J. Young)
	1974	The Betty Neuman Health-Care Systems Model: A total person approach to patient problems
Sr. C. Roy	1976	*Introduction to nursing: An adaptation model*
J. Paterson and L. T. Zderad	1976	*Humanistic nursing*
M. Newman	1979	*Theory development in nursing*
J. Watson	1979	*Nursing: The philosophy and science of caring*

TABLE 1–3. NURSING THEORIES OF 1980s

Theorist	Year	Title
	New Theories	
D. Johnson	1980	The behavioral system model for nursing
M. Leininger	1980	Caring: A central focus of nursing and health care services
	1981	The phenomenon of caring: Importance, research questions, and theoretical considerations
	1985	Transcultural Care Diversity and Universality: A theory of nursing
	1988	Leininger's theory of nursing: Culture care, diversity and universality
R. Parse	1981	*Man-living-health: A theory for nursing*
H. Erickson, E. Tomlin, and M. Swain	1983	*Modeling and role modeling*
	Revised/Evolving Theories	
D. Orem	1980	*Nursing: Concepts of practice,* 2nd ed.
	1985	*Nursing: Concepts of practice,* 3rd ed.
M. Rogers	1980	Nursing: A science of unitary man
	1983	Science of unitary human beings: A paradigm for nursing
	1989	Nursing: A science of unitary human beings
Sr. C. Roy	1980	The Roy Adaptation Model
	1981	*Theory construction in nursing: An adaptation model* (with S. Roberts)
	1984	*Introduction to nursing: An adaptation model,* 2nd ed.
	1989	The Roy Adaptation Model
I. King	1981	*A theory for nursing: Systems, concepts, process*
	1989	King's general systems framework and theory
B. Neuman	1982	*The Neuman Systems Model*
	1989	*The Neuman Systems Model,* 2nd ed.
M. Newman	1983	Newman's health theory
	1986	*Health as expanding consciousness*
R. Parse	1987	*Nursing science: Major paradigms, theories, critiques*
	1989	*Man–living–health: A theory of nursing*
J. Watson	1985/ 1988	*Nursing: Human science and human care: A theory of nursing*
	1989	Watson's philosophy and theory of human caring in nursing
M. Levine	1989	The conservation principles: Twenty years later

to meaning *mankind*. The assumptions and principles of the theory remain the same, only the language is new.

In 1993 Boykin and Schoenhofer published their theory of *Nursing as Caring*. They presented this theory as a grand theory with caring as a moral imperative for nursing.

From the mid-1990s to the present theorists have published commentary (and some revisions) about their theories. Selected publications are listed in Table 1–4.

TABLE 1–4. NURSING THEORIES 1990s

Theorist	Date	Title
		New Theory
A. Boykin & S. Schoenhofer	1993	*Nursing as Caring*
		Evolving Theories
I. M. King	1995a	A systems framework for nursing
	1995b	The theory of goal attainment
	1996	The theory of goal attainment in research and practice
	1997	King's theory of goal attainment in practice
M. Leininger	1996	Culture care theory, research, and practice
M. E. Levine	1996	The conservation principles: A retrospective
B. Neuman	1995	*The Neuman Systems Model*, 3rd ed.
	1996	The Neuman Systems Model in research and practice
M. A. Newman	1994	*Health as expanding consciousness*, 2nd ed.
	1997	Evolution of the theory of health as expanding consciousness
D. E. Orem	1991	*Nursing: Concepts of practice*, 4th ed.
	1995	*Nursing: Concepts of practice*, 5th ed.
	1997	Views of human beings specific to nursing
R. R. Parse	1992	Human becoming: Parse's theory of nursing
	1995b	*Illuminations: The human becoming theory in practice and research*
	1996	The human becoming theory: Challenges in practice
	1997	The human becoming theory: The was, is, and will be
	1998	*The human becoming school of thought*
H. E. Peplau	1997	Peplau's theory of interpersonal relations
M. Rogers	1990	Nursing: Science of Unitary, Irreducible, Human Beings: Update
	1992	Nursing science and the space age
Sr. C. Roy	1997	Future of the Roy model: Challenge to redefine adaptation
J. Watson	1997	The theory of human caring: Retrospective and prospective
	1999	*Postmodern nursing and beyond*

The Future

In 1992, Meleis predicted that six characteristics of the discipline of nursing would direct theory development in the twenty-first century. These predictions, which follow, are still valid today.

1. The human science underlying the discipline that "is predicated on understanding the meanings of daily lived experiences as they are perceived by the members or the participants of the science" (p. 112).
2. There is increased emphasis on the practice–orientation, or actual rather than "ought-to-be" practice.
3. Nursing's mission is to develop theories to empower nurses, the discipline, and clients.
4. "Acceptance of the fact that women may have different strategies and approaches to knowledge development than men" (p. 113).
5. Nursing's attempt to "understand consumers' experiences for the purpose of empowering them to receive optimum care and to maintain optimum health" (p. 114).
6. "The effort to broaden nursing's perspective includes efforts to understand the practice of nursing in third world countries" (p. 114).

Meleis (1992) forecasts that nursing theories will become theories for health, developed by nurses, physicians, occupational therapists, and others. She also forecasts that "the domain of nursing that focuses on environment–person interactions, energy levels, human responses, and caring will have long been accepted as a central and complementary perspective in providing health care to clients" (p. 115). She states that neglected aspects of care, such as advocacy, comfort, rest, access, sleep, trust, grief, symptom distress, harmony, and self-care will receive attention and will lead to collaborative programs of research and theory building. Contemporary nursing literature supports the validity of these predictions.

Research

Many contemporary authors state that qualitative and quantitative research are *equally* essential for the development of the discipline of nursing. The theories involved in this research may be single domain theories that describe, explain, or predict a phenomenon within a specific descriptive and explanatory context, or they may be prescriptive. Prescriptive theories reflect guidelines for caregivers and for providing appropriate actions. Meleis (1992) describes prescriptive theories of the future as having three components: levels and types of energy, mind–body wholeness, and environment–person connections.

ANALYSIS AND EVALUATION OF THEORY

Review of the Literature

Meleis (1997) suggests a model that defines theory evaluation as encompassing description, analyses, critique, testing, and support. This model also includes a unique aspect, which she calls the "contagiousness of the theory" (p. 264).

Fawcett (1993) has described theory analysis as the objective and systematic way of examining the content and structure of a theory *without* evaluating or making subjective value judgments about the theory. In her guidelines for *analysis*, the following objective questions are asked:

1. What is the scope of the theory?
2. How is the theory related to the metaparadigm of nursing?
3. What philosophical claims are reflected by the theory?
4. From what conceptual model was the theory derived?
5. What knowledge from other disciplines was used in the development of the theory?
6. What are the concepts of the theory?
7. What are the propositions of the theory? (p. 36).

In Fawcett's (1993) guidelines for theory *evaluation* the following subjective questions are asked:

1. Is the theory significant?
2. Is the theory internally consistent?
3. Is the theory parsimonious?
4. Is the theory testable?
5. Is the theory empirically adequate?
6. Is the theory pragmatically adequate? (p. 36).

A subquestion in Fawcett's sixth question for evaluation is very appropriate in today's health care arena—a question not suggested specifically by any other author in relation to theory evaluation—"Do the nursing actions lead to favorable outcomes?"

Walker and Avant (1995) state that they believe that it is not possible to separate the activities of analysis and evaluation, as analysis requires one to subjectively evaluate the different elements of content and to weight them differently. For example, if one finds the underlying assumptions of a theory to be unclear, unrealistic, or untrue, how one views the rest of the theory will be affected by this view—and this is subjectivity. For these authors, the purpose of theory analysis is to examine the theory for meaning, logical adequacy, usefulness, generality, parsimony, and testability (p. 133).

Barnum (1994) proposes analytic criteria of content, process, context, and goals. Her evaluative criteria of internal criticism include: clarity, consistency, adequacy, logical development, and level of theory development. Her criteria for external evaluation include reality convergence, utility, significance, discrimination, scope of theory, and complexity.

Fitzpatrick and Whall (1996) also propose guidelines for analysis and evaluation. These include analysis of the basic paradigm concepts and their definitions, and internal and external analysis and evaluation.

Alligood and Marriner-Tomey (1997) analyze theory by looking at its structure, its history and background, an overview of the concepts and relationships, and how it directs critical thinking in nursing practice and the nursing process. They do not specify a model or a framework for theory evaluation.

Chinn and Kramer (1999) offer a fairly pragmatic guide to critical reflection of theory. They suggest that one should consider the following five criteria: clarity, simplicity, generality, accessibility, and importance.

Guidelines for This Text

For the purposes of this text, theories will be critiqued using a synthesis of the analysis and evaluation frameworks of Meleis (1997), Fawcett (1993), Barnum (1994), Walker and Avant (1995), Fitzpatrick and Whall (1996), Alligood and Marriner-Tomey (1997), and Chinn and Kramer (1999), with the National League for Nursing Accrediting Commission's (NLNAC) Accreditation Standards and Criteria for Baccalaureate and Higher Degree Programs (1999). Critique, by definition, is the art of analyzing or evaluating a work of art or literature (Webster, 1991). It is assumed that there are both objective and subjective elements to the process of critiquing.

Currently, case management and integrated health care systems focus on the bottom-line, or the profit that can be realized from health care delivery. The system expects favorable outcomes to be delivered in increasingly shorter time frames in order to reduce costs. Advanced practice nurses are being utilized in many settings as physician extenders and nurse practitioner programs have grown rapidly. While this situation has put the discipline of nursing solidly into all realms of care as a primary provider of service, this focus has diverted attention away from nursing knowledge and toward medical knowledge as the base for nursing practice (Fawcett, 1997).

In order to analyze and evaluate nursing theory early in a new century, it seems appropriate to combine the best elements of the traditional academic sense of critique with those outcomes required by the NLNAC for graduates of baccalaureate and higher degree nursing programs. It is hoped that this synthesis blends academic critique with the reality of clinical education and clinical practice outcomes, and retains the important concept of nursing theory as the base for professional nursing practice. This synthesis recognizes nursing theory as a critical thinking structure, which guides the clinical decision-making process of professional practice (Alligood, 1997).

QUESTIONS FOR A NURSING THEORY CRITIQUE

1. What is the historical context of the theory? This first question requires the reader to look carefully at the assumptions on which the theory is built. Are the assumptions based on a specific philosophy and/or another theory—from nursing or a related discipline? Does one need additional study or information to understand the assumptions? Where does this theory fit in the history of nursing theory? Can it be identified as belonging within the totality or simultaneity paradigm or does it rest on a different metaparadigm entirely?

2. What are the basic concepts and relationships presented by the theory? Are the concepts of the theory defined and used in a consistent fashion? Are the relationships presented logically and based on the stated assumptions? Are the concepts and relationships clear to the reader?

3. What major phenomena of concern to nursing are presented? These phenomenon may include *but are not limited to:* human being, environment, health, interpersonal relations, caring, goal attainment, adaptation, and energy fields. Current literature in nursing theory suggests the presence of more than the "original" four metaparadigm concepts of man, health, environment, and nursing. A theory need not address all of the major phenomenon of concern to nursing, but for the purpose of critique it is important to identify those phenomena that *are* addressed by the theory.

4. To whom does this theory apply? In what situations? In what ways? What is the scope of the theory? Does it apply to all the recipients of nursing care in all possible situations? If not, to whom and where will the theory have meaning? Does the theory describe, explain, or predict phenomena?

5. By what method or methods can this theory be tested? Can the concepts and relationships of this theory be observed, measured, and tested using qualitative or quantitative methods? Has testing of this theory occurred? What findings have been presented in the literature?

6. Does this theory direct critical thinking in nursing practice? In what ways does the theory direct critical thinking in nursing practice? Has this aspect of the theory been tested by nursing research?

7. Does this theory direct therapeutic nursing interventions? In what ways does this theory direct therapeutic nursing interventions? Has this aspect of the theory been tested by nursing research?

8. Does this theory direct communication in nursing practice? In what ways does this theory direct communication in nursing practice? Has this aspect of the theory been tested by nursing research?

9. Does this theory direct nursing actions that lead to favorable outcomes? Does the research conducted about theory-directed practice demonstrate favorable client outcomes? With what frequency? In what situations?

10. How contagious is this theory? Who is using this theory? In what context? Is this theory directing nursing practice, nursing education, and/or administration?

SUMMARY

Nursing science provides the basis for professional nursing practice. Nursing theories provide the critical-thinking structures to direct the clinical decision-making process of professional nursing practice. Theory, research, and practice are circular in nature. As new knowledge and discoveries emerge in each of these realms, the cutting edge of the art and science of the discipline of nursing evolves.

Theory development in nursing began with Nightingale and was revived in the 1940s with publications beginning in the 1950s. Theory development has been described from the historical context, as well as current state-of-the-art theory development at the start of the new millennium.

A framework for the critique of a theory has been presented and will be used throughout this text for each of the theories presented. Please refer to chapters on the individual theories for these critiques.

REFERENCES

Abdellah, F. G., Beland, I. L., Martin, A., & Matheney, R. V. (1960). *Patient-centered approaches to nursing*. New York: Macmillan. (out of print)

Alligood, M. R. (1997). Models and theories: Critical thinking structures. In M. R. Alligood & A. Marriner-Tomey (Eds.). *Nursing theory: Utilization and application*. St. Louis: Mosby.

Alligood, M. R., & Marriner-Tomey, A. (Eds.). (1997). *Nursing theory: Utilization and application*. St. Louis: Mosby.

Barnum, B. J. S. (1994). *Nursing theory: Analysis, application, and evaluation* (4th ed.). Philadelphia: Lippincott.

Barrett, E. A. M. (1990). *Visions of Rogers' science based nursing* (Pub. No. 15-2285). New York: National League for Nursing.

Barrett, E. A. M., Cody, W. K., Daly, J., Millar, B., Mitchell, G. J., Takahasi, T., Toikanen, T., Willman, A. M. L., & Zanotti, R. (1997). What is nursing science? An international dialogue. *Nursing Science Quarterly, 10*, 8–13.

Boykin, A., & Schoenhofer, S. (1993). *Nursing as Caring: A model for transforming practice* (Pub. No. 15-2549). New York: National League for Nursing Press.

Chinn, P. L., & Kramer, M. K. (1999). *Theory and nursing: Integrated knowledge and development* (5th ed.). St. Louis: Mosby.

Cody, W. K. (1995). About all those paradigms: Many in the universe, two in nursing. *Nursing Science Quarterly, 8*, 144–147.

Cody, W. K. (1996). Response: On the requirements of a metaparadigm: An invitation to dialogue. *Nursing Science Quarterly, 9*, 97–99.

Dickoff, J., & James, P. (1968). A theory of theories: A position paper. *Nursing Research, 17*, 197–203.

Dickoff, J., James, P., & Wiedenbach, E. (1968). Theory in a practice discipline, Part 1—Practice-oriented theory. *Nursing Research, 17*, 415–435.

Erickson, H. C., Tomlin, E. M., & Swain, M. A. P. (1983). *Modeling and role-modeling*. Lexington, SC: Pine Press.

Fawcett, J. (1993). *Analysis and evaluation of nursing theories*. Philadelphia: Davis.

Fawcett, J. (1997). Conceptual models of nursing, nursing theories, and nursing practice: Focus on the future. In M. R. Alligood & A. Marriner-Tomey (Eds.). *Nursing theory: Utilization and application*. St. Louis: Mosby.

Fitzpatrick, J. J., & Whall, A. L. (1996). *Conceptual models of nursing: Analysis and application* (3d ed.). Stamford, CT: Appleton & Lange.

Haase, J. E., & Meyers, S. T. (1988). Reconciling paradigm assumptions of qualitative and quantitative research. *Western Journal of Nursing Research, 10*, 132.

Hall, L. (1959). Nursing . . . what is it? Published by the Virginia State Nurses Association.

Harmer, B., & Henderson, V. (1955). *Textbook of the principles and practice of nursing* (5th ed.). New York: Macmillan.

Henderson, V. (1960). *Basic principles of nursing care.* Geneva: International Council of Nurses.

Henderson, V. (1966). *The nature of nursing.* New York: Macmillan.

Johnson, D. E. (1980). The Behavioral System Model for nursing. In J. P. Riehl & C. Roy (Eds.), *Conceptual models for nursing practice* (2nd ed.) (pp. 207–216). New York: Appleton-Century-Crofts. (out of print)

Kim, H. S. (1989). Theoretical thinking in nursing: Problems and prospects. *Recent Advances in Nursing, 24*, 106–122.

King, I. (1971). *Toward a theory for nursing: General concepts of human behavior.* New York: Wiley. (out of print)

King, I. M. (1981). *A theory for nursing: System, concepts, process.* New York: Wiley. (Reissued 1991, Albany, NY: Delmar.)

King, I. M. (1989). King's general systems framework and theory. In J. Riehl-Sisca (Ed.), *Conceptual models for nursing practice* (3rd ed.) (pp. 149–158). Norwalk, CT: Appleton & Lange.

King, I. M. (1995a). A systems framework for nursing. In M. A. Frey & C. L. Sieloff (Eds.). *Advancing King's systems framework and theory of nursing* (pp. 14–22). Thousand Oaks, CA: Sage.

King, I. M. (1995b). The theory of goal attainment. In M. A. Frey & C. L. Sieloff (Eds.). *Advancing King's systems framework and theory of nursing* (pp. 23–32). Thousand Oaks, CA: Sage.

King, I. M. (1996). The theory of goal attainment in research and practice. *Nursing Science Quarterly, 9*, 61–66.

King, I. M. (1997). King's theory of goal attainment in practice. *Nursing Science Quarterly, 10*, 180–85.

Leininger, M. M. (1980). Caring: A central focus of nursing and health care services. *Nursing and Health Care, 1*, 135–143, 176.

Leininger, M. M. (1981). The phenomenon of caring: Importance, research questions, and theoretical considerations. In M. M. Leininger (Ed.), *Caring: An essential human need* (pp. 3–15). Thorofare, NJ: Slack. (out of print)

Leininger, M. M. (1985). Transcultural care diversity and universality: A theory of nursing. *Nursing and Health Care, 6*, 209–212.

Leininger, M. M. (1988). Leininger's theory of nursing: Culture care diversity and universality. *Nursing Science Quarterly, 1*, 152–160.

Leininger, M. (1996). Culture care theory, research, and practice. *Nursing Science Quarterly, 9*, 71–78.

Levine, M. E. (1967). The four conservation principles. *Nursing Forum, 6*, 45–59.

Levine, M. E. (1973). *Introduction to clinical nursing.* Philadelphia: Davis. (out of print)

Levine, M. E. (1989). The conservation principles: Twenty years later. In J. Riehl-Sisca (Ed.), *Conceptual models for nursing practice* (3rd ed.) (pp. 325–337). Norwalk, CT: Appleton & Lange.

Levine, M. E. (1996). The conservation principles: A retrospective. *Nursing Science Quarterly, 9*, 38–41.

Malinski, V. M. (1995). Response: Notes on book review of *Analysis and evaluation of nursing theories. Nursing Science Quarterly, 8*, 59.

Meleis, A. I. (1992). Directions for nursing theory development in the 21st century. *Nursing Science Quarterly, 5*, 112–117.

Meleis, A. I. (1997). *Theoretical nursing: Development and progress* (3rd ed.). Philadelphia: Lippincott.

National League for Nursing Accrediting Commission. (1999). *Interpretive guidelines for standards and criteria, Baccalaureate and higher degree programs in nursing.* New York: Author.

Neuman, B. (1974). The Betty Neuman Health Care Systems Model: A total person approach to patient problems. In J. P. Riehl & C. Roy (Eds.), *Conceptual models for nursing practice.* (pp. 99–114). New York: Appleton-Century-Crofts. (out of print)

Neuman, B. (1982). *The Neuman Systems Model.* Norwalk, CT: Appleton-Century-Crofts. (out of print)

Neuman, B. (1989). *The Neuman Systems Model* (2nd ed.). Norwalk, CT: Appleton & Lange. (out of print)

Neuman, B. (1995). *The Neuman Systems Model* (3rd ed.) Norwalk, CT: Appleton & Lange.

Neuman, B. (1996). The Neuman Systems Model in research and practice. *Nursing Science Quarterly, 9,* 67–70.

Neuman, B. M., & Young, R. J. (1972). A model for teaching total person approach to patient problems. *Nursing Research, 21,* 264–269.

Newman, M. A. (1979). *Theory development in nursing.* Philadelphia: Davis.

Newman, M. A. (1983). Newman's health theory. In I. W. Clements & F. B. Roberts (Eds.), *Family health: A theoretical approach to nursing care* (pp. 161–175). New York: Wiley. (out of print)

Newman, M. A. (1986). *Health as expanding consciousness.* St. Louis: Mosby.

Newman, M. A. (1994). *Health as expanding consciousness* (Pub. No. 14-2626). (2nd ed.), New York: National League for Nursing Press.

Newman, M. A. (1997). Evolution of the theory of health as expanding consciousness. *Nursing Science Quarterly, 10,* 22–25.

Nightingale, F. (1992). *Notes on nursing* (Com. ed.). Philadelphia: Lippincott. (Original work published in 1859.)

Orem, D. (1971). *Nursing: Concepts of practice.* New York: McGraw-Hill. (out of print)

Orem, D. (1980). *Nursing: Concepts of practice* (2nd ed.). New York: McGraw-Hill. (out of print)

Orem, D. (1985). *Nursing: Concepts of practice* (3rd ed.). New York: McGraw-Hill. (out of print)

Orem, D. (1991). *Nursing: Concepts of practice* (4th ed.). St. Louis: Mosby.

Orem, D. (1995). *Nursing: Concepts of practice* (5th ed.). St. Louis: Mosby-Yearbook.

Orem, D. E. (1997). Views of human beings specific to nursing. *Nursing Science Quarterly, 10,* 26–31.

Orlando, I. J. (1990). *The dynamic nurse-patient relationship: Function, process, and principles.* New York: National League for Nursing. (reprinted from 1961, New York: G. P. Putnam's Sons).

Parse, R. R. (1981). *Man–living–health: A theory of nursing.* New York: Wiley.

Parse, R. R. (1987). *Nursing science: Major paradigms, theories, and critiques.* Philadelphia: Saunders.

Parse, R. R. (1989). Man-Living-Health: A theory of nursing. In J. Riehl-Sisca (Ed.), *Conceptual models for nursing practice* (3rd ed.) (pp. 253–257). Norwalk, CT: Appleton & Lange.

Parse, R. R. (1992). Human Becoming: Parse's theory of nursing. *Nursing Science Quarterly, 5,* 35–42.

Parse, R. R. (1995a). Building a realm of nursing knowledge. *Nursing Science Quarterly, 8,* 51.

Parse, R. R. (1995b) *Illuminations: The human becoming theory in practice and research* (Pub. No. 15-2670). New York: National League for Nursing Press.

Parse, R. R. (1996). The human becoming theory: Challenges in practice and research. *Nursing Science Quarterly, 9,* 55–60.

Parse, R. R. (1997). The human becoming theory: The was, is, and will be. *Nursing Science Quarterly, 10,* 32–38.

Parse, R. R. (1998). *The human becoming school of thought.* Thousand Oaks, CA: Sage.

Paterson, J. G., & Zderad, L. T. (1976). *Humanistic nursing*. New York: Wiley. (Reissued 1988 (Pub. No. 41-2218), New York: National League for Nursing.)

Peplau, H. E. (1988). *Interpersonal relations in nursing*. New York: Springer. (Original work published 1952. New York: G. P. Putnam's Sons).

Peplau, H. E. (1997). Peplau's theory of interpersonal relations. *Nursing Science Quarterly, 10*, 162–167.

Polit, D. F., & Hungler, B. P. (1995). *Nursing research: Principles and methods* (5th ed.). Philadelphia: Lippincott.

Ray, M. A. (1998). Complexity and nursing science. *Nursing Science Quarterly, 11*, 91–93.

Rogers, M. E. (1970). *An introduction to the theoretical basis of nursing*. Philadelphia: Davis. (out of print)

Rogers, M. E. (1980). Nursing: A science of unitary man. In J. P. Riehl & C. Roy (Eds.), *Conceptual models for nursing practice* (2nd ed.) (pp. 329–337). New York: Appleton-Century-Crofts. (out of print)

Rogers, M. E. (1983). Science of unitary human beings: A paradigm for nursing. In I. W. Clements & F. B. Roberts (Eds.), *Family health: A theoretical approach to nursing care* (pp. 219–28). New York: Wiley. (out of print)

Rogers, M. E. (1989). Nursing: A science of unitary human beings. In J. Riehl-Sisca (Ed.), *Conceptual models for nursing practice* (3rd ed.) (pp. 181–188). Norwalk, CT: Appleton & Lange.

Rogers, M. E. (1990). Nursing: Science of unitary, irreducible human beings. In E. A. M. Barrett (Ed.), *Visions of Rogers' science based nursing* (pp. 5–11) (Pub. No. 15-2285). New York: National League for Nursing.

Rogers, M. E. (1992). Nursing science and the space age. *Nursing Science Quarterly, 5*, 27–34.

Roy, C. Sr. (1976). *Introduction to nursing: An adaptation model*. Upper Saddle River: Prentice-Hall, NJ. (out of print)

Roy, C. Sr. (1980). The Roy Adaptation Model. In J. P. Riehl & C. Roy (Eds.), *Conceptual models for nursing practice* (2nd ed.) (pp. 179–188). New York: Appleton-Century-Crofts. (out of print)

Roy, C. (1984). *Introduction to nursing: An adaptation model* (2d ed.). Norwalk, CT: Appleton-Century-Crofts.

Roy, C. (1989). The Roy Adaptation Model. In J. Riehl-Sisca (Ed.), *Conceptual models for nursing practice* (3rd ed.) (pp. 105–114). Norwalk, CT: Appleton & Lange.

Roy, C., & Roberts, S. (1981). *Theory construction in nursing: An adaptation model*. Upper Saddle River: Prentice-Hall, NJ. (out of print)

Streubert, H. J., & Carpenter, D. R. (1995). *Qualitative research in nursing*. Philadelphia: Lippincott.

Walker, L. O., & Avant, K. C. (1995). *Strategies for theory construction in nursing*. (3rd ed.). Norwalk, CT: Appleton & Lange.

Watson, J. (1979). *Nursing: The philosophy and science of caring*. Boston: Little, Brown. (out of print)

Watson, J. (1985). *Nursing: Human science and human care*. Norwalk, CT: Appleton-Century-Crofts. (Reissued 1988, New York: National League for Nursing.)

Watson, J. (1989). Watson's philosophy and theory of human caring. In J. Riehl-Sisca (Ed.), *Conceptual models for nursing practice* (3rd ed.) (pp. 219–236). Norwalk, CT: Appleton & Lange.

Watson, J. (1999). *Postmodern nursing and beyond*. Edinburgh, U.K.: Churchill Livingstone.

Webster's ninth new collegiate dictionary. (1991). Springfield, MA: Merriam.

Wiedenbach, E. (1964). *Clinical nursing—A helping art*. New York: Springer.

Wiedenbach, E. (1969). *Meeting the realities in clinical teaching*. New York: Springer.

CHAPTER 2

NURSING THEORY IN CLINICAL PRACTICE

Joan S. Reeves
Charlotte Paul

■ ■ ■

The purpose of this chapter is to provide the learner with some ways in which nursing theory may be applied in clinical practice. During the early development of nursing theories, most theorists focused on the clinical practice between an individual patient and a nurse. The focus was on the nurse planning the care for the patient. The locations and types of clinical practice have expanded and changed over the years. In addition, the norms about the relationship between nurse and client also have changed. For example, many current theorists write about partnerships with clients or nurse–client relationships based on human care. This chapter will present the classic nursing process and some of the current realities that have significantly changed the nurse's role in clinical settings. These changes in clinical practice have required nurses to consider new approaches in the application of theory to practice. Nursing theory may shape clinical practice when used within the nursing process, within a process developed by the theorist, or as the practice framework itself. The chapter also will address the approaches used in practice by theorists whose work is antithetical to the classic nursing process.

INTRODUCTION

The beginning texts that introduce students to the practice of nursing are very instructive in providing information about the way in which nursing theory has typically been included in clinical practice (Wilkinson, 2001). In general, theories are used to provide definitions for nursing practice, and the nursing process provides a thinking/doing approach to the provision of nursing care. However, Wilkinson encourages theory-based practice by integrating the use of nursing models/theories in explaining each phase of the nursing process. Although there is a basic assumption by practicing nurses that professional nursing practice is interpersonal in nature, the views of nurse theorists have often been seen to be peripheral to clinical practice. In reality, the nature of the interpersonal relationship is one key difference between nursing theorists. In the traditional theoretical view, the power or control in the relationship is primarily with the nurse; the nurse is the expert and the patient receives nursing care. Theorists such as Henderson (1991), Abdellah (Abdellah, Beland, Martin, & Matheney, 1960), or Orem (1995) would be proponents of this type of relationship. Other theorists such as Parse (1992), Boykin and Schoenhofer (1993), or Newman (1994) would characterize the relationship as "equal partners in process," which implies an equal view of power or control and emphasizes caring. Many theorists fall between these two positions.

Factors that have influenced changes in nursing theory and its use in practice include an increasingly diverse clientele, the move from hospital-based care to community-based care, and more opportunities for interdisciplinary practice. Traditionally, a large number of nurses have been Anglo-Americans who were unprepared to care for people from different cultural backgrounds. Leininger (1995) promotes culture-care based on her transcultural theory and research. Transcultural theories are essential in guiding nurses to provide culturally congruent care with individuals, families, groups, and communities. Transcultural nursing is beginning to have a major impact on clinical nursing practice both in the United States and in many areas of the world.

Over the years most nurses have practiced within hospital settings and are accustomed to providing care for individual patients. Major economic changes and restructuring of services within hospitals have placed a greater emphasis on the care of people in clinics and other community settings, such as group homes and shelters. The client's home has become another major setting for clinical practice. In addition to the nurse caring for an individual, some nurses also care for families, groups, aggregates (populations), and communities. An important question to ask is: "How useful is a nursing theory for various settings and types of clients?" The work of some nursing theorists can be used to guide practice with both individuals and groups, but the assumptions underlying other theories limit their application to specific situations. For example, Betty Neuman's Systems Model (1995) may be used to work with an individual client, or can be used to provide focus and direction in working with a community. The *Community-as-Partner* model developed by Anderson and McFarlene (1996) is based on Neuman's model. However, Orlando's theory (1990) is more useful with an individual client because of the focus on the interaction between a nurse and a patient.

In clinical practice, nurses often find it useful to combine one or more nursing theories with other theories. An example of this type of combination would be a planned change theory. Tiffany and Lutjens (1998) provide excellent critiques in their discussions about the worldviews foundational-to-nursing models/theories and planned change theories. By studying the theories and/or concepts upon which these theories depend, the practicing nurse can choose theories that are compatible and suitable for his or her work in a specific setting.

The practice of nursing is becoming more global (transcultural), more interdisciplinary, and is having a stronger focus on the caring relationship. The number of advanced practice nurses with blended roles is increasing, while at the same time, nursing is also losing power and becoming task oriented through managed care approaches.

This complex practice situation contributes to many theoretical views about the nature of nursing practice. In this changing practice world, it is very important for nurses to understand and use appropriate theories in their clinical work. Nurses also need to test theories in clinical practice settings to support, clarify, or refine theories. Most of the past and current theorists write from a Euro-American perspective or worldview, although nurses from other parts of the world have studied and critiqued their work. Nurse theorists with other worldviews add to our knowledge and practice.

In addition to theories, the classic nursing process, which is a planning and decision-making process, provides the structure for nursing care in a large percentage of practice settings. This process, however, has been simplified over the years by the use of generic care plans, charting by exception, and the use of computerized records. In the next section of this chapter this classic process will be presented and followed by a discussion of some of its current adaptations.

THE CLASSIC NURSING PROCESS

Since the 1970s the "nursing process" has been the label applied to an underlying scheme that provides order and direction to nursing care. Two basic assumptions— that nursing is interpersonal in nature and that human beings are holistic—give guidance and direction to the use of the nursing process, which is a "tool" used by practicing nurses to make decisions and to predict and evaluate the results of nursing actions. The deliberate intellectual activity of the nursing process guides the professional practice of nursing in providing care in an orderly, systematic manner.

As part of the movement toward identifying nursing as a profession, a scientific, or problem-solving, approach to nursing practice was identified as the nursing process (Christensen & Kenney, 1990; Oermann, 1996; Wilkinson, 2001). Nursing is not the only profession to claim a problem-solving approach. For example, health planners have long used a health-planning process that is a problem-solving approach aimed at planned social change (Blum, 1981), and physicians use a specific process of gathering assessment data to make a medical diagnosis. The nursing process deals with problems specific to nurses and their clients/patients. In nursing, the client/patient may be an individual, family, or community, and the nursing process has been adapted for use with each type of client/patient (Christensen & Kenney, 1990; Clark, 1998; Swanson & Nies, 1997).

Students of nursing use the nursing process as they learn to behave as professional nurses in practice behave. In many settings the nursing process is the tool (methodology) of professional nursing practice; therefore, students need to become familiar with it. The nursing process also can provide a means for evaluating the quality of nursing care given and thus be used in demonstrating nurses' accountability and responsibility to the client/patient.

PHASES OF THE NURSING PROCESS

In earlier writings about the nursing process, many authors agreed that four phases, components, steps, or stages were necessary: assessment, including nursing diagnosis or problem identification; planning, including outcome identification; intervention or implementation; and evaluation (Bower, 1977; Marriner, 1975; Mitchell,

1973; Yura & Walsh, 1973). However, in recent years, most authors have included nursing diagnosis as a separate phase (Christensen & Kenney, 1990; Lindberg, Hunter, & Kruszewski, 1994; Oermann, 1996; Wilkinson, 2001). Because of this acceptance, nursing diagnosis is considered an essential component of the nursing process and has been added as a separate phase or component. In 1991 the American Nurses' Association (ANA) published *Standards of clinical nursing practice* reflecting these five phases. In 1998, ANA's revised *Standards of clinical nursing practice* separated the identification of outcomes from the planning phase. Therefore the current nursing process includes six phases:

1. Assessment
2. Nursing diagnosis
3. Outcome identification
4. Planning
5. Implementation
6. Evaluation

Although these phases suggest movement from one discrete phase to the next, it is unusual for such linear movement to occur in the practice setting. In fact, most nurses move freely among the phases in their practice. The collection of data or information (assessment) begins the process. Data analysis leads to one or more nursing diagnoses. An obvious nursing diagnosis, such as altered nutrition in an extremely thin person, may be developed while data collection is ongoing. In emergent situations, implementation of such actions as cardiopulmonary resuscitation in which the desired outcome is obvious may have begun before the assessment, diagnosis, outcome identification, and planning phases could be verbalized. Throughout the phases, *reassessment* can lead to immediate changes in any of the last five phases. Reassessment, the further collection and analysis of data, is a continuous, ongoing process; it is not to be confused with evaluation, which measures outcomes. Reassessment may lead to a change in diagnosis, which could lead to a change in outcome identification, planning, implementation, and evaluation as the process continues (see Fig. 2–1).

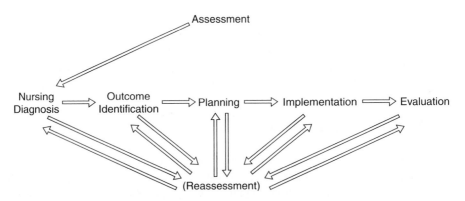

Figure 2–1. The nursing process.

Assessment

Assessment is the systematic and orderly collection and analysis of data about the past and present health status of the client/patient for the purpose of making the nursing diagnosis. It always leads to at least one nursing diagnosis. Inadequate or inaccurate assessment could lead to inappropriate nursing diagnoses, which could focus the rest of the nursing process in the wrong direction. Thus accurate assessment is vital and basic for the effectiveness of all other phases. While assessment is the first phase, the same activities will be carried out as reassessment during any other process phase as new data become available.

Collecting data in a systematic and orderly manner helps the nurse to identify that sufficient data have been collected. The theoretical framework (nursing model or theory, non-nursing model) that the nurse uses provides a scheme for organizing and analyzing the assessment information. Such organization also provides a method for quick retrieval of information needed for auditing professional practice and for doing nursing research. In addition, it serves as a means for communicating information to other health care providers. Several authors have included guidelines for the systematic collection of data (Christensen & Kenney, 1990; McFarland & McFarlane, 1996; Oermann, 1996; Wilkinson, 2001). ANA's (1998) *Standards of clinical nursing practice* also supports the systematic collection and organization of data. A holistic view during the assessment phase ensures that the total client is considered. All assessment guidelines should include the following:

- Biographical and demographic data
- A health history, including family members
- Subjective and objective data about the current health status, including physical examination and reasons for contact with health care professional, medical diagnosis if the client/patient has a medical problem, and results of diagnostic studies
- Generic or folk treatments and/or other treatments for the problem
- Social, cultural, spiritual, and environmental data
- Behaviors that may place a person at risk for potential disease or health problems

By using these guidelines, the data collected are classified into discrete areas that can be compared, contrasted for relationships, and clustered during the analysis of the data.

The biographical and demographic data are generally obtained during an interview with the client, the person responsible for the client, or from the health record (Christensen & Kenney, 1990; Wilkinson, 2001). These data provide a basis for assessing the individual and may provide clues to the client's health status. For example, the age of a client suggests the appropriate growth and development status, and where a client lives may suggest exposure to environmental toxins.

A health history is data about events from the past and present that have, or may have, an effect on the client's state of health now or in the future. The history is obtained through talking with the client or the person responsible for the client (i.e., parent or guardian) and from any available health records. The biographical and demographic data and health history forms may be completed by those clients who are able to do so. In addition, the time spent interviewing and observing the client provides an opportunity for collecting important data that gives direction for the rest of the nursing process, as well as for beginning to establish a therapeutic relationship. If possible, the health history of other family members should also be obtained. Note that the nurse who is initiating the nursing process during a home visit has an ideal opportunity to gain information about the client's usual environment.

Current health status is determined through the collection of objective data (e.g., physical examination, laboratory values) and subjective data (e.g., statements of feelings and beliefs made by the client). For example, a client's description of blurred vision is considered subjective data, whereas temperature, pulse, and respirations are examples of objective data (Marelli, 1992; Oermann, 1996; Wilkinson, 2001). When possible, objective data should be obtained to verify subjective data. For example, the client complains of having trouble breathing (subjective data), which the nurse verifies by observation of shallow respirations and auscultation of faint breath sounds at the bases of the lungs (objective data).

The transcultural nursing assessment also may be obtained during interviews and observations with the individual and/or family. Several assessment guides are available to assist the nurse in understanding the client (Andrews & Boyle, 1999; Giger & Davidhizar, 1995; Leininger, 1991, 1995; Spector, 1996). Information from the guides, along with research findings about a specific cultural group, should assist the nurse in organizing and analyzing the information.

Situation. Janet Carter has come to the ambulatory medical clinic because "I'm so tired." Her medical diagnosis is hypertension. An excerpt of the assessment data collected by the nurse for Mrs. Carter is presented in Table 2–1.

TABLE 2–1. ASSESSMENT OF MRS. CARTER

Biographical Data	Health History	Subjective Data	Objective Data
Client—Mrs. Carter	Spanish heritage	"Fingernails break easily"	Height: 5'1"
Age: 50	Client's parents both have "high blood"	Favorite foods are tacos, pizza, french fries, cheeseburgers.	Weight: 245 lbs.
Homemaker			B/P 172/96
Husband: John	"All my family are overweight"	Beverages are sweetened tea and diet Pepsi.	Skin pale, dry to touch
Age: 55	Shops at small local market		Nails ragged and broken
Day laborer		Dislikes milk, meats, vegetables, and fruits.	
Children:	Usually shops for food daily		Family income below the state poverty level
Judy 19	Responsible for cooking	Has financial problems paying bills and buying groceries.	
Jack 16	No regular eating schedule	States pants heavily after climbing one flight of stairs	

TABLE 2–2. COMPARISON AND RELATIONSHIP OF DATA FOR MRS. CARTER

Biographical Data	Health History	Current Health Status
50 years old	Parents have "high blood"	Height: 5'1" Weight: 245 lbs. B/P: 172/96

After collecting the data, the professional nurse organizes and analyzes the data. This analysis is necessary to form an accurate nursing diagnosis. Analysis of the data involves identifying, comparing, and contrasting each piece of data with the others. The data are also compared to societal norms, taking into consideration cultural differences. The purpose of this analysis is to identify actual or potential health problems. For example, a one year old who is unable to sit alone does not meet the developmental standards for one year olds; this is an illustration of an actual health problem. A 30 year old who smokes two packs of cigarettes a day may be physically fit by all subjective and objective measures today. However, there is a potential health problem of lung cancer or circulatory compromise related to smoking.

Theories are used during the assessment's analysis subphase to organize or cluster the collected data. Data are clustered by creating groups of data that are connected and show relationships in a way that makes sense and can be logically supported. These data lead to nursing diagnoses. The clustering of data in Table 2–2 indicates that the client has an actual health problem in relation to hypertension. The identification of this potential problem is based on age, family history, and obesity, as well as the medical diagnosis. When analyzing the age data, the nurse needs to know what is expected of people during each stage of development. There are a variety of sources in the literature that are useful references for appropriate expectations of development from birth to senescence.

During analysis, gaps in the data may be identified. Questions to be asked during the analysis include: Are additional data needed to logically support the relationships in one or more of the data clusters? Are the data logically organized? If clustered in a different way, would additional data be needed? It is vital that all relevant data be available to ensure the accuracy of the nursing diagnoses. For example, if a comatose person is assessed without the nurse talking with someone who knows the person or without gathering detailed information from the health record, the nurse can be certain there are gaps in the data.

Data analysis also should enable the nurse to begin to identify the client's behavior patterns that either promote health or place the client at risk for poor health. In the case of Mrs. Carter, there is a pattern of poor eating habits as well as poor selection of foods, which may be based on limited finances and cultural heritage. These patterns may have been handed down from generation to generation. In addition, the situation is complicated by the lack of financial resources.

Nursing Diagnosis

The second phase of the nursing process, nursing diagnosis, was recognized in the ANA's (1980, 1995) definition of nursing as "the diagnosis and treatment of human responses to actual or potential health problems" (p. 3). The North American Nursing

Diagnosis Association (NANDA) defined nursing diagnosis as "a clinical judgment about individual, family or community responses to actual or potential health problems/life processes. Nursing diagnoses provide the basis for selection of nursing interventions to achieve outcomes for which the nurse is accountable" (Kim, McFarland, & McLane, 1993, p. 395). The ANA Standards of Care in *Standards of clinical nursing practice* (1998) states that diagnoses are derived from the assessment data and are validated with the patient, family, and other health care providers, when possible and appropriate. The statement of nursing diagnosis identifies an actual or potential health problem, deficit, or area of concern that may be amenable to nursing actions. Models for these diagnostic statements have been provided by many authors, based on the taxonomy developed by NANDA (Berger & Williams, 1999; Cox, Hinz, Lubno, Ridenour, & Newfield, 1997; Craven & Hirnle, 1996; Doenges, Moorhouse, & Burley, 1995; Gordon, 1997; Kim & McFarland, 1997; McFarland & McFarlane, 1996; Potter & Perry, 1999; Sparks & Taylor, 1998; Wilkinson, 2001). It should be noted that the NANDA system is not well developed for family diagnoses so other systems, such as the Omaha System, may be used for diagnostic categorization when working with families as the client (Hitchcock, Schubert, & Thomas, 1999). For most clients, there will be more than one need to be stated as a nursing diagnosis.

The development of nursing diagnosis statements begins with the collected data. The nurse determines which data have been validated and organizes them according to the theoretical framework that is being used. The nurse's knowledge of nursing, science, and humanities concepts and theories is used in this analysis. As the analysis continues, patterns begin to emerge. These patterns can be connected to or associated with appropriate concepts and theories. As these patterns emerge, the nurse may refer to published examples of categories of nursing diagnosis. For example, nursing diagnoses organized by functional health patterns are available to aid nurses (Carpenito, 1999). The written diagnostic statement is based on the conclusions that are drawn from the data analysis. Each diagnosis is based on client behaviors and an area of need. The area of need may currently exist (actual) or be possible in the future (potential). The nursing diagnosis identifies the client's need for nursing. It is important to remember that diagnoses may relate to actual or potential problems arising from the totality of the client and the client's needs.

Situation. Mrs. Carter asks the nurse if having hypertension means she will need to make any changes in how she lives. She says she knows her parents have "high blood" but she is the first person in the family to have hypertension.

For Mrs. Carter, an actual problem affecting her health status can be identified as a lack of information regarding management of hypertension. This identification is based on data about her height, weight, personal nutrition patterns, financial problems, and the indication that she believes she is the first in her family to have hypertension. The nursing diagnosis for Mrs. Carter could be: *Knowledge deficit (management of hypertension) related to lack of information regarding cause, effect, and therapeutic action* (Craven & Hirnle, 1996; Kim & McFarland, 1997). This statement indicates that the client has inadequate information, as determined from assessed and validated data.

The nursing diagnosis may also indicate the areas where information is lacking. This style of nursing diagnosis assists the nurse in developing a plan of action. Following this style, a nursing diagnosis would be: *Nutrition, altered: high risk for more than body requirements* (Craven & Hirnle, 1996; Kim & McFarland, 1997). This statement identifies the need to investigate the client's eating habits, her motivation to change, her food buying and preparation patterns, and her knowledge of nutritional needs.

Other nursing diagnoses for Mrs. Carter may deal with potential problems that can be identified through patterns found in either the initial assessment data or that become evident during reassessment. These problems can be related to significant risk factors that can be modified to reduce the impact of the illness. In this case, a nursing diagnosis could be: *Activity intolerance, high risk of, related to weight as identified by respiratory distress with low level of exertion* (Craven & Hirnle, 1996; Kim & McFarland, 1997). This nursing diagnosis establishes the potential problem (risk of activity intolerance) and identifies the data that support the area of concern. Another way to state this diagnosis could be: *Knowledge deficit (hypertension and exercise)* (Craven & Hirnle, 1996; Kim & McFarland, 1997). This diagnosis implies the need to evaluate Mrs. Carter's knowledge base about exercise and hypertension. It is important to keep in mind that a nursing diagnosis is a statement of an actual or potential health problem that may be responsive to the actions of a professional nurse. It is a problem for which the nurse will assume responsibility and accountability regarding the outcome.

As the nursing diagnoses are identified, they should be ranked in order of priority, based on input from both the client and the nurse. The nursing diagnoses that have the greatest impact on the client, the family, or both and that the client is willing to work on should receive particular attention. The nurse will also consider past nursing experience and scientific knowledge of the needs and functions of human beings in establishing priorities. The prioritized list of nursing diagnoses should reflect the degree of threat each area of concern presents to the level of wellness of the client.

Outcome Identification

To begin the third stage, outcome identification, the nurse and client set realistic and measurable expected outcomes, which are derived from the diagnoses. These outcomes should be culturally appropriate and realistic in relation to the client's present and potential capabilities (ANA, 1998).

In a systematic review of the literature, Jennings, Staggers, and Brosch (1999) have identified four categories of outcome indicators: patient-focused, provider-focused, organization-focused, and population-focused. Of these four, only the first three were found in the literature reviewed. The authors indicate that while population-based measures are discussed in epidemiological literature, measures of population health have not yet been reported. Subcategories within patient-focused outcomes are diagnosis focused and holistically focused. Diagnosis-focused outcome indicators are typically quantitative indicators such as laboratory values, or clinical signs or symptoms. Examples given are CBC, Apgar scores, vital signs, dyspnea, or weight changes. Holistically focused outcome indicators are overall measures of health status or quality of life areas related to health. These are often measured through self-reports or performance on objective tests. Examples include mobility, ability to carry out activities of daily living, patient knowledge, patient satisfaction, or symptom management. Provider-focused outcome indicators may focus on the professional provider or on a family or significant other caregiver. Professional-provider outcome indicators deal with such areas as complication rates, interventions (e.g., appropriate use of medications), or profiles of providers. Examples include the appropriateness of treatment given, sentinel events, or technical proficiency. Family or significant-other caregiver outcome indicators focus on measures of family or caregiver burdens such as caregiver strain and caregiver interaction. Organization-focused outcome indicators involve measures across organizations and may focus on untoward events. Examples include access to care; cost of care; morbidity and mortality data; or rate-based information such as infections, falls, medication errors, and readmissions. Examples of outcome indicators throughout this book will be primarily patient-focused. Provider-focused outcome indicators will be discussed as appropriate for the theory.

The outcomes for Mrs. Carter will be individualized to take into consideration her Spanish cultural heritage, financial situation, and lack of knowledge about her nutritional and exercise needs. Outcome criteria should provide the information needed to evaluate attainment of the identified outcome. They should include who will take what actions under what conditions, how well it will be done, and a specified time frame for completing the actions (Craven & Hirnle, 1996). Many home care agencies use an outcome planner system to aid in the measurement of nursing care. The focus on quality improvement and prospective payment systems has forced nurses to use outcome planning systems (Smith & Maurer, 1999).

The client and his or her family should be consulted before formulating the client's outcomes, which should be realistic and attainable, supportive of the client's needs, and mutually acceptable. Client outcomes are different from outcome criteria. Client outcomes are broadly stated; outcome criteria specify the data needed for evaluating the results of nursing action. Outcomes can pertain to rehabilitation, prevention of complications associated with stressors, the ability of the client to adapt to these stressors, or all three. Other outcomes may deal with the achievement of the highest health potential for a client. A sample client outcome statement would be: "Mrs. Carter will have an adequate understanding of the elements of the food pyramid and their relationship to recommended daily allowance (RDA) requirements within one month." Outcome criteria would be "by (date one month from date of planning) Mrs. Carter will be able to (1) correctly identify foods in all elements of the food pyramid and (2) plan culturally appropriate meals that meet the nutritional needs of herself and her family."

Just as outcomes should be mutually set with a client whenever possible, it is also important for the nurse and client to mutually establish the criteria for evaluation. Criteria are determined from the outcomes and need to be stated in terms of observable behaviors. They may speak to end-behaviors or be used to identify step-by-step progress toward the desired outcome. Criteria are stated concisely in an "act-of-being" phrase. This phrase should contain a performer (the client), a performance (action), and a change in behavior to be accomplished (objective). This expected end-behavior needs to be identified and placed in the proper time frame, and can be used for evaluation. Criteria should define the conditions under which the expected end-behaviors are to occur and should specify the performance level and specific behaviors that will be accepted as evidence that desired outcomes have been met. The behaviors in question refer to observable responses.

Step-by-step criteria related to the identified outcome for Mrs. Carter could be that Mrs. Carter will be able to:

1. Identify the elements of the food pyramid from a chart by the end of Week 1.
2. Prepare a shopping list to include at least two necessary foods from each element by the end of Week 1.
3. Prepare family menus for three days using the elements of the food pyramid as a guide by Week 2.
4. Make substitutions in family menus for three days using the elements of the food pyramid as a guide by Week 3.
5. Evaluate eating patterns of family for one week using the elements of the food pyramid as a guide and identify at least two problem areas to discuss with her nurse by Week 4.

Criteria should be stated in a manner that everyone can understand without having to seek clarification. Robert Mager, in his classic book on preparing objectives, indicates that a meaningfully stated objective would be one that communicates the intent of the individual who stated it. "The statement which communicates best will be one which describes the terminal behavior of the learner well enough to prevent misinterpretation" (1962, p. 11). This statement is equally applicable to outcome criteria.

Time is another consideration when specifying desired outcomes and outcome criteria (both end-behavior and step-by-step criteria). The time frames should be specific enough to provide for evaluation purposes but should be flexible enough that needed changes can be made. Changes in time limits are based on reassessment of the priorities and desired outcomes. It is important to remember to state the outcomes in terms of client behaviors rather than nurse behaviors, which is in keeping with the standards of nursing practice developed by the ANA (1998).

Planning

Planning is the fourth phase of the nursing process, which can be described as the determination of what can be done to assist the client, and reflects nursing actions. The written plan identifies nursing actions designed to help the caregiver give quality client care, and contains relevant nursing diagnoses, expected outcomes and criteria, and evaluation information. In addition, it should become a permanent part of the client's record.

Planning involves the development of strategies to attain the expected outcomes: to resolve actual or potential problems (ANA, 1998; Craven & Hirnle, 1996; Wilkinson, 2001). The plan of care is developed from identified outcomes, which were derived from the nursing diagnoses and established for each nursing diagnosis.

Planning nursing care involves identifying actions to be taken for each nursing diagnosis. Each nursing action is based on scientific rationale and carefully thought out strategies. These actions specify what kind of nursing care is to be done to meet the client's need effectively. Nursing actions should be spelled out precisely, and may include supporting actions taken primarily by the client. Client actions are part of the scheme for providing good nursing care.

It is the responsibility of the nurse to work with the client, the family, or both to select appropriate actions to achieve the identified outcomes. Success will be enhanced when the available options are carefully analyzed and the probability of success in reaching the outcome is evaluated. Compromises may need to be made to provide the best care for the client. The nurse needs to be aware of this possibility when specifying nursing actions.

The nursing care plan deals with both actual and potential problems. The plan serves as a means for resolving problems and for reaching identified outcomes in an orderly fashion. It also provides a means for organization, giving direction and meaning to the nursing actions used in helping the client, the family, or both to resolve health problems. A plan of action is necessary to achieve efficient use of time.

Since the client's condition is continuously changing, the written nursing care plan needs to reflect these changes. Therefore, planning becomes a continuous process based on outcome criteria, evaluation, and reassessment. The written plan is the most efficient way to keep all individuals involved in the client's care informed of modifications in the plan of nursing care. It saves both time and energy by providing essential data for those individuals who are responsible for giving care.

Implementation

Implementation, the next, or fifth, phase of the nursing process occurs when the nurse implements the actions identified in the previous planning phase (ANA, 1998); in short, implementation is putting the plan into action. Other terms used to describe this part of the process are action or intervention. The words *implementation* and *intervention* are not synonymous. Implementation refers to putting a plan into action; intervention speaks to involvement in the affairs of another, a coming between the other and a problematic situation. Therefore, the term *implementation* seems more appropriate to describe this phase of the process since nursing actions flow from mutually established outcomes. The implementation phase encompasses all nursing actions taken toward resolving the problem and meeting the health care needs of the client. It is an ongoing process through which the nurse reassesses, reviews, and modifies the plan of care and, if necessary, seeks assistance in meeting the client's health care needs.

Since the nursing process is interpersonal in nature, it must take place between the nurse and the client. The client may be a person, a group, a family, or a community. The beliefs that the nurse and the client have about human beings, nurses, and clients, and about interactions between nurses and clients will affect the types of actions that both consider appropriate. If human beings are considered unique, then nursing actions should reflect this uniqueness. Therefore, the nurse's philosophy of nursing will affect the nursing actions used in meeting the needs of clients. Yura and Walsh (1973) indicated that the implementation phase of the nursing process draws heavily on the intellectual, interpersonal, and technical skills of the nurse.

Wilkinson (2001) supports the importance of critical thinking throughout the nursing process. Although the focus is on action, the action is intellectual, interpersonal, and technical in nature.

The implementation phase begins when the nurse selects those actions most suitable to achieve the identified outcomes. Just as diagnoses and outcomes have priorities in the plan, actions may also have priorities. The nurse who developed the nursing care plan, other nurses, nursing assistants, the client, or the client's family may carry out nursing actions. In the implementation phase, the nurse refers to the written plan for specific information about nursing actions. Nursing actions may fall into the broad categories of counseling, teaching, providing physical care, carrying out delegated medical therapy, coordinating resources, referring to other sources of help, therapeutic communication (verbal and nonverbal), and serving as a client advocate.

According to the outcomes and criteria for Mrs. Carter, as discussed earlier, several nursing actions could be implemented. For example, under the first step-by-step criterion (identify the elements of the food pyramid from a chart), the following actions could be considered:

1. Establish an agreed upon time when Mrs. Carter could meet with the nurse during the next week.
2. Establish baseline knowledge about Mrs. Carter's understanding of the elements of the food pyramid.
3. Give Mrs. Carter access to charts and booklets containing information about the elements of the food pyramid.
4. Teach Mrs. Carter about using the food pyramid for good nutrition in ways that meet family cultural preferences (base teaching on information gained from baseline knowledge).
5. Focus on the value of the elements of the food pyramid for each family member based on age, height, weight, and activity.
6. Request a return demonstration in which Mrs. Carter will identify foods by placing the food in each element of the food pyramid, and will state why each element is important.

In Campbell's (1980) study of nursing diagnoses and nursing actions, seven categories of nursing actions were developed: assertive, hygienic, rehabilitative, supportive, preventive, observational, and educative. Wilkinson (2001) speaks about preparing to act, action (doing or delegating), and recording. Both point out that almost all nursing actions are initiated by nurses without medical direction. Nurses initiate and carry out all activities that fall within the nursing domain. In the hospital setting, nurses are also asked to assist physicians in carrying out medical prescriptions, to follow institutional policies, and to work with other health care team members. Therefore, nurses need to be clear about their dependent, independent, and interdependent functions.

For every nursing action, the client responds as a total person; that is, as a whole. The concept of holism, which states that a person is more than and different from the sum of that person's parts, means that the nurse may be treating a person's leg but the person will respond as a whole person (Leddy & Pepper, 1998). The concept is useful in thinking about the consequences of any nursing action. For example, the simple action of turning the patient every two hours will have a variety of consequences. Some of these consequences could or should be: (1) increased circulation, (2) improved muscle tone, (3) improved breathing, (4) less flatus (gas) in the intestinal track, (5) prevention of pressure sores, (6) increased or decreased pain, (7) opportunity for communication with the caregiver, (8) increased ability to socialize with the patient in the next bed, and (9) increased or decreased ability to reach articles at the bedside. There may be other consequences that could not have been predicted, such as an opportunity to express values or beliefs. Therefore, in planning nursing actions, it is important to consider the cluster of consequences of both positive and negative value that can be expected to occur with and following each action (Oermann, 1991). Using this knowledge will help the nurse select the most appropriate actions. Although not all consequences are predictable for a specific client, it is possible to develop a general knowledge of expected consequences (outcomes). Knowledge of consequences is an important aspect of the implementation phase of the nursing process. The implementation phase is completed when the nursing actions are finished and the results are recorded against each diagnosis.

Evaluation

Evaluation is the sixth and final phase of the nursing process in which the client's progress toward attainment of outcomes are evaluated (ANA, 1998). Evaluation may be defined as the appraisal of the client's behavioral changes that are a result of the actions of the nurse (Christensen & Kenney, 1990; Leddy & Pepper, 1998; Wilkinson, 2001). Although evaluation is considered to be the final phase, it frequently does not end the process. As mentioned earlier in this chapter, evaluation may lead to reassessment, which in turn may result in the nursing process beginning all over again. The main questions to ask in evaluation are: Were the identified outcomes achieved? Were there identifiable changes in the client's behavior? If so, why? If not, why not? Were the consequences of nursing actions predicted? These questions help the nurse to determine which problems have been solved and which problems need to be reassessed and replanned. Unsolved problems cannot be assumed to reflect faulty or inadequate data collection; rather, each part of the nursing process may need to be evaluated to determine the cause of ineffective actions. The key to appropriate evaluation of nurse–client actions lies in the planning phase of the nursing process. When outcomes are described in behavioral terms with clearly stated outcome criteria, it is easy to determine whether or not the nurse–client actions were successful. These goals become the criteria for evaluating nurse–client actions.

According to Wilkinson (2001), evaluation consists of the following five steps:

1. Review the stated (predicted) outcomes.
2. Collect data about the client's responses to nursing interventions.
3. Compare actual outcomes to predicted outcomes and decide if goals have been met.
4. Record the conclusion.
5. Relate nursing plans and interventions to client outcomes.

The first three steps are specific to client outcomes. Step 1 has been briefly discussed in relation to the planning phase of the process. In addition to stating the desired behavior change, it is also important for the nurse to decide how the change will be measured (predicted outcome and related criteria) and when it will be measured.

Step 2 involves the collection of evidence (data). Although data are collected in both assessment and evaluation, the data collected during evaluation are used differently from data collected during assessment. In assessment, data are collected for the purpose of making a nursing diagnosis. In evaluation, data are collected as evidence to determine whether the goals and outcome criteria were met. This is an important difference to note in using the nursing process.

Step 3 in evaluation is often the most difficult because it is easy to use different measurements in making judgments. For example, if a nurse observed that a client "ate well," would this mean the same thing to the client or to another nurse? "Ate well" could be interpreted to mean that the client was able to chew, swallow, and digest the food with no difficulty, or it could refer to the amount and kind of food consumed. Therefore, in evaluation it is not only important to determine the criteria (objectives) and be specific in predicting outcomes, it is also important to determine the exact way(s) in which evidence is gathered and interpreted to ascertain whether the criteria were met.

In the situation regarding Mrs. Carter, criteria can be mutually set in measurable terms. Using Wilkinson's (2001) Step 1, it is possible to predict outcome criteria for measuring the first outcome (correctly identify foods in all elements of the food pyramid). The predicted outcome criteria could include 45 out of 50 foods correctly identified. If at the end of one month, Mrs. Carter can place 48 foods correctly in the food pyramid, then outcome 1 can be evaluated as "accomplished." Specific evidence has been collected (Step 2) and compared to the predicted outcome (Step 3). The actual outcome exceeded the predicted outcome.

Under outcome 2 (plan culturally appropriate meals that meet the nutritional needs of herself and her family), the outcome criteria could be the following:

1. Her shopping list will include all foods essential for preparing three meals per day for three days.
2. Two foods from each element of the food pyramid will be included on the shopping list.

In looking at the shopping list, the nurse may discover that no dairy foods are included, therefore creating a limited use of one element of the food pyramid. (Mrs. Carter revealed that she and her husband do not like dairy foods.) This information is then included as reassessment data, and the nurse collects information about foods containing calcium that the family can eat. By evaluating the family eating patterns (Objective 5), the nurse obtains information to help Mrs. Carter in choosing foods rich in vitamins and minerals, thereby meeting outcome 2. When predicted outcomes are not reached, reassessment should occur, and the process begins again. If the evaluation shows that the nurse–client objectives have been met, the nursing process is complete.

Evaluation based on behavioral changes is outcome evaluation. There are two other types of evaluation, both of which are reflected in Wilkinson's (2001) evaluation steps.

Structure evaluation relates to such things as appropriate equipment to assess the client or to carry out the plan and to record evaluation conclusions (Step 4). For example, if the scales were inaccurate, then correct data could not be obtained. Structure evaluation may also relate to the organization within which the nurse works. The nurse may be unable to carry out the nursing process appropriately because of agency-created limitations on time; this must be considered as part of the evaluation.

Process evaluation, which focuses on the activities of the nurse, can be done during each phase of the nursing process, or it may be carried out at the end of the process (Step 5). The following are examples of process evaluation questions that can be used in evaluating each phase of the process.

Assessment
1. Were historical data that might be related to health problems collected?
2. Was a physical examination carried out and the results recorded?
3. Were objective data collected by other members of the health care team included?
4. Was the analysis logical? Did it make use of the collected data? Were significant findings mentioned in the analysis?

Diagnosis
1. Was the diagnosis based on the analysis?
2. Is the diagnosis a logical conclusion from the data collected?
3. Were the diagnoses prioritized in a logical and realistic manner?

Outcome Identification
1. Were the predicted outcomes based on appropriate scientific rationales and nursing knowledge?
2. Were the outcomes clearly stated?

Planning
1. Are specific criteria stated?
2. Does the plan rationally follow from the diagnosis?
3. Were goals and objectives mutually established with the client?
4. Is a realistic time frame included?

Implementation
1. What activities did the nurse carry out?
2. What activities did the client carry out?
3. Were the activities consistent with the objectives?
4. What happened as a result of these activities?

Evaluation
1. Were the predicted outcomes achieved?
2. What evaluation methods were used?
3. Were the conclusions recorded?
4. If reassessment was needed, was it carried out?

The nurse and the client are responsible for carrying out outcome evaluation. The nurse, others in nursing administration, or both within an agency typically carry out structure and process evaluations.

NEW FOCI BASED ON THE NURSING PROCESS

The nursing process is a decision making tool by which nurses collect data to be used to support the provision of appropriate care to clients. With the advent of outcome-based care, critical pathways have been implemented as an extension of the nursing process. These pathways are generally developed for specific medical diagnoses in collaboration with other members of the health care team. This care management tool helps in describing how resources will be used to meet predetermined outcomes. It assists in establishing the sequencing of education, discharge planning, consultations, medication administration, diagnostics, therapeutics, and treatments under the guidance of the multidisciplinary team. The goals of critical pathways include: (a) Achievement of realistic and expected client and family outcomes based on norm criteria, (b) Promotion of professional and collaborative practice and care, (c) Establishment of continuity of care, (d) Reduction in cost and length of stay while, at the same time, guaranteeing appropriate use of resources, and (e) Establishment of a framework for continuous improvement in providing care to a group of clients (LeMone & Burke, 1996).

Today as quality is based on expected outcomes, case management models and quality circles have been implemented to improve the proficiency of nursing care through meeting the expected outcome criteria. As the traditional nursing role moves into the modern day of case managers, the nursing process remains the core by which decisions are made (Krul, 1998, Nov. 30). The case management team uses clinical pathways to assist in assessing, planning, implementing, and evaluating care. A clinical pathway provides nursing with a standard of care for a specific client population by which evaluation of care can occur. It also assists nurses in determining if the care being provided is meeting the standards as established (Gardner, Allhusen, Kann, & Tobin, 1997). These data assist nursing in improving care to clients, thus improving the allocation of resources and providing data for the justification of nursing workloads and cost factors.

In summary, the nursing process is the tool or methodology of professional nursing that assists nurses in arriving at decisions and helps them predict and evaluate consequences. To use the nursing process successfully, a nurse needs to apply concepts and theories from nursing; from biological, physical, and behavioral sciences; and from the humanities, to provide a rationale for decision making, judgments, interpersonal relationships, and actions. The six phases considered necessary to the nursing process are: assessment, nursing diagnosis, outcome identification, planning, implementation, and evaluation. As new foci evolve in health care today, clinical pathways have been implemented as a tool for case management models and quality circles. These models continue to use the nursing process as the core for decision making in determining if nursing care to clients is meeting the expected outcomes as established by the clinical pathways.

Students who are learning about the use of the nursing process need to use many references to augment their knowledge and skills as they proceed. The citations in this chapter reflect both historical and current materials.

Several nursing theorists have questioned the use of the nursing process. For example, Henderson (1980, 1982, 1987) has questioned if the problem-solving approach identified as the nursing process is truly unique to nursing, if problem solving is all there is to the practice of nursing, where the art of nursing fits in such a problem-solving approach, and how the process can be used in working with other members of the health care team. Parse (1981) states that the totality paradigm, and in particular her theoretical approach to nursing, is incompatible with the nursing process. Newman (1994) indicates disagreement with the concept of the nurse as the problem solver.

OTHER USE OF NURSING THEORY IN CLINICAL PRACTICE

Many nursing theorists have developed their own process or methodology for nursing practice. Orem (1995) describes a three-step process involving nursing diagnosis and prescription, nursing system design, and nursing system production and management. Orlando (1972) speaks to the disciplined process of nursing that involves patient behavior expressing a need for help, the nurse's reaction, and nurse action. Wiedenbach (1977) presents both a nursing process and a description of nursing practice. In her process she describes seven types of cognitive process in the nurse, each associated with an involuntary or voluntary action. Her description of nursing practice involves observation, ministration of help, and validation. These processes are presented in more detail in the appropriate theory chapters. In some cases, they will be demonstrated to be congruent with the nursing process.

There are several nursing theorists who find the classical nursing process incompatible with their theories. They take issue with the idea that the nurse is the problem solver and the focus on diagnosis, decision making, and problem solving, which are key components of the nursing process. Theorists who conceptualize care as the essence of nursing (Boykin & Schoenhofer, 1993; Leininger, 1995) or who believe that nursing's goal is based on a caring or "being with" process (Newman, 1994; Paterson & Zderad, 1988; Watson, 1987) take issue with the professionally controlled nursing process in which diagnostic categories and outcome criteria are standardized. For example, Leininger (1995) states the following:

> Currently, nursing diagnostic labels have been derived from Western nursing cultures and most fail to fit non-Western or underrepresented cultures such as minorities or subcultures. To label a client's behavior and needs in ways that are inaccurate creates ethical problems and leads to a host of other serious problems. Most nursing diagnostic taxonomies are still too biomedically focused, culture-bound, and do not reflect theory-based knowledge. They fail to include cultural language terms and specific emic cultural data. Many cultural knowledge deficits exist with the NANDA or modified nursing diagnoses. (p. 120)

Parse (1992) believes that clinical practice is being with a person and helping the person to gain harmony and to promote self-knowledge and self-healing. This clinical approach is based on a caring process, not a problem solving process, although the person may resolve problems through the interaction. Newman (1994) believes that the professional enters into a partnership with the client and that the client is seeking a partner for an authentic relationship where both people will emerge at a higher level of consciousness. Erickson, Tomlin, and Swain (1983) state that nursing requires a trusting relationship, the nurse needs to understand the client's world, and that individualized care needs to be based on the client's model of the world. Boykin and Schoenhofer (1993) describe nursing as caring and being with the other.

Both the theorists who see human caring as central to nursing and the theorists who focus on the relationship between the nurse and client strongly support partnerships where both the nurse and client (individual, family, or group) explore ideas and create meanings as they grow in their relationship together. Therefore, standardized outcomes cannot be established during a particular stage of the nursing process, but continue and may never be fully disclosed.

In examining much of current clinical practice, applying these theorists' views is a challenge when the bottom line is based on cost and time, except in specific situations such as hospice care. The nursing profession may miss valuable opportunities for meaningful clinical practice and clients may seek others who can provide care congruent with their needs, such as traditional healers or other holistic practitioners, if the profession does not continue to explore the relevance of theories in practice settings.

SUMMARY

Nursing theories may be used in clinical practice in a variety of ways. They may be used as the framework for practice by themselves, used in the practice methodology or process developed by the individual theorist, or used within the nursing process to guide and structure each of the phases of that process. This chapter has presented a general overview of the first two mechanisms and detailed review of the nursing process. Each of the theory chapters will present an application of the theory to a clinical case setting using one of these methods.

REFERENCES

Abdellah, F. G., Beland, I. L., Martin, A., & Matheney, R. V. (1960). *Patient-centered approaches to nursing.* New York: Macmillan. (out of print)

American Nurses' Association. (1991). *Standards of clinical nursing practice.* Washington, DC: American Nurses Publishing.

American Nurses' Association. (1998). *Standards of clinical nursing practice.* Washington, DC: American Nurses Publishing.

American Nurses' Association. (1980). *Nursing: A social policy statement.* Washington: American Nurses Publishing.

American Nurses' Association. (1995). *Nursing: A social policy statement.* Washington: American Nurses Publishing.

Anderson, E. T., & McFarlane, J. M. (1996). *Community as partner* (2nd ed.). Philadelphia: Lippincott.

Andrews, M. M., & Boyle, J. S. (1999). *Transcultural concepts in nursing care* (3rd ed.). Philadelphia: Lippincott.

Berger, K. J., & Williams, M. B. (1999). *Fundamentals of nursing: Collaborating for optimal health* (2nd ed.). Stamford, CT: Appleton & Lange.

Blum, H. L. (1981). *Planning of health* (2nd ed.). New York: Human Sciences.

Boykin, A., & Schoenhofer, S. (1993). *Nursing as caring: A model for transforming practice* (Pub. No. 15-2549). New York: National League for Nursing Press.

Bower, E. L. (1977). *The process of planning nursing care—A model for practice.* St. Louis: Mosby.

Campbell, C. (1980). *Nursing diagnosis and intervention in nursing practice.* New York: Wiley.

Carpenito, L. J. (1999). *Nursing diagnosis: Application to clinical practice* (8th ed.). Philadelphia: Lippincott Williams & Wilkins.

Christensen, P. J., & Kenney, J. W. (1990). *Nursing process—Application of conceptual models* (3rd ed.). St. Louis: Mosby.

Clark, M. J. (1998). *Nursing in the community* (2nd ed.). Stamford, CT: Appleton & Lange.

Craven, R. F., & Hirnle, C. J. (1996). *Fundamentals of nursing: Human health and function* (2nd ed.). Philadelphia: Lippincott.

Cox, H. C., Hinz, M. D., Lubno, M. A., Ridenour, N. A., & Newfield, S. A. (1997). *Clinical applications of nursing diagnosis* (3rd ed.). Philadelphia: Davis.

Doenges, M. E., Moorhouse, M. F., & Burley, J. T. (1995). *Application of nursing process and nursing diagnosis.* Philadelphia: Davis.

Erickson, H., Tomlin, E. M., & Swain, M. A. (1983). *Modeling and role modeling: A theory and paradigm for nursing.* Lexington, SC: Pine Press.

Gardner, G., Allhusen, J., Kamm, J., & Tobin, J. (1997). Determining the cost of care through clinical pathways. *Nursing Economics, 15* (4), 213.

Giger, J. N., & Davidhizar, R. E. (1995). *Transcultural nursing: Assessment and intervention* (2nd ed.). St. Louis: Mosby.

Gordon, M. (1997). *Manual of nursing diagnoses, 1997–1998.* St. Louis: Mosby Year Book.

Henderson, V. (1980). Nursing—Yesterday and tomorrow. *Nursing Times, 76,* 905–907.

Henderson, V. (1982). The nursing process—Is the title right? *Journal of Advanced Nursing, 7,* 103–109.

Henderson, V. (1987). Nursing process—A critique. *Holistic Nursing Practice, 1,* 7–18.

Henderson, V. (1991). *The nature of nursing: A definition and its implications for practice, research, and education. Reflections after 25 years* (Pub. No. 15-2346). New York: National League for Nursing Press.

Hitchcock, J. E., Schubert, P. E., & Thomas, S. A. (1999). *Community health nursing: Caring in action.* Albany: Delmar Publications.

Jennings, B. M., Staggers, N., & Brosch, L. R. (1999). A classification scheme for outcome indicators. *Image: Journal of Nursing Scholarship, 31,* 381–388.

Kim, M. J., McFarland, G. K., & McLane, A. M. (1993). *Pocket guide to nursing diagnoses* (5th ed.). St. Louis: Mosby.

Kim, M. J., & McFarland, G. K. (1997). *Pocket guide to nursing diagnoses* (7th ed.). St. Louis: Mosby.

Krul, R. (1998, November 30). Nurses as case managers: An evolution of the nursing process, *Nursing Spectrum,* 4.

Leddy, S., & Pepper, J. M. (1998). *Conceptual bases of professional nursing* (4th ed.). Philadelphia: Lippincott Williams & Wilkins.

Leininger, M. M. (Ed.). (1991). *Culture care diversity & universality: A theory of nursing* (Pub. No. 15-2402). New York: National League for Nursing Press.

Leininger, M. M. (1995). *Transcultural nursing: Concepts, theories, research & practices* (2nd ed.). New York: McGraw-Hill.

LeMone, P., & Burke, K. M. (1996). *Medical surgical nursing: Critical thinking in client care.* Menlo Park, CA: Addison-Wesley.

Lindberg, J. B., Hunter, M. L., & Kruszewski, A. Z. (1994). *Introduction to nursing: Concepts, issues, and opportunities* (2nd ed.). Philadelphia: Lippincott.

McFarland, G. K., & McFarlane, E. A. (1996). *Nursing diagnosis & intervention* (3rd ed.). St. Louis: Mosby Year Book.

Mager, R. (1962). *Preparing instructional objectives.* Palo Alto, CA: Fearon.

Marrelli, T. M. (1992). *Nursing documentation handbook.* St. Louis: Mosby.

Marriner, A. (1975). *The nursing process: A scientific approach to nursing care.* St.Louis: Mosby.

Mitchell, P. H. (1973). *Concepts basic to nursing.* New York: McGraw-Hill.

Neuman, B. (1995). *The Neuman Systems Model* (3rd ed.). Norwalk, CT: Appleton & Lange.

Newman, M. A. (1994). *Health as expanding consciousness* (2nd ed.) (Pub. No. 14-2626). New York: National League for Nursing Press.

Oermann, M. H. (1996). *Professional nursing practice: A conceptual approach* (2nd ed.). Philadelphia: Lippincott.

Orem, D. E. (1995). *Nursing: Concepts of practice* (5th ed.). St. Louis: Mosby Year Book.

Orlando, I. J. (1972). *The discipline and teaching of nursing process.* New York: G. P. Putnam's Sons. (out of print)

Orlando, I. J. (1990). *The dynamic nurse–patient relationship: Function, process and principles.* New York: National League for Nursing. (Reprinted from 1961, New York: G. P. Putnam's Sons).

Parse, R. R. (1992). Human becoming: Parse's theory of nursing. *Nursing Science Quarterly, 5,* 147.

Paterson, J., & Zderad, L. (1988). *Humanistic nursing* (Pub. No. 41-2218). New York: National League for Nursing. (Originally published, 1976, Wiley).

Potter, P. A., & Perry, A. G. (1999). *Basic nursing: A critical thinking approach.* St. Louis: Mosby.

Smith, C. M., & Maurer, F. A. (1999). *Community health nursing: Theory and practice* (2nd ed.). Philadelphia: Saunders.

Sparks, S. M., & Taylor, C. M. (1998). *Nursing diagnosis reference manual* (4th ed.). Springhouse, PA: Springhouse.

Spector, R. E. (1996). *Guide to heritage assessment and health traditions.* Stamford, CT: Appleton & Lange.

Swanson, J. M., & Nies, M. A. (1997). *Community health nursing* (2nd ed.). Philadelphia: Saunders.

Tiffany, C., & Lutjens, L. (1998). *Planned change theories for nursing: Review, analysis, and implications.* Thousand Oaks, CA: Sage.

Watson. J. (1987). Academic and clinical collaboration: Advancing the art and science of human caring. *Community Nursing Research, 20,* 1–16.

Wiedenbach, E. (1977). The nursing process in maternity nursing. In J. P. Clausen, M. H. Flook, & B. Ford. *Maternity nursing today* (2nd ed.) (pp. 39–51). New York: McGraw-Hill.

Wilkinson, J. M. (2001). *Nursing process: A critical thinking approach* (3rd ed.). Upper Saddle River, NJ: Prentice-Hall.

Yura, H., & Walsh, M. B. (1973). *The nursing process: Assessing, planning, implementing, evaluating* (2nd ed.). New York: Appleton-Century-Crofts.

CHAPTER 3

ENVIRONMENTAL MODEL
FLORENCE NIGHTINGALE

Marie L. Lobo

■ ■ ■

Florence Nightingale was born in Florence, Italy, on May 12, 1820, during one of her parents' extensive trips abroad. As she grew up, her father provided her with a very broad education, which was unusual for Victorian women. According to her biographer, Sir Thomas Cook, Nightingale was a linguist; had a broad knowledge of science, mathematics, literature, and the arts; was well read in philosophy, history, politics, and economics; and as well was knowledgeable about the workings of government. She wanted to do more with her life than become an idle wife of an aristocrat. She had a strong belief in God, and for a time believed she had a religious calling.

Nightingale became a heroine in Great Britain as a result of her work in the Crimean War. Her description of the very poor sanitary conditions in the hospital wards at Scutari is overwhelming. She fought the bureaucracy for bandages, food, fresh bedding, and cleaning supplies for the invalid soldiers. At times she bought supplies with her own money. She demonstrated great concern for the well-being of the English soldier—well, injured, or sick—including assisting with the establishment of a laundry, a library, assistance with letter writing, a banking system so the soldiers could save their pay, and a hospital for the families who accompanied the soldiers to war. As well, she provided comfort to the critically ill and dying. Her managerial skills were often greater than those of many officers in the army. She spent the years after the Crimea establishing schools of nursing and influencing public policy by lobbying her acquaintances about various of her concerns.

Nightingale was romanticized by Henry Wadsworth Longfellow in his poem The Lady with the Lamp. *Although this poem was meant to honor Nightingale, it may have done a great disservice to her because it ignored her superb management skills and ability to provide nursing care to both healthy and ill soldiers. Nightingale died on August 13, 1910, and she is honored each year in a commemorative service at St. Margaret's Church, East Wellow, Great Britain, where she is buried.*

Nightingale is viewed as the mother of modern nursing. She synthesized information gathered in many of her life experiences to assist her in the development of modern nursing. Her place in history has been established. To understand how Nightingale developed her conceptualization of nursing it is helpful to review her roots. As noted, she was highly educated for a woman of the Victorian era. In seeking to use her knowledge, she was frustrated by prevailing social norms. Her desire to have a position that was useful to society was incompatible with nineteenth-century upper class British society's expectations of women. While Nightingale was struggling with decisions about her life, the seeds of modern nursing were being planted in Germany.

Germany was the site of the first organized nursing school. In 1836 Pastor Theodor Fliedner, a protestant pastor in Kaiserswerth, Germany, opened a hospital in a "vacant textile factory with one patient, one nurse, and a cook" (Hegge, 1990, p. 74). When Fliedner realized there was no work force for the hospital, he designed a school of nursing. The physician for Fliedner's hospital spent one hour a week teaching the nursing students. Gertrude Reichardt, the physician's daughter, taught anatomy and physiology, although her only experience had been gained at her father's side. Reichardt became the first matron of the Deaconess School of Nursing. Local peasant girls were taught hygiene, manners, and ladylike behavior as well as how to read, write, and calculate. There were no textbooks for nursing until 1837, when a German physician prepared a handbook.

Nightingale visited Kaiserswerth for 14 days in 1850 after a trip to Egypt. She applied for admission to the school with a 12-page, handwritten "curriculum" stating her reasons for wanting to be a nurse and entered the nursing program July 6, 1851, as the 134th nursing student to attend the Fliedner School of Nursing. She left Kaiserswerth on October 7, 1851, and was deemed to be educated as a nurse (Hegge, 1990). During the three months she spent studying with the sisters of Kaiserswerth, she developed both nursing care and management skills, which she took back to England.

When Nightingale returned to England, she used the information from Kaiserswerth to champion her cause as a reformer for the health and well-being of the citizens. Her reform efforts occurred in part because she was frustrated with the conditions in England that limited women's life choices to "indolence, marriage, or servitude," as well as with the two existing social conditions of most of England's citizens: abject poverty and affluence (Nightingale, 1860).

In 1854 Nightingale went to the front of the Crimean War at the request of her friend, Sir Sidney Herbert, Secretary at War. She arrived in Scutari on November 5, 1854, accompanied by 38 nurses. Nightingale's 19-month stay at Scutari was difficult. The idea of women being involved in the affairs of the military was difficult for many to accept. The hospital barracks were infested with fleas and rats, and sewage flowed under the wards. The mortality rate at the hospital was 42.7 percent of those treated, a mortality rate that was higher from disease than from war injuries (Cohen, 1984). Six months after Nightingale came to Scutari the mortality rate at the hospital dropped to 2.2 percent. Nightingale achieved this drop in mortality by attending to the environment of the soldiers. One year and nine months after she landed at Scutari, on August 5, 1856, Nightingale returned from the Crimea. She sneaked into England to avoid a hero's welcome.

After her return to England, Nightingale used her knowledge of data concerning the health and well-being of soldiers to influence the decisions of the War Department by providing information to Sir Sidney Herbert. Many of the position papers and reports, although officially submitted by Sir Sidney Herbert, Secretary at War, were virtually intact manuscripts written by Nightingale. Because of the position of women in Victorian England, she was not permitted to submit her findings under her own name.

Nightingale was also a skilled statistician who used statistics to present her case for hospital reform. According to Cohen "the idea of using statistics for such a purpose—to analyze social conditions and the effectiveness of public policy—is commonplace today, but at that time it was not" (Cohen, 1984, p. 132). Nightingale was regarded as a pioneer in the graphic display of statistics and was elected a fellow of the Royal Statistical Society in 1858. In 1874 an honorary membership in the American Statistical Association was bestowed on her (Agnew, 1958; Nightingale, 1859/1992). Given her reliance on observable data to support her position, it can be said that Nightingale was the first nurse researcher.

NIGHTINGALE'S APPROACH TO NURSING

Nightingale used her broad base of knowledge, her understanding of the incidence and prevalence of disease, and her acute powers of observation to develop an approach to nursing as well as to the management and construction of hospitals. Nightingale's main focus was the control of the environment of individuals and families, both healthy and ill. She discussed the need for ventilation and light in sickrooms, proper disposal of sewage, and appropriate nutrition. Her most frequently cited work, *Notes on nursing*, was written not as a nursing text but to "give hints for thought to women who have personal charge of the health of others" (Nightingale, 1859/1992, preface). She did not intend for *Notes on nursing* to become a manual for teaching nurses to nurse. Rather, *Notes on nursing* is a thought-provoking essay on the organization and manipulation of the environment of those persons requiring nursing care. Nightingale stated that her purpose was "everyday sanitary knowledge, or the knowledge of nursing, or in other words, of how to put the constitution in such a state as that it will have no disease, or that it can recover from disease" (Nightingale, 1859/1992, preface). She wanted women to teach themselves to nurse and viewed *Notes on nursing* as hints to enable them to do this. Nightingale viewed disease as a reparative process, a thought that is reflected in the American Nurses' Association *Social Policy Statement* that nursing is the diagnosis and treatment of human responses to actual or potential health problems (American Nurses' Association, 1995).

Although *Notes on nursing* is Nightingale's most accessible work, she also wrote *Notes on hospitals* and *Introductory notes on lying-in institutions* (the first maternity centers), as well as numerous letters (Vicinus & Nergaard, 1990). In her volumes of writing she provided much information on the influence of the environment on the human being and the critical nature of balance between the human and his or her environment. For example, Nightingale did not view pregnancy as a disease and recommended facilities away from those treating diseases in which women could bear their babies. She analyzed data from the Midwifery Department of King's College Hospital concerning the mortality rate in childbearing and recommended environmental changes and handwashing to decrease puerperal fever, then the leading cause of maternal death (Nightingale, 1871).

NIGHTINGALE'S ENVIRONMENTAL MODEL

Webster (1991) defines environment as the surrounding matters that influence or modify a course of development. According to Miller (1978) the system must interact and adjust to its environment. Nightingale viewed the manipulation of the physical environment as a major component of nursing care. She identified health of houses, ventilation and warming, light, noise, variety, bed and bedding, cleanliness of rooms and walls, personal cleanliness, and nutrition as major areas of the environment the nurse could control. When one or more aspects of the environment are out of balance, the client must use increased energy to counter the environmental stress. These stresses drain the client of energy needed for healing. These aspects of the physical environment are also influenced by the social and psychological environment of the individual. Nightingale addressed these aspects of the environment in chapters titled "Chattering hopes and advices," "Petty management," "Observations of the sick," and "Variety." Although Nightingale did not address political activism in *Notes on nursing*, her life was a model of political involvement. She was very knowledgeable about current affairs and wrote many letters attempting to influence the health of individuals, families, and communities.

Health of Houses

In *Notes on nursing* Nightingale discussed the importance of the health of houses as being closely related to the presence of pure air, pure water, efficient drainage, cleanliness, and light. To support the importance of hospital-based nursing attending to these, Nightingale (1859/1992) said, "Badly constructed houses do for the healthy what badly constructed hospitals do for the sick. Once insure that the air is stagnant and sickness is certain to follow" (p. 15). Nightingale also noted that the cleanliness outside the house affected the inside. Just as Nightingale noted that dung heaps affected the health of houses in her time, so too can modern families be affected by toxic waste, contaminated water, and polluted air.

Ventilation and Warming

In her chapter on ventilation and warming, Nightingale (1859/1992) stated it was essential to "keep the air he breathes as pure as the external air, without chilling him" (p. 8). She urged the caregiver to consider the source of the air in the patient's room. The air might be full of fumes from gas, mustiness, or open sewage if the source was not the freshest. Nightingale believed that the person who repeatedly breathed his or her own air would become sick or remain sick. Today, we have buildings that are sealed in such a manner that fresh air is difficult to receive, and a new problem, labeled *building sickness*, has evolved.

Nightingale (1859/1992) was very concerned about "noxious air" or "effluvia" or foul odors that came from excrement. In many public places, as well as hospitals, raw sewage could be found near patients, in ditches under or near the house, or contaminating drinking water. Her concerns about "effluvia" also included bedpans, urinals, and other utensils used to discard excrement. She also criticized "fumigations," for she believed that the offensive source, not the smell, must be removed.

The importance of room temperature was stressed by Nightingale. The patient should not be too warm or too cold. The temperature could be controlled by appropriate balance between burning fires and ventilation from windows. Today buildings often are constructed to be climate-controlled in such a manner that the client or the nurse cannot control the temperature of the individual room. In shared rooms the climate control may not satisfy either patient, with one wanting the room colder and another wanting it warmer, as each individual interacts with the environment.

Light

Nightingale (1859/1992) believed that second to fresh air the sick needed light. She noted that direct sunlight was what patients wanted. Although acknowledging a lack of scientific information, she noted that light has "quite real and tangible effects upon the human body" (pp. 47–48). She noted that people do not consider the difference between light needed in a bedroom (where individuals sleep at night) and light needed in a sickroom. To a healthy sleeper it does not matter where the light is because he is usually in his room only during hours of darkness. She noted that the sick rarely lie with their face toward the wall but are much more likely to face the window, the source of the sun. Again, modern hospitals may be constructed in such a manner that daylight is rarely available. This is particularly the case in neonatal intensive care units, and for many years was also true in the construction of adult intensive care units. The lack of appropriate environmental stimuli can lead to intensive care psychosis or a confusion related to the lack of the accustomed cycling of day and night.

Noise

Noise was also of concern to Nightingale, particularly those noises that could jar the patient. She stated that patients should never be waked intentionally or accidentally during the first part of sleep. She asserted that whispered or long conversations about patients are thoughtless and cruel, especially when held so that the patient knows (or assumes) the conversation is about him. She viewed unnecessary noise, including noise from female dress, as cruel and irritating to the patient.

Nurses today do not wear crinoline petticoats, but they do wear jewelry and carry keys that jingle and make other noises. Other more modern noises include the snapping of rubber gloves, the clank of a stethoscope against metal bed rails, and radios and TVs. Modern health care facilities contain much equipment that issues alarms, beeps, and other noises that startle or jar a patient from sleep to wakefulness. Nightingale was very critical of noises that annoyed the patient, such as a window shade blowing against the window frame. She viewed it as the nurse's responsibility to assess and stop this kind of noise. While specific testing of the effects of noise has been done, it has not been under the framework of Nightingale. The exception is the work by McCarthy, Quimet, and Daun (1991) who extrapolated data from animal studies to support Nightingale's assertion that noise affects healing.

Variety

Nightingale believed that variety in the environment was a critical aspect affecting the patient's recovery. She discussed the need for changes in color and form, including bringing the patient brightly colored flowers or plants. She also advocated rotating 10 or 12 paintings and engravings each day, week, or month to provide variety for the patient. She wrote that "volumes are now written and spoken upon the effect of the mind upon the body. Much of it is true" (Nightingale, 1859/1992, p. 34). The increasing research being done on the interaction between mind and body has supported this observation. Nightingale also advocated reading, needlework, writing, and cleaning as activities to relieve the sick of boredom.

Bed and Bedding

Nightingale (1859/1992) viewed bedding as an important part of the environment. Although her view has not been substantiated by data, she noted that an adult in health exhales about three pints of moisture through the lungs and skin in a 24-hour period. This organic matter enters the sheets and stays there unless the bedding is changed and aired frequently. She believed that the bed should be placed in the lightest part of the room and placed so the patient could see out of a window. She reminded the caregiver never to lean against, sit upon, or unnecessarily shake the bed of a patient. In modern hospitals mattresses are usually covered with plastic or other materials that can be washed to remove drainage, excreta, or other matter. These mattresses often cause the patient to perspire, leading to damp bed clothing. Sheets also do not fit tightly on these mattresses, leading to wrinkles that can result in pressure points on the skin of the patient lying in bed. Modern technology may also interfere with providing a comfortable bed environment for the patient. Multiple intravenous pumps, ventilators, and monitors attached to a patient may impede comfort. It remains important for the nurse to keep bedding clean, neat, and dry and to position the patient for maximum comfort.

Cleanliness of Rooms and Walls

Nightingale (1859/1992) indicated that "the greater part of nursing consists in preserving cleanliness" (p. 49). She points out that even the best ventilation cannot freshen a room that is not first of all clean. She urges the removal of, rather than the relocation of, dust. This means using a damp cloth, not a feather duster. Floors should be easily cleaned rather than being covered with dust trapping carpets. Furniture and walls should be easily washed and not damaged by coming in contact with moisture. Some of Nightingale's restrictions against carpet, fabrics, and wallpaper can be offset today with current cleaning mechanisms, including vacuum cleaners. However, the concept that a clean room is a healthy room continues to be true.

Personal Cleanliness

Nightingale viewed the function of the skin as important, believing that many diseases "disordered," or caused breaks in the skin. She thought this was particularly true of children and that the excretion that comes from the skin must be washed away. She believed that unwashed skin poisoned the patient and noted that bathing and drying the skin provided great relief to the patient, saying, "Just as it is necessary to renew the air round a sick person frequently, to carry off morbid effluvia from the lungs and skin, by maintaining free ventilation, so is it necessary to keep the pores of the skin free from all obstructing excretions" (Nightingale, 1859/1992, p. 53). She also believed that personal cleanliness extended to the nurse and that "every nurse ought to wash her hands very frequently during the day" (p. 53).

Nutrition and Taking Food

Nightingale addressed the variety of food presented to the patient and discussed the importance of variety in the food presented. She found that the attention provided to the patient affected how the patient ate. She noted that individuals desire different foods at different times of the day and that frequent small servings may be more beneficial to the patient than a large breakfast or dinner. She observed that patients may desire a different pattern of taking foods, such as eating breakfast foods at lunch, and that chronically ill patients may be starved to death because their incapacitation can make them unable to feed themselves and attention is not given to what will enhance their ability to eat. She urged that no business be done with patients while they are eating because this was distraction. She also urged that the right food be brought at the right time and "be taken away, eaten or uneaten, at the right time" (p. 37).

Chattering Hopes and Advices

Nightingale did not speak to the social and psychological environment of the patient to the same degree that she addressed the physical environment. However, she included a chapter on "Chattering hopes and advices," which discussed what is said to the patient. She wrote that the chapter heading might seem "odd" but that to falsely cheer the sick by making light of their illness and its danger is not helpful. She considered it stressful for a patient to hear opinions after only brief observations had been made. False hope was depressing to patients, she felt, and caused them to worry and become fatigued. Nightingale encouraged the nurse to heed what is being said by visitors, believing that sick persons should hear good news that would assist them in becoming healthier.

Observation of the Sick

Nightingale (1859/1992) stated "the most important practical lesson that can be given to nurses is to teach them what to observe—how to observe—what symptoms indicate improvement—what is the reverse—which are of importance—which are of none—which are evidence of neglect—and what kind of neglect" (p. 59). She felt so strongly about the importance of obtaining complete and accurate information about patients that she said "if you cannot get the habit of observation one way or other, you had better give up being a nurse, for it is not your calling, however kind and anxious you may be" (p. 63). She urges precise, specific, and individualized questions and observations and warns against failure to observe and the use of averages to describe expectations of the individual. Finally, she urges that observation not be an end unto itself but a means for assuring that appropriate actions are taken.

Social Considerations

Nightingale (1859/1992) supported the importance of looking beyond the individual to the social environment in which he or she lived. She was an epidemiologist who looked at not only the numbers of people who died but also what was unique about a given house or street. She observed that generations of families lived and died in poverty. Using her statistical data, she wrote letters and position papers and sent them to her acquaintances in the government in an effort to improve undesirable living conditions. Nightingale was a role model for political activism by nurses.

Nightingale was also an excellent manager. She demonstrated her management skills at Scutari and wrote about them in many of her nursing-related books. In *Notes on nursing* (1859/1992), she discussed "petty management" or ways to assure that "what you do when you are there, shall be done when you are not there" (p. 20). She believed that the house and the hospital needed to be well managed—that is, organized, clean, and with appropriate supplies.

NIGHTINGALE'S ENVIRONMENTAL MODEL AND NURSING'S METAPARADIGM

Nightingale did not invent or define the four major concepts used to organize nursing theory. They evolved from an analysis of nursing curricula long after Nightingale did her initial work in nursing (Falco, 1989). Although we have applied our modern conventions to her framework, not all the concepts were addressed specifically by Nightingale. This is not a criticism of Nightingale's thinking but a reality of the development of nursing thought. Therefore, Nightingale's writings were analyzed to identify her definitions of these concepts.

Nursing. "What nursing has to do . . . is to put the patient in the best condition for nature to act upon him" (Nightingale, 1859/1992, p. 74). Nightingale viewed medicine and surgery as removing obstructions to health to allow nature to return the person to health. Nightingale stated that nursing "ought to signify the proper use of fresh air, light, warmth, cleanliness, quiet, and the proper selection and administration of diet—all at the least expense of vital power to the patient" (p. 6). She reflected the art of nursing in her statement that, "the art of nursing, as now practised, seems to be expressly constituted to unmake what God had made disease to be, viz., a reparative process" (p. 6).

   Based on her definition of nursing, the following definitions of human beings, environment, and health can be deduced.

Human Beings. Humans beings are not defined by Nightingale specifically. They are defined in relationship to their environment and the impact of the environment upon them.

Environment. The physical environment is stressed by Nightingale in her writing. As noted, she focused on ventilation, warmth, noise, light, and cleanliness. Nightingale's writings reflect a community health model in which all that surrounds human beings is considered in relation to their state of health. She synthesized immediate knowledge of disease with the existing sanitary conditions in the environment.

Health. Nightingale (1859/1992) did not define health specifically. She believed, however, that pathology teaches the harm disease has done, and nothing more. She stated, "We know nothing of health, the positive of which pathology is the negative, except from observation and experience" (p. 74). She believed "nature alone cures" (p. 74). Given her definition that of the art of nursing is to "unmake what God had made disease" (p. 6), then the goal of all nursing activities should be client health. She believed that nursing should provide care to the healthy as well as the ill and discussed health promotion as an activity in which nurses should engage.

   One way of organizing Nightingale's environmental model can be seen in Figure 3–1. Note that the client, the nurse, and the major environmental concepts are in balance; that is, the nurse can manipulate the environment to compensate for the client's response to it. The goal of the nurse is to assist the patient in staying in balance. If the environment of a client is out of balance, the client expends unnecessary energy. In Figure 3–2 the client is experiencing stress because of noise in the environment. Nursing observations focus on the client's response to noise; nursing interventions focus on reducing the noise and decreasing the client's unnecessary energy expenditure. The nurse's role is to place the client in the best position for nature to act upon him, thus encouraging healing.

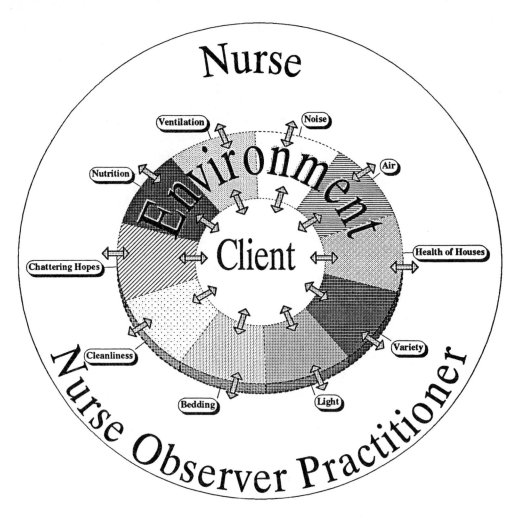

Figure 3–1. Client and environment in balance.

NIGHTINGALE AND THE NURSING PROCESS

In the *assessment* of clients Nightingale (1859/1992) advocated two essential behaviors by the nurse. The first is to ask the client what is needed or wanted. If the patient is in pain, ask where the pain is located. If the patient is not eating, ask *when* he or she would like to eat and *what* food is desired. Find out what the patient believes is wrong. Nightingale warned against asking leading questions and advocated asking precise questions. She recommended asking questions such as "How many hours' sleep has _____ had? and at what hours of the night?" (p. 61) instead of "Has he had a good night?" Nightingale also warned that the individual asking the questions needed to be concerned about the shyness of the patient in answering questions.

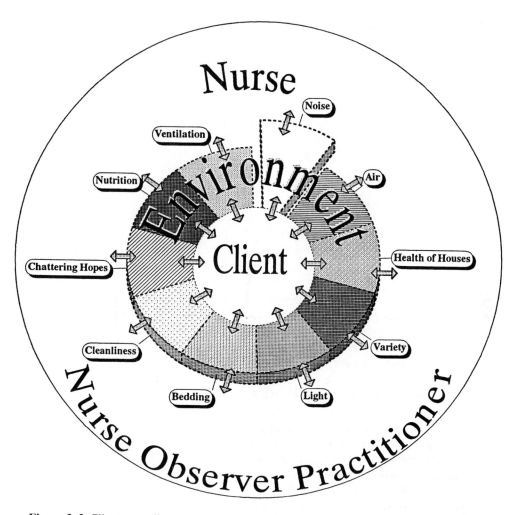

Figure 3–2. Client expending unnecessary energy by being stressed by environment (noise).

The second area of assessment that Nightingale (1859/1992) advocated was the use of observation. She used precise and specific observations concerning all aspects of the client's physical health and environment. Nurses must make the observations because clients may be too weak or shy to make them. Observations revolve around Nightingale's environmental model, that is, the impact of the environment on the individual. For example, how do light, noise, smells, and bedding affect the client?

An assessment guide can be structured from Nightingale's environmental model. The major environmental concepts guide the structure of the assessment tool, leading to examining the impact of the environment on clients and integrating the expanding body of scientific knowledge concerning the effects of a balanced or unbalanced environment.

Nursing diagnoses are based on an analysis of the conclusions gained from the information in the assessment. Nightingale believed data should be used as the basis for forming any conclusion. It is important that the diagnosis be the clients' response to their environment and not the environmental problem. Nursing diagnoses reflect the importance of the environment to the health and well-being of the client.

Outcomes and Planning includes identifying the nursing actions needed to keep clients comfortable, dry, and in the best state for nature to work on. "The value of informed action, based on extensive knowledge is well illustrated by the Nightingale personality" (Palmer, 1980). Planning is focused on modifying the environment to enhance the client's ability to respond to the disease process. The desired outcomes are derived from the environmental model—for example, being comfortable, clean, dry, in the best state for nature to work on.

Implementation takes place in the environment that affects the client and involves taking action to modify that environment. All factors of the environment should be considered, including noise, air, odors, bedding, cleanliness, light—all the factors that place clients in the best position for nature to work upon them.

Evaluation is based on the effect of the changes in the environment on the clients' ability to regain their health at the least expense of energy. Observation is the primary method of data collection used to evaluate the client's response to the intervention. Some have proposed using Nightingale to guide their practice (i.e., Gillette, 1996), however, these reviews are not data based, nor has any testing of the efficacy of using Nightingale's framework been done.

Application of Nightingale's Work in the Nursing Process

Assessment. Nancy Smith, a 10-year-old African American female from a rural area, was injured in an accident related to farm machinery. She had a head injury and although she was "conscious," she was not oriented to place and time. She had multiple abrasions, multiple bruises, and a deep leg wound containing dirt and debris from the farm equipment that injured her. She was transported to the regional children's hospital by helicopter. After triage in the emergency department and surgery, she was admitted to a crowded pediatric intensive care unit (PICU). In the PICU the lights were on 24 hours a day, noises from equipment permeated the unit, and visits by her parents were restricted. Today, after two days and nights of interrupted sleep, Nancy has become increasingly confused but does not have physiological evidence of increased intracranial pressure. Her leg has become infected, requiring increased intravenous antibiotics and dressing changes twice a day.

Analysis of Data. Data gaps include information about family structure; who lives in the household; who was present when the injury occurred; Nancy's school performance; economic resources available to the family, including insurance; Nancy's nutritional status; and evaluation of her growth and development in relation to developmental standards. Of primary concern are Nancy's lack of sleep and the infected wound.

Nursing Diagnosis. Sleep disruption related to environmental light and noise and separation from family.

Outcomes, Planning and Implementation. In relation to the nursing diagnosis, the desired outcome would be adequate sleep; overall the desired outcome is adaptation to the change in environment. Nursing actions focus on changing the environment to support more normal sleep patterns, that is, being awake during the day and sleeping at night. During the day, both natural and artificial light is plentiful around Nancy's bed. She is encouraged to listen to her favorite music or watch her favorite television show to expose her to normal sounds. Her parents are encouraged to visit more often and to talk with her about the future when she will return to home and school. The nurse teaches Nancy about her dressing change and encourages her to participate as much as possible to help her become more comfortable in this new environment. At night sleep is supported by dimming the lights, reducing noise including turning down the volume of alarms, and keeping to a minimum activities and procedures that would awaken Nancy.

Evaluation. Criteria for evaluation: After two nights of uninterrupted sleep, normal sounds, and parental encouragement, Nancy will demonstrate increased orientation to place by being able to identify that she is in the hospital. Nancy will begin participating in her dressing changes by the third day of the care plan.

CRITIQUE OF NIGHTINGALE'S ENVIRONMENTAL MODEL

1. What is the historical context of the theory? Florence Nightingale is the founder of modern nursing. Her work in the mid 1800s provided the basis for much of modern nursing, both education and practice. Her work in the Crimea led to the development of an epidemiological approach to improving the quality of the environment for the injured and ill at Scutari. Nightingale's work has had a worldwide influence, including the Far East, as well as North America and England.

Nightingale's environmental model fits neither the totality nor simultaneity paradigms. Primarily, the model is a view of the relationship between the health of human beings and the environments in which they function. It neither views the human as a sum of parts (totality paradigm) nor the human and environment as part of the same whole (simultaneity paradigm).

2. What are the basic concepts and relationships presented by the theory? Nightingale did not present her ideas as a theory, but as strategies to help women care for the ill in the home and in hostels for the ill. The major concepts covered in *Notes on Nursing* include: ventilation, noise, air, health of houses, variety in the environment, light, bedding, cleanliness, "chattering hopes" or talking over patients, and nutrition. Nightingale never articulates clearly the relationships or interrelationships of her ideas. However, she presents her ideas in a clear manner and the use of all of her ideas in caring for individuals puts them in the best place to become healthy. When nursing situations are viewed from a Nightingale perspective, using the basic concepts she presents, new insights into phenomena of interest to nursing can be identified. Examining environmental aspects, such as light, noise, or warmth, can provide new insight into human response to health and illness. For example, when a client in an isolation room becomes disoriented, obvious things to consider would be medical pathology and fluid and electrolyte balance. From Nightingale's perspective, the impact of the environment would be an initial concern. Thus the nurse would examine patterns of light, noise, ventilation, and interaction with other humans as potential sources or environmental stress on the client.

3. What major phenomena of concern to nursing are presented? These phenomenon may include *but are not limited to*: human being, environment, health, interpersonal relations, caring, goal attainment, adaptation, and energy fields. Nightingale's major focus is the environment and the manipulation of the environment by the nurse to put patients in the best place for nature to act upon the patients to assist them to getting to maximum health. Nightingale does not address interpersonal relations specifically but does talk about the need for the nurse to consider what she says when talking around the patient. Also the nurse must consider the noise level of the environment, especially sources of unnecessary noise. Cleanliness is also of major importance as it is discussed in 5 of the 13 canons—health of houses, personal cleanliness, cleaness of rooms and walls, and bed and bedding. The nurse is to consider all of these factors in applying the information to the patient.

4. To whom does this theory apply? In what situations? In what way? Nightingale's writings are simple, as is the articulation of her model. Nightingale's theory applies in all situations that nursing care is provided. All care is provided in some type of environmental interface. Structuring the environment to provide the best care for the patient is essential whether in the home, the intensive care unit, a day care center, or the community at large. At times Nightingale uses words that are no longer in common use to describe aspects of her model, however, the elegance of Nightingale's model is its generalizability, including its continued applicability today. Nightingale's model can be applied in the most complex hospital intensive care environment, the home, a work site, or the community at large. Concepts related to pure air, light, noise, and cleanliness can be applied across specific environments.

For example, noise, or noxious sound, can be found in any environment. The hospital has carts, monitors, and other machines that disrupt sleep and rest. The intensive care unit is noted for its number of staff members, machines, and alarms, all adding to the noise in the environment. A home may be near an interstate highway with loud truck noises, or an airport with planes taking off and landing day and night, or a home may be isolated in the country with outside noises being rare. A work site may be filled with machine noises, computer whine, or alarms on large machine. Finally, in our modern society a community may be involved in a war with shelling, bombing, and gunfire disrupting sleep, making it difficult to study or do other work.

Nightingale has been proposed as a model for the clinical nurse specialist role (Sparacino, 1994). Sparacino noted that Nightingale also lived in tumultuous times where she was required to make major changes in the manner in which care was delivered. The changes in care that she made in the Crimean War front resulted in a dramatic reduction of the mortality rate. She defined the issues and goals for her day. Such definition is a responsibility of the advanced practice nurse in the twenty-first century.

Nightingale's theory works well with ecological, systems, adaptation, and inter-personal theories. Systems theory discusses the relationships between various layers of the individual and his or her environment. This is precisely what Nightingale did in her discussions of the effects of the physical environment on the individual. She also discussed how individuals respond to their disease process and viewed nurs-ing's role as putting the client in the best position possible for nature to act upon. This allows clients to adapt or change in relation to their diseased state and maxi-mize their state of health.

5. By what method or methods can this theory be tested? While direct testing of Nightingale's theory has not been done, she has stimulated the development of nursing science with her work. For example, Nightingale did not believe in the germ theory. However the practices she recommended were not inconsistent with the scientific knowledge we have today. In fact many of her suggestions, which she based on observations of client responses to their environments, have been docu-mented as scientifically sound when tested with rigorous application of modern re-search methods.

Both quantitative and qualitative methods of research could be used to test rela-tionships in the environmental model. For example, qualitative methods could be used to investigate patient satisfaction in relation to continuity of care as a result of petty management. Nightingale herself supported the use of quantitative data in her use of statistics to demonstrate positive outcomes at Scutari.

6. Does this theory direct critical thinking in nursing practice? Nightin-gale's work has had a direct impact on critical thinking in nursing practice through the requirement to structure the environment to optimize the patient's health. Nightingale's work is often cited in discussions of the current political climate that affects nursing practice. Her focus on the environment has relevance to practitioners in today's global health care climate. Nurses are approaching care from a more scholarly perspective that includes manipulation of the envi-ronment to place the patient in the best possible position for nature to work on him. Nurses exposed to Nightingale's concepts have begun looking at their envi-ronment in a broader context.

Examples of how Nightingale continues to influence both modern nursing and health care can be seen in a number of articles. In a discussion on perinatal lessons from the past, Dunn (1996) discussed her impact on maternal mortality and the training of midwives. Her writings have influenced those who have written about the effects of noise on wound healing (McCarthy, Ouimet, & Daun,1991) and peri-operative nursing (Gillette, 1996). Whall, Shin and Colling (1999) used Nightingale to guide a model for dementia care in Korea.

Nightingale's work has also been used by individuals in management and leader-ship positions to influence the positions they have taken about issues affecting nurs-ing today around the world. Hisama (1996) examined Florence Nightingale's influ-ence on the development of professional nursing in Japan. Modern nursing was brought to Japan by a physician who had studied at St. Thomas Hospital in London and was impressed with Nightingale's training school.

7. Does this theory direct therapeutic nursing interventions? Reading her work raises a consciousness in the nurse about how the environment influences client outcomes. Considering the effect of noise may make a staff more aware of sounds that can be controlled. For example, the noise of placing a clipboard or other equipment on the top of an incubator is disruptive of an infant's sleep. Staff can choose to lay the clipboard elsewhere or to pad it to decrease the unnecessary noise. Or, after reading Nightingale's discussion of the importance of light to the well-being of clients and examining the scientific information on light waves, the importance of light and darkness in sleep–rest cycles and the release of growth hormone, the neonatal intensive care nurse may begin to turn the lights down at night to encourage a normal sleep–wake cycle in the developing premature infant. Nightingale's theory has directed interventions towards modulating the environment. Noise, light, and ventilation should be controlled and variety provided to maximize the patient's response to interventions.

8. Does this theory direct communication in nursing practice? While not as specific about the influence of the psychosocial environment on the client as she is about the influence of the physical environment, Nightingale observed that conversations about clients within their hearing or just out of their hearing but within their awareness could cause distress. She viewed clients as important persons to communicate with concerning their illness. While Nightingale did not define communication as clearly as Peplau or other interactionists, it was an important aspect of her organization of nursing care. Petty management depends upon clear communication of how patient needs are to be met.

9. Does this theory direct nursing actions that lead to favorable outcomes? Although Nightingale collected and organized the data to support the favorable outcomes of her work in the Crimea, her work has not been tested in a manner that proscribes nursing actions. However, her writings have helped nurses develop interventions that have resulted in restructuring the environment. By structuring the environment to provide an optimum place for patients to improve their health, the result is positive outcomes for the patients. Research on the intensive care unit environment and the effects of noise and light on the patient support the recommendations made by Nightingale in *Notes on nursing*. Nightingale's theory has not directly resulted in the development of those interventions.

10. How contagious is this theory? Nightingale has stimulated the development of nursing science with her influence on knowledge development in modern nursing. The majority of nursing theorists have used environment as a part of their theory. She has had a profound effect on many of the other nursing theorists cited in this book. These individuals have indicated the influence of Nightingale by citing her in their work or commenting on her influence in a commemorative edition of *Notes on nursing*. For example, Leininger (1992) analyzed what Nightingale did and did not say about caring, noting that although Nightingale never defined human care she did make inferences about treating the sick. Levine (1992) first wrote about Nightingale in 1962 and discussed the excitement she felt at holding notes written in Nightingale's own hand. Newman (1992) spoke of the timelessness of *Notes on* *nursing* and the impact it has had on her work. The research related to the impact of the environment on client health has been influenced by Nightingale. Hypotheses based on her work continue to be generated although often imbedded within the context of other theories. It should be noted that many of the theorists, such as Rogers, Roy, and others, consider the environment in their work.

SUMMARY

Nightingale has been called timeless by many of the individuals who have written about her. That Nightingale's writings are as meaningful now as they were in the nineteenth century is an indication of her genius. While her 13 canons (ventilation and warming, health of houses, petty management, noise, variety, taking food, what food?, bed and bedding, light, cleanliness of rooms and walls, personal cleanliness, chattering hopes and advices, and observation of the sick) may differ in the specifics of application today, the underlying principles provided by Nightingale remain sound. The example in this chapter applies Nightingale's concepts to a child in an intensive care unit, but they can also be applied to the senior citizen in a nursing home, the family in their inner city home, or the child in school. Although Nightingale spoke specifically to the health of human beings, she acknowledged that the health of the home and the community are critical components of the individual's health.

REFERENCES

Agnew, L. R. C. (1958). Florence Nightingale—Statistician. *American Journal of Nursing, 58,* 644–646.

American Nurses' Association. (1995). *Nursing: A social policy statement.* Washington: Author.

Cohen, I. B. (1984, March). Florence Nightingale. *Scientific American, 250,* 131–132.

Dunn, P. M. (1996). Florence Nightingale (1820–1910): Maternal mortality and the training of midwives. *Archives of Disease in Childhood, 74,* F219–F220.

Falco, S. M. (1989). Major concepts in the development of nursing theory. *Recent Advances in Nursing, 24,* 1–17.

Gillette, V. A. (1996). Applying nursing theory to perioperative nursing practice. *AORN Journal, 64,* 261–270.

Hegge, M. (1990). In the footsteps of Florence Nightingale: Rediscovering the roots of nursing. *Imprint, 37*(2), 74–79.

Hisama, K. K. (1996). Florence Nightingale's influence on the development of professionalization of modern nursing in Japan. *Nursing Outlook, 44,* 284–288.

Leininger, M. M. (1992). Reflections on Nightingale with a focus on human care theory and leadership. In F. Nightingale. *Notes on nursing: What it is and what it is not* (Com. ed.) (pp. 28–38). Philadelphia: Lippincott.

Levine, M. (1992). Nightingale redux. In F. Nightingale. *Notes on nursing: What it is and what it is not* (Com. ed.) (pp. 39–43). Philadelphia: Lippincott.

McCarthy, D. O., Ouimet, M. E., & Daun, J. M. (1991). Shades of Florence Nightingale: Potential impact of noise stress on wound healing. *Holistic Nursing Practice, 5,* 39–48.

Miller, J. G. (1978). *Living systems.* New York: McGraw-Hill.

Newman, M. A. (1992) Nightingale's vision of nursing theory and health. In F. Nightingale. *Notes on nursing: What it is and what it is not* (Com. ed.) (pp. 44–47). Philadelphia: Lippincott.

Nightingale, F. (1860). Vol. II, cited in Palmer, I. S. Florence Nightingale: Reformer, reactionary, researcher. *Nursing Research, 26,* 84–85.

Nightingale, F. N. (1871). *Introductory notes on lying-in institutions.* London: Longmans, Green.

Nightingale, F. N. (1992). *Notes on nursing: What it is, and what it is not* (Com. ed.). Philadelphia: Lippincott. (Original publication 1859.)

Palmer, I. S. (1980). Florence Nightingale: Reformer, reactionary, researcher. *Nursing Research, 26,* 84–85.

Sparacino, P. S. A. (1994). Florence Nightingale: A CNS role model. *Clinical Nurse Specialist, 8*(2), 64.

Vicinus, M., & Nergaard, B. (Eds.). (1990). *Ever yours, Florence Nightingale: Selected letters.* Cambridge, MA: Harvard University Press.

Webster's ninth new collegiate dictionary. (1991). Springfield, MA: Merriam.

Whall, A. L., Shin, Y. H., & Colling, K. B. (1999). A Nightingale-based model for dementia care and its relevance for Korean nursing. *Nursing Science Quarterly, 12,* 319–323.

ANNOTATED BIBLIOGRAPHY

It is important to note that much of the literature published in relation to Florence Nightingale focuses on her and her times rather than on the impact of her environmental model on nursing practice or in relation to practice today. The annotations that follow represent a selection of materials published in English that do relate Nightingale's work to nursing practice today.

Cohen, M. Z. (1984). Patients' experience of hospitalization for surgery: Implications for nursing care. *Dissertation Abstracts International, 45* (07B), 2099.
This doctoral dissertation recognizes that Florence Nightingale was among the first to recognize the importance of understanding the patient's view of the care received. Nightingale also pointed out the difficulty of obtaining this information. This study used a phenomenologically based method to identify three themes of patients' views (need to know and fear of knowing, fear of death, and impact of caring). The themes were confirmed through an analysis of 84 years of nursing literature.

Dennis, K. E., & Prescott, P. A. (1985). Florence Nightingale: Yesterday, today, and tomorrow. *Advances in Nursing Science, 7*(2), 66–81.
This qualitative research report supports the continued influence of Florence Nightingale's insight in today's good nursing practices as defined by nurses and physicians. It also indicates that her work is so much in the public domain, that her influence often is neither recognized nor documented.

Griffin, J. P. (1988). "The effect of progressive muscular relaxation on subjectively reported disturbance due to hospital noise." Unpublished dissertation, New York University.
Based upon Nightingale's identification of unnecessary noise as disturbing, this quantitative study investigated the effectiveness of progressive muscular relaxation in helping hospitalized patients deal with subjectively reported disturbance related to hospital noise. Patients were randomly assigned to the experimental or control groups. Results indicated no relationship between noise sensitivity and disturbance due to hospital noise. Patients in the coronary care unit reported significantly more noise disturbance than patients on telemetry units. The experimental group did demonstrate a significant decrease in noise disturbance after using progressive muscular relaxation at least twice daily for 24 hours.

CHAPTER 4

INTERPERSONAL RELATIONS IN NURSING

HILDEGARD E. PEPLAU*

Janice Ryan Belcher
Lois J. Brittain Fish

■ ■ ■

    Throughout her career, Dr. Hildegard Peplau was a pioneer in nursing. Born in Reading, Pennsylvania, Peplau (1909–1999) began her career in nursing in 1931 after graduating from a diploma nursing program in Pottstown, Pennsylvania. In 1943, Peplau received a B.A. degree in Interpersonal Psychology from Bennington College. This was followed in 1947 with an M.A. in Psychiatric Nursing and in 1953 an Ed.D. in Curriculum Development from Columbia University in New York. Peplau's nursing experience included private and general duty hospital nursing, the U.S. Army Nurse Corps, nursing research, and a private practice in psychiatric nursing. She taught the first classes in graduate psychiatric nursing at Columbia University before moving to Rutgers University where she continued to teach for 20 years and held the title of Professor Emeritus. Peplau influenced the development of many nursing programs, including the creation of the first postbaccalaureate nursing program in Belgium.

    Peplau published the book Interpersonal Relations in Nursing *in 1952. Although the manuscript was completed in 1949, it was not published until 1952 because it was initially considered to be too radical—it was the first theoretical textbook written by a nurse without having a physician as co-author. She also published numerous articles in professional journals on topics ranging from interpersonal concepts to current issues in nursing. Her work on anxiety, hallucinations, and the nurse as an individual therapist was especially groundbreaking. Her pamphlet "Basic Principles of Patient Counseling" was derived from her research and workshops ("Profile," 1974).*

Interpersonal relations in nursing, Peplau, 1988, Springer Publishing Company, Inc., New York 10012. Used with permission.

Dr. Peplau long held national and international recognition as a nurse and leader in health care. She participated in the development of the National Mental Health Act of 1946 and served with many organizations, including the World Health Organization, the National Institute of Mental Health, and the Nurse Corps. She was past executive director and past president of the American Nurses' Association and in 1998 was inducted into its Hall of Fame. A Fellow of the American Academy of Nursing, Peplau was also a board member of the International Council of Nurses, receiving in 1997 its highest honor, the Christianne Reimann Prize, for outstanding contributions in health care. She served as a nursing consultant to various foreign countries as well as to the Surgeon General of the Air Force. Although Peplau "retired" in 1974, she continued professional journal and book publications. Her 1952 book was reissued in 1988 by Springer, New York. Regretfully, Peplau died March 17, 1999. It is to this nurse, educator, administrator who was such a remarkable person that we dedicate this chapter. J.R.B. & L. J. B. F.

Hildegard Peplau (1952/1988) published *Interpersonal relations in nursing*, referring to her book as a "partial theory for the practice of nursing" (p. 261). It is quite remarkable that in 1952 Peplau referred to her book as a partial theory for nursing since this was before the thrust of nursing theory development. In her book, Peplau discussed the phases of the interpersonal process, roles for nursing, and methods for studying nursing as an interpersonal process. This chapter defines the crux of Peplau's nursing theory as the phases of the interpersonal process, and links her other concepts to this central core.

According to Peplau (1952/1988), nursing is therapeutic because it is a healing art, assisting an individual who is sick or in need of health care. Nursing can be viewed as an interpersonal process because it involves interaction between two or more individuals with a common goal. In nursing, this common goal provides the incentive for the therapeutic process in which the nurse and patient[†] respect each other as individuals, both of them learning and growing as a result of the interaction. An individual learns when she or he selects stimuli in the environment and then reacts to these stimuli.

The attainment of this goal, or any goal, is achieved through a series of steps following a sequential pattern. As the relationship of the nurse and patient develops in these steps, the nurse can choose how she or he practices nursing by using different skills and technical abilities, and by assuming various roles.

When the nurse and patient first identify a problem, they begin to develop a course of action to solve the problem. They approach this course of action from diverse backgrounds and with individual uniqueness. Each individual may be viewed as a unique biological-psychological-spiritual-sociological structure, one that will

---

[†]Patient will be used throughout this chapter since it is Peplau's definition of the individual who is in need of health care.

not react the same as any other individual. Both the nurse and the patient have learned their unique perceptions from different environments, mores, customs, and beliefs of that individual's given culture. Each person comes with preconceived ideas that influence perceptions, and it is these differences in perception that are so important in the interpersonal process. Furthermore, Peplau (1994b) states that these "perceptions vary with time, place, and experience" (p. 11). In addition, the nurse has a broad range of nursing knowledge such as stress–crisis management and developmental theories, which leads to a greater understanding of the nurse's professional role in the therapeutic process. Peplau (1992) states "In all encounters with patients, nurses observe, interpret what they notice, and then decide what needs to be done. This sequence occurs over and over again in any given nurse-patient interacton" (p. 16). As nurse and patient continue the relationship, they begin to understand one another's roles and the factors surrounding the problem. From this understanding, both the nurse and patient collaborate and share in mutual goals until the problem is resolved.

As the nurse and the patient work together, they become more knowledgeable and mature throughout the process. Peplau (1952/1988) views nursing as a "maturing force and an educative instrument" (p. 8). She believes nursing is a learning experience of oneself as well as of the other individual involved in the interpersonal action. This concept was supported by Genevieve Burton, another nursing author from the 1950s, who stated, "Behavior of others must be understood in light of self understanding" (Burton, 1958, p. 7). Thus, persons who are aware of their own feelings, perceptions, and actions are also more likely to be aware of another individual's reactions.

Each therapeutic encounter influences the nurse's and the patient's personal and professional development. As the nurse works with the patient to resolve problems in everyday life, the nurse's practice becomes increasingly more effective. Thus, the kind of person the nurse is and becomes has a direct influence on her or his skill in the therapeutic, interpersonal relationship. In fact, Peplau (1992) believes "the behavior of the nurse-as-a-person interacting with the patient as-a-person has significant impact on the patient's well-being and the quality and outcome of nursing care" (p. 14).

Peplau initially identified four sequential phases in interpersonal relationships: (1) orientation, (2) identification, (3) exploitation, and (4) resolution. Each of these phases overlaps, interrelates, and varies in duration as the process evolves toward a solution. However, in 1997, Peplau wrote that the nurse–patient relationship is composed of three phases: *orientation phase, working phase,* and *termination phase*—thus combining her two original phases, identification and exploitation, into the working phase. In this chapter, Peplau's original four phases will be discussed within the framework of the later three phases. Different nursing roles are assumed during the various phases. These roles can be broadly described as follows:

- **Teacher**   One who imparts knowledge concerning a need or interest
- **Resource**   One who provides specific, needed information that aids in understanding a problem or a new situation

- **Counselor**   One who, through the use of certain skills and attitudes, aids another in recognizing, facing, accepting, and resolving problems that are interfering with the other person's ability to live happily and effectively
- **Leader**   One who carries out the process of initiation and maintenance of group goals through interaction
- **Technical expert**   One who provides physical care by displaying clinical skills and operating equipment in this care
- **Surrogate**   One who takes the place of another

PEPLAU'S PHASES IN NURSING

Orientation

In the initial phase, *orientation*, the nurse and patient meet as two strangers. The patient and/or the family has a "felt need" (Peplau, 1952/1988, p. 18); therefore, professional assistance is sought. However, this need may not be readily identified or understood by the individuals who are involved. For example, a 16-year-old girl may call the community mental health center just because she feels "very down." It is in this phase that the nurse needs to assist the patient and family to realize what is happening to the patient. Peplau (1994b) states "Interpersonal relationships are important throughout the entire life span. The problems of adolescents, of young adults, and of the elderly are most often psychosocial or interpersonal" (p. 13).

Peplau (1995) emphasizes "Psychiatric nurses who practice in either hospital or community settings need to pay more attention to families" (p. 94). It is of the utmost importance that the nurse work collaboratively with the patient **and** family in analyzing the situation, so that together they can recognize, clarify, and define the existing problem. In the previous example the nurse, in the counselor's role, helps the teenaged girl who feels "very down" to realize that these feelings stem from an argument with her mother over last evening's date. As the nurse listens, a pattern evolves: The girl argues with her mother and then feels depressed. As these feelings are discussed, the girl recognizes that the arguing is the precipitating factor leading to the depression. Thus, the nurse and the patient have defined the problem. Later, the girl and her parents agree to discuss the issue with the nurse. Therefore, by mutually clarifying and defining the problem in the orientation phase, the patient can direct the accumulated energy from her anxiety about unmet needs and begin working with the presenting problem. Nurse–patient rapport is established and continues to be strengthened while concerns are being identified.

While the patient and family are talking to the nurse, a mutual decision needs to be made regarding what type of professional assistance the patient and family need. The nurse, as a resource person, may work with them. As an alternative, the nurse might, with the mutual agreement of all parties involved, refer the family to another source such as a nurse practitioner, psychologist, psychiatrist, family counselor, or social worker. In the orientation phase, the nurse, patient, and family decide what types of services are needed. Even though the nurse may work with the patient and family only a short time, Peplau (1994a) believes "Every professional contact with a patient, however brief, is an opportunity for educative input by nurses" (p. 5).

The orientation phase is directly affected by the patient's and nurse's attitudes about giving or receiving aid from a reciprocal person. In this beginning phase, the nurse needs to be aware of her or his personal reactions to the patient. For example, the nurse may react differently to the 40-year-old man with abdominal pain who enters the emergency department quietly in contrast to the 40-year-old man with abdominal pain who enters the emergency department boisterously after a few alcoholic drinks. The nurse's, as well as the patient's, culture, religion, race, educational background, experiences, and preconceived ideas and expectations all influence the nurse's reaction to the patient. In addition, the same factors influence the patient's reaction to the nurse (see Fig. 4–1). For example, the patient may have stereotyped the nurse as being able to perform only technical skills, such as giving medications or taking blood pressures, and therefore may not perceive the nurse as a resource person who can help define the problem. Nursing is an interpersonal process, and both the patient and nurse have an equally important part in the therapeutic interaction.

The nurse, the patient, and the family work together to recognize, clarify, and define the existing problem. Peplau (1995) discusses the need for the nurse to give not only "support but health teaching [to family members]. . . . They need time to talk with staff about their concern about the patient" (p. 94). This in turn decreases the tension and anxiety associated with the felt need and the fear of the unknown. Decreasing tension and anxiety prevents future problems that might arise as a result of repressing or not resolving significant events. Stressful situations are identified

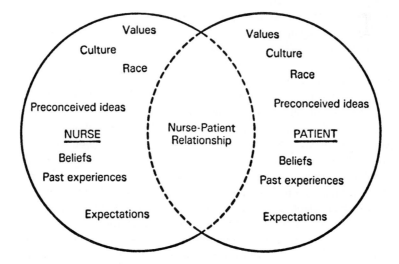

Figure 4–1. Factors influencing the blending of the nurse–patient relationship.

through therapeutic interaction. It is imperative that the patient recognize and begin to work through feelings connected with events before an illness.

In summary, in the beginning of the orientation phase, the nurse and the patient meet as strangers. At the end of the orientation phase, they are concurrently striving to identify the problem and are becoming more comfortable with one another. In addition, the patient becomes more comfortable in the helping environment. The nurse and the patient are now ready to logically progress to the next phase, the working phase.

Working Phase

The *working phase* encompasses the activities previously described in the identification and exploitation phases. As this phase begins, in what was formerly the identification phase, the patient responds selectively to people who can meet his or her needs. Each patient responds differently in this phase. For example, the patient might actively seek out the nurse or stoically wait until the nurse approaches. The response to the nurse is threefold: (1) participate with and be interdependent with the nurse, (2) be autonomous and independent from the nurse, or (3) be passive and dependent on the nurse (Peplau, 1952/1988). An example is that of a 70-year-old man who wants to plan his new 1,600 calorie diabetic diet. If the relationship is interdependent, the nurse and patient collaborate on the meal planning. Should the relationship be independent, the patient plans the diet himself with minimal input from the nurse. In a dependent relationship, the nurse does the meal planning for the patient.

Throughout the working phase, both the patient and nurse must clarify each other's perceptions and expectations (Peplau, 1952/1988). Past experiences of both the patient and the nurse will influence their expectations during this interpersonal process. As mentioned in the orientation phase, the initial attitudes of the patient and nurse are important in building a working relationship for identifying the problem and choosing appropriate assistance.

Psychiatric home care nurses need to progress to the working phase quickly because of their limited time with their clients. Peplau (1995) refers to psychiatric home care as "Hands-on care, health teaching, coordination of care, and supervision of home health aides are all nursing functions in psychiatric home care. Careful recording of nursing observations and services rendered is required" (p. 94). A broader scope includes these functions for all home health nurses. In home care, the patient responds to the nurse who can provide therapeutic support and individual counseling.

In the working phase, the perception and expectations of the patient and nurse are even more complex than in the orientation phase. The patient is now responding to the helper selectively. This requires a more intense therapeutic relationship.

To illustrate, a patient who has had a mastectomy may express to the home health nurse her conflict in understanding the importance of exercising the arm following surgery. The nurse observes that the affected arm is edematous (swollen). While the nurse is exploring possible reasons for the edema, the patient admits she is not doing her arm exercises because a friend told her that exercising after surgery delays healing. To facilitate the patient's understanding and subsequent resumption of the exercises, the nurse can identify additional professional people, such as the physical therapist and the physician, who will clarify the patient's misconceptions. Generally, it is best if the nurse objectively discusses each professional's role with the patient so that she will be aware of the advantages and disadvantages of consulting with each professional. However, in this case, the patient states that she does not care to discuss the exercises with the nurse or physical therapist because she perceives her physician to be the only one who has the appropriate information. Thus, previous perceptions of nursing and physical therapy can influence the patient's current decision on the selection of the professional person.

While moving through the working phase, the patient begins to have feelings of belonging and a capacity for dealing with the problem. These changes begin to decrease feelings of helplessness and hopelessness, creating an optimistic attitude from which inner strength ensues.

As the working phase continues, the patient moves into what was the exploitation phase, in which the patient takes advantage of all services available. The degree to which these services are used is based on the needs and interests of the patient. The individual begins to feel as though he or she is an integral part of the helping environment and begins to take control of the situation by extracting help from the services offered. In the previous example of the woman with an edematous arm, the patient begins to understand the information regarding the arm exercises. She reads pamphlets and watches videotapes describing the exercises; she discusses concerns with the nurse; and she may inquire about joining an exercise group through the physical therapy department.

During this phase some patients may make more demands than they did when they were seriously ill. They may make many minor requests or may use other attention-getting techniques, depending on their individual needs. These actions may often be difficult, if not impossible, for the health care provider to completely understand. The nurse may need to deal with the subconscious forces causing the patient's actions, and may need to use interviewing techniques as tools to explore, understand, and adequately deal with underlying patient problems. The nurse must convey an attitude of acceptance, concern, and trust in order to maintain a therapeutic relationship and prevent damage to the nurse–patient rapport that has been established to this point. Furthermore, she must encourage the patient to recognize and explore feelings, thoughts, emotions, and behaviors by providing a nonjudgmental atmosphere and a therapeutic emotional climate.

Peplau (1994a) states "There is a significant difference between taking responsibility for the care of patients and being therapeutically responsive to each patient. In taking responsibility, it is the scope of activities that can keep nurses busy, feeling important, and having a sense of some accomplishment at the day's end. However, the purpose of professional services and the expectation—indeed the need—is for patients to come to terms with their problems" (p. 5). Some patients may take an active interest in, and become involved in, self-care. Such patients become self-sufficient and demonstrate initiative by establishing appropriate behavior for goal attainment. In fact patients may wish to join a self-help group as described by Peplau (1997) when she says "many lay-oriented helping-each-other health related groups are forming" (p. 222). Through self-determination, patients progressively develop responsibility for self, belief in potentialities, and adjustment toward self-reliance and independence. These patients realistically begin to establish their own goals toward improved health status. They strive to achieve a direction in their lives that promotes a feeling of well-being. Patients who develop self-care become productive, they trust and depend on their own capabilities, and they also become responsible for their own actions. As a result of this self-determination, they develop sources of inner strength that allow them to face new challenges.

While in impaired health, most patients fluctuate between dependence on others and independent functioning at an optimal health level. This point is illustrated by using the previous example of the woman who had an edematous arm after surgery. Some days she wants to actively exercise on schedule; however, on other days she states she is too tired to exercise at all. When the patient does not exercise, the nurse needs to intervene by reminding the patient of her scheduled exercises.

This type of inconsistent behavior can be compared to the adjustment reaction of the adolescent in a dependency–independency conflict. The patient may temporarily be in a dependent role while having the simultaneous need for independence. Various stressors may trigger the onset of this psychological disequilibrium. The patient vacillates unpredictably between the two behaviors and appears confused and anxious, protesting dependence while fearing independence. In caring for patients who fluctuate between dependence and independence, the nurse must approach the specific behavior that is presented rather than trying to handle the composite problem of inconsistency. The nurse should provide an atmosphere of acceptance and support, one in which the person can become more self-aware and begin to use his or her strengths to minimize weaknesses. It is the nurse's responsibility to create a climate for the patient that is conducive to responsible self-growth.

Peplau (1994c) states "Conversations are too often serial monologues rather than interactions" (p. 58). In this phase, the nurse uses communication tools such as clarifying, listening, accepting, teaching, and interpreting to offer services to the patient. The patient then takes advantage of the services offered based on his or her needs and interests. Throughout this phase, the patient works collaboratively with the nurse to meet challenges and work toward maximum health. Thus, in the working phase, the nurse aids the patient in using services to help solve the problem. Progress is made toward the final step—the termination phase.

Termination

The last phase in Peplau's interpersonal process is *termination*. The patient's needs have already been met by the collaborative efforts between the patient and nurse. The patient and nurse now need to terminate their therapeutic relationship and dissolve the links between them.

Sometimes the nurse and patient have difficulty dissolving these links. Dependency needs in a therapeutic relationship often continue psychologically after the physiological needs have been met. The patient may feel that it "is just not time yet" to end the relationship. For example, a new mother has a desire to learn infant care. Readiness is one of the most important factors in the learning process and learning is initiated by a need or purpose. During the first home visit, the community health nurse and the new mother set their goal of having the mother properly demonstrate various facets of infant care by the third visit. The setting of these goals is important in order to evaluate whether or not the desired outcome has been achieved. After instruction and demonstration by the community health nurse on the first visit, the mother takes a more active role during the next home visits. In order for learning to become relatively permanent, it must be used in actual practice. By the third visit the mother demonstrates correctly all facets of infant care. Their goal is met. The relationship is ended because the mother's problem was solved. However, one week after the resolution, the mother telephones the community health nurse five times with minor questions on infant care. The mother has not dissolved the dependency link with the community health nurse.

The final resolution may also be difficult for the nurse. In the previous example, the mother may be willing to terminate the relationship; however, the community health nurse may continue to visit the home to watch the baby develop. The nurse may be unable to free herself or himself from this bond in their relationship. This may be, in part, due to the nurse's knowledge of the importance of the parent–child relationship. Peplau (1994b) refers to the "enormous influence which parents and significant caretakers have on the early development of infants, and in the shaping of behavior of growing children " (p.11). In termination, as in the other phases, anxiety and tension increase in the patient and the nurse if there is unsuccessful completion of the phase.

During successful termination, the patient drifts away from identifying with the helping person, the nurse. The patient then becomes independent from the nurse as the nurse becomes independent from the patient. As a result of this process, both the patient and nurse become stronger maturing individuals. The patient's needs are met, and movement can be made toward new goals. Termination occurs only with the successful completion of the previous phases. Table 4–1 indicates the focus of each phase.

PEPLAU'S THEORY AND NURSING'S METAPARADIGM

Nursing's metaparadigm includes the four concepts of human beings, health, society/ environment, and nursing. Peplau (1952/1988) defines *man* (used in generic terms) as an organism that "strives in its own way to reduce tension generated by needs" (p. 82). *Health* is defined as "a word symbol that implies forward movement of

TABLE 4–1. PHASES OF THE NURSE–PATIENT RELATIONSHIP

Phase	Focus
Orientation	Problem-definition
Working	Selection of appropriate professional assistance and Use of professional assistance for problem-solving alternatives
Termination	Termination of the professional relationship

personality and other ongoing human processes in the direction of creative, constructive, productive, personal, and community living" (p. 12).

Although Peplau (1952/1988) does not directly address *society/environment*, she does encourage the nurse to consider the patient's culture and mores when the patient adjusts to hospital routine. Today, the nurse reviews the patient's environment, and examines many more factors, such as cultural background and home and work environments, rather than considering only a patient's adjustment to the hospital. Peplau has a narrow perception of the environment, which is a major limitation of her theory.

Peplau (1952/1988) considers *nursing* to be a "significant, therapeutic, interpersonal process" (p. 16). She defines it as a "human relationship between an individual who is sick, or in need of health services, and a nurse especially educated to recognize and to respond to the need for help" (pp. 5–6). The nurse assists the patient in this interpersonal process. Major concepts within this process are nurse, patient, therapeutic relationship, goals, human needs, anxiety, tension, and frustration.

RELATIONSHIP BETWEEN PEPLAU'S PHASES AND THE NURSING PROCESS

Peplau's continuum of the three phases of *orientation, working,* and *termination* can be compared to the nursing process as discussed in Chapter 2 (see Table 4–2). The nursing process in Chapter 2 is defined as a "deliberate intellectual activity [that] guides the professional practice of nursing in providing care in an orderly, systematic manner" (see page 23).

There are similarities between the nursing process and Peplau's interpersonal phases. Both Peplau's phases and the nursing process are sequential and focus on therapeutic interactions. Both stress that the nurse and patient should use problem-solving techniques collaboratively, with the end purpose of meeting the patient's needs. Both emphasize assisting the patient to define general complaints more specifically so that specific patient needs can be identified. Both use observation, communication, and recording as basic tools for nursing practice.

Peplau's orientation phase parallels the beginning of the *assessment phase* in that both the nurse and patient come together as strangers. This meeting is initiated by the patient, who expresses a need, although the need is not always understood. Conjointly, the nurse and patient begin to work through recognizing, clarifying, and gathering facts important to this need. This step is presently referred to as data collection in the assessment phase of the nursing process.

In the nursing process the patient's need is not necessarily a felt need. For example, the nurse may be currently working in the community by assessing people who perceive themselves to be healthy. A school nurse screens for hearing impairment in school-aged children. A referral is initiated by the nurse if a deficit is found. Children do not usually seek out the nurse for this problem. In this situation, the need must be identified in order to persuade the parents to seek assistance for the child's hearing deficit. The nurse may send home a note about the hearing deficit so that the parents and child become aware of the problem. The nurse may also have to follow

TABLE 4–2. COMPARISON OF NURSING PROCESS AND PEPLAU'S PHASES

Nursing Process	Peplau's Interpersonal Process

Assessment
  Data collection and analysis
  Need not necessarily a "felt need"; may be nurse-initiated
	Orientation
	  Nurse and patient come together as strangers; meeting initiated by patient who expresses a "felt need"; work together to recognize, clarify, and define facts related to need. (Note: Data collection is continuous).

Nursing Diagnosis Summary statement based on nurse analysis, with possible patient involvement	Patient clarifies "felt need."

Outcomes and Planning
  Mutually set outcomes and goals
	Working
	  Interdependent goal setting. Patient has feeling of belonging and selectively responds to those who can meet his or her needs. Patient-initiated.

Implementation
  Plans initiated that move toward achievement of mutually set goals
  May be accomplished by patient, health care professional, or patient's family
	Working (cont'd)
	  Patient actively seeking and drawing on knowledge and expertise of those who can help. Patient-initiated.

Evaluation
  Based on mutually established expected behaviors
  May lead to termination of relationship or initiation of new plans
	Termination
	  Occurs after other phases are successfully completed.
	  Leads to termination of the relationship.

up the note with a telephone call or home visit. The nurse is actively helping the child and family to identify a need.

Orientation and assessment are not synonymous and must not be confused. Collecting data is continuous throughout Peplau's phases. In the nursing process, the initial collection of data is the nursing assessment, and further collection of data becomes an integral part of reassessment.

In the nursing process, the *nursing diagnosis* evolves once the health problems or deficits are identified. The nursing diagnosis is a summary statement of the data collected and analyzed. Peplau (1952/1988) writes that "during the period of orientation the patient clarifies his first, whole impression of his problem" (p. 30); whereas in the nursing process, the nurse's judgment forms the diagnosis from the data collected. The nurse and the patient may be mutual partners in identifying the nursing diagnosis.

Mutually set outcomes and goals evolve from the nursing diagnosis in the nursing process. These outcomes and goals give direction to the plan and indicate the appropriate helping resources. When the nurse and patient discuss helping resources, the patient can selectively identify with the resource persons. According to Peplau, the patient is then viewed as being in the working phase.

While collaborating on mutual outcomes and goals, the nurse and patient may have conflicts based on preconceptions and expectations of each person, as described earlier. The nurse and patient must resolve any discrepancies before mutual outcomes can be developed and mutual goals can be set. These decisions should be an interdependent activity between the patient and nurse.

The next phase in the nursing process is the *planning* phase. In this phase, the nurse must specifically formulate how the patient is going to achieve the mutually set outcomes and goals. The nurse actively seeks patient input so that the patient feels like an integral part of the plan. When the patient feels involved in the plan, outcomes are more likely to be achieved. The nurse is the facilitator but the teaching is a sharing process, a two-directional process of intercommunication with reciprocal feedback by which continuous responses are made between the nurse and the patient. In the planning phase, the nurse considers the patient's own skills for handling his or her problems. Peplau (1952/1988) stresses that the nurse wants to develop a therapeutic relationship so that the patient's anxiety will be constructively channeled into seeking resources, thus leading to decreased feelings of hopelessness and helplessness. Planning can be considered to be within Peplau's working phase.

The patient also begins to have a feeling of belonging within the therapeutic relationship because both patient and nurse must have mutual respect, communication, and interest. This feeling of belonging must be analyzed and should assist the patient to develop a healthier personality rather than imitative behavior. Peplau (1952/1988) states, "Some patients identify too readily with nurses, expecting that all of their wants will be taken care of and nothing will be expected of them" (p. 32). In Peplau's identification phase, the patient selectively responds to people who can meet his or her personal needs. Therefore, the identification phase is initiated by the patient.

The planning stage of the nursing process gives direction and meaning to the nursing actions to be taken toward resolving the patient's problems. Using nursing education, the nurse bases the nursing plan on scientific knowledge. In addition, the nurse incorporates the patient's individual strengths and weaknesses into the plan.

In the *implementation* phase, as in Peplau's working phase, the patient is finally reaping benefits from the therapeutic relationship by drawing on the nurse's knowledge and expertise. The individualized plans have already been formed, based on the patient's interest and needs. Similarly, the plans are geared toward completion of desired goals. However, there is a difference between the working phase and implementation. In the working phase, the patient is the one who actively seeks varying types of services to obtain the maximum benefits available, whereas in implementation there is a prescribed plan or procedure, holistic in nature, used to achieve predetermined goals or objectives based on nursing assessment. Thus, the working phase is oriented to the patient. In contrast, implementation can be accomplished by the patient or by other persons, including health professionals and the patient's family.

In Peplau's termination phase, all other phases have been successfully accomplished, the needs have been met, and resolution and termination are the end result. Although Peplau does not discuss *evaluation* per se, evaluation is an inherent factor in determining the readiness of the patient to proceed through the termination phase.

In the nursing process, evaluation is a separate step, and mutually established expected end-behaviors (goals) are used as evaluation tools. Time limits on attaining the goals are set for evaluation purposes, although these limits may change with reassessment. In evaluation, if the situation is clear-cut, the problem moves toward termination. If the problem is unresolved, outcomes, goals, and objectives are not met; if outcomes are not achieved or nursing care is ineffective, a reassessment must be done. New goals, planning, implementation, and evaluation are then established. An example of the application of Peplau's work in clinical practice may be found in Table 4–3.

TABLE 4–3. APPLICATION OF INTERPERSONAL RELATIONSHIPS IN CLINICAL PRACTICE

Orientation:

You are a staff nurse on the chemical dependency unit of your hospital. You note that Cecilia Bell, 32 years old, is assigned to you today. In reviewing her chart you note that she is admitted for alcohol abuse and this is her third admission for this diagnosis in the last nine months. Her first admission nine months ago occurred after she was found by the police wandering in the street. She had been drinking heavily and had lost her purse. Three months ago, she requested readmission after drinking heavily and feeling depressed. You remember her from this admission. She had attended all group therapy meetings, all Alcoholic Anonymous (AA) meetings, and seemed interested in her treatment and excited about being ready for discharge.

When Ms. Bell sees you, she recognizes you as a nurse whom she had seen during her previous admission. As you discuss why she is here now (seeking to identify her felt need), she reports she has been drinking a fifth of vodka and a "few" beers daily for the past several weeks. In tears, she says, "I'm a failure." Further discussion reveals that she attended AA regularly for about 6 weeks after her last discharge from the hospital. She returned to her employment as a high school English teacher and felt she did not have time to continue to go to daily meetings. She states she had too many papers to grade and her friends at work did not understand why she needed to go to meetings every day. She also says that her chemical dependency counselor never listened to her so she quit meeting with him. Her family lives in another state. The only friends she feels close to abuse alcohol and drugs. She agrees that she needs to once again feel in control of herself and her ability to not abuse alcohol.

Working:

Over the next few days, you explore with Ms. Bell what sources of help she believes will be most useful to her. She identifies that group therapy and AA really helped during her last admission and elects to participate in these activities again. The two of you also identify that she would feel more comfortable with a female chemical dependency counselor as a support person after she is discharged. She asks you to investigate if there is a counselor who works in the outpatient service who could meet with her while she is still hospitalized. She recognizes that she would feel better about meeting with someone in outpatient sessions whom she has gotten to know while in the security of the inpatient environment. She also requests help with how to share her needs for support with her fellow teachers in an effort to develop friends who are not abusing substances.

Termination:

As Ms. Bell's inpatient therapist and outpatient counselor agree with her that she has developed skills that will help her function without abusing alcohol, she prepares to be discharged from the chemical dependency unit to outpatient care. It is time to terminate the interpersonal relationship you have developed with Ms. Bell. You verify with her that she has practiced how to share her needs with her fellow teachers, and that she has selected two teachers to be the first people she will approach. She has also contacted her AA counselor who has made arrangements to pick her up at the hospital and provide her transportation home. She states she has made a commitment to attend AA meetings and has an appointment for tomorrow with her outpatient counselor. She shares with you that this counselor really listens to her and she believes she will receive the support she needs. They have begun discussing how she can use time management skills to meet the demands of her job and still have the time she needs to attend AA meetings and counseling sessions. You congratulate Ms. Bell on her progress and say "Good bye" as she is leaving.

CRITIQUE OF PEPLAU'S INTERPERSONAL RELATIONS

Peplau's work is now critiqued as a theory by the questions in this book's first chapter. Generally, Peplau's work is a theory of nursing.

1. What is the historical context of the theory? Peplau's theory was published in 1952 before the thrust of nursing theory development. Her work is a keystone in nursing practice focusing on the therapeutic relationship and theory development. Peplau identifies needs, frustration, conflict, and anxiety as important concepts in nursing situations. Furthermore, she states that these concepts must be addressed for patient and nurse growth to occur. These concepts can readily be identified as having been influenced by some theories of the time, especially Harry S. Sullivan's (1947) and Fromme's (1947) interpersonal theory and Sigmund Freud's (1936) theory of psychodynamics. Interpersonal theorists believe that behavior directly evolves from interpersonal relationships. Similar to Freudian theorists, interpersonal theorists believe that psychological development is critical in the evolution of a person. Even the name of two of her initial phases, identification and exploitation, were strongly influenced by interpersonal and psychodynamic theory.

Because Peplau focuses on the psychological tasks within the person, her theory does not examine the broad range of environmental influences on the person, a view that was timely in 1949 when the book was written (Sills, 1977, p. 202). In examining the historical trends in psychiatric nursing, this view is categorized as being "within the person," as later contrasted to views of "within the relationship" and "within the social system," both of which consider a broader range of environmental influences on the person (Sills, 1977).

Today's nurse evaluates many concepts such as intrafamily dynamics, socioeconomic forces (e.g., financial resources), personal space considerations, and community social service resources for each patient. These concepts provide a broader perspective for viewing the patient in his or her environment than do Peplau's concepts of needs, frustration, conflict, and anxiety.

Nurses have a broader perspective on nursing roles from that represented in Peplau's original 1952 publication. Nursing now assists the patient to reach a fuller health potential through health maintenance and promotion. As long ago as 1970, Martha Rogers wrote, "Maintenance and promotion of health, prevention of disease, nursing diagnosis, intervention, and rehabilitation encompass the scope of nursing's goals" (p. 86). Today, nurses actively seek to identify health problems in a variety of community and institutional settings.

Peplau's 1952 view does not support the current viewpoint of independent functioning by advanced practice nurses. Peplau (1952/1988) wrote that the physician's primary function was "recognizing the full import of the nuclear problem and the kind of professional assistance that is needed," which results, for the physician, in "the task of evaluating and diagnosing the emergent problem" (p. 23). Nursing functions, according to Peplau (1952/1988), include clarification of the information the physician gives the patient as well as collection of data about the patient that may point out other problem areas. In contrast, given today's expanded roles in nursing, advanced practice nurses may or may not refer the patient to the physician, depending on the patient's needs. Through expanded roles, nursing is becoming more accountable and responsible, giving professional nursing greater independence than previously. Peplau's view of nursing's role may well be an artifact of the era in which her book was originally published.

2. What are the basic concepts and relationships presented by the theory?
The phases of orientation, working, and termination interrelate the various components of each phase. This interrelationship creates a different perspective from which to view the nurse–patient interaction and the transaction of health care. The nurse–patient interaction can apply the concepts of human being, health, society/environment, and nursing. For example, in the phase of orientation there are components of nurse, patient, strangers, problem, and anxiety.

Peplau's theory provides a logical and systematic way of viewing nursing situations. The three progressive phases in the nurse–patient relationship are logical, beginning with initial contact in the phase of orientation and ending with the termination phase. Key concepts in the theory, such as anxiety, tension, goals, and frustration, are clearly defined with explicit relationships between them and the progressive phases.

The phases provide simplicity regarding the natural progression of the nurse–patient relationship. This simplicity leads to adaptability in any nurse–patient interaction, thus providing generalizability. The basic nature of nursing is still considered an interpersonal process even though Peplau and Forchuk have debated whether the interpersonal process should be four or three phases. Peplau (1992) refers to this when she states that Forchuk "has redefined the sometimes overlapping phases of the nurse–patient relationship as (a) the orientation phase, (b) the working phase, and (c) the resolution phase" (p.14). In 1997, Peplau reduced her four phases to (1) orientation phase, (2) working phase, and (3) termination phase.

3. What major phenomena of concern to nursing are presented? These phenomenon may include *but are not limited to:* human being, environment, health, interpersonal relations, caring, goal attainment, adaptation, and energy fields. As discussed in the section of this chapter on nursing's metaparadigm, Peplau's early work defines man in the generic use for human beings, health, and nursing. In later writings she emphasized the importance of including the family in the plan of care. However, with her interest in, and emphasis on interpersonal relations, she presented many more phenomena of interest to nursing. These include tension, anxiety, goals, frustration, therapeutic relationships, human needs, and mutual growth. All of these are defined and discussed by Peplau.

4. To whom does this theory apply? In what situations? In what ways?
Peplau's work has contributed greatly to nursing's body of knowledge, not only in psychiatric-mental health nursing but also in nursing in general. An example is the contributions made by her work on anxiety. Nursing is still defined as an interpersonal process built on the progressive nurse–patient phases. As Peplau proposed, communication and interviewing skills remain fundamental nursing tools. Peplau (1992) refers to several interrelated theoretical constructs such as "concepts, processes, patterns, and problems" that the nurse uses in the interpersonal process

(p.16). Also, her anxiety continuum is still used for nursing interventions in working with anxious patients.

In applying Peplau's theory in clinical practice, the focus is on assisting the patient to identify psychological and growth needs. This theory is not as useful for working with a patient with many physiological needs. Another limitation of this theory is in working with the unconscious patient. A major assumption in the theory is the ability of the nurse and patient to interact. For example, the phase of orientation begins when the patient has a felt need and initiates interaction between the nurse and the patient. This viewpoint is extremely limited in working with the unconscious patient.

5. By what method or methods can this theory be tested? Peplau's theory has generated both research questions and testable hypotheses. Early researchers focused on the concept of anxiety and used small samples. Hays (1961) examined teaching the concept of anxiety to six female patients in a group setting. Burd (1963) used Peplau's work on anxiety to develop a framework and to conduct a study of 25 nursing students who worked with anxious patients. Early research was mostly descriptive (see Table 4–4).

More recently, studies have focused on Peplau's nurse–patient relationship. In 1989, Forchuk and Brown created an instrument to assess Peplau's nurse–client relationship and tested the instrument on 132 clients. Later, Forchuk (1994a) used a prospective design with 124 newly formed nurse–client dyads to examine the orientation phase and found that preconceptions were an important factor. In 1998, Forchuk, et al. studied 10 client–nurse dyads to identify factors influencing the movement from the orientation phase to the working phase. The investigators found that nurses can help the clients move to the working phase by being available, consistent, and by promoting trust.

6. Does this theory direct critical thinking in nursing practice? and **7. Does this theory direct therapeutic nursing interventions?** Peplau's theory provides a framework for nurse self-assessment, a crucial component of critical thinking. Self-assessment is important to all nurses who interact with patients, regardless of clinical setting. Peplau asserts that the interpersonal process is directly affected by the nurse's preconceived ideas, values, culture, religion, race, past experiences, and expectations. By using this theory as a framework, the nurse assesses his or her thoughts and reactions to the patient and continually focuses on whether the relationship is therapeutic to the patient. This ongoing self-assessment is important to the professional growth of the nurse and enhances critical thinking, as well as direct therapeutic nursing interventions. The nurse–patient relationship is initiated by a felt need of the patient, the focus of the relationship is to meet that felt need, and the relationship ends when the need is met.

8. Does this theory direct communication in nursing practice? Peplau's interpersonal process directly improves communication. Communication and interviewing skills remain fundamental nursing tools. Peplau focused on observing a patient and using communication techniques based on patient needs. The thrust of her theory is improving the nurse–patient communication.

TABLE 4–4. SIGNIFICANT NURSING RESEARCH USING PEPLAU'S WORK AS A FRAMEWORK

Date and Author	Research	Findings
1961 Hays, D.	Provided a description of phases and steps of experiential teaching about anxiety to a patient group. Sample was six female psychiatric patients.	Verbal analysis of the group revealed that when taught by the experiential method the patients were able to apply the concepts of anxiety after the group was terminated.
1963 Burd, S. F.	Developed and tested a nursing intervention framework for working with anxious patients. Sample was 25 psychiatric nursing students consisting of 15 freshman and 10 graduate students.	Freshman students can develop beginning competency in interpersonal relationships. The earlier the student gains theoretical knowledge, the more the student is aware of his or her own anxiety. As students work with patients, patients respond by going through sequential phases including denial, ambivalence, and awareness of anxiety.
1989 Forchuk, C. and Brown, B.	Created an instrument to test Peplau's nurse–client relationship. Sample was 58 case management clients and 74 counseling/treatment clients.	The instrument provided an assessment of the nurse–patient relationship. Chronic schizophrenic clients had a long orientation phase.
1994a Forchuk, C.	Tested the orientation phase of Peplau's theory. Sample was 124 newly formed nurse–client dyads.	Client and nurse preconceptions were important in the development of the therapeutic relationship. Client and nurse anxieties were not significant in the relationship. Other interpersonal relationships were important for the clients but not for the nurses.
1996 Beeber, L. and Caldwell, C.	Collected data derived from clinical intervention over four month period with six women.	Behaviors were analyzed constituting pattern integrations for reciprocal interaction of nurses and patients.
1996 Morrison, E., Shealy, A, Kowalski, C., LaMont, J., and Range, B.	Used content analysis to identify nursing role behaviors with 31 RNs and 62 adult, child, and adolescent patients.	Counselor role was supported as being central to psychiatric nursing.
1998 Forchuk, C., Westwell, J., Martin, M., Azzapardi, W. B., Kosterewa-Tolman, D., and Hux, M.	Interviewed 10 nurse–client dyads until all parties agreed that they were in working phase.	In the working phase the relationship was described as being supportive and powerful. There were factors that enhanced and hindered the progression of the relationship.

9. Does this theory direct nursing actions that lead to favorable outcomes? Her theory does direct nursing actions that lead to favorable outcomes. However, Peplau does not discuss clinical outcomes per se since clinical outcomes was used in the 1980s and 1990s and Peplau's book was published in 1952. However, the timelessness of Peplau's theory is the focus on the patient and adjusting nursing interventions based on patient's needs. When nurses continuously assess and refine nursing actions to focus on meeting the patient's needs, there will be favorable outcomes.

10. How contagious is this theory? Much of Peplau's theory has become public domain or has been integrated into nursing practice without Peplau being overtly identified as being the author. For example, nursing is defined as an interpersonal process and self-awareness is presented as a critical component of being therapeutic with a patient without giving attribution to Peplau for these concepts. In every clinical setting, nurses continue to use Peplau's interventions in dealing with anxious patients.

Peplau's theory has spurred some research; however, research efforts have not been consistent since 1952. For example, two-thirds of the nursing research in the 1950s concentrated on the nurse–patient relationship and Peplau's theory (Sills, 1977). However, with the advent of other nursing theorists in the 1960s and 1970s, there was gap in using Peplau as a theorist in research. In the late 1980s, Forchuk et al. began using Peplau's theory as a model for research on the nurse–patient relationship.

Peplau's work is used internationally. Published works verify its use in Australia and New Zealand (Doncliff, 1994; Harding, 1995), Belgium (Gastmans, 1998), Canada (Forchuk 1992, 1994a, 1994b; Jewell & Sullivan, 1996; Yamashita, 1997), the United Kingdom and Ireland (Almond, 1996; Barker, 1998; Buswell, 1997; Chambers, 1998; Edwards, 1996; Fowler, 1994, 1995; Jones, 1995; Lambert, 1994; Lego, 1998; Price, 1998; Reynolds, 1997; Ryles, 1998; Vardy & Price, 1998) as well as in the United States. In addition to being used by psychiatric nurses, Peplau's theory has also been documented as useful in many other areas such as AIDS care, health education, moral issues of practice, palliative care, patients with strokes, pediatric oncology, postpartum care, reflective evaluation of practice, quality of life, and research (Almond, 1996; Edwards, 1996; Fowler, 1994, 1995; Gastmans, 1998; Hall, 1994; Harding, 1995; Jewell & Sullivan, 1996; Jones, 1995; Kelley, 1996; Peden, 1998; Peplau, 1994b).

SUMMARY

Peplau's (1952/1988) *Interpersonal relations in nursing* is still applicable in theory and practice. The core of Peplau's theory of nursing focuses on the interpersonal process, which is an integral part of present-day nursing. This process initially consisted of the sequential phases of orientation, identification, exploitation, and resolution. More recently, Peplau (1997) redefined the phases as the orientation phase, the working phase, and the termination phase. These phases overlap, interrelate, and vary in duration. The nurse and patient first clarify the patient's problems, and mutual expectations and goals are explored while deciding on appropriate plans for improving health status. This process is influenced by both the nurse's and patient's perceptions and preconceived ideas emerging from their individual uniqueness.

Peplau stresses that both the patient and nurse mature as the result of the therapeutic interaction. When two persons meet in a creative relationship, there is a continuing sense of mutuality and togetherness throughout the experience. Both individuals are involved in a process of self-fulfillment, which becomes a growth experience.

Peplau's nursing theory, the interpersonal process, has as its foundation theories of interaction. It has contributed to nursing in the areas of clinical practice, theory, and research, adding to today's base of nursing knowledge. Thus, Peplau's theory creates a unique view for understanding the nurse–patient relationship.

REFERENCES

Almond, P. (1996). How health visitors assess the health of postnatal women. *Health Visitor, 69,* 495–498.

Barker, P. (1998). The future of the Theory of Interpersonal Relations: A personal reflection on Peplau's legacy. *Journal of Psychiatric and Mental Health Nursing, 5,* 213–220.

Beeber, L., & Caldwell, C. (1996). Pattern integrations in young depressed women: Part 2. *Archives of Psychiatric Nursing, 10,* 157–164.

Burd, S. (1963). Effects of nursing interventions in anxiety of patients. In S. F. Burd & M. A. Marshall (Eds.), *Some clinical approaches to psychiatric nursing* (pp. 307–320). London: Macmillan. (out of print)

Burton, G. (1958). *Personal, impersonal, and interpersonal: A guide for nurses.* New York: Springer. (out of print)

Buswell, C. (1997). A model approach to care of a patient with alcohol problems . . . Peplau's model. *Nursing Times, 93,* 34–35.

Chambers, M. (1998). Interpersonal mental health nursing: Research issues and challenges. *Journal of Psychiatric and Mental Health Nursing, 5,* 203–211.

Doncliff, B. (1994). Putting Peplau to work. *Nursing New Zealand, 2*(1), 20–22.

Edwards, M. (1996). Patient–nurse relationships: Using reflective practice. *Nursing Standard, 10*(25), 40–43.

Forchuk, C. (1992). The orientation phase of the nurse–client relationship: How long does it take? *Perspectives in Psychiatric Care, 28*(4), 7–10.

Forchuk, C. (1994a). Preconceptions in the nurse-client relationship. *Journal of Psychiatric & Mental Health Nursing, 1,* 145–149.

Forchuck, C. (1994b). The orientation phase of the nurse–client relationship: Testing Peplau's theory. *Journal of Advanced Nursing, 20,* 532–537.

Forchuk, C., & Brown, B. (1989). Establishing a nurse–client relationship. *Journal of Psychosocial Nursing, 27,* 30–34.

Forchuk, C., Westwell, J., Martin, M., Azzapardi, W. B., Kosterewa-Tolman, D., & Hux, M. (1998). Factors influencing movement of chronic psychiatric patients from the orientation to the working phase of the nurse–client relationship on an inpatient unit. *Perspectives in Psychiatric Care: The Journal for Nurse Psychotherapists, 34*(1), 36–44.

Fowler, J. (1994). A welcome focus on a key relationship: Using Peplau's model in palliative care. *Professional Nurse, 10,* 194–197.

Fowler, J. (1995). Taking theory into practice: Using Peplau's model in the care of the patient. *Professional Nurse, 10,* 226–230.

Freud, S. (1936). *The problem of anxiety.* New York: Norton.

Fromme, E. (1947). *Man for himself.* New York: Rinehart.

Gastmans, C. (1998). Interpersonal relations in nursing: A philosophical-ethical analysis of the work of Hildegard E. Peplau. *Journal of Advanced Nursing, 28,* 1312–1319.

Hall, K. (1994). Peplau's model of nursing: Caring for a man with AIDS. *British Journal of Nursing, 3,* 418–422.

Harding, T. (1995). Exemplar . . . the essential foundation of nursing lies in the establishment of a therapeutic relationship. *Professional Leader, 2*(1), 20–21.

Hays, D. (1961). Teaching a concept of anxiety. *Nursing Research, 10,* 108–113.

Jewell, J. A., & Sullivan, E. A. (1996). Application of nursing theories in health education. *Journal of the American Psychiatric Nurses Association, 2*(3), 79–85.

Jones, A. (1995). Utilizing Peplau's psychodynamic theory for stroke patient care. *Journal of Clinical Nursing, 4*(1), 49–54.

Kelley, S. J. (1996). "It's just me, my family, my treatments, and my nurse . . . oh, yeah, and Nintendo": Hildegard Peplau's day with kids with cancer. *Journal of the American Psychiatric Nurses Association, 2*(1), 11–14.

Lambert, C. (1994). Depression: Nursing management, Part 2. *Nursing Standard, 8*(48), 57–64.

Lego, S. (1998). The application of Peplau's theory to group psychotherapy. *Journal of Psychiatric and Mental Health Nursing, 5,* 193–196.

Morrison, E. G., Shealy, A. H., Kowalsi, C., LaMont, J., & Range, B. A. (1996). Work roles of staff nurses in psychiatric settings. *Nursing Science Quarterly, 9,* 17–21.

Peden, A. R. (1998). The evolution of an intervention—the use of Peplau's process of practice-based theory development. *Journal of Psychiatric and Mental Health Nursing, 5,* 173–178.

Peplau, H. E. (n.d.). *Basic principles of patient counseling.*

Peplau, H. E. (1988). *Interpersonal relations in nursing.* NY: Springer. (Original work published 1952, New York: G. P. Putnam's Sons.)

Peplau, H. E. (1992). Interpersonal relations: A theoretical framework for application in nursing practice. *Nursing Science Quarterly, 5,* 13–18.

Peplau, H. E. (1994a). Psychiatric mental health nursing: Challenge and change. *Journal of Psychiatric and Mental Health Nursing, 1,* 3–7.

Peplau, H. E. (1994b). Quality of life: An interpersonal perspective. *Nursing Science Quarterly, 7,* 10–15.

Peplau, H. E. (1994c). The "Bridges of Madison County" has been on the best-seller list for more than 1 year. From a psycho-social perspective, what is the appeal of this popular book? *Journal of Psychosocial Nursing, 32,* 57–58.

Peplau, H. E. (1995). Some unresolved issues in the era of biopsychosocial nursing. *Journal of the American Psychiatric Nurses Association, 1,* 92–96.

Peplau, H. E. (1997). Peplau's theory of interpersonal relations. *Nursing Science Quarterly, 10,* 162–167.

Price, B. (1998). Explorations in body image care: Peplau and practice knowledge. *Journal of Psychiatric and Mental Health Nursing, 5,* 179–186.

Profile: Hildegard E. Peplau, R.N., Ed.D. (1974). *Nursing '74, 4,* 13.

Reynolds, W. J. (1997). Peplau's theory in practice. *Nursing Science Quarterly, 10,* 168–170.

Rogers, M. E. (1970). *An introduction to the theoretical basis of nursing.* Philadelphia: Davis. (out of print)

Ryles, S. (1998). Applying Peplau's theory in psychiatric nursing practice. *Nursing Times, 94,* 62–63.

Sills, G. (1977). Research in the field of psychiatric nursing, 1952–1977. *Nursing Research, 26,* 201–207.

Sullivan, H. S. (1947). *Conceptions of modern psychiatry*. Washington, D. C.: William Alanson White Psychiatric Foundation.

Vardy, C., & Price, V. (1998). Commentary. The utilization of Peplau's theory of nursing in working with a male survivor of sexual abuse. *Journal of Psychiatric and Mental Health Nursing, 5,* 149–155.

Yamashita, M. (1997). Family caregiving: Application of Newman's and Peplau's theories. *Journal of Psychiatric and Mental Health Nursing, 4,* 401–405.

BIBLIOGRAPHY

Beeber, L., Anderson, C. A., & Sills, G. M. (1990). Peplau's theory in practice, *Nursing Science Quarterly, 3,* 6–8.

Forchuk, C. (1991). Peplau's theory: Concepts and their relations. *Nursing Science Quarterly, 4,* 54–60.

Forchuk, C., & Dorsay, J. P. (1995). Hildegard Peplau meets family systems nursing: Innovation in theory-based practice. *Journal of Advanced Nursing, 21,* 110–115.

Peplau, H. E. (1969, March). Theory: The professional dimension. In *Proceedings from the First Nursing Theory Conference*. University of Kansas Medical Center. [Reprinted 1986 in L. H. Nicholl (Ed.), *Perspectives on nursing theory* (pp. 455–466). Boston: Little, Brown.]

Peplau, H. E. (1978). Psychiatric nursing: Role of nurses and psychiatric nurses. *International Nursing Review, 25,* 41–47.

Peplau, H. E. (1982). Some reflections on earlier days in psychiatric nursing. *Journal of Psychosocial Nursing and Mental Health Services, 20,* 17–24.

Peplau, H. E. (1985). Is nursing's self-regulatory power being eroded? *American Journal of Nursing, 85,* 140–143.

Peplau, H. E. (1985). The power of the dissociative state. *Journal of Psychosocial Nursing and Mental Health Services, 8,* 31–33.

Peplau, H. E. (1986). The nurse as counselor. *Journal of American College of Health, 35,* 11–14.

Peplau, H. E. (1987). Psychiatric skills, Tomorrow's world. *Nursing Times, 83,* 29–33.

Peplau, H. E. (1988). The art and science of nursing: Similarities, differences, and relations. *Nursing Science Quarterly, 1,* 8–15.

Peplau, H. E. (1989). Future directions in psychiatric nursing from the history. *Journal of Psychosocial Nursing, 2,* 18–21, 25–28.

Peplau, H. E. (1990). Evolution of nursing in psychiatric settings. In E. M. Varcarolis (Ed.), *Foundations of psychiatric mental health nursing*. Philadelphia: Saunders.

Peplau, H. E. (1997). Is healthcare a right? *Journal of Nursing Scholarship, 3,* 220–222.

Thompson, L. (1980). Peplau's theory: An application to short-term individual therapy. *Journal of Psychosocial Nursing, 24,* 26–31.

Trench, A. S. (Executive producer), Wallace, D. (Producer), & Coberg, T. (Director). (1988). *Hildegard Peplau—The nurse theorists: Portraits of excellence* [Videotape]. Oakland, CA: Studio Three Production, Samuel Merritt College of Nursing.

ANNOTATED BIBLIOGRAPHY

Beeber, L., & Caldwell, C. (1996). Pattern integrations in young depressed women: Part 1 and Part 2. *Archives of Psychiatric Nursing, 10*(3): 151–164.
Research in which 42 hours of clinical tapes were analyzed consisting of data derived from clinical interventions over a four month period with six depressed women. Analysis of clusters of

behaviors for nurse/client reciprocal interactions was made identifying four common pattern integrations of complementary, mutual, alternating, and antagonistic patterns as described by Peplau. Clinical illustrations and a model for intervention using the pattern integrations is discussed.

Forchuk, C. (1995). Development of nurse–client relationships: What helps. *Journal of the American Psychiatric Nurses Association, 1,* 146–153

This secondary analysis of data investigated factors that influence the progress of the therapeutic relationship during Peplau's orientation phase. Factors related to a shorter orientation phase included longer meetings between the nurse and patient, more cumulative time spent in such meetings, and a history of shorter previous hospitalizations. Factors that influenced the progression of the relationship in this phase included those that cannot be altered.

Forchuk, C., Beaten, S., Crawford, L., Ide, L., Voorberg, N., & Bethune, J. (1989). Incorporating Peplau's theory and case management. *Journal of Psychosocial Nursing, 2,* 35–38.

A case management program was established with a target client group of chronic mentally ill individuals who had no connection with the mental health system. Links were identified incorporating Peplau's theory and the case management model to develop a consistent approach. The importance of the interactive interpersonal relationship between the practitioner and the client became the main link. The combined model provided a basis for comprehensive permanent follow-up. Implementation is described in a case study.

Fowler, J. (1995). Taking theory into practice: Using Peplau's model in the care of patient. *Professional Nurse, 10*(4), 226–230.

The philosophy of palliative care and Peplau's Interpersonal Relations Model were reviewed for compatibility. A case study focused on the care of one terminally ill patient in a hospice setting as the model was applied to clinical practice.

Lego, S. (1998). The application of Peplau's theory to group psychotherapy. *Journal of Psychiatric and Mental Health Nursing, 5*(3), 193–196.

Portrayal of the phases of Peplau's Interpersonal Theory as they pertain to group psychotherapy is made. Clinical illustrations are discussed. Steps of the learning process are detailed as the patient moves through them in group therapy. Also, the nurse's roles are presented as they arise during group sessions.

Morrison, E. G., Shealy, A. H., Kowalski, C., LaMont, J., & Range, B. A. (1996). Work roles of staff nurses in psychiatric settings. *Nursing Science Quarterly, 9*(1), 17–21.

This research was conducted to authenticate the workroles of the psychiatric staff nurse as referenced by Peplau. Audiotaped one-to-one interactions were performed between 30 registered nurses and 62 patients. Overlapping behaviors were found between some roles. The most frequently occurring primary workrole was that of the counselor sustaining Peplau's view of the counselor's role.

Peden, A. R. (1998). The evolution of an intervention—the use of Peplau's process of practice-based theory development. *Journal of Psychiatric and Mental Health Nursing, 5*(3), 173–178.

Reviews Peplau's theories of nursing knowledge/practice. Peplau is credited for research methodology and is acknowledged as setting precedence in psychiatric nursing.

Peplau, H. E. (1997). Peplau's theory of interpersonal relations. *Nursing Science Quarterly, 10,* 162–167.

Peplau first presents other theories essential to nursing practice before describing her interpersonal relations theory. The remainder of the article's focus is on this interpersonal theory. Participant observation includes the nurse self analyzing overt and covert behaviors and ability to empathize. The nurse and patient progress through three phases of their relationship in the interpersonal process. These phases are discussed as well as the issues that occur throughout the interactions.

CHAPTER 5

DEFINITION AND COMPONENTS OF NURSING
VIRGINIA HENDERSON

Chiyoko Yamamoto Furukawa
Joan Swartz Howe

Virginia Henderson was born on March 19, 1897, in Kansas City, Missouri, and died on November 30, 1996. She was the fifth child of a family of eight children and lived most of her formative years in Virginia where the family lived during the period her father practiced law in Washington.

Henderson's interest in nursing evolved during World War I from her desire to help the sick and wounded military personnel. She enrolled in the Army School of Nursing in Washington, DC, and graduated in 1921. In 1926, Henderson began the continuation of her education at Columbia University Teachers College and completed her B.S. (1932) and M.A. (1934) degrees in nursing education. She taught clinical nursing courses with a strong emphasis on the use of the analytical process from 1934 to 1948 at Teachers College. From 1948 to 1953 she worked with Harmer on an extensive revision of the fifth edition of The Principles and Practice of Nursing. In 1953, she was appointed as faculty at Yale University School of Nursing. The Yale years were very productive with a number of Henderson's major publications copyrighted between 1955 and 1978 (McBride, 1996). From 1959 to 1971, Henderson directed the Nursing Studies Index Project, which clearly showed her interest in supporting nursing research (Henderson & Watt, 1983). Also, during 1953 to 1958, she was on the Survey and Assessment of Nursing Research staff, a project directed by Leo W. Simmons. In the 1980s Henderson (1982b) supported the idea that nursing must accept the responsibility for conducting investigations on nursing practice, and that the focus ought to be on measures of consumer welfare, satisfaction, and cost-effectiveness. Henderson also played an important role in the publication of The International Nursing Index, in 1966. The Index was the result and production of the promotional efforts of the Interagency on Library Resources in Nursing (Henderson, 1991). During retirement, she was Senior Research Associate Emeritus at Yale University.

Henderson was the recipient of numerous recognitions for her outstanding contributions to nursing including the Sigma Theta Tau International Nursing

Library, which bears her name. She received honorary doctoral degrees from the Catholic University of America, Pace University, University of Rochester, University of Western Ontario, Yale University, Old Dominion University, Boston College, Thomas Jefferson University, and Emery University.

Her writings are far-reaching and have made an impact on nursing throughout the world. In June 1985, the International Council of Nurses presented her with the first Christianne Reimann Prize in recognition of her influence as nursing consultant to the world (McBride, 1996). The publications The nature of nursing *(1966) and* Basic principles of nursing care *(1960, 1997) are widely known, and the latter has been translated into many languages for the benefit of non–English-speaking nurses. She clarified her beliefs about nursing, nursing education, and nursing practice in view of recent technological and societal advances in publications, interviews, and personal appearances (Henderson, 1978, 1979a, 1979b, 1982a, 1985, 1987). One of her last publications, in 1991, was* The nature of nursing—Reflections after 25 years. *The addendum to each chapter contains changes in her views and opinions relative to the 1966 first edition of* The nature of nursing.

Questions about the exclusive functions of nurses provided the impetus for Virginia Henderson to devote her career to defining nursing practice. Some of these questions were: What is the practice of nursing? What specific functions do nurses perform? What are nursing's unique activities? The development of her definition of nursing communicated her thoughts on these questions. She believed that an occupation that affects human life must outline its functions, particularly if it is to be regarded as a profession (Henderson, 1966, 1991). Her ideas about the definition of nursing were influenced by her nursing education and practice, by her students and colleagues at Columbia University School of Nursing, and by distinguished nursing leaders of her time. All these experiences and nursing practice were the dominating forces that gave her insight into nursing: what it is and what are its functions.

THE DEVELOPMENT OF HENDERSON'S DEFINITION OF NURSING

Two events are the basis for Henderson's development of a definition of nursing. First, she participated in the revision of a nursing textbook. Second, she was concerned that many states had no provision for nursing licensure to ensure safe and competent care for the consumer.

In the revision of *Textbook of the principles and practice of nursing*, written with Canadian nurse Bertha Harmer, Henderson recognized the need to be clear about the functions of the nurse (Harmer & Henderson, 1939; Safier, 1977). She believed a textbook that serves as a main learning source for nursing practice should present a sound and definitive description of nursing. Furthermore, the principles and practice of nursing must be built on and derived from the definition of the profession.

Henderson was committed to the process of regulating nursing practice through state licensure. She believed that to accomplish this, nursing must be explicitly defined in Nurse Practice Acts that would provide the legal parameters for nurses' functions in caring for consumers, and to safeguard the public from unprepared and incompetent practitioners.

Although official statements on the nursing function were published by the American Nurses' Association (ANA) in 1932 and 1937, Henderson (1966, 1991) viewed these statements as nonspecific and unsatisfactory definitions of nursing practice. Then, in 1955, the earlier ANA (1962) definition was modified to read as follows:

> The practice of professional nursing means the performance for compensation of any act in the observation, care, and counsel of the ill, injured, or infirm, or in the maintenance of health or prevention of illness of others, or in the supervision and teaching of other personnel, or the administration of medications and treatment as prescribed by a licensed physician or dentist; requiring substantial specialized judgment and skill and based on knowledge and application of the principles of biological, physical, and social science. The foregoing shall not be deemed to include acts of diagnosis or prescription of therapeutic or corrective measures (p. 7).

This statement was seen as an improvement because nursing functions were identified, but the definition still was thought to be very general and too vague. In the new statement, the nurse could observe, care for, and counsel the patient and could supervise other health personnel without herself or himself being supervised by the physician. The nurse was to give medications and do treatments ordered by the physician but was prohibited from diagnosing, prescribing treatment for, or correcting nursing care problems. Thus, Henderson viewed the statement as another unsatisfactory definition of nursing.

Henderson's extensive experiences as a student, teacher, practitioner, author, and participant in conferences on the nurse's function contributed to the development of her definition of nursing. She regretted that publications of conference debates and investigations were not widely circulated. Only a few nurses were privy to the information published about the outcomes of these conferences.

In 1955, Henderson's first definition of nursing was published in Bertha Harmer's revised nursing textbook (Harmer & Henderson, 1955). It reads as follows:

Henderson's First (1955) Definition

Nursing is primarily assisting the individual (sick or well) in the performance of those activities contributing to health, or its recovery (or peaceful death) that he would perform unaided if he had the necessary strength, will, or knowledge. It is likewise the unique contribution of nursing to help the individual to be independent of such assistance as soon as possible (p. 4).

This statement on nursing conveys the essence of Henderson's definition of nursing as it is known today. Since there was collaboration, it is instructive to compare Henderson's definition with Harmer's 1922 definition, which follows:

Harmer's 1922 Definition

Nursing is rooted in the needs of humanity and is founded on the ideal of service. Its object is not only to cure the sick and heal the wounded but to bring health and ease, rest and comfort to mind and body, to shelter, nourish, and protect and to minister to all those who are helpless or handicapped, young, aged or immature. Its object is to prevent disease and to preserve health. Nursing is, therefore, linked with every other social agency which strives for the prevention of disease and the preservation of health. The nurse finds herself not only concerned with the care of the individual but with the health of a people (p. 3).

Some similarities can be seen between the two definitions of nursing. Henderson's definition abbreviated and consolidated portions of Harmer's beliefs about nursing. Harmer's definition highlighted disease prevention, health preservation, and the need for linkages with other social agencies to strive for preventive care. Harmer stressed that nursing's role in society was oriented toward the community and wellness. Henderson placed more emphasis on the care of sick and well individuals and did not mention nursing's concern for the health and welfare of the aggregate. However, there is brief mention in *Basic principles of nursing* that at times nurses do function with families or other aggregates rather than solely with individuals (Henderson, 1997).

Henderson's focus on individual care is evident in that she stressed assisting individuals with essential activities to maintain health, to recover, or to achieve peaceful death. She proposed 14 components of basic nursing care to augment her definition (Henderson, 1966, 1991), as follows:

[The individual can]
1. Breathe normally.
2. Eat and drink adequately.
3. Eliminate body wastes.
4. Move and maintain desirable postures.
5. Sleep and rest.
6. Select suitable clothes—dress and undress.
7. Maintain body temperature within normal range by adjusting clothing and modifying the environment.

8. Keep the body clean and well groomed and protect the integument.
9. Avoid dangers in the environment and avoid injuring others.
10. Communicate with others in expressing emotions, needs, fears, or opinions.
11. Worship according to one's faith.
12. Work in such a way that there is a sense of accomplishment.
13. Play or participate in various forms of recreation.
14. Learn, discover, or satisfy the curiosity that leads to normal development and health and use the available health facilities (pp. 16–17).

In 1966, Henderson's ultimate statement on the definition of nursing was published in *The nature of nursing*. This statement was viewed as "the crystallization of my ideas" (p. 15):

> The unique function of the nurse is to assist the individual, sick or well, in the performance of those activities contributing to health or its recovery (or to peaceful death) that he would perform unaided if he had the necessary strength, will or knowledge. And to do this in such a way as to help him gain independence as rapidly as possible (p. 15).

Except for slight wording changes, the 1955, 1966, and more recent 1978 definitions are quite similar, indicating that her definition of nursing, conceived earlier, remains intact (Harmer & Henderson, 1955; Henderson, 1966; Henderson & Nite, 1978). Henderson's definition of nursing in itself fails to fully explain her main ideas and views. To appreciate the breadth of her thoughts about nursing functions and the 14 components of basic nursing care, it is necessary to study *Basic principles of nursing care*, a publication of the International Council of Nurses (Henderson, 1960, 1997). This textbook eloquently describes each of the basic nursing care components so that they can be used as a guide to delineate the unique nursing functions. The definition of nursing and the 14 components together outline the functions the nurse can initiate and control. Further understanding of these components can be gained through study of the sixth edition of *Principles and practice of nursing*. This edition was organized according to the 14 components and also includes citations from the work of nurses around the world.

Henderson (1966, 1991) expects nurses to carry out the therapeutic plan of the physician as a member of the medical team. The nurse is the prime helper to the ill person in assuring that the medical prescriptions are instituted. This nursing function is believed to foster the therapeutic nurse–client relationship. As a member of an interdisciplinary health team, the nurse assists the individual to recovery or provides support in dying. The ideal situation for a nurse is full participation as a team member with no interference with the nurse's unique functions. The nurse serves as a substitute for whatever the patient lacks in order to make him or her "complete," "whole," or "independent," considering his or her available physical strength, will, or knowledge to attain good health.

The nurse is cautioned about tasks that detract from the professional role and the need to give priority to the nurse's unique functions. However, Henderson encourages the nurse to assume the role and functions of other health workers if the need is apparent and the nurse has expertise. On a worldwide basis, nursing functions differ from country to country, or even within countries. The ratio of nurses to physicians and to other health care providers affects what nurses do. Consequently, the public is confused about the nurse's role, particularly since the creation of nurse practitioners.

In one of her last publications, Henderson (1991) acknowledged that the efforts to define nursing had been unsuccessful: "In spite of the fact that generations of nurses have tried to define it, 'the nature of nursing' remains a question" (p. 7). In her opinion, nurses were no closer to consensus on the official definition of nursing than in 1966. She stated the only difference now is that nursing education offers courses on nursing theory and nursing process. If *The nature of nursing* were to be written in the 1990s, she felt she would be obliged to include a discussion of both nursing theory and the nursing process.

Furthermore, with respect to a universal definition of nursing, Henderson (1991) concluded that there is difficulty in promoting the notion of universality. She based her view on her numerous visits to countries worldwide where she observed the variations in nursing education coupled with differing nursing practices used to serve the needs of various populations.

HENDERSON'S THEORY AND NURSING'S METAPARADIGM

In viewing the concept of the *human* or individual, Henderson considered the biological, psychological, sociological, and spiritual components. Her 14 components of nursing functions can be categorized in the following manner: The first nine components are physiological; the tenth and fourteenth are psychological aspects of communicating and learning; the eleventh component is spiritual and moral; and the twelfth and thirteenth components are sociologically oriented to occupation and recreation. She referred to humans as having basic needs that are included in the 14 components. However, she further stated, "It is equally important to realize that these needs are satisfied by infinitely varied patterns of living, no two of which are alike" (Henderson, 1997, p. 27). Henderson (1966, 1991) also believed that mind and body are inseparable. It is implied that the mind and body are interrelated.

Henderson emphasized some aspects of the concept of *society/environment*. In her writings, she primarily discussed individuals. She saw individuals in relation to their families but minimally discussed the impact of the community on the individual and family. In the book cowritten with Harmer (Harmer & Henderson, 1955), she supported the tasks of private and public agencies in keeping people healthy. She believed that society wants and expects the nurse's service of acting for individuals who are unable to function independently (Henderson, 1966, 1991). In return, she expected society to contribute to nursing education:

> The nurse needs the kind of education that, in our society, is available only in colleges and universities. Training programs operated on funds pinched from the budgets of service agencies cannot provide the preparation the nurse needs (p. 69).

This generalized education gives the nurse a better understanding of the consumers of nursing care and the various environmental factors that influence people.

Henderson's beliefs about *health* were related to human functioning. Her definition of health was based on the individual's ability to function independently, as outlined in the 14 components. Because good health is a challenging goal for individuals, she argued that it is difficult for the nurse to help the person reach it (Henderson, 1997). She also referred to nurses stressing promotion of health and prevention and cure of disease (Henderson, 1966). Henderson (1997) explained how the factors of age, cultural background, physical and intellectual capacities, and emotional balance affect one's health. These conditions are always present and affect basic needs. Because of her concern for the welfare of people, Henderson (1989) believed that nurses "should be in the forefront of those who work for social justice, for a healthful environment, for access to adequate food, shelter, and clothing, and universal opportunities for education and employment, realizing that all of these as well as preventive and creative health care are essential to the well-being of citizens" (p. 82). By working on various social issues, nurses can have an impact on people's health.

Henderson's concept of nursing is interesting from the perspective of time. She was one of the earlier leaders who believed nurses need a liberal education, including knowledge of sciences, social sciences, and humanities. Aside from using the definition of nursing and the 14 components of basic nursing care, the nurse is expected to carry out the physician's therapeutic plan. Individualized care is the result of the nurse's creativity in planning for care. Furthermore, the nurse is expected to improve patient care by using the results of nursing research:

> ... the nurse who operates under a definition that specifies an area of independent practice, or an area of expertness, *must* assume responsibility for identifying problems, for continually validating her function, for improving the methods she uses, and for measuring the effect of nursing care. In this era research is the name we attach to the most reliable type of analysis (Henderson, 1966, p. 38).

For Henderson, the nurse must be knowledgeable, have some base for practicing individualized and humane care, and be a scientific problem solver. In her update of

The nature of nursing, Henderson (1991) viewed "research in nursing as *essential* to the validation and improvement of practice" (p. 58). Even though she believed that caring for patients "is an important, really essential element of nurses' service," she also emphasized that "nursing practice and nursing education should nevertheless be based on research" (p. 58). It is important that nursing care be improved by implementing valid research results.

HENDERSON AND THE NURSING PROCESS

Henderson (1980a) viewed the nursing process as "really the application of the logical approach to the solution of a problem. The steps are those of the scientific method" (p. 906). With this approach, each person can receive individualized care. Likewise, with the nursing process, individualized care is the result.

In Henderson's later writings, she raised some issues regarding the nursing process. One of the issues questioned whether the problem-solving approach of the nursing process is peculiar to nursing. She compared the nursing process to the traditional steps of the medical process: "the nursing history parallels the medical history; the nurse's health assessment, the physician's medical examination; the nursing diagnosis corresponds to the physician's diagnosis; nursing orders to the plan of medical management; and nursing evaluation to medical evaluation" (Henderson, 1980a, p. 907). It looks as if the language has been changed to fit nursing's purpose. Could other health care workers use the steps of the nursing process to fit their practice? If so, then what makes the nursing process peculiar to nursing?

Another issue Henderson raised also dealt with problem solving. But now she asked if problem solving is all there is to nursing. Henderson (1987) stated, "this makes it so specific that activities outside those in the problem solving steps of the process cannot be peculiar to or characteristic of nursing" (p. 8). She questioned where intuition, experience, authority, and expert opinion fit into the nursing process since they are not stressed. She further commented, "Expert opinion or authority is also, by implication, discredited as a basis for practice" (Henderson, 1982a, p. 108). Does the "the" in the nursing process make it too limiting for effective practice?

A third issue Henderson raised flows from the problem-solving approach. She asks where the art of nursing fits into the nursing process. If one views science as objective with little left undefined and art as subjective with some parts hard to define, then where does intuition fit? Henderson (1987) argued that "The nursing process now weighted so heavily on the scientific side, seems to belittle the intuitive, artistic side of nursing" (p. 8). She also claimed, "nursing process stresses the science of nursing rather than the mixture of science *and art* on which it seems effective health care services of any kind is based" (Henderson, 1987, p. 9). Does the nursing process disregard the subjective and intuitive qualities used in nursing?

The fourth concern Henderson raised about the nursing process deals with the lack of collaboration among health care workers, the patient, and the family. She stated, "As currently defined, nursing process does not seem to suggest a collabora-tive approach on diagnosis, treatment, *or* care by health care workers, nor does it suggest the essential rights of patients and their families in all of these questions" (Henderson, 1982a, p. 109). Henderson (1987) thought the nursing process stressed an independent function for the nurse rather than a collaborative one with other health professionals, the patient, and the patient's family. Does the nursing process focus more on independent nursing functions than on interdependent functions?

Perhaps it is semantics that is a problem with the nursing process. The real value of the nursing process depends on one's understanding, interpretation, integration, and use of it. The nursing process discussed in Chapter 2 is now examined with Henderson's definition of nursing.

Even though Henderson's definition and explanation of nursing do not fit di-rectly with the steps of the nursing process, a relationship between the two can be demonstrated. Although Henderson did not refer directly to assessment, she implied it in her description of the 14 components of basic nursing care. The nurse uses the 14 components to assess the individual's needs. For example, in assessing the first component, "breathe normally," the nurse gathers all pertinent data about the per-son's respiratory status. The nurse then moves to the next component and gathers data in that area. The gathering of data about the person continues until all compo-nents have been assessed.

To complete the assessment phase of the nursing process, the nurse needs to ana-lyze the data. According to Henderson, the nurse must have knowledge about what is normal in health and disease. Using this knowledge base, then, the nurse com-pares the assessment data with what was known about that area. For example, if res-pirations were observed to be 40 per minute in an adult aged 50, the nurse would conclude that this person's respiratory rate is faster than normal. Or if a laboratory report showed that the urine was highly concentrated, the nurse would know this "means that the patient's fluid intake is inadequate, unless he is losing body fluids by other routes" (Henderson, 1997, p. 51). With a scientific knowledge base, the nurse can draw conclusions from the assessment data. Henderson (1997) stated the following:

> . . . the nursing needed by the individual is affected by age, cultural background, emotional balance and the patient's physical and intellec-tual capacities. All of these should be considered in the nurse's evalua-tion of the patient's needs for help (p. 31).

Following the analysis of the data according to these factors, the nurse then de-termines the nursing diagnosis. Henderson did not specifically discuss nursing diag-noses. She believed the physician makes the diagnosis, and the nurse acts on that diagnosis or that both could make the same diagnosis and there was no need for a separate nursing diagnosis. However, if one looks at Henderson's definition, the nursing diagnosis deals with identifying the individual's ability to meet human needs with or without assistance, taking into account that person's strength, will, and knowledge. Given the assessment data and its analysis, the nurse *can* identify actual problems such as abnormal respirations. In addition, potential problems may be identified. For example, with Component 11, about one's faith, a potential problem could develop because of hospitalization and a change in the person's normal activities of daily living. If, based on the nurse's assessment and analysis of the data, a person was unable to meet this need, then a nursing diagnosis regarding an actual problem would be made.

Once the nursing diagnosis is made, the nurse proceeds to the outcomes and planning phase of the nursing process, about which Henderson (1997) stated:

> All effective nursing care is planned to some extent. A written plan *forces* those who make it to give some thought to the individual's needs—unless the person's regimen is made to fit into the routines of the institution (p. 37).

She also contended that *discharge planning* was influenced by the other members of the family (Henderson, 1997). Furthermore, plans need continuing modification that is based on the individual's needs. Henderson advocated written nursing care plans so others giving care can follow the planned sequence. She emphasized that "nursing care is always arranged around, or fitted into, the physician's therapeutic plan" (p. 38). Henderson outlined the planning phase as making the plan fit the individual's needs, updating the plan as necessary on the basis of those needs, being specific so others can implement it, and fitting with the physician's prescribed plan. Written nursing care plans, in essence, identify the nursing needs of the person. Even though Henderson does not apply the current terminology about nursing plans, she uses the same ideas. The ideal outcome would be the complete return to independence.

Implementation follows the planning of nursing care. For Henderson (1966, 1991), nursing implementation was based on helping the patient meet the 14 components. For example, in helping the individual with sleep and rest, the nurse tries known methods of inducing sleep and rest before giving drugs. Henderson summarized, "I see nursing as primarily complementing the patient by supplying what he needs in knowledge, will, or strength to perform his daily activities and to carry out the treatment prescribed for him by the physician" (p. 21). Henderson also stated, "This primary function of the practicing nurse, of course, must be performed in such a way that it promotes the physician's therapeutic plan" (p. 27). So the nurse needs to carry out the physician's orders of treatment along with her nursing care.

Another important aspect of implementation that Henderson (1966, 1991) discussed is the relationship between nurse and patient. The nurse gets "inside the skin" of the patient to better understand the patient's needs and carry out measures to meet those needs. Henderson (1997) also spoke about the quality of nursing care:

> The danger of turning over the physical care of the patient to relatively unqualified nurses is twofold. They may fail to assess the patient's needs adequately but, perhaps more important, the qualified nurse, being deprived of the opportunity while giving physical care to assess the patient's needs, may not find any other chance to do so. In this connection it should also be pointed out that it is easier for any person to

develop an emotional supportive role with another if he can perform a tangible service (p. 36).

This statement clearly supports the idea that the competent nurse uses both the interpersonal process and assessment while giving care.

Henderson (1966) bases the evaluation of each person "according to the speed with which, or the degree to which, he performs independently the activities that make, for him, a normal day" (p. 27). This notion is outlined in the definition of and the unique function of the nurse. For evaluation purposes, changes in a person's level of functioning need to be observed and recorded. A comparison of the data about the person's functional abilities is done pre- and postnursing care. All changes are noted for evaluation.

To summarize the stages of the nursing process as applied to Henderson's definition of nursing and to the 14 components of basic nursing care, refer to Table 5–1. Furthermore, the case study in Table 5–2 demonstrates the application of the nursing process to Henderson's definition and 14 components.

TABLE 5–1. A SUMMARY OF THE NURSING PROCESS AND OF HENDERSON'S 14 COMPONENTS AND DEFINITION OF NURSING

Nursing Process	Henderson's 14 Components and Definition of Nursing
Nursing assessment	Assess need of human being based on the 14 components of basic nursing care: 1. Breathe normally 2. Eat and drink adequately 3. Eliminate body wastes 4. Move and maintain posture 5. Sleep and rest 6. Suitable clothing, dress or undress 7. Maintain body temperature 8. Keep body clean and well-groomed 9. Avoid dangers in environment 10. Communicate 11. Worship according to one's faith 12. Work accomplishment 13. Recreation 14. Learn, discover, or satisfy curiosity Analysis: Compare data to knowledge base of health and disease
Nursing diagnosis	Identify individual's ability to meet own needs with or without assistance, taking into consideration strength, will, and knowledge.
Outcomes	Establish desired outcomes based on return to independence.
Planning	Document how the nurse can assist the individual, sick or well.
Implementation	Assist the sick or well individual and the family in the performance of activities in meeting human needs to maintain health, recover from illness, or to aid in peaceful death. Implementation based on physiological principles, age, cultural background, emotional balance, and physical and intellectual capacities. Carry out treatment prescribed by the physician.
Evaluation	Use the acceptable definition of nursing and appropriate laws related to the practice of nursing—can the person now meet the basic human needs? The quality of care is drastically affected by the preparation and native abilities of the nursing personnel rather than the number of hours of care. Successful outcomes of nursing care are based on the speed with which or the degree to which the patient performs independently the activities of daily living that are normal to him.

TABLE 5–2. THE NURSING PROCESS FOR MR. L., USING HENDERSON'S 14 COMPONENTS

Case Study: Mr. L. is 25 years old, married, and the father of two preschool-age children. His wife is 6 months pregnant. Mr. L. quit school in the 10th grade. He works 8 hours a day as a skilled laborer in a factory and holds a second job washing dishes at a restaurant for an additional 8 hours in order to meet family expenses.

Nursing Process	Data and Relevant Information
Assessment (Assess needs of Mr. L. based on the 14 components of basic nursing care)	Assessment
1. Breathe normally.	1. Respiration rate—18, regular; smokes 2 packs of cigarettes/day; dry cough in A.M.; no shortness of breath. (Data about work environment needed.)
2. Eat and drink adequately.	2. Height 5 ft., 10 in.; weight 164 lbs.; skin turgor good. Takes sandwich, fruit, potato chips for lunch; skips breakfast; buys soft drink; eats evening meals at restaurant. (Results of 72 hours diet recall needed.)
3. Elimination of body wastes.	3. Reports no problems related to elimination.
4. Move and maintain posture.	4. Reports pain in both legs after 8 hours of washing dishes. No problems with mobility.
5. Sleep and rest.	5. Reports 5 to 6 hours sleep/night. "Feels tired most of the time."
6. Suitable clothing, dress/undress.	6. Wears jeans and shirt to work—both jobs. Owns ski jacket and boots for cold weather wear. (Work environment data needed.)
7. Maintain body temperature.	7. Temperature 98.6° F. Reports no problem with being hot or cold.
8. Keep body clean and well-groomed.	8. Showers and shampoos hair daily.
9. Avoid environmental hazards.	9. Wears clothes to match weather conditions. (Home environment safety—need more data.)
10. Communication.	10. Able to speak and be understood. (Communication with family—need further data.)
11. Worship according to faith.	11. Attends church (Baptist) with family every other Sunday.
12. Work accomplishment.	12. Reports happy with jobs.
13. Recreation.	13. "Need more time to spend with family."
14. Learn, discover, or satisfy curiosity.	14. Reports interested in finishing high school. Plans to pursue college education.
Analysis	According to Erikson's (1963) developmental theory, Mr. L. is in the intimacy stage. He is able to support his family and take care of most of their needs, except for recreational needs. Physiologically, Mr. L. is functioning within the normal range. Three concerns are: his smoking, pains in his legs, the inadequate sleep and rest pattern. Mr. L. plans for the future to upgrade his education and to seek better employment.

TABLE 5–2. (*CONT.*)

Nursing Process	Data and Relevant Information
Nursing diagnosis	1. Inadequate sleep and rest pattern resulting in feeling tired and no time to spend with family. 2. Knowledge deficit regarding cigarette smoking resulting in potential health hazard for self and family. 3. Leg pain resulting from standing 8 hours on the job.
Outcomes	Long range plan for stable family income that will allow for rest and recreation. Decreased smoke exposure for himself and his family. Decreased leg pain.

Nursing plan	1. Explore with Mr. L. and his wife:
	  a. alternatives to his working two jobs.
	  b. adjusting schedule to include family recreation.
	2. Assure that Mr. L. is fully aware of the hazards of smoking and of resources to help him quit smoking.
	3. Teach Mr. L. isometric exercises for his legs.

Nursing implementaion	1. Discuss with Mr. L. and his wife:
	  a. feasible alternatives to his working two jobs.
	  b. schedule changes that would allow for more family recreation.
	2. With Mr. L. and his wife:
	  a. discuss pros and cons of smoking.
	  b. teach the health hazards of smoking, including the effects of second-hand smoke on the family.
	  c. discuss options available to help Mr. L. stop smoking.
	3. Teach Mr. L.
	  a. isometric exercises for his legs.
	  b. to walk around or march in place instead of standing in one position.
	  c. to elevate his feet when sitting.

Evaluation	The outcomes of nursing care were successful because Mr. L. demonstrated his independence in making changes in his activities of daily living by: Deciding to work toward his GED so he can meet his long-range goal of going to college; Mrs. L. will go to work when the children are all in school so Mr. L. can quit his second job. Working with his employers to adjust his work shifts so at least 2 days of the week he works only one job. This allows him to get more sleep and to participate in family recreation. The family is taking walks together on the evenings he is home. Not smoking in the house, cutting back to 1 pack a day, and he is considering using a nicotine patch or nicotine gum to help him quit completely. Doing leg exercises regularly. He reports his legs feel better and that makes the shift go faster.

CRITIQUE OF HENDERSON'S DEFINITION AND COMPONENTS OF NURSING

1. What is the historical context of the theory? Henderson was one of the earliest "theorists" who attempted to describe the practice of nursing. She began to develop her definition of nursing prior to 1920 as a student in the Army School of Nursing. This is clearly demonstrated by the analysis she made of each student experience; this analysis continued after her graduation in 1921. The assumptions for the definition of nursing are implicit in the process by which it evolved. Henderson recognized the need to focus on the functions that were exclusively the domain of nursing and, therefore, did not rely on any other discipline's philosophy as a basis for nursing. Henderson's (1966, 1991) interpretation of the nurse's function was the synthesis of many positive and negative influences. She was a pioneer in her mission to identify the components of nursing practice. A review of Henderson's educational preparation and nursing practice furnishes the basis on which to examine the history of the development of her definition of nursing.

A major influence was her basic nursing education in a general hospital affiliated with the Army School of Nursing, which emphasized learning by doing, speedy performance, technical competence, and successful mastery of nursing procedures (e.g., catheterization, making beds, changing dressings). As a result, an impersonal approach to care emerged and was interpreted as professional behavior. Although the importance of ethics in nursing and a compassionate attitude toward humanity were stressed, these were not given as high a priority as the nursing procedures were.

Physician lectures were the major portion of classroom learning for the nursing students. The lectures used a cut-and-dried approach to learning and were a simplified version of medical education. The focus was disease, diagnosis, and treatment regimens. Henderson was discontented with the regimentalized care based on medical teaching. She recognized that this kind of nursing was merely an extension of medical practice (Henderson, 1966, 1991). Her dean, Annie W. Goodrich, agreed with this evaluation of nursing education.

Another educational concern for Henderson was a lack of an appropriate role model to emulate in giving nursing care. She yearned to observe patient care given by either her teacher or graduate nurses, which was impossible because students staffed the hospital in return for their nursing education. Thus, clinical practice was viewed as a self-learned process while students cared for the sick and wounded soldiers. She perceived this atmosphere to be one of indebtedness to the patients for having served the country in time of war. The nurse–patient relationship was described as warm and generous. The soldiers asked for little, and the nurses wanted to do all they could. This experience was believed to be unique and special, for the opportunity to express indebtedness to military patients did not exist in a civilian hospital.

Henderson's next educational experience, psychiatric nursing, was disappointing because the human relations skills that could have been learned in this setting failed to materialize. As in her previous experiences, the approach to psychiatric patient care continued to focus on disease entities and treatment. There was a lack of understanding about the nurse's role in the prevention of mental illness or in the curative aspects of care for the psychiatric patient. Her experience resulted in a sense of fail-ure as a nurse. The only value of the psychiatric affiliation was the opportunity to gain some appreciation of mental illness.

The pediatric nursing experience at the Boston Floating Hospital was more posi-tive and introduced three concepts of care: patient-centered, continuity of, and ten-der, loving care. The task-oriented and regimented approach to care was discarded in this setting. However, other shortcomings were identified, such as the failure to use family-centered care. Parents were not allowed to visit a sick child. Therefore, the child was isolated from parental support when it was most needed. Furthermore, Henderson saw little or no effort to assess the home environment to identify the needs of the child and family.

The final student experience at the Henry Street Visiting Nurse Agency in New York introduced her to community nursing care. The formal approach to patient care learned earlier was replaced with care that considered the sick person's life style. Henderson was concerned about discharging patients to the same environ-ment that originally led them to hospitalization. She believed that the hospital care only served as a stopgap measure without getting to the cause of the problem. She recognized that this type of care failed to consider the person living outside the be-havioral controls of the institutional setting.

As a graduate nurse, Henderson worked for several years in Visiting Nursing Services in Washington, DC, and New York, because she deplored the hospital sys-tem of nursing and did not want to be in it. This experience was rewarding and of-fered the opportunity to try out her ideas about nursing.

Her next position was teaching nursing students at the Norfolk Protestant Hospi-tal diploma program in Virginia. She accepted this five-year responsibility without further education, a situation that was not uncommon because many diploma schools at that time did not require academic credentials for teaching. Despite this, she recognized the need for more knowledge and for clarification of the functions of nursing. Subsequently, she enrolled at Columbia University Teachers College to learn about the sciences and humanities relevant to nursing. These courses enabled Henderson to develop an inquiring and analytical approach to nursing.

After graduation, she briefly accepted the position of teaching supervisor at Strong Memorial Hospital's clinics in Rochester, New York. Next, she returned to Columbia, where her distinguished teaching career continued until 1948. While at this university, Henderson implemented several ideas about nursing in her medical-surgical nursing courses. The concepts taught were a patient-centered approach, the nursing problem method replacing the medical model, field experience, family follow-up care, and chronic illness care. She also established nursing clinics and en-couraged coordinated multidisciplinary care.

With her appointment to the faculty at Yale University School of Nursing, Hen-derson continued to develop her concepts that supported her evolving definition of nursing. She was influenced by her colleagues, Ernestine Wiedenbach and Ida Orlando, in the areas of observing and interpreting patient behavior and the nurses' role in meeting the patients' needs. Henderson acknowledged faculty discussion on these topics, which continued to assist her in clarifying her own notions about nurs-ing. In return, her colleagues also benefitted by Henderson's discussion on not only her definition of nursing, but also the concepts outlined in her publications *Basic principles of nursing care* and the *Principles and practice of nursing.*

2. What are the basic concepts and relationships presented by the theory?

Henderson used the concepts of fundamental human needs, bio-physiology, culture, and interaction-communication. These concepts are borrowed from other disciplines rather than being unique to nursing; it is how they are used that makes them unique to nursing. These concepts are not defined as one now expects in the process of theory development, therefore the relationships of the concepts as currently known are not presented as based on stated assumptions. Much of Henderson's work may be considered to be descriptive statements to convey the definition and unique functions of nursing.

However, Maslow's (1970) hierarchy of human needs fits well with the basic 14 components. The first nine components are physiological and safety needs. The remaining five components deal with love and belonging, social esteem, and self-actualization needs.

Henderson used the biophysiological concept when she stressed the importance of physiology and physiological balances in making decisions about nursing care. Biological knowledge was deemed to be the basis on which the nurse helped the patient with the necessary activities to get well or to assist in peaceful death. To Henderson, the information provided by physiology, anatomy, and microbiology about how the human body functions was important. This then can be used by the nurse to determine appropriate care needed to alleviate the illness or injury.

The concept of culture as it affects human needs is learned from the family and other social groups. Because of this, Henderson suggests that a nurse is unable to fully interpret or supply all the requirements for the individual's well-being. At best the nurse can merely assist the individual in meeting human needs.

The concept of interaction-communication can be seen in Henderson's writings. She believed sensitivity to nonverbal communication is essential to encourage the expression of feelings (Henderson, 1966). Henderson supported the works of her colleagues, Ernestine Wiedenbach and Ida Orlando (Pelletier), in their work in interaction of patients and nurses. Wiedenbach and Orlando clearly identified "what the nurse observes, what she thinks or feels, what she says or does in response to this thought or feeling, and how the patient responds, how he affirms or denies the nurse's interpretation of his problems and needs, and finally how the nurse evaluates her successes in helping the patient to solve his problem or meet his need" (Henderson, 1991, p. 36). In addition, interaction-communication includes the opportunities to see and talk with the patient's friends and family to increase understanding of needs to be addressed by the nurse. Furthermore, a prerequisite to validate a patient's needs is a constructive nurse–patient relationship. It can be seen that from the social sciences, Henderson believed that understanding the background of the individual was important. An individual's nursing needs must include the context in which the person lives. A person's cultural background, including his or her socioeconomic status, beliefs, and values must be taken into account to meet nursing care needs.

It can be seen that the concepts of human needs, biophysiology, culture, and interaction-communication are interrelated. Put into the context of Henderson's definition of nursing, all of these concepts are identified and incorporated to describe what the nurse is expected to provide to those in need of his/her services. These concepts are clearly in support of the 14 components of basic nursing. The first five components are biophysical needs that the nurse/patient must attend to for sustaining life. The next four components focus on biophysical, human needs, and some aspects of cultural needs. The final five components include interaction-communication aspects as well as cultural and human needs. Therefore, one can surmise that the concepts underlying Henderson's components of basic nursing care are interrelated and addressed the care that nurses ought to provide to their clients/patients.

3. What major phenomenon of concern to nursing are presented? These phenomena may include *but are not limited to:* **human being, environment, health, interpersonal relations, caring, goal attainment, adaptation, and energy fields.** Henderson's definition of nursing, along with the statement of the 14 components of basic nursing, provide the basis for identifying the phenomena she believed are of concern to nursing. The phenomenon of concern are human being, environment, health, interpersonal relations, caring, goal attainment, and adaptation and are explicit and implicit in these sources.

In terms of concern for human beings, Henderson viewed nursing as helping patients with the necessary activities they are unable to perform to make them "complete," "whole," or "independent." She emphasized the patient is the central figure to be served or assisted by the nurse. This enables persons to care for themselves as soon as possible and be better off because they have achieved independence (Henderson, 1991).

The phenomenon of environment is the ninth component of basic nursing, "avoid dangers in the environment and avoid injuring others." Early in her experiences as a student, she recognized the importance of assessment of the home environment of sick children and their families to identify their needs after hospitalization. Then again, in her experience with the Henry Street Visiting Nurse Agency, she was concerned about discharging patients to the same environment that precipitated admission to the hospital.

When the 14 components of basic nursing are taken together, all contribute to the health of the individual. Henderson stated, "in talking about nursing, we tend to stress promotion of health and prevention and cure of disease" (1991, p. 25).

Interpersonal relations between the nurse and individual to facilitate care were a key factor in the performance of the unique functions of nursing. Henderson believed the process for the nurse to "get inside the skin" of the patient is always difficult and only relatively successful. However, in the tenth component of nursing functions (communicate with others in expressing emotions, needs, fears or opinions) she stressed there is a need for a "listening ear and constant observation and interpretation of nonverbal behavior" (Henderson, 1991, p. 34). It is also important for the nurse to have a self-understanding and recognition of her own emotions that hinder concentrating on the patient's needs and to respond to these needs appropriately. For a mutual understanding to develop between the patient and nurse, the nurse must be willing to selectively express what she is feeling and thinking. The nurse who tries to put herself or himself in the patient's position is assisted by the use of unlimited knowledge of the general laws underlying human behavior and specific information about people in different cultures and walks of life. Henderson acknowledged the contributions of Orlando and Wiedenbach in relation to the interactions of patients and nurses. Furthermore, she thought the involvement of the patient and family to develop an individualized plan required interactions with the health care team as well.

The concept of caring is heavily emphasized in Henderson's definition of nursing. She saw the concept of the nurse as a substitute for what the patient lacks to make him or her "complete," "whole," or "independent." The nurse is "temporarily the consciousness of the unconscious, love of life for the suicidal, the leg of the amputee, the eyes of the newly blinded, a means of locomotion for the infant, knowledge and confidence for the young mother, the mouth-piece for those too weak or withdrawn to speak and so on" (Henderson, 1991, p. 22).

The phenomenon of goal attainment is quite clearly stated within Henderson's (1991) definition of nursing in the final sentence: "And to do this in such a way as to help him gain independence as rapidly as possible" (p. 21). The nurse is the master to initiate and control the care of individuals and helps the patient carry out the treatment plan ordered by the physician. Also, as a team member, the nurse assists other members who in turn assist the nurse to plan and carry out the total health care plan whether for improvement of health, recovery from illness, or support in death. Henderson (1997) expected all team members to view the recipient of care as the central figure and provide assistance for understanding, acceptance, and participation in the plan of care. Ultimately, the sooner the person can care for himself or herself, find health information, or carry out prescribed treatments, the better off the person is. It is hoped that the recipients of care feel that the choice is their own. "In the last analysis it is the patient's self-understanding and desire to adopt a healthful regimen that is the critical factor" (Henderson, 1997, p. 23). Although Henderson presented the 14 components of basic nursing as the nurses' function, the outcome is to enable patients to achieve the "normal" basic human functions, physiologically, psychologically, sociologically, and spiritually.

Although Henderson does not explicitly use the concept of adaptation in her definition of nursing or in the 14 components of basic nursing care, there is evidence that the adaptation process is an expectation for recipients of nursing care in which the nurse assists. Examples are components 4, move and maintain desirable postures; 6, select suitable clothes; 9, avoid dangers in the environment and avoid injuring others; 12, work in a way that there is a sense of accomplishment; and 14, learn, discover, or satisfy the curiosity that leads to normal development and health. These examples give indication that the individual needs to adjust to changes in response to the environmental, physiological, social, cultural, and educational factors that challenge the human system. Adaptation is a constant phenomenon that humans and other living creatures must face on a daily basis and to adjust for survival. Both sick and well individuals must adapt to daily needs in different ways depending on the degree of illness or health or compromising status.

4. To whom does this theory apply? In what situations? In what ways? The far-reaching impact of Henderson's work, particularly her definition of nursing and the *Basic principles of nursing care*, on nurses throughout the world is well-known and celebrated. McBride (1996) eloquently stated, "in the last quarter century, Miss Henderson used her emeritus years to serve as nursing consultant to the world . . . her elegant definition of nursing, with its emphasis on complementing the patient's capabilities, provides a clear direction for what nursing should be—a wonderful counter force to the confusion that surrounds a health care system increasingly pre-occupied with bottom line rather than the enduring values" (p. 23).

Basic principles of nursing care was originally published by the International Council of Nurses in 1960 and was reprinted numerous times: 1961, second printing; 1966, third printing; 1968, fourth printing; 1969, fifth revised printing; 1970, sixth printing; 1972, seventh printing; and 1997, second revised printing. Clearly, this indicates the acceptance of Henderson's notions about nursing functions.

In 1960, Bridges noted in the forward of *Basic principles of nursing care* that this publication would provide its worldwide membership with a number of diverse activities to assist in maintaining the highest standards of nursing or improve their nursing care by education, legislation, and through professional organizations. Furthermore, it was hoped that this publication on the fundamentals of nursing would provide a stimulus to further progress for nursing in many countries through the benefits experienced by patients and the encouragement given to nurses to provide the best possible care.

Basically, Henderson was interested in defining nursing, and the 14 components of nursing care were not intended to explain or predict phenomena. Rather, her intent was to describe fully the function of nursing in the care of individuals, families, and communities. Thus, her work applies in any situation where a person lacks the strength, will, or knowledge to perform those activities that contribute to health, its recovery, or a peaceful death.

5. By what method or methods can this theory by tested? Henderson's definition of nursing cannot be viewed as theory, given today's understanding of theories. Therefore, it is impossible to generate testable hypotheses from it. However, some questions that investigate the definitions of nursing and the 14 components may be useful. Some examples of these questions include:

1. Is the sequence of the 14 components followed by nurses in the United States? In other countries?
2. What priorities are evident in the use of the basic nursing functions?
3. Do nurses give care to presenting medical problems initially and then use the unique functions, or do they first use the unique functions?
4. Which clinical specialty areas of nursing practice include or exclude components 10 through 14?

Henderson (1977) was an advocate for conducting research in nursing. She favored studies directed to improving practice rather than those conducted as an academic or theoretical endeavor.

In one of her last publications, support for the application of research in nursing practice is emphasized and encouraged (Henderson, 1991). Henderson acknowledged that "research is identified as one of the eight processes nurses use in arriving at a valid reason for their actions" (p. 56). However, there are no suggestions made regarding the testing of her concepts that underlie her 1966 definition of nursing. The reason for this may be that Henderson saw the research process as time-consuming and inappropriate to use for minute-by-minute life decisions. She believed that research is not a substitute for instinctive and intuitive reactions to situations but that these reactions are influenced by the nurse's knowledge of the sciences that guide human behavior in the society of which nursing is an integral part.

6. Does this theory direct critical thinking in nursing practice? If one accepts that the definition of critical thinking involves identifying the problem, assessing resources, and generating possible solutions, then these activities assist in finding a reasonable solution after considering other alternative solutions that affect the end results (Nicoteri, 1998). Although Henderson did not explicitly state that a critical-thinking process is required in the nursing functions, the use of critical thinking is demonstrated throughout her writings. For example:

> Although the nurse seeks to help the patient meet his needs during a period of dependency, she also tries to shorten this period. Before she carries out any act for him, she asks herself what part of it he could himself perform. If he is unable to act at all, she tries to identify what he lacks and to help him develop, as rapidly as possible, the necessary will, strength, or knowledge required for the act (Henderson, 1991, p. 37).

From an earlier publication, another example of critical-thinking activities by the nurse to meet the patient's needs:

> During periods of prostration or of coma and irreversible illness, when dependence and death are believed inevitable, the nurse's goal changes. She remains, under such conditions, indispensable. Her object as I implied earlier, is to protect the patient from loss of dignity during this period of inescapable dependence. The nurse will be alert to what gives the patient physical and spiritual comfort and will seek out for him the persons he needs, if it is possible, and will do what she can to see that they are not barred from his presence (Henderson, 1966, p. 27).

Indeed these two examples demonstrate that Henderson expected that nursing functions require critical-thinking skills. Finally, when the 14 components of nursing are examined, the nurse must be able to ascertain the problems faced by the patient, which the nurse must address in providing appropriate care.

To date, whether Henderson's theory directs critical thinking in nursing practice has not been tested by nursing research. Possibly, it never will be.

7. Does this theory direct therapeutic nursing intervention? Ideally, the nurse would improve nursing practice by using Henderson's definition and 14 components to improve the health of individuals and thus reduce illness. The final desirable outcome would be a measure of recovery rate, health promotion and maintenance, or a peaceful death.

With respect to Henderson's (1991) most recent thought on the use of theories, she stated, "application of general principles should be part of any effort to improve or advance a profession" (p. 98). However, she disagreed with the current nursing education practice that encourages students to adopt and practice the theory of others. If she were to write *The nature of nursing* today, she would stress to students not only the need to study the existing theories but also the need to recognize that the guiding concepts should be their own, for the reason that the mixture of concepts studied may differ from those concepts uniquely suited to that individual nurse.

8. Does this theory direct communication in nursing practice? In addition to component 10, "Communicate with others," the impact of Henderson's work on communication in nursing can be seen in the worldwide use of her publications. A number of major publications were copyrighted between 1955 and 1978 (McBride, 1996). Henderson began her conceptualization of nursing functions when she found the professional organization's definition of nursing to be unsatisfactory. She believed the definition was vague and very general. Her 1955 definition was intended to describe the practice of nursing. She believed her statement of nursing conveyed the essence of nursing practice. Also, Henderson (1980b) warned that in incorporating the use of high technology in nursing one must be mindful that the unique function of nursing not be compromised.

In relation to the use of her name for the Sigma Theta Tau International library, "Virginia Henderson was arguably the most famous nurse of our century. . . . She was only willing to permit use of her name if the electronic networking system to be developed would advance the work of staff nurses by getting to them current and jargon-free information wherever they were based. She was proud of that living testimonial to nursing excellence" (McBride, 1996, p. 23). This attests to Henderson's commitment to disseminate relevant information about nursing practice to the majority of nurses who give day-to-day care in a variety of health care settings. It is important to reiterate here that Henderson was truly a pioneer following Nightingale to communicate what she believed was the essence of nursing practice to her definition.

Henderson's belief of the importance of open communication with patients was supported in her opinion that the record of care should be the patient's record, not the medical record. She also believed the information in that record should be for the patient, not just about the patient, and should be shared with the patient.

9. Does this theory direct nursing actions that lead to favorable outcomes? A search of the literature did not reveal any research conducted about Henderson's work directing practice to demonstrate favorable client outcomes. If one may surmise, given the numbers of the publication, *Basic principles of nursing practice*, used by practicing nurses, educators, and administrators, the possibility exists that anecdotal or other information about improved outcomes on patient care is attributable to using information from this book. Despite the fact that there is a belief that a number of underdeveloped countries use Henderson's book as a guide for nursing education and practice, sadly thus far the outcome information is unavailable or unpublished.

On the other hand, the goal of nursing using Henderson's ideas is to do for the person what that person lacks the strength, will, or knowledge to do until that person can return to independence. Nursing actions are directed to do only what the person cannot do, thus supporting the individual in continuing to do as much as possible. The directed outcome is a return to independence. This must be considered a favorable outcome!

10. How contagious is this theory? Those who have used Henderson's work and the extent to which they have used it cannot be precisely determined, as these details have not appeared in publications. It is likely that many nurses have used this work without attribution. However, from the information about the numbers of reprints by the International Council of Nurses (ICN) for *Basic principles of nursing care*, it may be concluded that nursing practice, nursing education, and nursing administration have benefited by this worldwide publication. ICN resources indicated that the publication has been translated into more than 30 languages since 1960 (S. Patel, personal communication, February, 1999). Also, the textbooks written with Harmer (1939, 1955) and with Nite (1978) provide further evidence about the influence of Henderson's notion of nursing functions on nursing education and practice. More recently, a literature review identified four publications that demonstrate Henderson's worldwide influence.

First, Miller and Beckett (1980), in their survey of randomly selected general practitioners about their support for the extended role of nurses in British primary care, cited Henderson's contribution to defining the skills of the practice nurse and the need for educational aims of a special training program.

Halloran and Halloran (1985) in their publication on exploring the DRG/Nursing equation, credited Henderson's definition and the American Nurses Association definition that "most nurses' practice today reflects the concepts of both of these definitions" (p. 1093). However, these authors viewed Henderson's definition as being the more eloquent.

Swedish investigators cited Henderson's 1980 publication on the effect of technology on the essence of nursing. They investigated the elderly intensive care unit patients' experiences of pain and distress as well as interventions aimed at reducing these conditions by nurses and assistant nurses (Hall-Lord, Larrson, & Steen, 1998). They concluded that Henderson's notion of nursing function about the need for assessing the total needs of ICU patients is desirable.

Lastly, authors from Sydney, Australia, in their literature review on the impact of technological care environment on the nursing role cite Henderson (1980b) for her contribution to resolve the issue of conflict between the humane and the technological aspects of nursing (Pelletier, Duffield, Adams, Crisp, Nagy, & Murphy, 1996). Henderson acknowledged that the essence of nursing would be difficult to preserve in the high technology environment of the health care system. However, if effective nursing is to prevail it is essential to incorporate high technology to successfully treat the most critically ill and to extend the life span of those who are in need of such care. "Nursing has never been more important than in this age when the comforting, caring presence and touch of the nurse enable institutionalized patients to tolerate invasive, often frightening and sometimes painful technology" (Henderson, 1985, p. 7).

These four examples support Henderson's worldwide influence on nursing practice. Her original definition of nursing continues to have influence, particularly in the changing nursing practice scene with high technology, expanded roles, and the evolving health care system.

LIMITATIONS AND STRENGTHS

Henderson based her ideas about nursing care on fundamental human needs and the physical and emotional aspects of the individual. A major shortcoming in her work is the lack of a conceptual linkage between physiological and other human characteristics. The concept of the holistic nature of human beings does not clearly emerge from her publications. However, it must be kept in mind that Henderson wrote her ideas about nursing before the emergence of the holism concept. If the assumption is made that the 14 components are stated in their order of priority, the relationship among the components is unclear. Each component does affect the next one on the list. In later publications, however, Henderson did indicate her acceptance of the holistic approach to nursing.

If priority according to individual needs is implied in the listing of the components, does a presenting emotional problem take a backseat to physical care? Is the emotional area of care deferred until the physiological needs have been given proper attention? Henderson specifies that the nurse must consider such factors as age, temperament, social or cultural status, and physical and intellectual capacity in the use of the components, thus emphasizing differences among individuals. How these factors interrelate and influence nursing care is vague, except individualized care must emerge when all factors of a person are taken into account in the process of nursing.

In a critique of a major international conference on primary care, Henderson (1989) offered some conclusions about the weaknesses of today's nurses. She thought that the basic sciences (e.g., biophysical sciences) as well as the scientific method and its application to nursing were neglected in the presentations. Other areas in which a lack of knowledge by the presenters was of concern to Henderson included budgeting and financial management, holistic family-centered and community-based approaches to health care, policy making and planning processes, roles of leaders as change agents, taking risks with unpopular actions, and being assertive. These concerns underscore the currency of Henderson's thinking and views about nursing; many of these concerns were not reflected in her earlier writings.

In fairness to Henderson, her effort to define nursing evolved before the discussions of a theoretical basis for the profession emerged. Therefore, the lack of theory in her definition of nursing should not lessen her contribution to nurses and nursing. Her pioneering spirit to lead nursing toward a profession and accountability to the public for competent care were enormous contributions to society as well as to nursing.

Last, in assisting the individual in the dying process, Henderson contended that the nurse helps, but she gave little explanation of what the nurse does. In her definition of nursing, the placing of a parenthesis around the words "peaceful death" is curious. It leads one to wonder why the parentheses were used—perhaps it was merely to single out this event as an important one in which nursing has a significant role. However, in her later writings, she provided more information about this process. In 1991, she reflected on her earlier thinking about the role of the nurse in helping people have a good death when death is inevitable. She wrote that she would emphasize the "question of prolonging life beyond the period of usefulness" (p. 33). She supported working with families and the patient over the issues of "right to die" or dying with dignity that have become an increasingly important part of nursing care. Henderson explained the development of hospice care has influenced the philosophy of care for the dying. This may not have been reflected in her 1966 definition of nursing. Finally, it must be noted that in 1966 she eloquently described the nurse's role in the final stages of life and this description supported much of her thinking expressed in her 1991 publication.

SUMMARY

The concept of nursing formulated by Henderson in her definition of nursing and the 14 components of basic nursing is uncomplicated and self-explanatory. Therefore, it could be used without difficulty as a guide for nursing practice by most nurses. Many of the ideas she presented continue to be used worldwide in both developed and undeveloped countries to guide nursing curricula and practice, which is validated by the demand for her ICN publication that in 1972 was in its seventh printing, has been printed in more than 30 languages and in 1997 was re-released in a second revised printing.

If a suggestion can be made to improve Henderson's concept of nursing, it is the delineation of a theoretical basis and having it tested by research. For example, it would be interesting to see how holism or general systems theory might explain the relationship of the components of basic nursing care to each other. Confirmation of whether or not the list of components are prioritized is needed to clarify what the nurse ought to do if the presenting problem is other than a physical one.

In view of the time in which Henderson published her definition of nursing, she deserves much credit as a leader in the development of nursing practice, education, and licensure. Her work ought to be considered a beginning and impetus for nurses to pursue the highest academic degree. This is critical for analyses of nursing practice and for identifying and testing the theoretical bases for patient care.

In conclusion, Henderson provides the essence of what she believes is a definition of nursing as follows:

> I believe that the function the nurse performs is primarily an independent one—that of acting for the patient when he lacks knowledge, phys-

ical strength, or the will to act for himself as he would ordinarily act in health, or in carrying out prescribed therapy. This function is seen as complex and creative, as offering unlimited opportunity for the application of the physical, biological, and social sciences, and the development of skills based on them (Henderson, 1966, p. 68).

REFERENCES

ANA Statement on Auxiliary Personnel in Nursing Service. (1962). *The American Journal of Nursing, 62,* 7.

Erikson, E. H. (1963). *Childhood and society* (2nd ed.) (pp. 247–274). New York: Norton & Company.

Hall-Lord, M. L., Larrson, G., & Steen, B. (1998). Pain and distress among elderly intensive care unit patients: Comparison of patient's experiences and nurses' assessment. *Heart & Lung, 27,* 123–132.

Halloran, E., & Halloran, C. D. C. (1985). Exploring the DRG/Nursing equation. *American Journal of Nursing, 85,* 1090–1095.

Harmer, B. (1922). *Textbook of the principles and practice of nursing.* New York: Macmillan. (out of print)

Harmer, B., & Henderson, V. (1939). *Textbook of the principles and practice of nursing* (4th ed.). New York: Macmillan. (out of print)

Harmer, B., & Henderson, V. (1955). *Textbook of the principles and practice of nursing* (5th ed.). New York: Macmillan. (out of print)

Henderson, V. (1960). *Basic principles of nursing care.* Geneva: International Council of Nurses.

Henderson, V. (1966). *The nature of nursing.* New York: Macmillan. (out of print)

Henderson, V. (1977). We've "come a long way" but what of the direction? *Nursing Research, 26,* 163–164.

Henderson, V. (1978). The concept of nursing. *Journal of Advanced Nursing, 3,* 16–17.

Henderson, V. (1979a). Preserving the essence of nursing in a technological age, Part I. *Nursing Times, 75,* 2012–2013.

Henderson, V. (1979b). Preserving the essence of nursing in a technological age, Part II. *Nursing Times, 75,* 2056–2058.

Henderson, V. (1980a) Nursing—Yesterday and tomorrow. *Nursing Times, 76,* 905–907.

Henderson, V. (1980b). Preserving the essence of nursing in a technological age, *Journal of Advanced Nursing, 5,* 245–260.

Henderson, V. (1982a). The nursing process—Is the title right? *Journal of Advanced Nursing, 7,* 103–109.

Henderson, V. (1982b). Speech at History of Nursing Museum, Philadelphia, May 1982.

Henderson, V. (1985). The essence of nursing in high technology. *Nursing Administration Quarterly, 9,* 1–9.

Henderson, V. (1987). Nursing process—A critique. *Holistic Nursing Practice, 1,* 7–18.

Henderson, V. (1989). Countdown to 2000: A major international conference for the primary health care team, 21–23 September 1987, London. *Journal of Advanced Nursing, 14,* 81–85.

Henderson, V. (1991). *The nature of nursing: A definition and its implications for practice, research, and education. Reflections after 25 years.* (Pub. No. 15-2346). New York: National League for Nursing Press.

Henderson, V. (1997). *Basic principles of nursing care (Revised).* Geneva: International Council of Nurses.

Henderson, V., & Nite, G. (1978). *Principles and practice of nursing* (6th ed.). New York: Macmillan.

Henderson, V., & Watt, S. (1983). 70+ and going strong. Virginia Henderson: A nurse for all ages. *Geriatric Nursing, 4*, 58–59.

Maslow, A. (1970). *Motivation and personality* (2nd ed.). New York: Harper & Row.

McBride, A. B. (1996). In celebration of Virginia Avenuel Henderson. *Reflections, 22*(1), 22–23 or *http://sttiweb.iupuil.edu//stti/virginia.html*

Miller, D. S., & Beckett, E. M. (1980). A new member of the team? Expanding the role of the nurse in British primary care. *The Lancet, 2*, 358–361.

Nicoteri, J. A. (1998). Critical thinking skills. *American Journal of Nursing, 98*(10), 62, 64–65.

Pelletier, D., Duffield, C. M., Adams, A., Crisp, J., Nagy, S., & Murphy, J. (1996). The impact of the technological care environment on the nursing role. *International Journal of Technology Assessment in Health Care, 12*, 358–366.

Safier, G. (1977). *Contemporary American leaders in nursing*. New York: McGraw-Hill.

BIBLIOGRAPHY

Campbell, C. (1985). Virginia Henderson: The definitive nurse. *Nursing Mirror, 160*, 12.

Fulton, J. S. (1987). Virginia Henderson: Theorist, prophet, poet. *Advances in Nursing Science, 10*, 1–9.

Halloran, E. J. (1996). Virginia Henderson and her timeless writings. *Journal of Advanced Nursing, 23*(1), 17–24.

Halloran, E. J., & Wald, F. S. (1996). Professionally speaking: Virginia Henderson, the nursing profession and the reform of health services. *Nursing Leadership Forum, 2*(2), 58–63.

Henderson, V. (1977). *Reference resource for research and continuing education in nursing.* Kansas City: American Nurses Association Publication No. 6125.

Henderson, V. (1982). Is the study of history rewarding for nurses? *Society for Nursing History Gazette, 2*, 1–2.

Henderson, V. (1986). Some observations on health care by health services or health industries (editorial). *Journal of Advanced Nursing, 1*, 1–2.

Henderson, V., & Watt, S. (1983). Epidermolysis bullosa. *Nursing Times, 79*, 43–46.

McCarty, P. (1987). How can nurses prepare for year 2000? (A response from Virginia Henderson). *The American Nurse, 19*, 3, 6.

Shamansky, S. L. (1964). CHN revisited: A conversation with Virginia Henderson. *Public Health Nursing, 1*, 193–201.

Shamansky, S. L. (1984). Virginia Henderson: A national treasure. *Focus Critical Care, 11*, 60–61.

ANNOTATED BIBLIOGRAPHY

Fulton, J. S. (1987). Virginia Henderson: Theorist, prophet, poet. *Advances in Nursing Science, 10*(1), 1–9.

A journey, using nursing's metaparadigm as guideposts, that looks at the esthetics and character of Virginia Henderson's work. The major work considered is *The nature of nursing*. Unique in the translation of selected materials into poetry.

Halloran, E. J. (1995). *A Virginia Henderson reader: Excellence in nursing.* NY: Springer.

A compliation of 22 of Henderson's works, spanning a 30-year period. This volume organizes these into the categories of patient care, nursing education, nursing research, and nursing in society. Included are 12 chapters from the 1978 edition of *Principles and practice of nursing*.

Hardin, S. R. (1997). Virginia Henderson: Universality & individuality. *Journal of Multicultural Nursing and Health, 3*(3), 6–9.

This article summarizes Henderson's definition of nursing and her thoughts on culture. It addresses Henderson's work in relation to culturally competent care.

Hargrove-Huttel, R. A. (1988). Virginia Henderson's nature of nursing theory and quality of life for the older adult. *Dissertation Abstracts International,* 49–08B, 3104.

A descriptive study that investigated the relationship between Henderson's basic care needs and the quality of life for 174 older adults living in a rural area. Findings supported that meeting the basic care needs is positively associated with the quality of life for older adults.

Lindell, M. E., & Olsson, H. M. (1989). Lack of care givers' knowledge causes unnecessary suffering in elderly patients. *Journal of Advanced Nursing, 14,* 976–979.

This study investigated the personal hygiene of women over the age of 65; 35 of these women were healthy and 28 were residents of long-term care wards. Those in long-term care required assistance with daily hygiene activities. Results indicated that those who required assistance with personal hygiene were likely to have abnormal genital problems. It was concluded that their caregivers lacked knowledge about the normal physiological aging process in women and thus were hindered in carrying out basic component 8, "Keep the body clean and well groomed and protect the integument."

Smith, J. P. (1989). *Virginia Henderson: The first ninety years.* Harrow, Middlesex, England: Scutari. This biography is based on information obtained during interviews with Virginia Henderson and several of those who knew her well. James Smith spent several weeks as Henderson's guest in New Haven, CT, with the support of Trevor Clay, Royal College of Nursing, United Kingdom, and Vernice Ferguson, Deputy Assistant Medical Director for Nursing Programs, Veterans Administration, Washington, DC. This volume adds to our information about who Virginia Henderson was, as well as what she did.

CHAPTER 6

CARE, CORE, AND CURE
LYDIA E. HALL

Julia B. George

■ ■ ■

Lydia E. Hall (1906–1969) received her basic nursing education at York Hospital School of Nursing in York, Pennsylvania, and graduated in 1927. Both her B.S. in Public Health Nursing (1937) and M.A. in teaching Natural Sciences (1942) are from Teachers College, Columbia University, New York.

Lydia Hall was the first director of the Loeb Center for Nursing and Rehabilitation and continued in that position until her death in 1969. Her experience in nursing spans the clinical, educational, research, and supervisory components. Her publications include several articles on the definition of nursing and quality of care. Lydia Hall articulated what she considered a basic philosophy of nursing upon which the nurse may base patient care.

LOEB CENTER FOR NURSING AND REHABILITATION

As a nurse theorist, Lydia Hall is unique in that her beliefs about nursing were demonstrated in practice with relatively little documentation in the literature. Hall originated the philosophy of care of Loeb Center at Montefiore Hospital, Bronx, New York. Loeb Center opened in January 1963 to provide professional nursing care to persons past the acute stage of illness. The center's functioning concept was that the need for professional nursing care increases as the need for medical care decreases.

Those in need of continued professional care who were 16 years of age or older and who were no longer experiencing an acute biological disturbance were transferred from the acute care hospital to Loeb Center. Good candidates for care at Loeb were those who had a desire to come to Loeb, were recommended by their physicians, and possessed a favorable potential for recovery and return to the community.

As physically designed by Hall, Loeb Center had a capacity of 80 beds and was attached to Montefiore Hospital. The rooms were arranged with patient comfort and maneuverability as the first priority. The patients also had access to a large

111

communal dining room. The primary care givers were registered professional nurses. Nonpatient care activities were supplied by messenger–attendants and ward secretaries. The center's philosophy, as stated by Bowar-Ferres (1975), was as follows:

> Loeb's primary purpose was and is to demonstrate that high quality nursing care given by registered nurses, in a non-directive setting, offers a supportive setting to people in the post-acute phase of their illness that enables them to recover sooner, and to leave the center able to cope with themselves and what they must face in the future (p. 810).

To create a nondirective setting, there are very few rules or routines, no schedules, and no dictated mealtimes or specified visiting hours (Bower-Ferres, 1975). The nurses at Loeb strive to help the patient determine and clarify goals and, with the patient, work out ways to achieve the goals at the individual's pace, consistent with the medical treatment plan and congruent with the patient's sense of self. At Loeb Center, the nurses were in charge, and Hall, as director of the Center, hired and fired the physicians who were employed there (Hall, 1955, 1969).

LYDIA HALL'S THEORY OF NURSING

Lydia Hall presented her theory of nursing by drawing three interlocking circles, each circle representing a particular aspect of nursing: *care, core,* and *cure.*

The Care Circle

The care circle (Fig. 6–1) represents the nurturing component and is exclusive to nursing. Nurturing involves using the factors that make up the concept of mothering (care and comfort of the person) and provide for teaching–learning activities. The professional nurse provides bodily care for the patient and helps the patient to com-

Figure 6–1. The care circle of patient care. (*From Hall, L.* Nursing—What is it? *p. 1. Publication of the Virginia State Nurses' Association, Winter 1959. Used with permission.*)

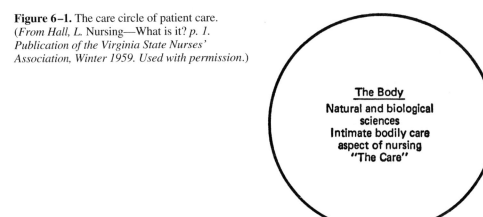

The Body
Natural and biological sciences
Intimate bodily care
aspect of nursing
"The Care"

plete such basic daily biological functions as eating, bathing, elimination, and dressing. When providing this care, the nurse's goal is the comfort of the patient.

Providing care for a patient at the basic needs level presents the nurse and patient with an opportunity for closeness. As closeness develops, the patient can share and explore feelings with the nurse. This opportunity to explore feelings represents the teaching–learning aspect of nurturing.

When functioning in the care circle, the nurse applies knowledge of the natural and biological sciences to provide a strong theoretical base for nursing implementations. In interactions with the patient the nurse's role needs to be clearly defined. A strong theory base allows the nurse to maintain a professional status rather than a mothering status, while at the same time incorporating closeness and nurturance in giving care. The patient views the nurse as a potential comforter, one who provides care and comfort through the laying on of hands.

The Core Circle

The core circle (Fig. 6–2) of patient care is based in the social sciences, involves the therapeutic use of self, and is shared with other members of the health team. The professional nurse, by developing an interpersonal relationship with the patient, is able to help the patient verbally express feelings regarding the disease process and its effects, as well as discuss the patient's role in recovery. Through such expression the patient is able to gain self-identity and further develop maturity. As Hall (1965) says:

> To look at and listen to self is often too difficult without the help of a significant figure (nurturer) who has learned how to hold up a mirror and sounding board to invite the behaver to look and listen to himself. If he accepts the invitation, he will explore the concerns in his acts and as he listens to his exploration through the reflection of the nurse, he may uncover in sequence his difficulties, the problem area, his problem, and eventually the threat which is dictating his out-of-control behavior.

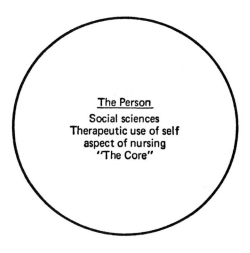

Figure 6–2. The core circle of patient care. (*From Hall, L. Nursing—What is it? p. 1. Used with permission.*)

The Person
Social sciences
Therapeutic use of self
aspect of nursing
"The Core"

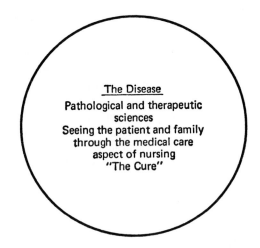

Figure 6–3. The cure circle of patient care. (*From Hall, L.* Nursing—What is it? *p. 1. Used with permission.*)

The professional nurse, by use of the reflective technique (acting as a mirror for the patient), helps the patient look at and explore feelings regarding his or her current health status and related potential changes in life style. The nurse uses a freely offered closeness to help the patient bring into awareness the verbal and nonverbal messages being sent to others. Motivations are discovered through the process of bringing into awareness the feelings being experienced. With this awareness the patient is now able to make conscious decisions based on understood and accepted feelings and motivations. The motivation and energy necessary for healing exist within the patient, rather than in the health care team.

The Cure Circle

The cure circle of patient care (Fig. 6–3) is based in the pathological and therapeutic sciences and is shared with other members of the health team. The professional nurse helps the patient and family through the medical, surgical, and rehabilitative prescriptions made by the physician. During this aspect of nursing care, the nurse is an active advocate of the patient.

The nurse's role during the cure aspect is different from the care circle because many of the nurse's actions take on a negative quality of avoidance of pain rather than a positive quality of comforting. This is negative in the sense that the patient views the nurse as a potential cause of pain, one who is involved in such actions as administering injections, versus the potential comforter who provides care and comfort in the care circle.

Interaction of the Three Aspects of Nursing

Because Hall emphasizes the importance of a total person approach, it is important that the three aspects of nursing (see Fig. 6–4) not be viewed as functioning independently but as interrelated. The three aspects interact, and the circles representing them change size, depending on the patient's total course of progress.

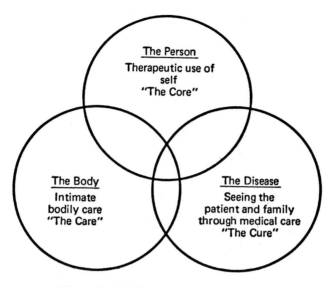

Figure 6–4. Hall's three aspects of nursing.

In the philosophy of Loeb Center, the professional nurse functions most therapeutically when patients have entered the second stage of their hospital stay (i.e., they are recuperating and are past the acute stage of illness). During this recuperation stage, the care and core aspects are the most prominent, and the cure aspect is less prominent (see Fig. 6–5). The size of the circles represents the degree to which the patient is progressing in each of the three areas. The professional nurse at this time is able to help the patient reach the core of his problem through the closeness provided by the care aspect of nursing. Unfortunately, in today's managed care environment all too often this stage occurs posthospitalization and the patients' access to nursing care is limited.

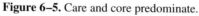

Figure 6–5. Care and core predominate.

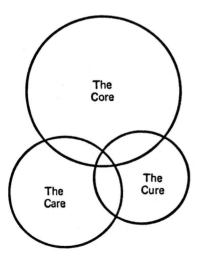

HALL'S THEORY AND NURSING'S METAPARADIGM

Although the concept of nursing is identified by Hall, she does not speak directly to the other three concepts: human, health, and society/environment. However, inferences can be made from her work, as noted below.

The *individual* human who is 16 years of age or older and past the acute stage of a long-term illness is the focus of nursing care in Hall's work. The source of energy and motivation for healing is the individual care recipient, not the health care provider. Hall emphasizes the importance of the individual as unique, capable of growth and learning, and requiring a total person approach.

Health can be inferred to be a state of self-awareness with conscious selection of behaviors that are optimal for that individual. Hall stresses the need to help the person explore the meaning of his or her behavior to identify and overcome problems through developing self-identity and maturity.

The concept of *society/environment* is dealt with in relation to the individual. Hall is credited with developing the concept of Loeb Center because she assumed that the hospital environment during treatment of acute illness creates a difficult psychological experience for the ill individual (Bowar-Ferres, 1975). Loeb Center focuses on providing an environment that is conducive to self-development. In such a setting, the focus of the action of nurses is the individual, so that any actions taken in relation to society or environment are for the purpose of assisting the individual in attaining a personal goal.

Nursing is identified as consisting of participation in the care, core, and cure aspects of patient care. Care is the sole function of nurses, whereas core and cure are shared with other members of the health care team. However, the major purpose of care is to achieve an interpersonal relationship with the individual that will facilitate the development of core (i.e., the development of self-identity and self-direction by the patient).

HALL'S THEORY AND THE NURSING PROCESS

Hall places the motivation and energy needed for healing within the patient. This aspect of her theory influences the nurse's total approach to the six phases of the nursing process: assessment, diagnosis, outcomes, planning, implementation, and evaluation.

The *assessment* phase involves collection of data about the health status of the individual. According to Hall, the process of data collection is directed for the benefit of the patient rather than for the benefit of the nurse. Data collection should be directed toward increasing the patient's self-awareness. Through use of observation and reflection, the nurse is able to assist the patient in becoming aware of both verbal and nonverbal behaviors. In the individual, increased awareness of feelings and needs in relation to health status increases the ability for self-healing. The assessment phase also pertains to guiding the patient through the cure aspect of nursing. The health team collects biological data (physical and laboratory) to help the patient and family understand and progress through the medical regimen.

The second phase is the *nursing diagnosis*, or statement of the patient's need or problem area. How a nurse envisions the nursing role influences the interpretation of assessment data and conclusions reached. Viewing the patient as the power for self-healing directs conclusions differently than if the healing power rests in the physician or nurse. The patient is the one in control, the one who identifies the need.

Outcomes and *planning* involves setting priorities and mutually establishing patient-centered outcomes and goals. The patient decides what is of highest priority and also what outcomes and goals are desirable.

The core is involved in outcomes and planning. The role of the nurse is to use reflection to help the patient become aware of and understand needs, feelings, and motivations. Once motivations are clarified, Hall indicates that the patient is the best person to identify outcomes, set goals, and arrange priorities. The nurse seeks to increase patient awareness and to support decision making based on the patient's new level of awareness. The nurse works with the patient to help keep the goals consistent with the medical prescription. The nurse needs to draw on a knowledge base in the social and scientific areas to present the patient with creative alternatives from which to choose.

Implementation involves the actual institution of the plan of care. This phase is the actual giving of nursing care. In the care and core circles, the nurse works with the patient, helping with bathing, dressing, eating, and other care and comfort needs. The professional nurse uses a "permissive non-directive teaching–learning approach" to implement nursing care, thus helping the patient reach the established goals (Bowar-Ferres, 1975, p. 813). This includes "helping the patient with his feelings, providing requested information and supporting patient-made decisions" (Brown, 1970, p. 159). The nurse also helps the patient and family through the cure aspect of nursing, working with the patient and family to help them understand and implement the medical plan.

Evaluation is the process of assessing the patient's progress toward the health goals. The evaluation phase of the process is directed toward deciding whether or not the patient is successful in reaching the established goals. The following questions apply to the use of Hall's theory in the evaluation phase:

1. Is the patient learning "who he is, where he wants to go, and how he wants to get there"? (Bowar-Ferres, 1975, p. 813)
2. Is the patient learning to understand and explore the feelings that underlie behavior?
3. Is the nurse helping the patient see motivations more clearly?
4. Are the patient's goals congruent with the medical regime? Is the patient successful in meeting the goals?
5. Is the patient physically more comfortable?

Whether or not a person is growing in self-awareness regarding his or her feelings and motivations can be recognized through changes in his or her outward behavior.

The application of Hall's work is demonstrated in the following case study:

Assessment: Ned J. is a 17-year-old high school senior. He is a star on the football team and has aspirations for a football college scholarship. Last week he was involved in an automobile accident in which his left arm was crushed and his right foot was injured. While there was initial concern about possible internal injuries, there have been no internal sequelae. The required surgeries have been completed for his arm and foot; he is now in physical therapy to deal with the effects of the accident and his recent immobility.

CARE: Physically, the remarkable findings are his left arm is in an orthopedic device to stabilize it and encourage bone healing; he is left handed but has learned to compensate with his right hand for most activities of daily living. He needs minor assistance with dressing (help putting his shirt on). His family has brought in a slip-on shoe for him to wear on his left foot so he does not need to worry about tying shoelaces. He is rapidly gaining confidence in his ability to provide for his own physical care.

CORE: Ned, looking at the floor, tells you, his nurse, that he is going home tomorrow. You respond, "You're going home tomorrow?" and share your observation that he is not looking very happy about the prospect. Ned says, "Yes . . . I'm doing OK here but I'm scared about going back to school. How will I take notes and tests? It looks like I've totally messed up my chances for a football scholarship so now I really need to do well with my grades. If I mess those up too I may never get to college."

CURE: The surgical incision on his right foot has healed and he is beginning to bear weight on the foot. There are no problems with hydration or elimination, skin is intact with good turgor, all vital signs and lab values are within normal limits. His neurological signs stabilized within 24 hours of admission to the hospital. He is finishing his course of antibiotics.

Nursing Diagnosis: Reluctant to be discharged associated with concerns about abilities to successfully meet academic expectations.

Outcome: College admission with a scholarship

Goals:

1. Regain use of left arm as much as possible. (Care and Cure Circles)
2. Successful completion of high school with academic performance at level to support an academic scholarship. (Core circle)

Implementation: (The school nurse is the most likely nurse to be involved at this point.)

1. Arrange physical therapy sessions around school schedule.
2. Take notes with right hand; possibly use computer to do so.
3. Arrange to have extra time for taking written tests.
4. Provide a listening ear to help Ned deal with the frustrations that are bound to arise.

Evaluation: (using Hall's five questions)

1. Yes, he wants to go to college and now is not likely to get a football scholarship so he has changed his focus to academics. (Core)
2. He has verbalized his anger at "the stupid accident" and at the possibility that he may not regain full use of his dominant arm. He has also recognized that his initial resistance to physical therapy was based in fear. (Core)
3. The nurse at the hospital helped him explore his concerns about being discharged. The school nurse helped him decide to ask for extra time for tests since he writes slower with his right hand (at first he was too embarrassed to do this). Now, Ned talks about how he needs to do whatever he can to do well scholastically. He says he was "coasting" academically because he counted on football to get him to college. (Core)
4. His goals are congruent with the medical regimen and he is meeting those goals. Physical therapy has been arranged for after school; he has learned to use a laptop computer with one hand to take notes, do homework, and take tests; his teachers have been accommodating about testing time, some have been willing to give oral tests for him. (Cure and Core)
5. Physically, his arm continues to be uncomfortable and his foot aches at times. As a total person, he is comfortable that he is successfully refocusing his efforts to meet his objective of attending college on a scholarship. (Care and Core)

CRITIQUE OF HALL'S CARE, CORE, AND CURE

Hall's work can be compared to the characteristics of a theory as presented in Chapter 1.

1. What is the historical context of the theory? In observing what happened during hospitalization, Hall became convinced that as persons moved past the acute stage of illness, the need for professional nursing care increased while the need for medical care decreased. It is important to note that this was during the time of retrospective payment systems when patients typically remained hospitalized until they were nearly ready to fully resume their usual activities. Thus, patients who were past the acute stage of their illness had access to 24 hours of nursing care and the full services of a hospital setting as needed. Hall's underlying assumption was that the person who had an increased need for professional nursing care could be best served in a setting that focused on his or her needs and encouraged participation.

She interrelated the concepts of care, core, and cure, and in 1963 provided a different way of looking at the phenomenon of care of the individual with a long-term illness, which was an acute social problem of those times. Although other developments in health care have altered the need to some extent, her ideas are still relevant and useful, particularly if some of the limitations she imposed are removed. For example, care, core, and cure needs exist in acute and ambulatory settings and in individuals younger than 16.

Also, Hall recognized the importance of knowledge of validated theories, laws, and principles. She indicated the theoretical base for each of the aspects of patient care: the care aspect is based in the natural and biological sciences, core in the social sciences, and cure in the pathological and therapeutic sciences. The specific applications of these sciences provide a source of unanswered questions to be investigated.

2. What are the basic concepts and relationships presented by the theory?
The use of the terms *care, core,* and *cure* is unique to Hall. On first reading, Hall's work appears to be completely and simply logical with clear relationships among these three concepts. However, closer scrutiny reveals that although Hall indicates that care, the bodily laying on of hands, is the only aspect that is solely nursing—implying that it is the major focus for nursing—her major emphasis is on core. The care aspect is a means for achieving core rather than an end in itself (Barnum, 1994). Although this is not illogical, the initial impression is not the true logic of the work.

3. What major phenomena of concern to nursing are presented? These phenomena may include *but not are limited to***: human being, environment, health, interpersonal relations, caring, goal attainment, adaptation, and energy fields.** The major phenomena are intimate care needs (the body in the care circle), therapeutic use of self and the use of reflective techniques (the person in the core circle) and pathology and the therapeutic sciences (the disease in the cure circle).

4. To whom does this theory apply? In what situations? In what ways? Hall indicated the theory applies to persons who are 16 years of age or older, past the acute stage of illness, and interested in recovering. While these limitations served her well in establishing the Loeb Center, it is feasible to apply the theory to persons in other circumstances. Certainly, those under 16 are capable of self-reflection. Those in the acute stage of illness would need much more emphasis on the cure circle but could still be functioning in both the care and core circles. When the circles are conceptualized as changing in size as the person's needs change, it is possible to apply this theory in caring for almost any individual who is interested in working towards recovery.

However, core cannot really meet its goals with the very young and is very difficult to use with the comatose, unless the view is a very large care and cure circles and a very small core circle. This would be incongruent with Hall's emphasis on core.

Hall's work is simple in its presentation. However, the openness and flexibility required for its application may not be so simple for nurses whose personality, educational preparation, and experience have not prepared them to function with minimal structure.

5. By what method or methods can this theory be tested? Hall tested her theory through demonstrating its use in a practice setting and conducting quantitative research to evaluate the effectiveness of Loeb Center. This research was conducted at

Hall's insistence, in spite of the enthusiastic acceptance of her philosophy by those in the Montefiore health care community (Brown, 1970). This research is evidence that hypotheses can be developed and tested. In addition, the sharing of a report about the Loeb Center in a Congressional hearing is evidence of an increase in the general body of knowledge (Loeb Center, 1963). Quantitative methods can be used to test the impact of the use of Hall's theory on length of stay, readmission rates, and other quantitative measures of the outcomes of health care. Qualitative measure could be used to investigate the quality of life achieved by those who received care from those practicing Hall's theory as compared to those who received care in another manner.

6. Does this theory direct critical thinking in nursing practice? Critical thinking is absolutely necessary for the nurse to use reflection effectively, as well as to provide optimum nursing care in any of the circles. The use of critical thinking will also facilitate the communication needed for interdisciplinary practice in the core and cure circles.

7. Does this theory direct therapeutic nursing interventions? The care circle especially directs therapeutic nursing interventions. This circle is solely the nurse's and involves nurturing and providing comfort and education as well as meeting other bodily needs. It provides support in helping the person move toward recovery. Therapeutic nursing interventions may be part of the other circles or the actions that would be identified as nursing interventions may be carried out by other members of the health care team.

8. Does this theory direct communication in nursing practice? Communication is an important component of all of the circles—care, core, and cure. In the care circle communication is primarily with the patient and will focus on comforting and education. In the core circle communication will occur with the patient and with other team members. In the cure circle, the family may be added to those who are involved in communication.

9. Does this theory direct nursing actions that lead to favorable outcomes? The importance of favorable outcomes is apparent in the five evaluation questions posed by Hall. Questions 1, 2, 4, and 5 focus on the outcomes for the patient, while question 3 focuses on the nurse's role in achieving these outcomes. Thus, nursing actions are directly linked with the resulting outcomes. Whether or not these outcomes are favorable is decided by what the patient wants to achieve. The outcomes and goals are selected from the various options by the patient, not the nurse.

10. How contagious is this theory? The Loeb Center continues to function at Montefiore Hospital, the primary demonstration of Hall's theory. An electronic search of CINAHL and Medline found a very limited number of articles related to Hall or Loeb Center. One of these discusses Hall's induction into the ANA Hall of Fame (Loose, 1994). Others are those listed in the reference list of this chapter that speak to Loeb Center. A third grouping is discussion by Griffiths (1997) and Griffiths and Willis-Barnett (1998) about nurse-led centers in the United Kingdom.

APPLICATION AND LIMITATIONS OF THE THEORY

Hall's theory of nursing has several areas that limit its application to patient care. The first of these areas is the stage of illness. Hall applies her ideas of nursing to a patient who has passed the acute stage of biological stress—that is, the patient who is experiencing the acute stage of illness is not included in Hall's approach to nursing care. However, it is possible to apply the care, core, and cure ideas to the care of those who are acutely ill. The acutely ill individual often needs care in relation to basic needs, as well as core awareness of what is going on and, in cure, understanding of the plan of medical care.

A second limiting factor is age. Hall refers only to adult patients in the second stage of their illness, thus eliminating all younger patients. On the basis of this theory, Loeb Center admits only patients 16 years of age and older. However, it would be possible to apply Hall's theory with younger individuals. Certainly adolescents younger than 16 are capable of seeking self-identity.

A third limiting factor is the description of how to help a person toward self-awareness. The only tool of therapeutic communication Hall discusses is reflection. By inference, all other techniques of therapeutic communication are eliminated. This emphasis on reflection arises from the belief that both the problem and the solution lie in the individual and that the nurse's function is to help the individual find them. But reflection is not always the most effective technique to be used. Other techniques, such as active listening and nonverbal support, may be used to facilitate the development of self-identity.

Fourth, the family is mentioned only in the cure circle. This means that the nursing contact with families is used only in regard to the patient's own medical care. It does not allow for helping a family increase awareness of the family's self and limits the use of the theory to the individual as the unit of care.

Finally, Hall's theory relates only to those who are ill. This would indicate no nursing contact with healthy individuals, families, or communities, and it negates the concept of health maintenance and health care to prevent illness.

Basically, Hall's theory can be readily applied within the confines of the definition of adults past the acute stage of illness. However, this is too confining for a total view of nursing, which includes working with individuals, families, and communities throughout the life cycle and in varying states of health.

However, it should be noted that the nurse who uses Hall's theory functions in a manner similar to the method of assignment known as primary nursing. Considering that Hall instituted Loeb Center in the early 1960s, her ideas certainly provided leadership and innovation in nursing practice. She also deserves praise for having the courage to create a new environment in which to put her ideas into practice.

SUMMARY

Hall's theory of nursing involves three interlocking circles, each representing one aspect of nursing. The care aspect represents intimate bodily care of the patient. The core aspect deals with the innermost feelings and motivations of the patient. The cure aspect tells how the nurse helps the patient and family through the medical aspect of care. The main tool the nurse uses to help the patient realize his or her motivations and to grow in self-awareness is that of reflection.

Of the major concepts in nursing's metaparadigm, only nursing is defined as the function necessary to carry out care, core, and cure. Hall presents a philosophical view of humans as having the energy and motivation for self-awareness and growth. Definitions of health and society or environment must be inferred.

Lydia Hall's theory may be used in the nursing process. The core, care, and cure aspects are all applicable to each phase of the nursing process. The limitations of Hall's theory—illness orientation, age, restrictions on family contact, and use of reflection only—can be overcome by taking a broader view of care, core, and cure and by emphasizing the aspects that are most appropriate for a particular situation.

REFERENCES

Barnum, B. J. S. (1994). *Nursing theory: Analysis, application, evaluation* (4th ed.). Philadelphia: Lippincott.

Bowar-Ferres, S. (1975). Loeb Center and its philosophy of nursing. *The American Journal of Nursing, 75,* 810–815.

Brown, E. L. (1970). *Nursing reconsidered: A study of change, Part 1: The professional role in institutional nursing.* Philadelphia: Lippincott.

Griffiths, P. (1997). In search of the pioneers of nurse led care. . . . The Loeb Centre. *Nursing Times, 93*(21), 46–48.

Griffiths, P., & Willis-Barnett, J. (1998). The effectiveness of 'nursing beds': A review of the literature. *Journal of Advanced Nursing, 27,* 1184–1192.

Hall, L. (1955). Quality of nursing care. *Public Health News, New Jersey State Department of Health, 36,* 212–215.

Hall, L. (1959). *Nursing—What is it?* Publication of the Virginia State Nurses Association.

Hall, L. (1965). Another view of nursing care and quality. Address given at Catholic University Workshop, Washington, DC.

Hall, L. (1969). The Loeb Center for Nursing and Rehabilitation at Montefiore Hospital and Medical Center. *International Journal of Nursing Studies, 6,* 81–95.

Loeb Center for Nursing and Rehabilitation Project Report, Congressional Record, May-June 1963, pp. 1515–1562.

Loose, V. (1994). Lydia E. Hall: Rehabilitation nursing pioneer in the ANA Hall of Fame. *Rehabilitation of Nursing, 19,* 174–176.

BIBLIOGRAPHY

Alfano, G. (1984). Administration means working with nurses. *American Journal of Nursing, 64,* 83–85.

Alfano, G. (1969). Loeb Center. *Nursing Clinics of North America, 4,* 3.

Bernardin, E. (1964). Loeb Center—As the staff nurse sees it. *American Journal of Nursing, 64,* 85–86.

Hall, L. (1963). A center for nursing. *Nursing Outlook, 2,* 805–806.

Hall, L. (1964). Can nursing care hasten recovery? *American Journal of Nursing, 64,* 6.

Isler, C. (1964). New concepts in nursing therapy: More care as the patient improves. *RN, 27,* 58–70.

CHAPTER 7

SELF-CARE DEFICIT NURSING THEORY
DOROTHEA E. OREM

Peggy Coldwell Foster
Agnes M. Bennett

■ ■ ■

Dorothea E. Orem, M.S.N.Ed., D.Sc., R.N., was born in 1914 in Baltimore, Maryland. She began her nursing education at Providence Hospital School of Nursing in Washington, DC. After receiving her diploma in the early 1930s, she earned her Bachelor of Science in Nursing Education in 1939 and her Master of Science in Nursing Education in 1945 from the Catholic University of America.

She has received several honorary degrees including a Doctor of Science from Georgetown University in 1976; Doctor of Science from the Incarnate World College, San Antonio, Texas, in 1980; and Doctor of Humane Letters from Illinois Western University, Bloomington, Illinois, in 1988. Orem is a member of Sigma Theta Tau and Pi Gamma Mu. She has received several national awards, including the Catholic University of America's Alumni Achievement Award for Nursing Theory in 1980, and the Linda Richards Award from the National League for Nursing in 1991. Orem was named an Honorary Fellow of the American Academy of Nursing in 1992.

During her professional nursing career, she has worked as a staff nurse, private duty nurse, nurse educator, nurse administrator, and nursing consultant. Orem continues to work as a nurse consultant and to refine her nursing theory.

During 1958–1959, as a consultant to the Office of Education, Department of Health, Education, and Welfare, Dorothea E. Orem participated in a project to improve practical (vocational) nurse training. This work stimulated her to consider the question, "What condition exists in a person when judgments are made that a nurse(s) should be brought into the situation (i.e., that persons should be under nursing care)?" (Orem, 2001, p. 20). Her answer encompassed the idea that a nurse is "another self." This idea evolved into her nursing concept of "self-care." That is, when they are able, individuals care for themselves. When the person is unable to care for himself or herself, the nurse provides the assistance needed. For children, nursing care is needed when the parents or guardians are unable to provide the amount and quality of care needed.

Orem's concept of nursing as the provision of self-care was first published in 1959. She joined with several faculty members from the Catholic University of America in 1965 to form a Nursing Model Committee. In 1968, a portion of the Nursing Model Committee, including Orem, continued their work through the Nursing Development Conference Group (NDCG). This group was formed to produce a conceptual framework for nursing and to establish the discipline of nursing. The NDCG published *Concept formalization in nursing: Process and product* in 1973 and 1979.

Orem continued to develop her nursing concept of self-care and in 1971 published *Nursing: Concepts of practice*. The second, third, fourth, fifth, and sixth editions of this book were published in 1980, 1985, 1991, 1995, 2001, respectively. The first edition focused on the individual. The second edition was expanded to include multiperson units (families, groups, and communities). The third edition presented Orem's general theory of nursing as it is constituted from three related theoretical constructs: self-care, self-care deficits, and nursing systems. The fourth edition more fully developed the ideas presented in earlier editions. In the fifth edition her writing (with a chapter contributed by Susan Taylor and Kathie McLaughlin Renpenning) provided an increased emphasis on multiperson situations, family and community groups in our society. The sixth edition continues the development of Orem's ideas, provides a prologue to understanding nursing, increases emphasis on the interpersonal aspects of nursing, and adds an emphasis on positive mental health.

OREM'S GENERAL THEORY OF NURSING

Orem (2001) states her general theory as follows:

> The condition that validates the existence of a **requirement for nursing** in an adult is *the health-associated absence of the ability to maintain continuously that amount and quality of self-care that is therapeutic in sustaining life and health, in recovering from disease or injury, or in coping with their effects.* With children, the condition is the *inability of the parent (or guardian) associated with the child's health state to maintain continuously for the child the amount and quality of care that is therapeutic* (p. 82).

Orem developed the Self-Care Deficit Theory of Nursing (her general theory), which is composed of three interrelated theories: (1) the theory of self-care, (2) the theory of self-care deficit, and (3) the theory of nursing systems. Incorporated within these three theories are six central concepts and one peripheral concept. Understanding these central concepts of self-care and dependent care, self-care agency and dependent care agency, therapeutic self-care demand, self-care deficit, nursing

TABLE 7–1. RELATIONSHIP OF OREM'S CONCEPTS TO THE THREE THEORIES

Theory of Self-Care	Theory of Self-Care Deficit	Theory of Nursing Systems

Self-care
Self-care agency
Self-care requisites
  Universal
  Developmental
  Health deviation
Therapeutic self-care demand
	When therapeutic self-care demand exceeds self-care agency, a self-care deficit exists and nursing is needed	Nursing agency
		Nursing systems
		  Wholly compensatory
		  Partly compensatory
		  Supportive-educative

← ————————————— Basic conditioning factors ————————————— →

(*From Julia B. George, California State University, Fullerton, 1997. Used with permission.*)

agency, and nursing systems, as well as the peripheral concept of basic conditioning factors, is essential to understanding her general theory. See Table 7–1 for the relationship of these concepts to the three interrelated theories.

The Theory of Self-Care

To understand the theory of self-care one must first understand the concepts of self-care, self-care agency, basic conditioning factors, and therapeutic self-care demand. *Self-care* is the performance or practice of activities that individuals initiate and perform on their own behalf to maintain life, health, and well-being. When self-care is effectively performed, it helps to maintain structural integrity and human functioning, and contributes to human development (Orem, 2001, p. 43).

Self-care agency is the human's aquired ability or power to engage in self-care. This ability to engage in self-care is affected by basic conditioning factors. These *basic conditioning factors* are age, gender, developmental state, health state, sociocultural factors, health care system factors (i.e., diagnostic and treatment modalities), family system factors, patterns of living (e.g., activities regularly engaged in), environmental factors, and resource adequacy and availability. "Normally, adults voluntarily care for themselves. Infants, children, the aged, the ill, and the disabled require complete care or assistance with self-care activities" (Orem, 2001, p. 43). The *therapeutic self-care demand* is the totality of "care measures necessary at specific times or over a duration of time for meeting an individual's self-care requisites by using appropriate methods and related sets of operations and actions" (p. 523). The therapeutic self-care demand is modeled on deliberate action—that is, actions deliberately performed by some members of a society to benefit themselves or others (p. 61).

An additional concept incorporated within the theory of self-care is *self-care requisites*. Self-care requisites can be defined as "the reasons for which self-care is undertaken; they express the intended or desired results" (Orem, 2001, p. 522). Orem presents three categories of self-care requisites, or requirements, as: (1) universal, (2) developmental, and (3) health deviation. *Universal self-care requisites* are associated with life processes, the maintenance of the integrity of human structure and functioning, and with general well-being (p. 48). They are common to all human beings during all stages of the life cycle and should be viewed as interrelated factors, each affecting the others. A common term for these requisites is the activities of daily living. Orem identifies self-care requisites as follows:

1. The maintenance of a sufficient intake of air.
2. The maintenance of a sufficient intake of water.
3. The maintenance of a sufficient intake of food.
4. The provision of care associated with elimination processes and excrements.
5. The maintenance of a balance between activity and rest.
6. The maintenance of a balance between solitude and social interaction.
7. The prevention of hazards to human life, human functioning, and human well-being.
8. The promotion of human functioning and development within social groups in accord with human potential, known human limitations, and the human desire to be normal. *Normalcy* is used in the sense of that which is essentially human and that which is in accord with the genetic and constitutional characteristics and the talents of individuals (p. 225).

"*Developmental self-care requisites* are associated with human growth and developmental processes and with conditions and events occurring during various stages of the life cycle . . . and events that can adversely affect development" (Orem, 2001, p. 48). Examples would be adjusting to a new job or adjusting to body changes such as facial lines or hair loss.

Health deviation self-care requisites are related to "genetic and constitutional defects and human and structural and functional deviations" (Orem, 2001, p. 48). They may be performed when there are medical measures used to diagnose and/or correct a certain condition (e.g., right upper quadrant abdominal pain when foods with a high fat content are eaten, or learning to walk using crutches following the casting of a fractured leg) and may deal with the effects of the defects or deviations and the effects of efforts to diagnose and treat them. The health deviation self-care requisites are as follows:

1. Seeking and securing appropriate medical assistance . . .
2. Being aware of and attending to the effects and results of pathologic conditions and states . . .
3. Effectively carrying out medically prescribed diagnostic, therapeutic, and rehabilitative measures . . .
4. Being aware of and attending to or regulating the discomforting or deleterious effects of prescribed medical care measures . . .
5. Modifying the self-concept (and self-image) in accepting oneself as being in a particular state of health and in need of specific forms of health care

6. Learning to live with the effects of pathologic conditions and states and the effects of medical diagnostic and treatment measures in a life-style that promotes continued personal development (Orem, 2001, p. 235).

In the theory of self-care, Orem explains *what* is meant by self-care and lists the various factors that affect its provision. In the self-care deficit theory, she specifies *when* nursing is needed to assist individuals in the provision of self-care.

The Theory of Self-Care Deficit

The theory of self-care deficit is the basic element of Orem's (2001) general theory of nursing because it delineates when nursing is needed. Nursing is required when adults (or in the case of a dependent, the parent or guardian) are incapable of or limited in their ability to provide continuous effective self-care. Nursing may be provided if the "care abilities are less than those required for meeting a known self-care demand . . . [or] self-care or dependent-care abilities exceed or are equal to those required for meeting the current self-care demand, but a future deficit relationship can be foreseen because of predictable decreases in care abilities, qualitative or quantitative increases in the care demand, or both" (p. 147). Nursing may be needed when individuals need "to incorporate newly prescribed, complex self-care measures into their self-care systems, the performance of which requires specialized knowledge and skills to be acquired through training and experience" (p. 283); or when the individual needs help "in recovering from disease or injury, or in coping with their effects" (p. 82). It is important to note that the first category includes universal, developmental, and health-deviation self-care needs whereas the other categories focus on health-deviation self-care.

Orem (2001) identifies the following five methods of helping that nurses may use:

1. Acting for or doing for another
2. Guiding and directing
3. Providing physical or psychological support
4. Providing and maintaining an environment that supports personal development
5. Teaching (p. 56).

The nurse may help the individual by using any or all of these methods to provide assistance with self-care.

The relationship between Orem's concepts is demonstrated in Figure 7–1. From this model it can be seen that at any given time an individual has specific self-care abilities as well as therapeutic self-care demands. If there are more demands than abilities, nursing is needed. The activities in which nurses engage when they provide nursing care can be used to describe the domain of nursing. Orem (2001) has identified work operations of nurses in clinical nursing practice:

• Entering into and maintaining nurse–patient relationships with individuals, families, or groups

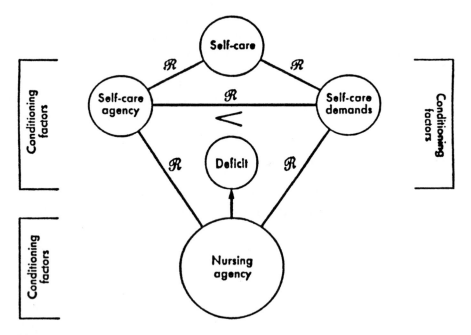

Figure 7–1. A conceptual framework for nursing. (R = relationship; < = deficit relationship, current or projected.) (*Used with permission from Orem, D. E. (1991). Nursing: Concepts of practice (4th ed.). St. Louis: Mosby, p. 64.*)

- Designing, planning for, instituting, and managing systems of nursing care
- Responding to patients' requests, desires, and needs for nurse contact and assistance
- Coordinating nursing care
- Establishing the kind and amount of immediate and continuing care needed
- Coordinating the care with other services such as other health care, social, or educational services needed or being received
- Discharging patients from nursing care when they have regained their abilities to perform their own self-care needs (p. 19).

Self-care has been defined and the need for nursing explained in the first and second theories. In Orem's third theory of nursing systems, she outlines *how* the patient's self-care needs will be met by the nurse, the patient, or both.

The Theory of Nursing Systems

The nursing system, designed by the nurse, is based on the assessment of an individual's self-care needs and on the assessment of the abilities of the patient to perform self-care activities. If there is a self-care deficit, that is, if there is a deficit between what the individual can do (self-care agency) and what needs to be done to maintain optimum functioning (therapeutic self-care demand), then nursing is required.

Nursing agency is a complex property or attribute of people educated and trained as nurses that enables them to act, to know, and to help others meet their therapeutic self-care demands by exercising or developing their own self-care agency. Nursing agency is similar to self-care agency in that both symbolize characteristics and abilities for specific types of deliberate action. They differ in that nursing agency is carried out for the benefit and well-being of others, and self-care agency is employed for one's own benefit (Orem, 2001, p. 289).

Orem (2001) has identified three classifications of nursing systems to meet the self-care requisites of the patient (see Fig. 7–2). These systems are the wholly compensatory system, the partly compensatory system, and the supportive-educative system.

The design and elements of the nursing system make clear "(1) the scope of the nursing responsibility in health care situations; (2) the general and specific roles of nurses, patients, and others; (3) reasons for nurses' relationships with patients; and (4) the kinds of actions to be performed and the performance patterns and nurses' and patients' actions in regulating patients' self-care agency and in meeting their therapeutic self-care demand" (Orem, 2001, p. 348). All nurses must have some skills in designing or in making adjustments in the design of nursing systems.

The *wholly compensatory nursing system* is represented by a situation in which the individual is unable "to engage in those self-care actions requiring self-directed and controlled ambulation and manipulative movement or the medical prescription to refrain from such activity. . . . Persons with these limitations are socially dependent on others for their continued existence and well-being" (Orem, 2001, p. 352). Subtypes of the wholly compensatory system are nursing systems for people who are: "[1] unable to engage in any form of deliberate action, for example, persons in a coma, . . . [2] aware and who may be able to make observations, judgments, and decisions about self-care and other matters but cannot or should not perform actions requiring ambulation and manipulative movements, . . . [and 3] unable to attend to themselves and make reasoned judgments and decisions about self-care and other matters but who can be ambulatory and may be able to perform some measures of self-care with continuous guidance and supervision" (p. 352). Examples of persons in the second subtype could include those with C3–C4 vertebral fractures, and of those in the third subtype, persons who are severely mentally retarded.

The *partly compensatory nursing system* is represented by a situation in which "both nurse and patient perform care measures or other actions involving manipulative tasks or ambulation. . . . [Either] the patient or the nurse may have the major role in the performance of care measures" (Orem, 2001, p. 354). An example of a person needing nursing care in the partly compensatory system would be an individual who has had recent abdominal surgery. This patient might be able to wash his or her face and brush his or her teeth but needs the nurse to change the surgical dressing or for help in ambulating and bathing.

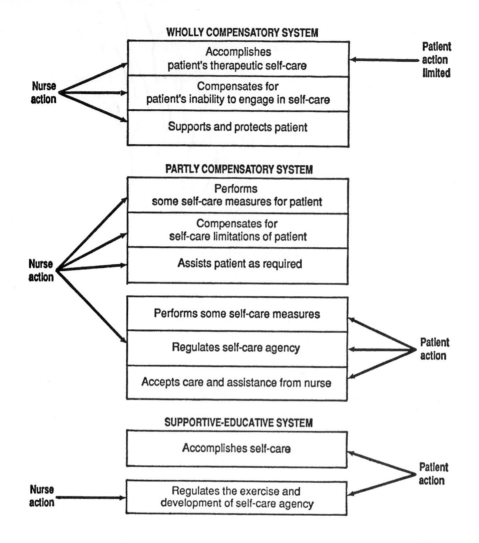

Figure 7–2. Basic nursing systems. (*Adapted with permission from Orem, D. E. (1991). Nursing: Concepts of practice (4th ed.), St. Louis: Mosby, p 288.*)

The third nursing system is the *supportive-educative system*. In this system, the person "is able to perform or can and should learn to perform required measures of externally or internally oriented therapeutic self-care but cannot do so without assistance" (Orem, 2001, p. 354). This is also known as a supportive-developmental system. In this system the patient is doing all of the self-care. The "patient's requirements for help are confined to decision making, behavior control, and acquiring knowledge and skills" (p. 354). The nurse's role, then, is to promote the patient as a self-care agent. An example of a person in this system would be a 16-year-old who is requesting birth control information. The nurse's role in this system is primarily that of a teacher or consultant.

One or more of the three types of systems may be used with a single patient. For example, a woman in labor may move from a supportive-educative system while she is in early labor to a partly compensatory system as her labor advances. If she requires a cesarean delivery, her care might require her to be in a wholly compensatory system. She would then progress to a partly compensatory system as she recovers from the anesthetic. Later, as she prepares to go home, a supportive-educative system would again be appropriate.

OREM'S THEORY AND NURSING'S METAPARADIGM

Orem discusses each of the four major concepts of human beings, health, society, and nursing in her work. *Human beings* "are distinguished from other living things by their capacity (1) to reflect upon themselves and their environment, (2) to symbolize what they experience, and (3) to use symbolic creations (ideas, words) in thinking, in communicating, and in guiding efforts to do and to make things that are beneficial for themselves or others" (Orem, 2001, p. 182). Integrated human functioning includes physical, psychological, interpersonal, and social aspects. Orem believes that individuals have the potential for learning and developing. The way an individual meets self-care needs is not instinctual but is a learned behavior. Factors that affect learning include age, mental capacity, culture, society, and the emotional state of the individual. If the individual cannot learn self-care measures, others must learn the care and provide it.

In the sixth edition of *Nursing: Concepts of practice*, Orem (2001) considers human beings from two different perspectives. The first is as persons viewed as moving "toward maturation and achievement of the individual's human potential" (p. 187). Orem stresses that this development is a dynamic, ever-changing concept. "*Self-realization* and *personality development* are terms used at times to refer to the process of personalization" (p. 188). The second perspective "focuses on structural and functional differentiations within the unity that is a human being . . . developed by various human and life sciences . . . [including] genetics, biochemistry, biophysics, human anatomy, and human physiology, . . . psychology, psychophysiology, and social psychology" (p. 188). Orem emphasizes, however, that both perspectives need to be integrated for effective nursing care.

Orem (2001) supports the World Health Organization's definition of *health* as "a state of physical, mental, and social well-being and not merely the absence of disease or infirmity" (p. 184) as well as speaking to the relationship between health, well-being, and being whole or sound. She states that "the physical, psychologic[al], interpersonal and social aspects of health are inseparable in the individual" (p. 182). Orem also presents health based on the concept of preventive health care. This health care includes the promotion and maintenance of health (primary prevention), the treatment of disease or injury (secondary prevention), and the prevention of complications (tertiary prevention).

About *nursing*, Orem (2001) states:

In modern society, adults are expected to be self-reliant and responsible for themselves and for the well-being of their dependents. Most

societies accept that persons who are helpless, sick, aged, handicapped, or otherwise deprived should be helped in their immediate
distress and helped to attain or regain responsibility within their existing capacities. Thus, both self-help and help to others are valued by
society as desirable activities. Nursing as a specific type of human
service is based on both values. In most communities people see nursing as a desirable and necessary service (p. 81).

Nursing is required whenever the maintenance of continuous self-care
requires the use of special techniques and the application of scientific
knowledge in providing care or in designing it (Orem, 2001, p. 83).

Orem speaks to several factors related to the concept of nursing. These are the art
and prudence of nursing, nursing as a service, role theory related to nursing, and
technologies in nursing. "The art of nursing is the intellectual quality of individual
nurses that allows them to make creative investigations, analyses, and syntheses of
the variables and conditioning factors within nursing situations in order to work toward the goal of the production of effective systems of nursing assistance for individuals or multiperson units" (p. 293). These decisions require a theoretical base in
the discipline of nursing and in the sciences, arts, and humanities. This base directs
decisions when designing nursing systems within the nursing process. *"Nursing
prudence* is the quality of nurses that enables them (1) to seek and take counsel in
new or difficult nursing situations, (2) to make correct judgments . . . , (3) to decide
to act in a particular way, and (4) to take action" (p. 293). Unique life and nursing
experiences affect the development of the individual nurse's art and prudence.

Orem (2001) further defines nursing as a human service. Nursing is distinguished from other human services by its focus on persons with inabilities to maintain the continuous provision of health care. Nursing is needed when the adult is
unable "to maintain continuously that amount and quality of [health-associated]
self-care that is therapeutic in sustaining life and health, in recovering from disease
or injury, or in coping with their effects" (p. 82). With children, nursing is needed
when the parent or guardian associated with the child's health state is unable "to
maintain continuously for the child the amount and quality of care that is therapeutic" (p. 82). For children, nursing may be needed to assist with development or
maturation.

The nurse's and the patient's roles define the expected behaviors for each in the
specific nursing situation. Various factors that influence the expected role behaviors
are culture, environment, age, sex, the health setting, and finances. The roles of
nurse and patient are complementary. That is, a certain behavior of the patient elicits
a certain response in the nurse, and vice versa. Both work together to accomplish
the goal of self-care.

In the nurse–patient relationship, the nurse or patient may experience role conflict because each is performing concurrent roles. For example, the patient has expected behaviors from his roles as father, husband, Cub Scout leader, soccer coach,
and librarian. The nurse has expected behaviors from her roles as wife, mother,
daughter, choir director, and PTA president. Thus, the conflict in the behaviors

required for the various roles may affect the performance of self-care by the patient and by the nurse.

It is important to note that although Orem (2001) recognizes that specialized technologies are usually developed by members of the health professions, she emphasizes the need for social and interpersonal dimensions in nursing. The effective integration of social and interpersonal technologies with regulatory technologies promotes quality professional nursing. She states, "Treatment or regulatory operations are the practical activities through which what is prescribed is executed and through which the diagnosed condition or problem is treated in order to remove it, control it, or keep it within boundaries compatible with human life, health, and well-being" (p. 308).

OREM'S THEORY AND THE NURSING PROCESS

According to Orem (2001), "*Nursing process* is a term nurses use to refer to nurses' performance of the professional-technologic operations of nursing practice" (p. 309). Other activities associated with nursing process are planning and evaluation. A process is a continuous and regular sequence of goal achieving, deliberately performed actions taking place or carried out in a definite manner.

Orem (2001) discusses a three-step nursing process, which she labels the professional-technologic operations of nursing practice. These steps are shown in Table 7–2 as:

- *Step 1.* Nursing diagnosis and prescription—that is, determining why nursing is needed; analysis and interpretation—making judgments regarding care, also labeled case management operations.
- *Step 2.* Designing the nursing system and planning for delivery of care.
- *Step 3.* The production and management of nursing systems, also labeled planning and controlling.

Orem (2001) states that nursing process is "constituted from nurses' performance of diagnostic, prescriptive, and regulatory or treatment operations, with associated control operations including evaluation" (p. 309).

TABLE 7–2. COMPARISON OF OREM'S NURSING PROCESS AND THE NURSING PROCESS

Nursing Process	Orem's Nursing Process
1. Assessment 2. Nursing diagnosis 3. Outcomes	Step 1. Diagnosis and prescription; determine why nursing is needed. Analyze and interpret—make judgments regarding care.
4. Plans with scientific rationale	Step 2. Design of a nursing system and plan for delivery of care.
5. Implementation 6. Evaluation	Step 3. Production and management of nursing systems.

Nursing Diagnosis and Prescription (Step 1)

"Nursing diagnosis necessitates investigation and the accumulation of data about patients' self-care agency and their therapeutic self-care demand and the existent or projected relationships between them" (Orem, 2001, p. 310). The goal defines the direction and nature of the actions. Prescriptive operations specify the means (course of actions, care measures) to be used to meet particular self-care requisites, or to meet all components of the therapeutic self-care demand. Orem emphasizes that, in nursing's diagnostic and prescriptive operations and in the regulatory or treatment operations, patients' and families' abilities and interests in collaboration affect what nurses can do.

Designs for Regulatory Operation (Step 2)

Designing an effective and efficient system of nursing involves choosing suitable ways to help the patient. This design includes nurse and patient roles in relation to which self-care tasks will be performed when modifying the therapeutic self-care demands, controlling the implementation of self-care agency, shielding the already developed powers of self-care agency, and assisting with new developments in self-care agency (Orem, 2001, p. 319).

Planning is the movement from designing the nursing systems to identifying the mechanisms of their production. "A plan sets forth the organization . . . of essential tasks to be performed in accordance with role responsibilities" (Orem, 2001, p. 321). "The planning for implementation of the design and related procurement activities . . . determine[s] when nurses should be with patients and when essential materials and equipment will be available and ready for use" (p. 322).

Production/Management of Nursing Systems (Step 3)

"Regulatory nursing systems are produced when nurses interact with patients and take consistent action to meet their prescribed therapeutic self-care demands and to regulate the exercise or development of their capabilities for self-care" (Orem, 2001, p. 322). In this, the third step of the professional-technologic nursing process, nurses act to produce and manage nursing systems.

During the interactions of nurses and patients, nurses do the following:

1. Perform and regulate the performance of self-care tasks for patients or assist patients with their performance of self-care tasks
2. Coordinate self-care task performance so that a unified system of care is produced and coordinated with other components of health care
3. Help patients, their families, and others bring about systems of daily living for patients that support the accomplishment of self-care and are, at the same time, satisfying in relation to patients' interest[s], talents, and goals
4. Guide, direct, and support patients in their exercise of, or in withholding the exercise of, their self-care agency

5. Stimulate patients' interest in self-care by raising questions and promoting discussions of care problems and issues when conditions permit; be available to patients at times when questions are likely to arise
6. Support and guide patients in learning activities and provide cues for learning as well as instructional sessions
7. Support and guide patients as they experience illness or disability and the effects of medical care measures and as they experience the need to engage in new measures of self-care or change their ways of meeting ongoing self-care requisites
8. Monitor patients and assist patients to monitor themselves to determine if self-care measures were effectively performed and to determine the effects of self-care, the results of efforts to regulate the exercise or development of self-care agency, and the sufficiency and efficiency of nursing action directed to these ends
9. Make characterizing judgments about the sufficiency and efficiency of self-care, the regulation of the exercise or development of self-care agency, and nursing assistance
10. Make judgments about the meaning of the results derived from nurses' performance of the preceding two operations for the well-being of patients and make or recommend adjustments in the nursing care system through changes in nurse and patient roles (Orem, 2001, pp. 322–323).

The first seven operations constitute direct nursing care. The last three are for the purpose of deciding if the care provided should be continued in the present form or be changed. This comprises the evaluation component of the nursing process.

The case study demonstrates the use of Orem's theory and the nursing process (see Tables 7–3, page 138, and 7–4, pages 140–141).

Step 1. Orem defines Step 1 as the diagnosis and prescription phase, determining if nursing is needed. In this assessment phase, the nurse collects data in six areas:

1. The person's health status
2. The physician's perspective of the person's health
3. The person's perspective of his or her health
4. The health goals within the context of life history, life style, and health status
5. The person's requirements for self-care
6. The person's capacity to perform self-care

Specific data are gathered in the areas of the individual's universal, developmental, and health-deviation self-care needs and their interrelationship. Data are also collected about the individual's knowledge, skills, motivation, and orientation. Orem is careful to point out that the data to be collected should be limited to those needed to come to legitimate conclusions about the person's needs (Orem, 2001, p. 310).

TABLE 7–3: APPLICATION OF OREM'S THEORY TO NURSING PROCESS

Basic Conditioning Factors	Universal Self-Care	Developmental Self-Care	Health Deviations	Medical Problem and Plan	Self Care Deficits
Age Sex Height Weight Culture Race Marital status Religion Occupation	Air, water, food Excrements Activity and rest Solitude and social interaction Hazards to life and well-being Promotion of human functioning and development	Specialized needs for developmental processes New requisites from a condition Requisites associated with an event	Conditions of illness or injury Treatments to correct the condition	Physician's perspective of condition Medical diagnosis Medical treatment	Difference between self-care needs and self-care capabilities

Nursing Diagnosis	Outcomes and Plan	Implementation
Based on self-care deficits	Outcomes, nursing goals, and objectives: a. Congruent with nursing diagnosis b. Based on self-care demands c. Promote patient as self-care agent Designing the nursing system: a. Wholly compensatory b. Partly compensatory c. Supportive-educative Appropriate methods of helping: a. Guidance b. Support c. Acting or doing for d. Providing developmental environment	Nurse-patient actions to: a. Promote patient as self-care agent b. Meet self-care needs c. Decrease self-care deficit Effectiveness of nurse-patient actions to: a. Promote patient as self-care agent b. Meet self-care needs c. Decrease self-care deficits

Adapted from Pinnell, N. N., & de Meneses, M. (1986). *The nursing process—Theory, application and related processes*. Norwalk, CT: Appleton-Century-Crofts, p. 66. Used with permission.

Within Step 1, the nurse seeks answers to the following questions:

1. What is the patient's therapeutic care demand? Now? At a future time?
2. Does the patient have a deficit for engaging in self-care to meet the therapeutic self-care demand?
3. If so, what is its nature and the reasons for its existence?
4. Should the patient be helped to refrain from engagement in self-care or to protect already developed self-care capabilities for therapeutic purposes?
5. What is the patient's potential for engaging in self-care at a future time period? Increasing or deepening self-care knowledge? Learning techniques of self-care? Fostering willingness to engage in self-care? Effectively and consistently incorporating essential self-care measures (including new ones) into the systems of self-care and daily living? (Orem, 1985, pp. 225–226).

Once the assessment data have been gathered, they must be analyzed. In the category of universal self-care needs, Ms. M. demonstrates a deficit in adequate air, water, and food intake because she is 5 feet 2 inches, weighs 175 pounds, and consumes excessive calories, fat, and cholesterol from fast food and late-night meals. Ms. M. shows an imbalance between activity and rest because she has minimal exercise. There is also an imbalance between her solitude and social interaction since her husband's death, which is a significant loss for her in the mid-life developmental needs category. Ms. M.'s elevated cholesterol levels, when interrelated with her family history of stroke and heart attack, present a hazard to her life, functioning, and well-being. The physician's perspective is that Ms. M. needs to lose 40 pounds because of her family history and elevated blood cholesterol but that she has limited nutritional knowledge. However, Ms. M. has a motivational deficit to lose weight because her Italian cultural tradition associates food with family and love.

Based on the analysis of Ms. M.'s data, she has potential hazards to her health related to obesity, high cholesterol, smoking, social isolation, and decreased exercise. The analysis of the collected data leads to the nursing diagnosis, enabling the nurse to prioritize self-care deficits. The nursing diagnosis must include the response and etiology pattern. Within Orem's framework, the nursing diagnosis would be stated as an inability to meet the self-care demand (the response) related to the self-care deficit (etiology) (Ziegler, Vaughn-Wrobel, & Erlen, 1986). For Ms. M. the response pattern would be "potential for impaired cardiovascular functioning," and the etiology would be "lack of knowledge about how her current life style increases her risk for heart attack and stroke."

Step 2. Orem defines Step 2 as designing the nursing systems and planning for the delivery of nursing. The nurse designs a system that is wholly compensatory, partly compensatory, or supportive-educative. "The actual design of a concrete nursing system emerges as nurses and patients interact and take action to calculate and meet patient's therapeutic self-care demands, to compensate for or overcome

TABLE 7–4: APPLICATION OF OREM'S THEORY USING MRS. M'S CASE STUDY WITHIN THE NURSING PROCESS

Assessment

Basic Conditioning Factors	Universal Self-Care	Developmental Self-Care	Health Deviations	Medical Problem and Plan	Self-Care Deficits
48 y.o.	Smokes 1.5 packs/day	Loss of husband	Family history:	Diagnoses of obesity with potential for cardiac disease and low motivation for weight loss	Difference between healthy life style and Ms. M.'s knowledge base and life style which increases her risk of heart attack or stroke
Female	Frequently eats fast food; high fat diet; drinks 48 oz. of water daily	Loss of social activity	F—heart attack, age 50	Prescription to:	
5'2"	Largest meal of day is late evening	Finds work as university faculty fulfilling	M—died of stroke, age 53	Monitor cholesterol levels and vital signs	
175 lbs.	No difficulties with elimination	Works 12-hour days	Cholesterol 260 mg.; other lab values WNL	Decrease cholesterol and fat intake	
Italian	No regular exercise	Well groomed	Lacks knowledge of risk factors and cardiovascular functioning	Increase exercise	
White	Sleeps 6 to 7 hours nightly		B/P 142/88	Decrease or stop smoking	
Widowed for 6 months after 25 yrs of happy marriage	Decreased social interaction × 6 months—no longer plays bridge with group she and her husband played with		T 98.4° F.	Re-evaluate and if needed prescribe medication to lower cholesterol	
Catholic			P 92		
University faculty			R 26, not SOB		
			Potential for cardiac disease related to obesity, smoking, elevated cholesterol, lack of exercise, and family history		

Nursing Diagnosis	Outcomes and Plan	Implementation	Evaluation
Potential for impaired cardiovascular functioning related to lack of knowledge about relationship between current life style and risk of heart attack or stroke	OUTCOME: Lowered cholesterol Healthier lifestyle with regular exercise, decreased smoking, and balanced nutrition NURSING GOALS AND OBJECTIVES: Goal: To decrease risk for cardiac impairment Objectives: Ms. M. will state that high cholesterol levels increase her risk for cardiac impairment Ms. M. will recognize the relationship between smoking and cardiovascular risk DESIGN OF NURSING SYSTEM: Supportive-educative METHODS OF HELPING: Guidance, support, teaching, and provision of a developmental environment	Jointly develop contract related to: 1. CHOLESTEROL REDUCTION. Ms. M. will keep a 3-day food diary Ms. M. will learn about cholesterol and its effects on cardiovascular functioning Ms. M. will request/obtain cholesterol and fat content of fast foods Ms. M. will learn about low cholesterol and fast foods, foods that decrease cholesterol and restaurants that serve low cholesterol and fat-free foods Jointly analyze food diary and decide how to decrease cholesterol/fat intake to reduce Ms. M's weight Jointly determine Italian foods that are low in cholesterol and fat, and how recipes may be adapted. Ms. M's accomplishments will be reinforced Ms. M. will seek advice from her physician re: medication to reduce cholesterol 2. REDUCTION OF SMOKING Ms. M. will identify when she smokes and what initiates the desire for a cigarette. Ms. M. will plan ways to replace smoking with other activities (exercising, chewing gum).	Does Ms. M. understand that, with her present life style, her risk of heart attack or stroke is high? Did Ms. M. select low cholesterol, low fat foods? Did Ms. M.'s self care deficit decrease? Is Ms. M.'s cholesterol lower? Did Ms. M. lose weight? Has Ms. M. decreased the number of cigarettes smoked daily? Was the supportive-educative system effective in promoting Ms. M. as a self-care agent?

the identified action limitations of patients, and to regulate the development and exercise of patients' self-care abilities" (Orem, 2001, p. 348).

Using Orem's model, the outcomes and goals are congruent with the nursing diagnosis to enable the patient to become an effective self-care agent. Outcomes and goals are directed by the response statement of the nursing diagnosis and are focused on health. The outcome for Ms. M. would be: Decrease her risk of cardiovascular impairment. The goals would be: lowered blood cholesterol level, healthier lifestyle that includes regular exercise, decreased smoking, and balanced nutrition.

Once the outcomes and goals have been determined, the objectives can be stated. An example of an objective for Ms. M. would be: Ms. M. will state that high cholesterol levels increase her risk for cardiac impairment. Other objectives might relate to the risk factors of obesity, lack of exercise, smoking, and family history. The designed nursing system for Ms. M. would be the supportive-educative nursing system.

Step 3. Within Orem's (2001) nursing process, Step 3 includes the production and management of the nursing system. In this step, the nurse performs and regulates the patient's self-care tasks, or assists the patient in doing so; coordinates the performance of self-care with other components of health care; helps patients, families and others create and use systems of daily living that meet self-care needs in a satisfying way; guides, directs, and supports patients in exercising, or not exercising, self-care agency; stimulates patient's interest in care problems; supports learning activities; supports and guides the patient in adapting the needs arising from medical measures; monitors and assists in self-monitoring the performance and effects of self-care measures; judges the sufficiency and efficiency of self-care, self-care agency, and nursing agency; adjusts the nursing care system as needed.

The nurse and patient actions are directed by the etiology component of the nursing diagnosis. "Lack of knowledge about how her current life style increases her risk for heart attack and stroke" is the etiology component of Ms. M.'s nursing diagnosis. When the nurse and patient implement this supportive-educative system, each has specific roles. Examples of these roles might be: Together they would develop a contract relating to the goal of blood cholesterol reduction. Ms. M. would keep a three-day food diary. The nurse would provide information about cholesterol and its effects on cardiovascular function. Ms. M. would request and obtain the fat and cholesterol content of the fast-food menu items from the restaurants she frequents. The nurse would provide information about specific foods that are low in fat and cholesterol, those food items that help reduce cholesterol, and a list of fast-food restaurants that offer low-fat and low-cholesterol food items. Together they would analyze the three-day food diary and decide how Ms. M. might modify her diet to reduce her fat and cholesterol intake. They would determine which Italian dishes are low in fat and cholesterol or how these recipes can be adapted. As her blood cholesterol levels decrease, Ms. M. would be praised for her accomplishments. During this implementation, the nurse would teach, guide, and support Ms. M. while providing a developmental environment.

Step 3 includes evaluation. The nurse and patient together do the evaluation. Questions they might ask are: When evaluating some of Ms. M.'s plans, does she understand that her present life style may increase her risk of developing a heart attack or stroke? Did she select low-fat and low-cholesterol fast foods? Did she attain her goal of reducing her blood cholesterol levels? Did she lose weight? The results must then be communicated with the physician and any further medical interventions needed then obtained. Were the plans effective in decreasing the self-care deficit? Was the nursing system effective in promoting the patient as a self-care agent?

Evaluation is an ongoing process. It is essential that the nurse and patient continually evaluate any changes in the data that would affect the self-care deficit, the self-care agent, and the nursing system.

CRITIQUE OF OREM'S SELF CARE DEFICIT THEORY OF NURSING

Orem presented a conceptual framework in 1959. Since then her work has continued to evolve. Orem's General Theory of Nursing was formulated and expressed in 1979–1980. This Self-Care Deficit Theory of Nursing is comprised of three interrelated theories: the theory of self-care, the theory of self-care deficit, and the theory of nursing systems. These three interrelated theories are the basis of the following discussion.

1. What is the historical context of the theory? Orem began her work in the late 1950s while working with licensed practical nurses. She continued the development of her theory throughout the twentieth century and into the twenty-first century. Her work initially focused on the individual inpatient, but in her fifth and sixth editions (1995, 2001) discusses the multiperson unit, the person at home, and positive mental health. She has indicated that the theory is derived from clinical practice and that its evaluation is dependent on continued contact and exchange with clinicians.

2. What are the basic concepts and relationships presented by the theory? Orem discusses persons as needing to have self-care needs met in order to live and develop. When persons are unable to care for themselves (self-care needs are greater than self-care abilities or self-care agency), then someone else must provide that care and nursing is needed. The basic concepts are "self-care," "universal, developmental, and health deviation self-care requisites," "basic conditioning factors," "therapeutic self-care demand," "self-care deficit," "supportive-educative, partly compensatory, and wholly compensatory nursing systems," "self-care agency," and "nursing agency." When a person's self-care agency is adequate to meet the therapeutic self-care demand created by the self-care requisites and basic conditioning factors, then self-care needs are met by the person. When the therapeutic self-care demand is greater than the self-care agency, then a self-care deficit exists and nursing is needed. Nursing agency supports the person in meeting self-care needs through the design and delivery of supportive-educative, partly compensatory, and wholly compensatory nursing systems.

3. What major phenomena of concern to nursing are presented? These phenomena may include *but are not limited to*: **human beings, environment, health, interpersonal relations, caring, goal attainment, adaptation, and energy fields.** Orem (2001) discusses human beings as "distinguished from other living things by their capacity (1) to reflect upon themselves and their environment, (2) to symbolize what they experience, and (3) to use symbolic creations (ideas, words) in thinking, in communicating, and in guiding efforts to do and to make things that are beneficial for themselves or others" (p. 182).

Within Orem's theory, the environment directly influences the patient. Orem (2001) discusses the individuals' needs for air, water, and food. She also discusses that "prevention of hazards to life, functioning and well-being contributes to the maintenance of human integrity and, therefore, to the effective promotion of human functioning and development" (p. 226).

Orem's discussion of health and the supportive-educative system is relevant in today's society since she supports health promotion and health maintenance. Self-care in Orem's theory likewise supports the premises of holistic health in that both promote the individual's responsibility for health care.

Orem's discussion of interpersonal relations would involve the nurse acting for or doing for the patient, but also relying on the other (patient or nurse) in the partly compensatory and wholly compensatory systems. She incorporates the care of the patient with the abilities of the family members and recognizes that they may be the ones providing the "self-care" for the patient. She also discusses the need to determine what the physician's perspective is on the patient's illness.

Nursing is needed according to Orem whenever the maintenance of continuous self-care requires the use of special techniques and the application of scientific knowledge to provide or design care. The requirements occur when there is a self-care deficit. The design of nursing systems involves consideration of the areas in which, and the degree to which, support is needed.

Orem (2001) states: "The interpersonal features of nursing are based on existent contractual relationships of nurses and patients" (p. 99). She recognizes that "ideally, the interpersonal relationship between a nurse and a patient contributes to the alleviation of the patient's stress and that of the family, enabling the patient and the family to act responsibly in matters of health and health care" (p. 101). Orem's theory refers to "care" from a more physical provision of nursing care with the interpersonal relationships discussed, rather than feeling the emotional perspective of "caring."

4. To whom does this theory apply? In what situations? In what ways? Orem's theory applies to all of those who need nursing care. The theory applies to situations in which individuals (including children) cannot meet all of their self-care needs. One of the unique characteristics of Orem's theory is that she recognizes that normal life and human development necessitates adjustments, which might be improved by supportive-educative care from the nurse. Orem's theory has been expanded by Susan Taylor and Kathie McLaughlin Renpenning to include multiperson units, families, and communities. However, Orem (2001) has recommended that, based on current knowledge, the nursing systems be limited to use with individuals as units of service.

A search of the literature supports the use of this theory in a wide variety of settings and with a variety of patients. A partial list includes:

> multiperson units (Chevannes, 1997; DeMoutigny, 1995; Geden & Taylor, 1999; Logue, 1997; Taylor & McLaughlin, 1991);
>
> caregivers (Baker, 1997; Fawdry, Berry, & Rajacich, 1996; Schott-Baer, Fisher, & Gregory, 1995);
>
> culture (Hartweg & Berbiglia, 1996; Lee, 1999; Roberson & Kelley, 1996; Sonderhamm, Evers, & Hamrin, 1996; Villarruel & Denyes, 1997; Wang, 1997);
>
> health education (Jewell & Sullivan, 1996);
>
> multiple age groups (Anderson & Olnhausen, 1999; Brock & O'Sullivan, 1985; Chang, Cuman, Linn, Ware, & Kane, 1985; Clark, 1998; Dahlen, 1997; Denyes, 1982; Foote, Holcombe, Piazza, & Wright, 1993; Harper, 1984; Reed, 1986; Roy & Collin, 1994; Smith, 1996; Vesely, 1995; Villarruel & Denyes, 1991);
>
> framework for inpatient care (Laurie-Shaw & Ives, 1988a, 1988b);
>
> various clinical areas (Ailinger & Dear, 1997; Aish, 1996; Aish & Isenberg, 1996; Anastasio, McMahan, Daniels, Nicholas, & Paul-Simon, 1995; Beach, Smith, Luthringer, Utz, Ahrens, & Whitmire, 1996; Fitzgerald, 1980; Frey & Denyes, 1989; Fujita, & Dungan, 1994; Gulick, 1987; Hagopian, 1996; Jaarsma, Halfens, Senten, AbuSaad, & Dracup, 1998; Keohane, & Lacey, 1991; Logue, 1997; Mack, 1992; Orem & Vardiman, 1995; Tolentino, 1990; Zinn, 1986); and
>
> long-term care (Norris, 1991).

Concepts of the theory that have received specific focus include:

> self-care deficit (Gaffney & Moore, 1996);
>
> self-care agency (Allan, 1990; Baker, 1997; Denyes, 1988; Gast, Denyes, Campbell, Hartweg, Schott-Baer, & Isenberg, 1989; Hart & Foster, 1998; Jirovic & Kasno, 1993; Kearney & Fleischer, 1979; McDermott, 1993; Ulbrich, 1999; Utz, Shuster, Merwin, & Williams, 1994);
>
> dependent-care agency (Moore & Gaffney, 1989);
>
> conditioning factors (Ailinger & Dear, 1997; Anatasio, McMahan, Daniels, Nicholas, & Paul-Simon, 1995; Carroll, 1995; Conner-Warren, 1996; Freston, Young, Calhoun, Fredericksen, Salinger, Malchodi, & Edan, 1997; Frey & Denyes, 1989; Gaffney & Moore, 1996; Geden & Taylor, 1991; Hanucharurnkul, 1989; Jirovec & Kasno, 1990; Lawrence & Schank, 1995; Mapanga & Andrews, 1995; Marz, 1988; Moore, 1993; Moore & Mosher, 1997; Zadinsky & Boyle, 1996); and
>
> therapeutic self-care demand (Kubricht, 1984).

5. By what method or methods can this theory be tested? Orem's theory is one of the most readily applied theories. An electronic search by Taylor, Geden, Isaramalai, and Wongvatunyu (2000) found 143 journal articles (unpublished dissertations are not included) that used Orem's theory. The search was limited to those written in English and identified as being research articles. Of these, 66 were identified as clearly testing relationships within the theory. The others used Orem's work as part of the organizing framework or to provide a definition of self-care. The studies reviewed included both quantitative and qualitative research methods. Taylor, Geden, Isaramalai, and Wongvatuny identified four instruments that have been developed and validated to measure aspects of Orem's theory. Self-care agency was the focus of Denyes (1982) in the Denyes Self-Care Agency Instrument; Kearney and Fleischer (1979) in their tool, Exercise of Self-Care Agency; and Evers, Isenberg, Philipsen, Senten, & Brouns (1989) in their tool, Assessment of Self-Care Agency. Geden and Taylor (1991) developed the Self-Care Inventory.

6. Does this theory direct critical thinking in nursing practice? This theory does direct critical thinking in nursing practice. Orem's concepts are simple, yet complex, so beginning as well as advanced practitioners can use them. Practitioners are stimulated to apply the concepts of partly compensatory nursing systems and supportive-educative systems to their care as they recognize that their patients are improving, or that everyone meets developmental and situational life events in which they need education and support in order to maintain optimum health.

7. Does this theory direct therapeutic nursing intervention? Orem's theory does direct therapeutic nursing interventions. Orem's concepts of self-care needs, therapeutic self-care demands, self-care agency, self-care deficit, and nursing systems provide a framework for the nurse to consider the individual, what is needed to meet self-care needs, determine what the difference is between these needs and self-care abilities, design the nursing system that would best meet the needs, provide the nursing care, evaluate the care, and then as the individual recovers, discharge the person from the nursing care system. These steps may also be used to generate therapeutic nursing interventions for multiperson units.

8. Does this theory direct communication in nursing practice? Orem's theory does direct communication in nursing practice mostly from a physical perspective. She recognizes that interpersonal communications are essential, but the theory looks more at the physical relationships of *what* acts must be done, and *how* physically to accomplish those actions with lesser emphasis on the emotional *way* that the needs are met. Orem also discusses that nursing care must be designed, implemented, and coordinated, and then later that the person must be discharged from the nursing system. This would imply that communication is needed but one does not get a warm, nurturing feeling tone from these descriptions, but rather a more factual presentation.

9. Does this theory direct nursing actions that lead to favorable outcomes? Orem's theory definitely directs nursing actions that lead to favorable outcomes. The individual is recognized as having self-care needs that the person (if a healthy adult) has the ability or self-care agency to meet. These needs develop and change as the person grows, develops, and experiences life events. Orem's theory recognizes that if there are more needs than abilities, then there is a self-care deficit.

Nursing is then needed. A nursing system can be designed to help the person meet those needs. When the nurse and patient work together in that designed system, the patient's self-care needs can be met.

10. How contagious is this theory? Orem's theory is extremely contagious. The easily understood concepts are simple, yet complex and may be used by practitioners at all levels (beginning through advanced) and in all areas of practice. Taylor, Geden, Isaramalai, and Wongvatunyu (2000) found 143 research-related journal articles published in English. There is an additional body of literature related to application of the theory in practice, unpublished dissertation reports, and articles published in languages other than English. Orem's work is used internationally. Its use in Canada, Norway, Sweden, Switzerland, Thailand, and Pakistan is also supported by reports in the literature (Aish 1996; Aish & Isenberg, 1996; Dahlen, 1997; Hanucharurnkul, 1989; Jewell & Sullivan, 1996; Laurie-Shaw & Ives, 1988a, 1988b; Lee, 1999; Soderhamm, Evers, & Hamrin, 1996; Spirig & Willhelm, 1995). Further support is demonstrated by the existence of the International Orem Society.

STRENGTHS AND LIMITATIONS

In the preface to the sixth edition of *Nursing: Concepts of practice*, Orem (2001) outlines the following six broad themes: why persons need and can be helped by nursing, the relationship between persons needing and producing nursing, the unitary nature of humans, the selection and performance of deliberate actions to achieve desired results, assistive methods, and nursing as a practical science. In the text she describes her general theory, which is supported by three interrelated theories. Within these theories, six central concepts and one peripheral concept are identified. These provide the learner with a blueprint for the structure of Orem's Self-Care Deficit Theory of Nursing.

Orem's theory is derived from a clinical base. She states that "in working on the components of [her] theory [she] needs to work with other people—utilizing data from clinicians" (Trench, Wallace, & Coberg, 1988). She incorporates a chapter by Susan Taylor and Kathie McLaughlin Renpenning, which includes the position of family involvement within the self-care deficit nursing theory (Orem, 2001). Also, the Self-Care Deficit Theory of Nursing has been supported by clinical case-study data (Orem & Taylor, 1986).

Orem's theory of nursing provides a comprehensive base for nursing practice. It has utility for professional nursing in the areas of education, clinical practice, administration, research, and nursing information systems. A major strength of Orem's theory is that it is applicable for nursing by the beginning practitioner as well as the advanced clinician. The terms *self-care, nursing systems*, and *self-care deficit* are easily understood by the beginning nursing student and can be explored in greater depth as the nurse gains more knowledge and experience.

Another strength of Orem's (2001) theory is that she specifically defines when nursing is needed: Nursing is needed when the individual cannot maintain continuously that amount and quality of self-care necessary to sustain life and health, recover from disease or injury, or cope with their effects. And, "nursing is required whenever the maintenance of continuous self-care requires the use of special techniques and the application of scientific knowledge in providing care or in designing it" (p. 83).

Orem (2001) promotes the concepts of professional nursing. She defines the roles of vocational, technical, and professional nurses, and recognizes the importance of each. She indicates that thinking nursing and conceptualizing the dynamics and structure of nursing situations is distinct from viewing nursing as skilled performance of tasks.

Her self-care premise is contemporary with the concepts of health promotion and health maintenance. Self-care in Orem's theory is comparable to holistic health in that both promote the individual's responsibility for health care. This is especially relevant with today's emphasis on early hospital discharge, home care, and outpatient services. Orem (2001) recognizes the term *client* as a regular seeker of services but prefers the term *patient* for one who is "under the care of a health care professional at this time" (p. 70).

According to Orem (2001), "nurses should select the type of nursing system or sequential combination of nursing systems that will have an optimum effect in achieving the desired regulation of patients' self-care agency and the meeting of their self-care requisites" (p. 355). Some practitioners have found Orem's theory to be more clinically applicable when more than one system is used concurrently (Knust & Quarn, 1983).

Another strength is Orem's delineation of three identifiable nursing systems. These are easily understood by the beginning nursing student. Orem's use of the term *system* has developed to include entities that behave as a whole and in which a change in a part affects the whole (Orem, 2001, p. 155). This definition is congruent with the general system theory view of a system as a dynamic, flowing process.

Orem (2001) has expanded her initial focus of individual self-care to include multiperson units (families, groups, and communities). She notes that when multiperson units are served by nurses, the resulting nursing systems combine the features of partly compensatory and supportive-educative nursing systems. However, an incongruence is present because she suggests that "it is advisable at this stage of the development of nursing knowledge to confine the use of the three nursing systems to situations in which individuals are the units of care or service" (p. 351).

Orem's theory is simple yet complex. However, the essence is clouded by ancillary descriptions. The term *self-care* is used with numerous configurations. This multitude of terms, such as self-care agency, self-care demand, self-care premise, self-care deficit, self-care requisites, and universal self-care, can be very confusing initially until the essence of each concept is understood.

Other limitations include her discussion of health. Health is often viewed as dynamic and ever changing. Orem's model of the boxed nursing systems (see Fig. 7–2) implies three static conditions of health. She refers to a "concrete nursing system," which connotes rigidity. Another impression from the model of nursing systems is that a major determining factor for placement of a patient in a system is the individual's capacity for physical movement. Throughout her work there is limited acknowledgment of the individual's emotional needs.

SUMMARY

Orem presents her general theory of nursing, the self-care deficit theory of nursing, which is composed of the three interrelated theories of self-care, self-care deficit, and nursing systems. Incorporated within and supportive of these theories are the six central concepts of self-care, self-care agency, therapeutic self-care demand, self-care deficit, nursing agency, and nursing system, as well as the peripheral concept of basic conditioning factors.

Nursing is needed when the self-care demands are greater than the self-care abilities. The nurse designs nursing systems when it has been determined that nursing care is needed. The systems of wholly compensatory, partly compensatory, and supportive-educative specify the roles of the nurse and the patient.

Throughout Orem's work, she interprets nursing's metaparadigm of human beings, health, nursing, and society. She defines three steps of nursing process as (1) diagnosis and prescription, (2) design of a nursing system and planning for the delivery of care, and (3) production and management of nursing systems. This process parallels the nursing process of assessment, diagnosis, outcomes, planning, implementation, and evaluation.

Orem's theory of self-care has pragmatic application to nursing practice. It has been applied by nursing clinicians in a variety of settings. The theory has been used as the basis for nursing school curricula and the base for a nursing information system.

Orem's Self-Care Deficit Theory of Nursing continues to evolve and its impact is international. The widespread use of this theory reflects its utility for professional nursing. Orem's theory offers a unique way of looking at the phenomenon of nursing. Her work contributes significantly to the development of nursing theories for this generation and the next.

REFERENCES

Ailinger, R. L., & Dear, M. R. (1997). An examination of the self-care needs of clients with rheumatoid arthritis. *Rehabilitation Nursing, 22*(3), 13–14.

Aish, A. (1996). A comparison of female and male cardiac patients' responses to nursing care promoting nutritional self-care. *Canadian Journal of Cardiovascular Nursing, 7*(3), 4–13.

Aish, A. E., & Isenberg, M. (1996). Effects of Orem-based nursing intervention on nutritional self-care of myocardial infarction patients. *International Journal of Nursing Studies, 33*, 259–270.

Allan, J. D. (1990). Focusing on living, not dying: A naturalistic study of self-care among seropositive gay men. *Holistic Nursing Practice, 4*(2), 56–63.

Anastasio, D., McMahan, T., Daniels, A., Nicholas, P. K., & Paul-Simon, A. (1995). Self-care burden in women with Human Immunodeficiency Virus. *Journal of the Association of Nurses for AIDS Care, 6*(3), 31–42.

Anderson, J. A., & Olnhausen, K. S. (1999). Adolescent self-esteem: A foundational disposition. *Nursing Science Quarterly, 12*, 62–67.

Baker S. (1997). The relationships of self-care agency and self-care actions to caregiver strain as perceived by female family caregivers of elderly parents. *Journal of New York State Nurses Association, 28*(1), 7–11 .

Beach, E. K., Smith, A., Luthringer, L., Utz, S. K., Ahrens, S., & Whitmire, V. (1996). Self-care limitations of persons after acute myocardial infarction. *Applied Nursing Research, 9*(1), 24–28.

Brock, A. M., & O'Sullivan, P. (1985). A study to determine what variables predict institutionalization of the elderly. *Journal of Advanced Nursing, 10*, 533–537.

Carroll, D. (1995). The importance of self-efficacy expectations in elderly patients recovering from coronary artery bypass. *Heart & Lung, 24*(1), 50–59.

Chang, B. L., Cuman, G., Linn, L. S., Ware, J. E., & Kane, R. L. (1985). Adherence to health care regimens among elderly women. *Nursing Research, 34*, 27–31.

Chevannes, J. (1997). Nurses caring for families—Issues in a multiracial society. *Journal of Clinical Nursing, 6*(2), 161–167.

Clark, C. C. (1998). Wellness self-care by healthy older adults. *Image: Journal of Nursing Scholarship, 30*, 351–355.

Conner-Warren, R. (1996). Pain intensity and home pain management of children with sickle cell disease. *Issues in Comprehensive Pediatric Nursing, 19*, 183–195.

Dahlen, A. (1997). Health status of elderly—67 years and older in a community—and their need of nursing care. A survey. *Vard I Norden. Nursing Science and Research in the Nordic Countries, 17*(3), 36–42.

De Moutigny, F. (1995). Family nursing interventions during hospitalization. *Canadian Nurse, 91*(10), 38–42 .

Denyes, M. J. (1982). Measurement of self-care agency in adolescents (abstract). *Nursing Research, 31*, 63.

Denyes, M. J. (1988). Orem's model used for health promotion: Directions from research. *Advances in Nursing Science, 11*(1), 13–21.

Evers, G. C., Isenberg, M. A., Philipsen, H., Senten, M., & Brouns, G. (1989). *Validity testing of the Dutch translation of the appraisal of the self-care agency A.S.A. scale.* Assen, the Netherlands: Van Gorcum.

Fawdry, M. K., Berry, M. L., & Rajacich, D. (1996). The articulation of nursing systems with dependent care systems of intergenerational caregivers. *Nursing Science Quarterly, 9*, 22–26.

Fitzgerald, S. (1980). Utilizing Orem's Self-Care Model in designing an educational program for the diabetic. *Topics in Clinical Nursing, 2*, 57–65.

Foote, A., Holcombe, J., Piazza, D., & Wright, P. (1993). Orem's theory used as a guide for the nursing care of an eight-year-old child with leukemia. *Journal of Pediatric Oncology Nursing, 10*(1), 26–32.

Freston, M., Young, S., Calhoun, S., Fredericksen, T., Salinger, L., Malchodi, C., & Egan, J. (1997). Responses of pregnant women to potential preterm labor symptoms. *Journal of Obstetric, Gynecologic, and Neonatal Nursing, 26*(1), 35–41.

Frey, M. A., & Denyes, M. J. (1989). Health and illness self-care in adolescents with IDDM: A test of Orem's theory. *Advances in Nursing Science, 12*(1), 67–75.

Fujita, L. Y., & Dungan, J. (1994). High risk for ineffective management of therapeutic regimen: A protocol study. *Rehabilitation Nursing, 19*, 75–79, 126.

Gaffney, K. F., & Moore, J. B. (1996). Testing Orem's theory of self-care deficit: Dependent care agent performance for children. *Nursing Science Quarterly, 9*, 160–164.

Gast, H. L., Denyes, M. J., Campbell, J. C., Hartweg, D. L., Schott-Baer, D., & Isenberg, M. (1989). Self-care agency: Conceptualizations and operationalizations. *Advances in Nursing Science, 12*(1), 26–38.

Geden, E., & Taylor, S. G. (1991). Construct and empirical validity of the self-as-carer inventory. *Nursing Research, 40*, 47–50.

Geden, E. A., & Taylor, S. G. (1999). Theoretical and empirical description of adult couples' collaborative self-care systems. *Nursing Science Quarterly, 12*, 329–334.

Gulick, E. E. (1987). Parsimony and model confirmation of the ADL Self-Care Scale for Multiple Sclerosis persons. *Nursing Research, 36*, 278–283.

Hagopian, G. A. (1996). The effects of informational audiotapes on knowledge and self-care behaviors of patients undergoing radiation therapy. *Oncology Nursing Forum, 23*, 697–700.

Hanucharurnkl, S. (1989). Predictors of self-care in cancer patients receiving radiotherapy. *Cancer Nursing, 12*(1), 21–27.

Harper, D. C. (1984). Application of Orem's theoretical constructs to self-care medication behaviors in the elderly. *Advances in Nursing Science, 6*(3), 29–46.

Hart, J. A., & Foster, S. N. (1998). Self-care agency in two groups of pregnant women. *Nursing Science Quarterly, 11*, 167–171.

Hartweg, D. L., & Berbiglia, V. A. (1996). Determining the adequacy of a health promotion self-care interview guide with healthy, middle-aged, Mexican-American women: A pilot study. *Health Care for Women International, 17*(1), 57–68.

Jaarsma, T., Halfens, R., Senten, M., AbuSaad, H. H., & Dracup, K. (1998). Developing a supportive-educative program for patients with advanced heart failure within Orem's General Theory of Nursing. *Nursing Science Quarterly, 11*, 79–85.

Jewell, J. A., & Sullivan, E. A. (1996). Application of nursing theories in health education. *Journal of the American Psychiatric Nurses Association, 2*(3), 79–85.

Jirovec, M., & Kasno, J. (1990). Self-care agency as a function of patient-environmental factors among nursing home residents. *Research in Nursing and Health, 13*, 303–309.

Jirovec, M. M., & Kasno, J. (1993). Predictors of self-care abilities among the institutionalized elderly. *Western Journal of Nursing Research, 15*, 314–326.

Kearney, B., & Fleischer, B. (1979). Development of an instrument to measure self-care agency. *Research in Nursing and Health, 2*, 25–34.

Keohane, N. S., & Lacey, L. A. (1991). Preparing the woman with gestational diabetes for self-care. *Journal of Obstetrics Gynecologic and Neonatal Nursing, 20*, 189–193.

Knust, S. J., & Quarn, J. M. (1983). Integration of self-care theory with rehabilitation nursing. *Rehabilitation Nursing*, 26–28.

Kubricht, D. W. (1984). Therapeutic self-care demands expressed by outpatients receiving external radiation therapy. *Cancer Nursing 7*, 43–52.

Laurie-Shaw, B., & Ives, S. M. (1988a). Implementing Orem's self-care deficit theory . . . Part I. *Canadian Journal of Nursing Administration, (1)*1, 9–12.

Laurie-Shaw, B., & Ives, S. M. (1988b). Implementing Orem's self-care deficit theory . . . Part 2. *Canadian Journal of Nursing Administration, (1)*2, 16–19.

Lawrence, D., & Schank, M. (1995). Health care diaries of young women. *Journal of Community Health Nursing, 12*(3), 171–182.

Lee, M. B. (1999). Power, self-care and health in women living in urban squatter settlements in Karachi, Pakistan: A test of Orem's theory. *Journal of Advanced Nursing. 30* (1), 248–259.

Logue, G. A. (1997). An application of Orem's Theory to the nursing management of pertussis. *Journal of School Nursing. 13*(4), 20–25.

Mack, C. J. (1992). Assessment of the autologous bone marrow transplant patient according to Orem's self-care model. *Cancer Nursing, 15*, 429–436.

Mapanga, K., & Andrews, C. (1995). The influence of family and friends' basic conditioning factors and self-care agency on unmarried teenage primiparas' engagement in contraceptive practice. *Journal of Community Health Nursing, 12*(2), 89–100.

Marz, M. S. (1988). Effect of differentiated practice, conditioning factors and nursing agency on performance and strain of nurses in hospital settings. *Dissertation Abtracts International, 50–05B*, 1856.

McDermott, M. A. N. (1993). Learned helplessness as an interacting variable with self-care agency: Testing a theoretical model. *Nursing Science Quarterly, 6*, 28–38.

Moore, J. B. (1993). Predictors of children's self-care performance: Testing the theory of self-care deficit. *Scholarly Inquiry for Nursing Practice: An International Journal, 7*, 199–212.

Moore, J. B., & Gaffney, K. F. (1989). Development of an instrument to measure mother's performance of self-care activities for children. *Advances in Nursing Science, 12*(1), 76–84.

Moore, J. B., & Mosher, R. (1997). Adjustment responses of children and their mothers to cancer: Self-care and anxiety. *Oncology Nursing Forum, 24*(3), 519–525.

Norris, M. K. G. (1991). Applying Orem's theory to the long-term care of adolescent transplant recipients. *American Nephrology Nurses Association Journal, 18*(1), 45–47, 53.

Nursing Development Conference Group. (1973). *Concept formalization in nursing: Process and product.* Boston: Little, Brown.

Nursing Development Conference Group. (1979). *Concept formalization in nursing: Process and product* (2nd ed.). Boston: Little, Brown.

Orem, D. E. (1959). *Guides for developing curricula for the education of practical nurses.* Washington, DC: Government Printing Office.

Orem, D. E. (1971). *Nursing: Concepts of practice.* New York: McGraw-Hill. (out of print)

Orem, D. E. (1980). *Nursing: Concepts of practice* (2nd ed.). New York: McGraw-Hill. (out of print)

Orem, D. E. (1985). *Nursing: Concepts of practice* (3rd ed.). New York: McGraw-Hill. (out of print)

Orem, D. E. (1991). *Nursing: Concepts of practice* (4th ed.). St. Louis: Mosby.

Orem, D. E. (1995). *Nursing: Concepts of practice* (5th ed.). St. Louis: Mosby.

Orem, D. E. (1997). Views of human beings specific to nursing. *Nursing Science Quarterly, 10,* 26–31.

Orem, D. E. (2001). *Nursing: Concepts of Practice* (6th ed.). St. Louis: Mosby.

Orem, D. E., & Taylor, S. G. (1986). Orem's General Theory of Nursing. In P. Winstead-Fry (Ed.), *Case studies in nursing theory* (pp. 37–71) (Pub. No. 15-2152). New York: National League for Nursing.

Orem, D. E., & Vardiman, E.M. (1995). Orem's nursing theory and positive mental health: Practical considerations. *Nursing Science Quarterly, 8,* 165–173.

Reed, P. G. (1986). Developmental resources and depression in the elderly. *Nursing Research, 35,* 368–374.

Roberson, M. R., & Kelley, J. H. (1996). Using Orem's theory in transcultural settings: A critique. *Nursing Forum, 31*(3), 22–28.

Roy, O., & Collin, F. (1994). The aged patient with dementia. *Canadian Nurse, 90*(1), 39–42.

Schott-Baer, D., Fisher, L., & Gregory, C.(1995). Dependent care, caregiver burden, hardiness, and self-care agency of caregivers. *Cancer Nursing, 18,* 299–305.

Smith, C. (1996) Care of the older hypothermic patient using a self-care model. *Nursing Times, 92*(3), 29–31.

Soderhamm, O., Evers, G., & Hamrin, E. (1996). A Swedish version of the Appraisal of Self-Care Agency (ASA) Scale. *Scandinavian Journal Caring Science, 10*(1), 3–9.

Spirig, R., & Willhelm, A. B. (1995). Bibliography on the subject of Dorothea Orem's nursing theory [German]. *Pflege, 9,* 213–220.

Taylor, S. G., Geden, E., Isaramalai, S., & Wongvatunyu, S. (2000). Orem's Self-Care Deficit Nursing Theory: Its philosophic foundation and the state of the science. *Nursing Science Quarterly, 13,* 104–110.

Taylor, S. G., & McLaughlin, K. (1991). Orem's General Theory of Nursing and community nursing. *Nursing Science Quarterly, 4,* 153–160.

Tolentino, M. B. (1990). The use of Orem's self-care model in the neonatal intensive-care unit. *Journal of Obstetric, Gynelogic, and Neonatal Nursing, 19,* 496–500.

Trench, A. S. (Executive producer), Wallace, D. (Producer), & Coberg, T. (Director). (1988). *Dorothea E. Orem—The nurse theorists: Portraits of excellence.* Oakland, CA: Studio Three Production, Samuel Merritt College of Nursing.

Ulbrich, S. L. (1999). Nursing practice theory of exercise as self-care. *Image—The Journal of Nursing Scholarship. 31*(1), 65–70.

Utz, S. W., Shuster, G. F., Merwin, E., & Williams, B. (1994). A community based smoking-cessation program: Self-care behaviors and success. *Public Health Nursing, 11*, 291–299.

Vesely, C. (1995). Pediatric patient-controlled analgesia: Enhancing the self-care construct. *Pediatric Nursing, 21*(2), 124–128.

Villarruel, A. M., & Denyes, M. J. (1991). Pain assessment in children: Theoretical and empirical validity. *Advances in Nursing Science, 14*, 32–41.

Villarruel, A. M., & Denyes, N. J. (1997). Testing Orem's theory with Mexican Americans. *Image—The Journal of Nursing Scholarship, 29*, 283–288.

Wang, C. Y. (1997). The cross cultural applicability of Orem's conceptual framework. *Journal of Cultural Diversity. 4*(2), 44–48.

Zadinsky, J., & Boyle, J. (1996). Experiences of women with chronic pelvic pain. *Healthcare of Women International, 17*, 223–232.

Ziegler, S. M., Vaughn-Wrobel, B. C., & Erlen, J. A. (1986). *Nursing process, nursing diagnosis, nursing knowledge—Avenues to autonomy.* Norwalk, CT: Appleton-Century-Crofts.

Zinn, A. (1986). A self-care program for hemodialysis patients based on Dorothea Orem's concepts. *Journal of Nephrology Nursing, 3*, 65–77.

ANNOTATED BIBLIOGRAPHY

Aish, A. (1996). A comparison of female and male cardiac patients' responses to nursing care promoting nutritional self-care. *Canadian Journal of Cardiovascular Nursing, 7*(3), 4–13.
This study investigated gender-based response to an Orem-based nursing care plan that focused on nutrition. The care was provided to 62 men and 42 women who had suffered myocardial infarctions in the patients' homes within a week of discharge from the hospital. A three-day diet record was obtained seven weeks after discharge. Both men and women in the treatment group had changed their dietary habits by lowering the intake of both total and saturated fat.

Aish, A. E., & Isenberg, M. (1996). Effects of Orem-based nursing intervention on nutritional self-care of myocardial infarction patients. *International Journal of Nursing Studies, 33*, 259–270.
This study investigated the effect of an Orem-based nursing care measure on the nutrition of patients who had experienced myocardial infarction. The major variables of interest were the impact of self-care agency and self-efficacy on healthy eating. The treatment took place during the first six weeks after discharge for 104 patients who were randomly assigned to treatment and control groups. Findings supported that the nursing care influenced self-care agency but did not have an impact on self-efficacy in healthy eating.

Anderson, J. A., & Olnhausen, K. S. (1999). Adolescent self-esteem: A foundational disposition. *Nursing Science Quarterly, 12*, 62–67.
After conducting a concept synthesis and concept derivation, the authors argue that self-esteem is a foundational disposition within the self-care deficit theory. As such, self-esteem is also a component of self-care agency.

Baker, S. (1997). The relationships of self-care agency and self-care actions to caregiver strain as perceived by female family caregivers of elderly parents. *Journal of the New York State Nurses Association, 28*(1), 7–11.
This descriptive correlational study investigated caregiver strain in 131 primary caregivers. Findings included an inverse relationship between self-care agency and caregiver strain; mediation effects of self-care actions on the relationships between household tasks, emotional support, and caregiver strain; that multiple roles increased caregiver strain and that personal-care tasks had a moderator effect on self-care actions that decreased caregiver strain. The author suggests that nurses need to educate caregivers of the importance of self-care.

Dennis, C. M. (1997). *Self-care deficit theory of nursing: Concepts and applications.* St. Louis: Mosby.

This text provides a basic introduction to Orem's theory, based on work done by faculty at Illinois Wesleyan University. It seeks to define the concepts and terminology associated with the theory in ways that are useful to beginning students of nursing and aid them in the practical application of the theory.

Taylor, S. G., Geden, E., Isaramalai, S., Wongvatunyu, S. (2000). Orem's Self-Care Deficit Nursing Theory: Its philosophic foundation and the state of the science. *Nursing Science Quarterly, 13,* 104–110.

Reviews the published research relating to Orem's theory, using the five stages of theory development identified by Orem. Most of the studies reviewed were descriptive research and served to increase the knowledge base about self-care but provided little indication of sustained research programs based on the theory. The authors conclude that "the bricks are piling up around the framework, but only a few scholars are working on building the walls" (p. 108).

CHAPTER 8

BEHAVIORAL SYSTEM MODEL DOROTHY E. JOHNSON

Marie L. Lobo

Dorothy Johnson was born in Savannah, Georgia, in 1919, the last of seven children. Her Bachelor of Science in Nursing was from Vanderbilt University, Nashville, Tennessee, and her Masters in Public Health from Harvard. She began publishing her ideas about nursing soon after graduation from Vanderbilt. Most of her teaching career was in pediatric nursing at the University of California, Los Angeles. She retired as Professor Emeritus, January 1, 1978, and currently lives in Florida.

Dorothy Johnson has influenced nursing through her publications since the 1950s. Throughout her career, Johnson has stressed the importance of research-based knowledge about the effect of nursing care on clients. Johnson was an early proponent of nursing as a science as well as an art. She also believed nursing had a body of knowledge reflecting both the science and the art. From the beginning, Johnson (1959) proposed that the knowledge of the science of nursing necessary for effective nursing care included a synthesis of key concepts drawn from basic and applied sciences.

In 1961, Johnson proposed that nursing care facilitated the client's maintenance of a state of equilibrium. Johnson proposed that clients were "stressed" by a stimulus of either an internal or external nature. These stressful stimuli created such disturbances, or "tensions," in the patient that a state of disequilibrium occurred. Johnson identified two areas of foci for nursing care that are based on returning the client to a state of equilibrium. First, nursing care should reduce stimuli that are stressors, and second, "nursing care should provide support of the client's 'natural' defenses and adaptive processes" (p. 66).

In 1992, Johnson articulated that much of her thinking was influenced by Florence Nightingale. Johnson related that she was first exposed to Nightingale in the mid-1940s. While reading Nightingale's (1859/1992) *Notes on nursing* she found that Nightingale focused on the "fundamental needs" of people rather than on the disease process. She also noted that Nightingale focused on the relationship of the person to the environment rather than the disease to the person. In the 1950s and 1960s, as Johnson developed her model, an increasing number of observational studies on child and adult behavior patterns were published. During these same years, general system theory was also discussed frequently. All these experiences influenced Johnson (1992) in the development of her Behavioral Systems Model.

In 1968, Johnson first proposed her model of nursing care as the fostering of "the efficient and effective behavioral functioning in the patient to prevent illness" (Johnson, 1968, April, p. 2). The patient is identified as a behavioral system with multiple subsystems. At this point Johnson began to integrate concepts related to systems models into her work. Johnson's (1968) integration of systems concepts into her work was further illustrated by her statement of belief that nursing was "concerned with man as an integrated whole and this is the specific knowledge of order we require" (p. 207). Not only did nurses need to care for the "whole" client, but the generation of nursing knowledge needed to take a course in the direction of concern with the entire needs of the client.

In the mid- to late-1970s, several nurses published conceptualizations of nursing based on Johnson's behavioral systems model. Some of these were revised in the 1980s. Auger (1976), Damus (1980), Grubbs (1980), Holaday (1980), and Skolny and Riehl (1974) are authors who have interpreted Johnson. Roy (1989), Wu (1973), and others were sharing their beliefs about nursing at the same time, and Johnson's influence, as their professor, is clearly reflected in their works. In 1980, Johnson published her conceptualization of the Behavioral System Model for Nursing. This is the first work published by Johnson that explicates her definitions of the Behavioral System Model. The evolution of this complex model is clearly demonstrated in the progression of Johnson's ideas from works published in the 1950s to her latest available work published in 1990.

DEFINITION OF NURSING

Johnson (1980) developed her Behavioral System Model for nursing from a philosophical perspective "supported by a rich, sound, and rapidly expanding body of empirical and theoretical knowledge" (p. 207). From her early beliefs, which focused on the impaired individual, Johnson evolved a much broader definition of nursing. By 1980, she defined nursing as "an external regulatory force which acts to preserve the organization and integration of the patient's behavior at an optimal level under those conditions in which the behavior constitutes a threat to physical or social health, or in which illness is found" (p. 214). Based on this definition, the following four goals of nursing are to assist the patient to become a person:

1. Whose behavior is commensurate with social demands
2. Who is able to modify his behavior in ways that support biologic imperatives
3. Who is able to benefit to the fullest extent during illness from the physician's knowledge and skill
4. Whose behavior does not give evidence of unnecessary trauma as a consequence of illness (p. 207).

ASSUMPTIONS OF THE BEHAVIORAL SYSTEM MODEL

Johnson makes several layers of assumptions in the development of her conceptualization of the Behavioral System Model. Assumptions are made about the system as a whole as well as about the subsystems. Another set of assumptions deals with the knowledge base necessary to practice nursing.

As with Rogers (1970) and Roy (1989), Johnson believes that nurses need to be well grounded in the physical and social sciences. Particular emphasis should be placed on knowledge from both the physical and social sciences that is found to influence behavior. Thus, Johnson believes it would be of equal importance to have information available about endocrine influences on behavior as well as about psychological influences on behavior.

In developing assumptions about behavioral systems, Johnson was influenced by Buckley, Chin, and Rapport, early leaders in the development of systems concepts. Johnson (1980) cites Chin (1961) as the source for her first assumption about systems. In constructing a behavioral system, the assumption is made that there is "'organization, interaction, interdependency, and integration of the parts and elements' (Chin, 1961) of behavior that go to make up the system" (p. 208). It is the interrelated parts that contribute to the development of the whole.

The second assumption about systems also evolves from the work of Chin. A system "'tends to achieve a balance among the various forces operating within and upon it' (1961), and that man strives continually to maintain a behavioral system balance and steady states by more or less automatic adjustments and adaptations to the 'natural' forces impinging upon him" (Johnson, 1980, p. 208). The individual is continually presented with situations in everyday life that require adaptation and adjustment. These adjustments are so natural that they occur without conscious effort by the individual. Johnson says:

> The third assumption about a behavioral system is that a behavioral system, which both requires and results in some degree of regularity and constancy in behavior, is essential to man; that is to say, it is functionally significant in that it serves a useful purpose both in social life and for the individual. (p. 208)

The patterns of behavior characteristic of the individual have a purpose in the maintenance of homeostasis by the individual. The development of behavioral patterns that are acceptable to both society and the individual foster the individual's ability to adapt to minor changes in the environment.

The final assumption about the behavioral system is that the "system balance reflects adjustments and adaptations that are successful in some way and to some degree" (Johnson, 1980, p. 208). Johnson acknowledges that the achievement of this balance may and will vary from individual to individual. At times this balance may *not* be exhibited as behaviors that are acceptable or meet society's norms. What may be adaptive for the individual in coping with impinging forces may be disruptive to society as a whole. Most individuals are flexible enough, however, to be in some state of balance that is "functionally efficient and effective" for them (p. 209).

The integration of these assumptions by the individual provides the behavioral system with the patterns of action to form "an organized and integrated functional unit that determines and limits the interaction between the person and his environment and establishes the relationship of the person to the objects, events, and situations in his environment" (Johnson, 1980, p. 209). The function of the behavioral system, then, is to regulate the individual's response to input from the environment so that the balance of the system can be maintained.

Four assumptions are made about the structure and function of each subsystem. These four assumptions are the "structural elements" common to each of the seven subsystems. The first assumption is "from the form the behavior takes and the consequences it achieves can be inferred what *drive* has been stimulated or what *goal* is being sought" (Johnson, 1980, p. 210). The ultimate goal for each subsystem is expected to be the same for all individuals. However, the methods of achieving the goal may vary depending on culture or other individual variations.

The second assumption is that each individual has a "predisposition to act, with reference to the goal, in certain ways rather than in other ways" (Johnson, 1980, pp. 210–11). This predisposition to act is labeled "set" by Johnson. The concept of "set" implies that despite having only a few alternatives from which to select a behavioral response, the individual will rank those options and choose the option considered most desirable.

The third assumption is that each subsystem has available a repertoire of choices or "scope of action" alternatives from which choices can be made. Johnson (1980) subsumes under this assumption that larger behavioral repertoires are available to more adaptable individuals. As life experiences occur, individuals add to the number of alternative actions available to them. At some point, however, the acquisition of new alternatives of behavior decreases as the individual becomes comfortable with the available repertoire. The point at which the individual loses the desire or ability to acquire new options is not identified by Johnson.

The fourth assumption about the behavioral subsystems is that they produce observable outcomes—that is, the individual's behavior (Johnson, 1980). The observable behaviors allow an outsider—in this case the nurse—to note the actions the individual is taking to reach a goal related to a specified subsystem. The nurse can then evaluate the effectiveness and efficiency of these behaviors in assisting the individual in reaching one of these goals.

In addition, each of the subsystems has three functional requirements. First, each subsystem must be "*protected* from noxious influences with which the system cannot cope" (Johnson, 1980, p. 212). Second, each subsystem must be "*nurtured* through the input of appropriate supplies from the environment" (p. 212). Finally, each subsystem must be "*stimulated* for use to enhance growth and prevent stagnation" (p. 212). As long as the subsystems are meeting these functional requirements, the system and the subsystems are viewed as self-maintaining and self-perpetuating. The internal and external environments of the system need to remain orderly and predictable for the system to maintain homeostasis or remain in balance. The interrelationships of the structural elements of the subsystem are critical for each subsystem to function at a maximum state. The interaction of the structural elements allows the subsystem to maintain a balance that is adaptive to that individual's needs.

An imbalance in a behavioral subsystem produces tension, which results in disequilibrium. The presence of tension resulting in an unbalanced behavioral system requires the system to increase energy use to return the system to a state of balance (Johnson, 1968, April). Nursing is viewed as a part of the external environment that can assist the client to return to a state of equilibrium or balance.

Johnson's Behavioral System Model

Johnson (1980) believes each individual has patterned, purposeful, repetitive ways of acting that comprise a behavioral system specific to that individual. These actions or behaviors form an "organized and integrated functional unit that determines and limits the interaction between the person and his environment and establishes the relationship of the person to the objects, events, and situations in his environment" (p. 209). These behaviors are "orderly, purposeful and predictable . . . [and] sufficiently stable and recurrent to be amenable to description and explanation" (p. 209). Johnson identifies seven subsystems within the Behavioral System Model, an identification that is at variance with others who have published interpretations of Johnson's model. Johnson (1980) states that the seven subsystems identified in her 1980 publication are the only ones to which she subscribes, and she recognizes they are at variance with Grubbs. These seven subsystems were originally identified in Johnson's 1968 paper presented at Vanderbilt University. The seven subsystems are considered to be interrelated, and changes in one subsystem affect all the subsystems.

Johnson has never produced a schematic representation of her system. Conner, Harbour, Magers and Watt (1994); Loveland-Cherry and Wilkerson (1989); and Torres (1986) have produced similar schematic representations of Johnson's model (see Fig. 8–1).

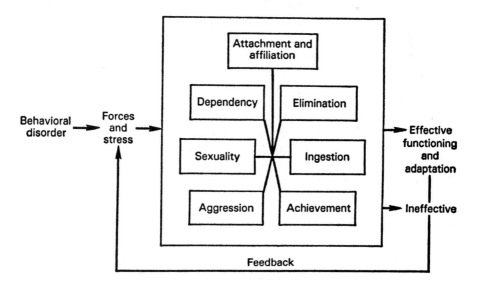

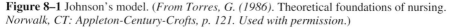

Figure 8–1 Johnson's model. (*From Torres, G. (1986). Theoretical foundations of nursing. Norwalk, CT: Appleton-Century-Crofts, p. 121. Used with permission.*)

Johnson's Seven Behavioral Subsystems

The *attachment* or *affiliative* subsystem is identified as the first response system to develop in the individual. The optimal functioning of the affiliative subsystem allows "social inclusion, intimacy, and the formation and maintenance of a strong social bond" (Johnson, 1980, p. 212). Attachment to a significant caregiver has been found to be critical for the survival of an infant. As the individual matures, the attachment to the caretaker continues and there are additional attachments to other significant individuals as they enter both the child's and the adult's network. These "significant others" provide the individual with a sense of security.

The second subsystem identified by Johnson is the *dependency* subsystem. Johnson (1980) distinguishes the dependency subsystem from the attachment or affiliative subsystem. Dependency behaviors are "succoring" behaviors that precipitate nurturing behaviors from other individuals in the environment. The result of dependency behavior is "approval, attention or recognition, and physical assistance" (p. 213). It is difficult to separate the dependency subsystem from the affiliative or attachment subsystem because without someone invested in or attached to the individual to respond to that individual's dependency behaviors, the dependency subsystem has no animate environment in which to function.

The *ingestive* subsystem relates to the behaviors surrounding the intake of food. It is related to the biological system. However, the emphasis for nursing, from Johnson's (1980) perspective, is the meanings and structures of the social events surrounding the occasions when food is eaten. Behaviors related to the ingestion of food may relate more to what is socially acceptable in a given culture than to the biological needs of the individual.

The *eliminative* subsystem relates to behaviors surrounding the excretion of waste products from the body. Johnson (1980) admits this may be difficult to separate from a biological system perspective. However, as with behaviors surrounding the ingestion of food, there are socially acceptable behaviors for the time and place for humans to excrete waste. Human cultures have defined different socially acceptable behaviors for excretion of waste, but the existence of such a pattern remains from culture to culture. Individuals who have gained physical control over the eliminative subsystem control those subsystems rather than behave in a socially unacceptable manner. For example, biological cues are often ignored if the social situation dictates that it is objectionable to eliminate wastes at a given time.

The *sexual* subsystem reflects behaviors related to procreation (Johnson, 1980). Both biological and social factors affect behaviors in the sexual subsystem. Again, the behaviors are related to culture and vary from culture to culture. Behaviors also vary according to the gender of the individual. The key is that the goal in all societies has the same outcome—behaviors acceptable to society at large.

The *aggressive* subsystem relates to behaviors concerned with protection and self-preservation. Johnson (1980) views the aggressive subsystem as one that generates defensive responses from the individual when life or territory is threatened. The aggressive subsystem does not include those behaviors with a primary purpose of injuring other individuals, but rather those whose purpose is to protect and preserve self and society.

Finally, the *achievement* subsystem provokes behaviors that attempt to control the environment. Intellectual, physical, creative, mechanical, and social skills are some of the areas that Johnson (1980) recognizes. Other areas of personal accomplishment or success may also be included in this subsystem.

JOHNSON'S BEHAVIORAL SYSTEM MODEL AND NURSING'S METAPARADIGM

Johnson views *human beings* as having two major systems: the biological system and the behavioral system. It is the role of medicine to focus on the biological system, whereas nursing's focus is the behavioral system. There is recognition of the reciprocal actions that occur between the biological and behavioral systems when some type of dysfunction occurs in one or the other of the systems.

Society relates to the environment in which an individual exists. According to Johnson, an individual's behavior is influenced by all the events in the environment. Cultural influences on the individual's behavior are viewed as profound. However, it is felt that there are many paths, varying from culture to culture, that influence specific behaviors in a group of people, although the outcome for all the groups or individuals is the same.

Health is an elusive state that is determined by psychological, social, biological, and physiological factors (Johnson, 1978). Johnson's behavioral model supports the idea that the individual is attempting to maintain some balance or equilibrium. The individual's goal is to maintain the entire behavioral system efficiently and effectively but with enough flexibility to return to an acceptable balance if a malfunction disrupts the original balance.

Nursing's primary goal is to foster equilibrium within the individual, which allows for the practice of nursing with individuals at any point in the health–illness continuum. Nursing implementations may focus on alterations of a behavior that is not supportive to maintaining equilibrium for the individual. In earlier works, Johnson focused nursing on impaired individuals. By 1980, she stated that nursing is concerned with the organized and integrated whole, but that the major focus is on maintaining a balance in the behavioral system when illness occurs in the individual.

JOHNSON'S BEHAVIORAL SYSTEM AND THE NURSING PROCESS

Johnson's Behavioral System Model easily fits the nursing process model. Grubbs (1980) developed an assessment tool based on Johnson's seven subsystems, plus a subsystem she labeled "restorative," which focused on activities of daily living. Activities of daily living are considered to include such areas as patterns of rest, hygiene, and recreation. A diagnosis can be made related to insufficiencies or discrepancies within a subsystem or between subsystems. Planning for the implementation of nursing care should start at the subsystem level with the ultimate outcome of effective behavioral functioning of the entire system. Implementations by the nurse present to the client an external force for the manipulation of the subsystem back to the state of equilibrium. Evaluation of the result of this implementation is readily possible if the state of balance that is the outcome has been defined during the planning phase before the implementation.

Assessment

In the assessment phase of the nursing process, questions related to specific subsystems are developed. Holaday (1980), Damus (1980), and Small (1980) propose that the assessment focus on the subsystem related to the presenting health problem. An assessment based on the behavioral subsystems does not easily permit the nurse to gather detailed information about the biological system. Assessment questions related to the affiliative subsystem might focus on the presence of a significant other or on the social system of which the individual is a member. In the assessment of the dependency subsystem, attention is placed on understanding how the individual makes needs known to significant others so that the significant others in the environment can assist the individual in meeting those needs. Assessment of the ingestive subsystem examines patterns of food and fluid intake, including the social environment in which the food and fluid are ingested. The eliminative subsystem generates questions related to patterns of defecation and urination and the social context in which the patterns occur. The sexual subsystem assessment includes information about sexual patterns and behaviors. The aggressive subsystem generates questions about how individuals protect themselves from perceived threats to safety. Finally, the achievement subsystem allows for assessment of how the individual changes the environment to facilitate the accomplishment of goals.

There are many gaps in information about the whole individual if only Johnson's Behavioral System Model is used to guide the assessment. There are few physiological data on the individual's present or past health status. The exception might be when an impaired health state is demonstrated in the ingestive or eliminative subsystems. Family interaction and patterns are touched on only in the affiliative and dependency subsystems. Basic information relating to education, socioeconomic status, and type of dwelling is tangentially related to most of the subsystems. However, these factors are not clearly identified as an important aspect of any of the subsystems.

Diagnosis

Diagnosis using Johnson's Behavioral System Model becomes cumbersome. Diagnosis tends to be general to a subsystem rather than specific to a problem. Grubbs (1980) has proposed four categories of nursing diagnoses derived from Johnson's Behavioral System Model, as follows:

> 1. *Insufficiency*—a state which exists when a particular subsystem is not functioning or developed to its fullest capacity due to inadequacy of functional requirements . . .

2. *Discrepancy*—a behavior that does not meet the intended goal. The incongruity usually lies between the action and the goal of the subsystem, although the set and choice may be strongly influencing the ineffective action . . .

3. *Incompatibility*—the goals or behaviors of two subsystems in the same situation conflict with each other to the detriment of the individual . . .

4. *Dominance*—the behavior in one subsystem is used more than any other subsystem regardless of the situation or to the detriment of the other subsystems (pp. 240–241).

Since Johnson has never written about the use of nursing diagnosis with her model, it is difficult to know whether these diagnostic classifications are Johnson's or if they are an extension of Johnson's work by Grubbs.

Outcomes, Planning, and Implementation

Planning for implementation of the nursing care related to the diagnosis may be difficult because of the lack of client input into the plan. The plan focuses on the nurse's action to modify client behavior. These plans, then, have a desired outcome: to bring about homeostasis in a subsystem that is based on the nurse's assessment of the individual's drive, set, behavioral repertoire, and observable behavior. The plan may include protection, nurturance, or stimulation of the identified subsystem.

Planning and implementation for clients that are based on Johnson's Behavioral System Model focus on maintaining or returning an individual's subsystem to a state of equilibrium. Implementation focuses on achieving the goals of nursing as identified by Johnson (1980). Although Johnson refers to the biological system in her goals of nursing, it is not included in her Behavioral System Model and can and does produce incongruities for the planning and implementation of nursing care in relation to a specific diagnosis.

Evaluation

Evaluation is based on the attainment of the desired outcome of balance in the identified subsystems. If baseline data are available for the individual, the nurse may have a goal for the individual to return to the baseline behavior. If the alterations in behavior that are planned do occur, the nurse should be able to observe the return to previous behavior patterns.

There is little or no recognition by either Johnson (1980) or Grubbs (1980) of the client's input into plans for nursing implementation. They use the term *nursing intervention*. Holaday's (1980) example of implementation also does not contain strong client input. Using Johnson's Behavioral System Model with the nursing process is a nurse-centered activity, with the nurse determining the client's needs and the state of behavior appropriate to those needs.

Holaday (1980) demonstrates the flexibility available in the use of the Johnson Behavioral System Model with the nursing process by using a very specific assessment tool to determine appropriate interventions. Holaday uses tests of cognitive development developed by Piaget to determine the level of information to present to a child during a preoperative teaching session.

Situation. An example of the use of the nursing process with Johnson's Behavioral System Model is demonstrated with Johnny Smith, age 6 weeks, brought into the clinic for a routine checkup. He presents with no weight gain since his checkup at age 2 weeks. His mother states that she feeds him but that he does not seem to eat much. He sleeps 4 to 5 hours between feedings. His mother holds him in her arms without making trunk-to-trunk contact. As the assessment is made, the nurse notes that Mrs. Smith never looks at Johnny and never speaks to him. She states that he was a planned baby but that she never "realized how much work an infant could be." She says her mother has told her she is not a good mother because Johnny is not gaining weight as he should. She states that she has not called the nurse when she knew Johnny was not gaining weight because she thought the nurse would think she is a "bad mother" just as her own mother thinks she is a "bad mother."

Based on the information available and using the Johnson Behavioral System Model, assessment focuses on the affiliative and dependency subsystems between mother and Johnny. Further assessment of Mrs. Smith's relationship with her own mother needs to be done. The critical need is for Johnny to begin gaining weight. The secondary need is for Mrs. Smith to resolve her conflict with her own mother. The assessment of the affiliative subsystem focuses on the specific behaviors manifested by Johnny to indicate attachment to his mother. The assessment of the dependency subsystem focuses on the specific behaviors manifested by Johnny to cue his mother to his needs. Because of the nature of his problem, a decision is made to use a tool that specifically focuses on parent–infant interaction during a feeding situation. Thus, the Nursing Child Assessment Feeding Scale (NCAFS) (Barnard, 1978) is used during a feeding that takes place at a normal feeding time for Johnny. Johnny cries at the beginning of the feeding and turns toward his mother's hand when she touches his cheek. Mrs. Smith does not speak to Johnny or in any verbal way acknowledge his hunger. When Johnny slightly chokes on some formula, she does not remove the bottle from his mouth. Mrs. Smith does not describe any of the environment to Johnny, nor does she stroke his body or make eye contact with him. Johnny does not reach out to touch his mother nor does he make any vocalizations. The assessment scale indicates that both mother and baby are not cueing each other at a level at which they can respond appropriately.

The diagnoses based on this assessment, using Johnson's Behavioral System Model, are, "insufficient development of the affiliative subsystem" and "insufficient development of the dependency subsystem." Based on these diagnoses, the desired outcomes are adequate development of the affiliative and dependency subsystems for Johnny. Goals include adequate weight gain and higher scores on the NCAFS. Nursing implementation focuses on increasing Mrs. Smith's awareness of the meaning of Johnny's infrequent cues. By increasing her awareness of the meaning of his cues, she can begin to reinforce them so that he begins to know there is someone in the environment who cares about him, thus fostering his attachment to her. Further assistance needs to be given in helping Mrs. Smith in communicating with her infant. If further assessment indicates Mrs. Smith is uncomfortable talking with an infant who does not respond with words, it may be suggested that she read to Johnny from a book, thus providing him with needed verbal stimulation. Another implementation may include the nurse placing herself in Johnny's role and "talking" for him to his mother. The nurse may sit, watching Mrs. Smith hold Johnny, and say such things as "I like it when you pat me," "It feels good when you cuddle me," "When I turn my head like this, I'm hungry."

Evaluation of these implementations are based on two criteria. First, Johnny's weight gains or losses are carefully assessed. Not gaining weight places him in a life-threatening situation; therefore, it is critical that a pattern of weight gain be initiated. Second, the mother–infant interaction can be reassessed, again using the Nursing Child Assessment Feeding Scale (Barnard, 1978), which allows for comparison of the first observation with a series of subsequent observations.

CRITIQUE OF JOHNSON'S BEHAVIORAL SYSTEM MODEL

Johnson states that she is presenting a model related to subsystems of the human being that have observable behaviors leading to specific outcomes, although the method of attaining the specific outcomes may vary according to the culture of the individual. Using the critique of a theory discussed in Chapter 1 as a guide, it is clear that Johnson has indeed developed a model. Johnson's Behavioral System Model is based on general system concepts. However, the definitions related to the terms used to label her concepts have not been made explicit by Johnson. Grubbs (1980) has presented her definitions of Johnson's terms, and those are the definitions most often reflected in the literature of other investigators claiming to use Johnson's model.

1. What is the historical context of the theory? Johnson developed her model in the 1950s while teaching at the University of California, Los Angeles (UCLA). At that time increasing numbers of observational studies on child and adult behavior patterns were being published and general system theory was generating much discussion. All of these experiences influenced Johnson in the development of her Behavioral Systems Model. In the 1960s and 1970s Johnson taught many of the nursing leaders of today in her nursing theory classes at UCLA.

2. What are the basic concepts and relationships presented by the theory? The basic concepts are the seven behavioral subsystems of affiliative, dependency, ingestive, eliminative, sexual, aggressive, and achievement; the four structural characteristics of drive, set, choices, and observable behaviors; and the three functional requirements of protection, nurturance, and stimulation as well as tensions and balance. Johnson does not clearly interrelate these concepts of the Behavioral System Model. The lack of clear interrelationships among the concepts creates difficulty in following the logic of Johnson's work. The definitions of the concepts are so abstract that they are difficult to use. For example, intimacy is identified as an aspect of the affiliative subsystem, but the concept is not defined or described. An advantage of the abstract definition is that individuals using the model may identify an assessment tool that most specifically fits a problem and use it in their work. There are two major disadvantages. First, the abstract level and multiplicity of definitions make it difficult to compare the same subsystem across studies. Second, the lack of clear definitions for the interrelationships among and between the subsystems makes it difficult to view the entire behavioral system as an entity.

3. What major phenomena of concern to nursing are presented? These phenomenon may include *but are not limited to*: human being, environment, health, interpersonal relations, caring, goal attainment, adaptation, and energy fields. The major phenomenon of concern to nursing in Johnson's work is behavior. Johnson's Behavioral System Model provides a framework for organizing human behavior. However, it is a different framework from that provided by other nursing theorists, such as Roy (1989) or Rogers (1970). Johnson believes that she is the first person to view "man as a behavioral system." Others have viewed the behavioral subsystem as just one piece of the biopsychosocial human being. Johnson's framework does contribute to the general body of nursing knowledge but needs further development.

4. To whom does this theory apply? In what situations? In what way? Johnson's behavioral model can be generalized across the lifespan and across cultures. However, the focus on the behavioral system may make it difficult for nurses working with physically impaired individuals to use the model. Johnson's model is also very individual oriented, so that nurses working with groups of individuals with similar problems would have difficulty using the model. The subsystems in Johnson's Behavioral System Model are individual oriented to such an extent that the family can be considered only as the environment in which the individual presents behaviors and not as the focus of care. The model has been used to guide psychiatric nursing practice (Dee, 1990; Poster, Dee, & Randell, 1997). Derdiarian and Schobel (1990) used the model as a strategy to measure, describe, and classify major changes related to a diagnosis of acquired immune deficiency syndrome. Herbert (1989) used the model to guide the nursing care of a 75-year-old stroke patient. However, rigorous research to validate the premises or the findings presented in these publications has not been done.

5. By what method or methods can this theory be tested? It is difficult to test Johnson's model by the development of hypotheses. Subsystems of the model can be examined because relationships within the subsystems can be identified. The lack of definitions and connections between the subsystems creates a barrier for stating relationships in the form of hypotheses to be tested. Although such relationships may be predicted, the lack of definitions in the original work makes it impossible to identify whether it is Johnson's work or someone's interpretation of her work that is being tested.

6. Does this theory direct critical thinking in nursing practice? Decision making for nursing practice using the Johnson model would involve critical thinking. As noted above, a few individuals have written about the use of Johnson's model for nursing practice. Dee (1990) reported on the practical issues that arose in the course of implementing the Johnson Behavioral Model at a psychiatric institution. They revised the definitions of the subsystems and included a restorative subsystem. Others have used Johnson's model to assist in the understanding of the family member's adjustment to Alzheimer's disease (Freuhwirth, 1989). Riegel (1989) used the model to guide the review of literature related to social support of individuals with coronary heart disease, although she did not test her model. While these authors used the model to guide their thinking about particular practiced issues, they did not test the model. It is unclear whether others have used the information they have shared to further develop their practice.

7. Does this theory direct therapeutic nursing interventions? Johnson does not clearly define the expected outcomes when one of the subsystems is being affected by nursing implementation. An implicit expectation is made that all humans in all cultures will attain the same outcome—homeostasis. Because of the lack of definitions, the model does not allow for control of the areas of interest, so it is difficult to use the model to guide practice. The authors reportedly using the model to guide practice have not integrated the subsystems to the degree necessary to label this model a theory. In fact, Reynolds and Cormack (1991) reported that there was an inability to prescribe specific nursing interventions using this model.

8. Does this theory direct communication in nursing practice? While Johnson's model does not directly address communication in nursing practice, it does address the behavioral patterns of affiliation which affects patterns of relating to others. Relating to others involved communication. The model refers to communication rather than directing it.

9. Does this theory direct nursing actions that lead to favorable outcomes? In contrast to Reynolds and Cormack (1991) who indicated they could not prescribe specific nursing interventions, Dee (1990) reported that using the Johnson model provided "a comprehensive and systematic method of assessing patient behavior" (p. 38). Dee found that the Johnson model could be used to "explain, predict, and control clinical phenomena for the purpose of achieving desired patient outcomes" (p. 41). The implementation of the Johnson model to guide practice in one specific institution is unusual in that few clinical institutions select just one theory or model to guide the practice in their institution.

10. How contagious is this theory? Johnson's Behavioral System Model has a limited following when compared to Callista Roy and Martha Rogers. There is a limited body of literature on the use of the Behavioral System Model in clinical practice or to provide the framework for nursing research. The majority of individuals using the Johnson Behavioral System Model studied with her in their master of science in nursing program or were colleagues with her at UCLA.

SUMMARY

Although Johnson's Behavioral System Model has many limitations, she does provide a frame of reference for nurses concerned with specific client behaviors. It must also be noted that Johnson, through her work at the University of California, Los Angeles, has had a profound influence on the development of nursing models and nursing theories. Through her position as a faculty member she influenced Roy, Grubbs, Holaday, and others. As a peer, she influenced Riehl, Neuman, Wu, and others, scholars who have generated many ideas about nursing concepts and theories.

Johnson's Behavioral System Model is a model of nursing care that advocates the fostering of efficient and effective behavioral functioning in the patient to prevent illness. The patient is identified as a behavioral system composed of seven behavioral subsystems: affiliative, dependency, ingestive, eliminative, sexual, aggressive, and achievement. Each subsystem is composed of four structural characteristics: drive, set, choices, and observable behaviors. The three functional requirements for each subsystem include protection from noxious influences, provision for a nurturing environment, and stimulation for growth. An imbalance in any of the behavioral subsystems results in disequilibrium. It is nursing's role to assist the client to return to a state of equilibrium.

REFERENCES

Auger, J. R. (1976). *Behavioral systems and nursing*. Upper Saddle River, NJ: Prentice-Hall.

Barnard, K. E. (1978). *Nursing Child Assessment Feeding Scale*. Seattle: University of Washington.

Chin, R. (1961). The utility of system models and developmental models for practitioners. In K. Benne, W. Bennis, & R. Chin (Eds.), *The planning of change*. New York: Holt.

Conner, S. S., Harbour, L. S., Magers, J. A., & Watt, J. K. (1994). Dorothy E. Johnson: Behavioral System Model. In A. Marriner-Tomey (Ed.), *Nursing theorists and their work* (3rd ed.). (pp. 231–245). St Louis: Mosby.

Damus, K. (1980). An application of the Johnson Behavioral System Model for nursing practice. In J. P. Riehl & C. Roy (Eds.), *Conceptual models for nursing practice* (2nd ed.) (pp. 274–289). New York: Appleton-Century-Crofts.

Dee, V. (1990). Implementation of the Johnson Model: One hospital's experience. In M. E. Parker (Ed.), *Nursing theories in practice* (pp. 33–44) (Pub. No. 15-2350). New York: National League for Nursing.

Derdiarian, A. K., & Schobel, D. (1990). Comprehensive assessment of AIDS patients using the behavioural systems model for nursing practice instrument. *Journal of Advanced Nursing, 15*, 436–446.

Freuhwirth, S. E. S. (1989). An application of Johnson's Behavioral Model: A case study. *Journal of Community Health Nursing, 6*, 61–71.

Grubbs, J. (1980). An interpretation of the Johnson Behavioral System Model for nursing practice. In J. P. Riehl & C. Roy (Eds.), *Conceptual models for nursing practice* (2nd ed.) (pp. 217–254). New York: Appleton-Century-Crofts.

Herbert, J. (1989). A model for Anna. *Nursing—Oxford, 3*(42), 30–34.

Holaday, B. (1980). Implementing the Johnson Model for Nursing Practice. In J. P. Riehl & C. Roy (Eds.), *Conceptual models for nursing practice* (2nd ed.) (pp. 255–263). New York: Appleton-Century-Crofts.

Johnson, D. E. (1959). The nature of a science of nursing. *Nursing Outlook, 7,* 291–294.

Johnson, D. E. (1961). The significance of nursing care. *American Journal of Nursing, 61*, 63–66.

Johnson, D. E. (1968, April). *One conceptual model of nursing.* Paper presented at Vanderbilt University, Nashville, Tennessee.

Johnson, D. E. (1968). Theory in nursing: Borrowed and unique. *Nursing Research, 17*, 206–209.

Johnson, D. E. (1974). Development of theory: A requisite for nursing as a profession. *Nursing Research, 23*, 372–377.

Johnson, D. E. (1978). State of the art of theory development in nursing. In *Theory development: What, why, how?* (pp. 1–10) (Pub. No. 15-1708). New York: National League for Nursing.

Johnson, D. E. (1980). The Behavioral System Model for Nursing. In J. P. Riehl & C. Roy (Eds.), *Conceptual models for nursing practice* (2nd ed.) (pp. 207–216). New York: Appleton-Century-Crofts.

Johnson, D. E. (1990). The behavioral system model for nursing. In M. E. Parker (Ed.), *Nursing theories in practice* (pp. 23–32) (Pub. No. 15-2350. New York: National League for Nursing.

Johnson, D. E. (1992). The origins of the Behavioral Systems Model. In F. Nightingale, *Notes on nursing: What it is, and what it is not* (Com. ed.). Philadelphia: Lippincott. (Originally published, 1859).

Loveland-Cherry, C., & Wilkerson, S. A. (1989). Dorothy Johnson's Behavioral System Model. In J. Fitzpatrick & A. Whall (Eds.), *Conceptual models of nursing: Analysis and application* (2nd ed.) (pp. 147–164). Norwalk, CT: Appleton & Lange.

Nightingale, F. (1992). *Notes on nursing: What it is, and what it is not* (Com. ed.). Philadelphia: Lippincott. (Originally published, 1859).

Poster, E. C., Dee, V., & Randell, B. P. (1997). The Johnson Behavioral Systems Model as a framework for patient outcome evaluation. *Journal of the American Psychiatric Nurses Association, 3*, 73–80.

Reynolds, W., & Cormack, D. F. S. (1991). An evaluation of the Johnson Behavioral System Model for nursing. *Journal of Advanced Nursing, 16*, 1122–1130.

Riegel, B. (1989). Social support and psychological adjustment to chronic coronary heart disease: Operationalization of Johnson's Behavioral System Model. *Advances in Nursing Science, 11*(2), 74–84.

Rogers, M. (1970). *The theoretical basis for nursing.* Philadelphia: Davis.

Roy, C. (1989). The Roy Adaptation Model. In J. Riehl-Sisca (Ed.), *Conceptual models for nursing practice* (3rd ed.) (pp. 105–114). Norwalk, CT: Appleton & Lange.

Skolny, M. A., & Riehl, J. P. (1974). Hope: Solving patient and family problems by using a theoretical framework. In J. P. Riehl & C. Roy (Eds.), *Conceptual models for nursing practice* (pp. 206–217). New York: Appleton-Century-Crofts.

Small, B. (1980). Nursing visually impaired children with Johnson's Model as a conceptual framework. In J. P. Riehl & C. Roy (Eds.), *Conceptual models for nursing practice* (2nd ed.) (pp. 264–273). New York: Appleton-Century-Crofts.

Torres, G. (1986). *Theoretical foundations of nursing.* Norwalk, CT: Appleton-Century-Crofts.

Wu, R. (1973). *Behavior and illness.* Upper Saddle River, NJ: Prentice-Hall.

CHAPTER 9

PATIENT-CENTERED APPROACHES
FAYE GLENN ABDELLAH

Suzanne M. Falco

■ ■ ■

Faye Glenn Abdellah was born in New York City. She graduated magna cum laude from Fitkin Memorial Hospital School of Nursing in Neptune, New Jersey, in 1942 and received her B.S. (1945), M.A. (1947), and Ed.D. (1955) from Teachers College, Columbia University. She also did graduate work in the sciences at Rutgers. As a new graduate, she taught at Yale. The frustrations that arose from this teaching experience led to the beginnings of her pursuit of the scientific basis of nursing practice (McAuliffe, 1998).

Dr. Abdellah served as Deputy Surgeon General and as Chief Nurse Officer for the U.S. Public Health Service (USPHS), Department of Health and Human Services, Washington, DC. She retired from the USPHS with the rank of rear admiral. In 1993 she became Dean of the newly formed Graduate School of Nursing, Uniformed Services University of the Health Sciences. She has more than 140 publications related to nursing care, education for advanced practice in nursing, health care administration, and nursing research. Some of these have been translated into six languages.

She has been granted 11 honorary doctorates by various institutions, including Case Western Reserve, Rutgers, University of Akron, Catholic University of America, Eastern University, and Monmouth College. These honors recognized her work in nursing research, development of the first nurse scientist training program, expertise in health policy, as well as her outstanding contributions to the health of the nation.

Her international service includes delegation member to the USSR, Yugoslavia, France, and the Peoples Republic of China; coordinator of the US–Argentina Cooperation in Health and Medicine Research Project; consultant to Portugal for program development for the disabled and the elderly, to Tel Aviv University on long-term care and nursing research, the Japanese Nursing Association in relation to nursing education and research, and in Australia and New Zealand in relation to nursing home care, nursing education, and research. She has also been a research consultant to the World Health Organization.

Dr. Abdellah is a Charter Fellow of the American Academy of Nursing, has served as this organization's vice president and president, and received its Living Legend Award. She has been recognized by Sigma Theta Tau as a Distinguished Research Fellow, and recipient of the Excellence in Nursing award, and the first Presidential Award. She was awarded the Allied Signal Award for her groundbreaking research in aging. The Institute of Medicine presented her with the Gustav O. Lienhard award in recognition of her contributions to the environment and healthier lifestyles. In addition she has received the following military awards: Surgeon General's Medallion and Medal; two Distinguished Service Medals; Uniformed Services University of the Health Sciences Distinguished Service Medal; Meritorious Service Medal; the Secretary of Department of Health Education and Welfare Distinguished Service Award; as well as two Founders Medals from the Association of Military Surgeons of the United State (McFadden, 2000).

In 1960, influenced by the desire to promote patient-centered comprehensive nursing care, Abdellah described nursing as a service to individuals, to families, and, therefore, to society. According to Abdellah, nursing is based on an art and science that mold the attitudes, intellectual competencies, and technical skills of the individual nurse into the desire and ability to help people, sick or well, cope with their health needs. Nursing may be carried out under general or specific medical direction. As a comprehensive service, nursing includes the following:

1. Recognizing the nursing problems of the patient;
2. Deciding the appropriate courses of action to take in terms of relevant nursing principles;
3. Providing continuous care of the individual's total health needs;
4. Providing continuous care to relieve pain and discomfort and provide immediate security for the individual;
5. Adjusting the total nursing care plan to meet the patient's individual needs;
6. Helping the individual to become more self-directing in attaining or maintaining a healthy state of mind and body;
7. Instructing nursing personnel and family to help the individual do for himself that which he can within his limitations;
8. Helping the individual to adjust to his limitations and emotional problems;
9. Working with allied health professions in planning for optimum health on local, state, national, and international levels; and
10. Carrying out continuous evaluation and research to improve nursing techniques and to develop new techniques to meet the health needs of people (Abdellah, Beland, Martin, & Matheney, 1960, pp. 24–25).

These original premises have undergone an evolutionary process. As a result, in 1973, Item 3—"providing continuous care of the individual's total health needs"—was eliminated (Abdellah, Beland, Martin, & Matheney, 1973). Although no reason was given, it can be hypothesized that the words *continuous* and *total* render that service virtually impossible to provide. From these premises, Abdellah's theory was derived.

ABDELLAH'S THEORY

Although Abdellah's writings are not specific as to a theoretical statement, such a statement can be derived by using her three major concepts of health, nursing problems, and problem solving. Abdellah's theory would state that nursing is the use of the problem-solving approach with key nursing problems related to the health needs of people. Such a theoretical statement maintains problem solving as the vehicle for the nursing problems as the patient is moved toward health—the outcome. It is also a relatively simple statement and can be used as a basis for nursing practice, administration, education, and research.

Health

Although Abdellah never defined it per se, her concept of health may be inferred to be the dynamic pattern of functioning whereby there is a continued interaction with internal and external forces that results in the optimal use of necessary resources that serve to minimize vulnerabilities (Abdellah & Levine, 1986; Torres & Stanton, 1982). Emphasis should be placed on prevention and rehabilitation with wellness as a lifetime goal. By performing nursing services through a holistic approach to the patient, the nurse helps the patient achieve a state of health. However, to effectively perform these services, the nurse must accurately identify the lacks or deficits regarding health that the patient is experiencing. These lacks or deficits are the patient's health needs.

Nursing Problems

The patient's health needs can be viewed as problems, which may be *overt* as an apparent condition, or *covert* as a hidden or concealed one. Because covert problems can be emotional, sociological, and interpersonal in nature, they are often missed or perceived incorrectly. Yet, in many instances, solving the covert problems may solve the overt problems as well (Abdellah, et al., 1960).

Such a view of problems implies a patient-centered orientation. Abdellah, however, seems to imply a different viewpoint (Abdellah et al., 1960). In an effort to differentiate them from medical problems, she says a nursing problem presented by a patient is a condition faced by the patient or patient's family that the nurse, through the performance of professional functions, can assist them to meet. Abdellah's use of the term *nursing problems* can be interpreted as more consistent with "nursing functions" or "nursing goals" than with patient-centered problems. This viewpoint could lead to an orientation that is more nursing-centered than patient-centered (Nicholls & Wessells, 1977).

Such a nursing-centered orientation to patient care seems contrary to the patient-centered approach that Abdellah professes to uphold (Abdellah et al., 1960). The apparent contradiction can be explained by her desire to move away from a disease-centered, overt problem, procedural orientation for nursing. In her attempt to bring nursing practice into its proper relationship with restorative and preventive measures for meeting total patient needs, she seems to swing the pendulum to the opposite pole, from the disease orientation to a nursing orientation, while leaving the patient somewhere in the middle (see Fig. 9–1). However, while the problems are labeled nursing problems, it is clear that the problems are those being experienced by the patient that the nurse can help meet. The problems identify where nursing can help. In her typology of basic nursing problems presented by patients, she includes three columns: basic nursing problem presented by the patient, specific problem of patient, and common conditions. An example may be found in Table 9–1. This focus would bring the pendulum back to the patient orientation.

It is noted that Abdellah recognized the need to shift from nursing problems to patient outcomes (Abdellah & Levine, 1986). However, there has been no further development of the framework to provide guidance in doing this.

Problem Solving

Quality professional nursing care requires that nurses be able to identify and solve overt and covert nursing problems. These requirements can be met by the problem-solving approach. The problem-solving process involves identifying the problem, selecting pertinent data, formulating hypotheses, testing hypotheses through the col-

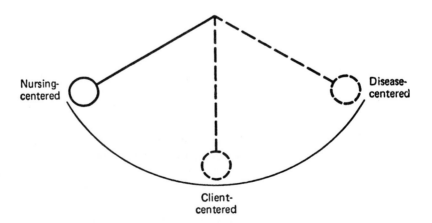

Figure 9–1. The focus of care pendulum.

TABLE 9–1. EXAMPLE OF TYPOLOGY OF BASIC NURSING PROBLEMS PRESENTED BY PATIENTS

Basic Nursing Problem Presented by Patient	Specific Problem of Patient	Common Conditions
5. To facilitate the maintenance of a supply of oxygen to all body cells	Supply of oxygen	Anesthesia High altitudes
	Clear airway	Asthmatic Postoperative Chest surgery Foreign bodies Unconscious patient
	Adequate functioning of neuromuscular system	Bulbar poliomyelitis Medulla damage Myasthenia gravis Muscular dystrophy
	Adequate absorbing surface	Far-advanced tuberculosis Congestive heart failure Pulmonary edema Pneumonia
	Ability to transport oxygen	Anemia Congestive heart failure Occlusive arterial disease Carbon monoxide poisoning
	Ability to utilize oxygen	Cyanide poison Moribund state
	Nursing care to decrease patient's need for oxygen and to supply higher concentration of oxygen	Through control of his environment Through reducing his activity

Source: Reprinted with permission of Simon & Schuster from PATIENT-CENTERED APPROACHES TO NURSING by Faye G. Abdellah, Martin Almeda, Irene L. Beland, Ruth V. Matheney. Copyright © 1960 Macmillan Publishing Company.

lection of data, and revising hypotheses when necessary on the basis of conclusions obtained from the data (Abdellah & Levine, 1986).

Many of these steps parallel the steps of the nursing process of assessment, diagnosis, outcomes, planning, implementation, and evaluation. The problem-solving approach was selected because of the assumption that the correct identification of nursing problems influences the nurse's judgment in selecting the next steps in solving the patient's nursing problems (Abdellah & Levine, 1986). The problem-solving approach is also consistent with such basic elements of nursing practice espoused by Abdellah as observing, reporting, and interpreting the signs and symptoms that comprise the deviations from health and constitute nursing problems, and with analyzing the nursing problems and selecting the necessary course of action (Abdellah et al., 1960). Note also that Abdellah supported the use of the problem-solving process before the nursing process was developed.

THE TWENTY-ONE NURSING PROBLEMS

The crucial element within Abdellah's theory is the correct identification of nursing problems. To assist in identification, the need was defined for a systematic classification of nursing problems presented by the patient. It was believed that such problems could be classified into the following three major categories.

1. Physical, sociological, and emotional needs of the patient;
2. Types of interpersonal relationships between the nurse and the patient; and
3. Common elements of patient care (Abdellah, et al., 1960, p. 11).

Over a five-year period, several studies were carried out to establish the classification. As a result of this research, 21 groups of common nursing problems were identified (see Table 9–2). It is these 21 common nursing problems of Abdellah's that are most widely known, and they are the focus of the rest of the chapter.

These 21 nursing problems focus on the physical, biological, and sociopsychological needs of the patient and attempt to provide a more meaningful basis for

TABLE 9–2. ABDELLAH'S 21 NURSING PROBLEMS

1. To maintain good hygiene and physical comfort.
2. To promote optimal activity; exercise, rest, and sleep.
3. To promote safety through the prevention of accident, injury, or other trauma and through the prevention of the spread of infection.
4. To maintain good body mechanics and prevent and correct deformities.
5. To facilitate the maintenance of a supply of oxygen to all body cells.
6. To facilitate the maintenance of nutrition of all body cells.
7. To facilitate the maintenance of elimination.
8. To facilitate the maintenance of fluid and electrolyte balance.
9. To recognize the physiological responses of the body to disease conditions—pathological, physiological, and compensatory.
10. To facilitate the maintenance of regulatory mechanisms and functions.
11. To facilitate the maintenance of sensory functions.
12. To identify and accept positive and negative expressions, feelings, and reactions.
13. To identify and accept the interrelatedness of emotions and organic illness.
14. To facilitate the maintenance of effective verbal and nonverbal communication.
15. To promote the development of productive interpersonal relationships.
16. To facilitate progress toward achievement of personal spiritual goals.
17. To create and/or maintain a therapeutic environment.
18. To facilitate awareness of self as an individual with varying physical, emotional, and developmental needs.
19. To accept the optimum possible goals in the light of limitations, physical and emotional.
20. To use community resources as an aid in resolving problems arising from illness.
21. To understand the role of social problems as influencing factors in the cause of illness.

Source: Abdellah, F. G., et al. (1960). *Patient-centered approaches to nursing*. New York: Macmillan, pp. 16–17. Used with permission.

organization than the categories of systems of the body. The most difficult problems were thought to be Numbers 12, 14, 15, 17, 18, and 19 (Abdellah et al., 1973). Although a rationale is not provided for this conclusion, it is interesting that all these problems fall into the realm of sociopsychological needs and tend to be covert in nature. The challenge of covert problems is supported in the discussion that such problems are often overlooked or misinterpreted. This discussion includes reference to Florence Nightingale's emphasis on the importance of accurate observations (Abdellah, et al., 1960, p. 7).

Within the practice of nursing, it was anticipated that these 21 problems as broad groupings would encourage the generalization of principles and would thereby guide care and promote the development of the nurse's judgmental ability. In each of the broad nursing problems are numerous specific overt and covert problems. It was also anticipated that the constant relating of the broad basic nursing problems to the specific problems of the individual patient and vice versa would encourage the development of increased ability to use theory in clinical practice. Thus, a greater understanding of the relationship between theory and practice would strengthen the usefulness of the nursing problems (Abdellah et al., 1960).

ABDELLAH'S THEORY AND NURSING'S METAPARADIGM

Abdellah does not clearly specify each of the four major concepts—the individual or human, health, environment/society, and nursing. She does describe the recipients of nursing as *individuals* (and families, and thus, society), although she does not delineate her beliefs or assumptions about the nature of human beings. Her 21 nursing problems deal with biological, psychological, and social areas of individuals and can be considered to represent areas of importance to them.

Health, or the achieving of it, is the purpose of nursing services. Although Abdellah does not give a definition of health, she speaks to "total health needs" and "a healthy state of mind and body" in her description of nursing as a comprehensive service (Abdellah et al., 1960).

Society is included in "planning for optimum health on local, state, national, and international levels" (Abdellah et al., 1960). However, as Abdellah further delineates her ideas, the focus of nursing service is clearly the individual. Society is negated when she discusses implementation of care to the individual. She indicates that by providing a service to individuals and families, society is served but does not discuss society as patient or define society.

Nursing is broadly grouped into the 21 problem areas to guide care and promote the use of nursing judgment. Abdellah considers nursing to be a comprehensive service that is based on an art and science and aims to help people, sick or well, cope with their health needs. The ten original areas of this service (became 9 in 1973) are listed in the beginning of this chapter.

USE OF THE TWENTY-ONE PROBLEMS IN THE NURSING PROCESS

Use of the 21 nursing problems in the nursing process serves primarily to direct the nurse in identifying the areas in which the patient needs the nurse's help. If the nurse helps the patient reach all the goals stated in the nursing problems, then the patient will be moved toward health.

Within the *assessment* phase, the nursing problems provide guidelines for the collection of data. A principle underlying the problem-solving approach is that for each identified problem, pertinent data are collected. Thus, for each of the identified 21 nursing problems, relevant data are collected. The overt or covert nature of the problems necessitates a direct or indirect approach, respectively. For example, the overt problem of nutritional status can be assessed by direct measures of weight, food intake, and body size, whereas the covert problem of maintaining a therapeutic environment requires more indirect approaches to data collection. These might include observations of such aspects as situations in which the patient is tense and those in which the patient is relaxed.

The nursing problems can be divided into those that are basic to all patients and those that reflect sustenal, remedial, or restorative care needs, as seen in Table 9–3. By facilitating data collection, such a classification promotes investigating those problems consistent with the patient's ability to provide self-help. If patients are holistic, then they can have needs in any and all areas regardless of the stage of illness. A multitude of nursing problems could then exist. Abdellah emphasized the importance of the total person so it is important not to "divide up" the person by categories of problems.

The results of the data collection would determine the patient's specific overt and/or covert problems. These specific problems would be grouped under one or more of the broader nursing problems. This step is consistent with that involved in *nursing diagnosis*. Within this framework, the nursing diagnoses are derived from the exhibited nursing problems.

The 21 nursing problems can have a great impact on the *outcome* and *planning* phases of the nursing process. The statements of the nursing problems contain the basis for desired outcomes and most closely resemble goal statements. Therefore, once the problem has been diagnosed, the outcomes can be identified and the goals have been established. Many of the nursing problem statements can be considered goals for either the nurse or the patient. Given that these problems are called *nursing problems*, then it could be reasonable to conclude that these goals are basically nursing goals. However, Abdellah's emphasis on moving care from a disease and procedure-centered approach to a patient-centered approach indicates that the term *nursing problems* identifies those areas of patient needs with which the patient needs nursing assistance.

Using the goals as the framework, a plan is developed and appropriate nursing implementations are determined. Table 9–3 summarizes the kinds of interventions that would be appropriate for the categories of nursing problems. Again, holism could be negated in *implementation* because of the isolated, particulate nature of the nursing problems. However, if one views the problem as the area in which the client needs assistance in order to function as a whole again, Abdellah's total person view is supported.

Following implementation of the plan, *evaluation* takes place. According to the American Nurses' Association's (1998) *Standards of clinical nursing practice*, the plan is evaluated in terms of the patient's progress or lack of progress toward the achievement of the stated outcomes and goals. If Abdellah's nursing problems are viewed as *nursing* goals, not *patient* goals, the most appropriate evaluation would be the *nurse's* progress or lack of progress toward the achievement of the stated goals. If the nursing problems are seen as areas in which the nurse can assist the patient, then the patient's ability to provide self-help in the identified areas must be evaluated.

Abdellah postulates that criterion measures can be determined from the groupings of the nursing problems, as shown in Table 9–3. A criterion is a value-free name of a measurable variable believed or known to be a relevant indicator of the quality of patient care (Bloch, 1977). Criteria can be used to measure patient care. Although it is not clear in her writings, the measurement of criteria may be related to the measurement of the achievement of the desired outcomes. Abdellah has suggested the following criteria might be used to determine the effectiveness of patient-centered care:

1. The patient is able to provide for the satisfaction of his own needs.
2. The nursing care plan makes provision to meet four needs—sustenal care, remedial care, restorative care, and preventive care.
3. The care plan extends beyond the patient's hospitalization and makes provision for continuation of the care at home.
4. The levels of nursing skills provided vary with the individual patient care requirements.
5. The entire care plan is directed at having the patient help himself.
6. The care plan makes provision for involvement of members of the family throughout the hospitalization and after discharge. (Abdellah & Levine, 1965, pp. 77–78)

The use of Abdellah's 21 nursing problems in an example might be beneficial.

Assessment data: Consider the case of Ron, who experienced severe crushing chest pain following a board meeting at his place of business. In addition to the pain, he experienced shortness of breath, tachycardia, and profuse diaphoresis. Upon admission to the hospital, assessment indicated that Ron might have sustained some cardiac damage. Investigation into his history revealed that he had been having episodes of chest pain for the past two months.

Nursing Diagnoses and Outcomes: With this as the data base, the specific problems of pain, impaired cardiac functioning, work-related stress, and failure to seek medical assistance can be identified. These specific problems can be related to selected nursing problems defined by Abdellah, and the nursing problems can be related to the categories of Ron's needs and desired outcomes identified.

TABLE 9–3. THE RELATIONSHIPS AMONG THE CLASSIFICATION AND APPROACH OF THE 21 NURSING PROBLEMS AND THE CATEGORIES OF NEEDS, NURSING IMPLEMENTATIONS, AND CRITERION MEASURES

Categories of Needs[1]	Nursing Problems	Classification and Approach[2]	Nursing Implementations[3]	Criterion Measures[1]
Basic to all patients	1. To maintain good hygiene and physical comfort. 2. To promote optimal activity; exercise, rest, and sleep. 3. To promote safety through the prevention of accident, injury, or other trauma and through the prevention of the spread of infection. 4. To maintain good body mechanics and prevent and correct deformities.	Overt problems, covert problems, or both Direct methods, indirect methods, or both	Measures necessary to maintain hygiene, physical comfort, activity, rest and sleep, safety, and body mechanics.	Related to preventive care needs and present to some degree in all patients.
Sustenal care needs	5. To facilitate the maintenance of a supply of oxygen to all body cells. 6. To facilitate the maintenance of nutrition of all body cells. 7. To facilitate the maintenance of elimination. 8. To facilitate the maintenance of fluid and electrolyte balance. 9. To recognize the physiological responses of the body to disease conditions—pathological, physiological, and compensatory. 10. To facilitate the maintenance of regulatory mechanisms and functions. 11. To facilitate the maintenance of sensory functions.	Usually overt problems Direct methods	Measures necessary to maintain oxygen supply, nutrition, elimination, fluid and electrolyte balance, regulatory mechanisms, and sensory functions. Implementations imply recognition of body's response to disease.	Related to sustenal and restorative care needs—the normal and disturbed physiological body processes that are vital to sustaining life.

		Usually covert problems Indirect methods	Measures that are helpful to the patient and his/her family during their emotional reactions to the patient's illness.	Related to rehabilitation needs, particularly those involving emotional and interpersonal difficulties.
Remedial care needs	12. To identify and accept positive and negative expressions, feelings, and reactions.			
	13. To identify and accept the interrelatedness of emotions and organic illness.			
	14. To facilitate the maintenance of effective verbal and nonverbal communication.			
	15. To promote the development of productive interpersonal relationships.			
	16. To facilitate progress toward achievement of personal spiritual goals.			
	17. To create and/or maintain a therapeutic environment.			
	18. To facilitate awareness of self as an individual with varying physical, emotional, and developmental needs.			
	19. To accept the optimum possible goals in the light of limitations, physical and emotional.			
Restorative care needs	20. To use community resources as an aid in resolving problems arising from illness.	Cover problems, covert problems, or both	Measures that will assist the patient and his/her family to cope with the illness and necessary life adjustment.	Related to sociological and community problems affecting patient care.
	21. To understand the role of social problems as influencing factors in the cause of illness.	Direct methods, indirect methods, or both		

[1]From Abdellah, F. G., & Levine, E. (1965). *Better patient care through nursing research*. New York: Macmillan, pp. 78–79, 280–281.
[2]From Abdellah, F. G., et al (1960). *Patient centered approaches to nursing*. New York: Macmillan, pp. 81–82.
[3]From Carter, J. H., et al (1976). *Standards of nursing care*. New York: Springer, pp. 8–9.

TABLE 9–4. AN ILLUSTRATION OF THE IMPLEMENTATION OF ABDELLAH'S FRAMEWORK IN RON'S CARE

Classification of Needs	Selected Abdellah Nursing Problems	Classification and Approach	Selected Nursing Implementations	Criterion Measures
Basic care	1. To maintain good hygiene and physical comfort	Overt problem of pain Direct and indirect methods	1. Administer oxygen 2. Elevate headrest 3. Reposition Ron 4. Administer prescribed analgesic 5. Remain with Ron	Amount of pain or degree of physical comfort
Sustenal care needs	5. To facilitate the maintenance of a supply of oxygen to all body cells	Overt problem of impaired cardiac functioning Direct methods	1. Promote rest 2. Place in sitting position 3. Promote deep breathing and coughing 4. Implement exercise program as tolerated	Vital signs Skin color
Remedial care needs	13. To identify and accept the interrelatedness of emotions and organic illness	Covert problem of effects of work-related stress on cardiac functioning Indirect methods	1. Investigate the nature of his job and the activities involved 2. Explore his work-related goals 3. Explore the kinds of stress associated with his job and his response to them	Knowledge of relationship between stress and his illness
Restorative care needs	20. To use community resources as an aid in resolving problems arising from illness	Overt problem of failure to seek medical assistance when needed Direct methods	1. Teach early warning signs and symptoms of cardiac distress 2. Teach course of action should specific symptoms occur	Knowledge of appropriate use of certain community resources

Planning and Implementation: Nursing strategies and criterion (outcomes) measures can then be determined. Table 9–4 illustrates the implementation of Abdellah's framework. The possibilities for fractionalizing care can be readily seen by the repetition of implementation strategies for the two problems of pain and impaired cardiac functioning. The repetition of implementation strategies may also be seen as indicative of the multifaceted response of the human being to any given action.

Evaluation: The evaluation would be based on the desired outcomes and goals—can Ron once again perform all of the activities in the 21 nursing problems by himself? More specifically, is his pain controlled, does he express knowledge and understanding about the interactive effects of stress and cardiac functioning, is he making a commitment to make appropriate lifestyle changes, including seeking medical assistance when symptoms occur? (Table 9–4 is in no way designed to be inclusive. Rather, it is offered as an attempt to make the theory operational.)

CRITIQUE OF ABDELLAH'S PATIENT CENTERED APPROACHES

1. What is the historical context of the theory? An examination of the 21 problems yields similarities to other theories. Most notable is their similarity to Henderson's (1991) 14 components of basic nursing care (see Table 9–5). As can be seen in this table, Abdellah has consolidated some components (such as Number 7—Select suitable clothing, and Number 8—Keep body clean and well groomed) and has expanded others (most notably Number 14—Learn, discover, and satisfy curiosity). The strong similarity may be the result of both Henderson's and Abdellah's exposure to the same environment—Teachers College, Columbia University, New York. It might be hypothesized that Abdellah moved from the rather simplistic form of Henderson's theory to a more complex structure.

Despite the noted similarity, a major difference is evident. Henderson's components are written in terms of patient behaviors, whereas Abdellah's problems are formulated in terms of the nursing services that should be incorporated into the determination of the patient's needs (DeYoung, 1976). Henderson seems to have maintained the patient orientation, whereas Abdellah seems to have moved beyond it (see Table 9–5).

Abdellah's nursing problems are also comparable to Maslow's (1954) hierarchy of needs. In contrast to Henderson's components, which have a strong physiological orientation, Abdellah's expansion in the area of *esteem needs* provides a more balanced set of nursing problems between the physical and nonphysical areas (Table 9–5). As with Henderson's components, Abdellah's problems do not meet the self-actualization needs of Maslow. This is not surprising, for self-actualization is not a goal to be accomplished but a process that is ongoing—the dynamic process of becoming. To place elements in this area would negate the dynamism of self-actualization. From a different viewpoint, if Henderson's components and Abdellah's problems are fulfilled, then the patient will move toward becoming and self-actualization.

TABLE 9–5. COMPARISON OF MASLOW'S, HENDERSON'S, AND ABDELLAH'S FRAMEWORKS

Maslow	Henderson	Abdellah
1. Physiological needs	1. Breathe normally	5. To facilitate the maintenance of a supply of oxygen to all body cells
	2. Eat and drink adequately	6. To facilitate the maintenance of nutrition to all body cells
		8. To facilitate the maintenance of fluid and electrolyte balance.
	3. Eliminate body waste	7. To facilitate the maintenance of elimination
	4. Move and maintain desirable posture	4. To maintain good body mechanics and prevent and correct deformities
	5. Sleep and rest	2. To promote optimal activity; exercise, rest, and sleep.
	6. Select suitable clothing	10. To facilitate the maintenance of regulatory mechanisms and functions
	7. Maintain body temperature	
	8. Keep body clean and well groomed and protect the integument	1. To maintain good hygiene and physical comfort
2. Safety needs	9. Avoid environmental dangers and avoid injuring others	3. To promote safety through the prevention of accidents, injury, or other trauma and through the prevention of the spread of infection
		11. To facilitate the maintenance of sensory function
3. Belonging and love needs	10. Communicate with others	14. To facilitate the maintenance of effective verbal and nonverbal communication
		15. To promote the development of productive interpersonal relationships
	11. Worship according to faith	16. To facilitate progress toward achievement of personal spiritual goals
4. Esteem needs	12. Work at something providing a sense of accomplishment	19. To accept the optimum possible goals in the light of limitations, physical and emotional
	13. Play or participate in various forms of recreation	
	14. Learn, discover, or satisfy curiosity	9. To recognize the physiological responses of the body to disease conditions— pathological, physiological, and compensatory
		12. Identify and accept positive and negative expressions, feelings, and reactions
		13. To identify and accept the interrelatedness of emotions and organic illness
		17. To create and/or maintain a therapeutic environment
		18. To facilitate awareness of self as an individual with varying physical, emotional, and developmental needs
		20. To use community resources as an aid in resolving problems arising from illness
		21. To understand the role of social problems as influencing factors in the case of illness
5. Self-actualization needs		

While Abdellah included discussion of the 21 nursing problems in her research texts written with Levine, she has not extended this particular area of her work. Her more recent publications have focused on advanced practice (Abdellah, 1997), management (Abdellah, 1995), graduate education (Abdellah, 1993), and research (Abdellah 1991a, 1991b, 1991c, 1991d).

Abdellah's theory is grounded in need theory, and is related to the frameworks of Maslow's hierarchy of needs and Henderson's basic needs. The expansion from Maslow's five needs and Henderson's 14 needs to Abdellah's 21 nursing problems demonstrates an effort to try to identify the totality of patient needs. Thus, the framework is compatible with the totality paradigm.

2. What are the basic concepts and relationships presented by the theory? Abdellah's theory has interrelated the concepts of health, nursing problems, and problem solving in an attempt to create a different way of viewing nursing phenomena. The resulting relationship is the use of the problem-solving approach with key nursing problems related to the health needs of people.

3. What major phenomena of concern to nursing are presented? The major phenomena of concern to nursing are the 21 nursing problems and patient-centered care.

4. To whom does this theory apply? In what situations? In what ways? Abdellah's theory provides a basis for determining and organizing nursing care. If all 21 problems are investigated, the patient would be likely to be thoroughly assessed. The problems also provide a basis for organizing appropriate nursing strategies. It is anticipated that by solving the nursing problems, the patient would be moved toward health. This theory applies to any persons who cannot meet any of the activities in the 21 nursing problems by themselves or who are in need of preventive care to avoid becoming unable to meet those needs. Abdellah clearly states that the nurse must be competent in working with patients' health needs both within the hospital and outside of it.

5. By what method or methods can this theory be tested? This theory was developed through multiple research projects conducted over a five-year period. Testing of the theory in the clinical environment has not been undertaken, possibly because Abdellah's presentations of the nursing problems have focused on nursing education and hospital organization. Research questions and hypotheses generated from the theory would determine the research approach to be used. Abdellah used methodological research to identify the nursing problems of patients (Abdellah, & Levine, 1965, p. 490).

Abdellah has indicated that current nursing research needs are to "focus on evidence based research . . . identify clinical practice guidelines that identify indicators that measure quality of care . . . and identify methods or instruments that monitor the extent to which actions of health care practitioners conform to practice guidelines, medical review criteria, or standards of quality, and then point out the policy implications of the research" (Abdellah, 1998, p. 216). These are compatible with investigations using the 21 nursing problems—what evidence is needed that the problems have been solved? What related guidelines indicate quality of care? She also says nursing research needs to be linked to "practice, cost, or policy" as well as to have interdisciplinary and collaborative aspects (Abdellah, 1998, p. 216).

6. Does this theory direct critical thinking in nursing practice? This theory places heavy emphasis on problem solving, an activity that is considered essential to critical thinking. The broad groups of the 21 nursing problems have the potential to encourage generalization of the principles, to promote the development of the nurse's judgmental ability, and to strengthen the relationship between theory and practice.

7. Does this theory direct therapeutic nursing interventions? The statements of the 21 nursing problems most closely resemble goal statements, and as such have the ability to directly influence nursing interventions. The interrelationships between the nursing problems and categories of needs make a great contribution to nursing practice with patients with specific needs. The theory focuses quite heavily on nursing practice with individuals, thereby limiting the potential scope of therapeutic interventions in relation to families and communities.

8. Does this theory direct communication in nursing practice? Given that the theory is nursing-problem based, it has great potential for facilitating communication in nursing practice. Indeed, problem 14 is "to facilitate the maintenance of effective verbal and nonverbal communication."

9. Does this theory direct nursing actions that lead to favorable outcomes? Abdellah's theory clearly directs the nurse to investigate and take appropriate action in the 21 nursing problem areas. Emphasis is on the identification of the areas in which nursing help is needed rather than specifying what the patient is to achieve. Thus, it is assumed that if the nursing problem is resolved, then a favorable patient outcome has been achieved, since the resolution of the problem would indicate the patient is once again able to meet the need.

10. How contagious is this theory? At this time, Abdellah's theory is not in popular use as a field of study. Its uses may be seen more in the organization of teaching content within educational programs, the evaluation of a student's performance for providing total care in the clinical area, and the grouping of patients in clinical settings according to anticipated nursing needs. However, as indicated in the biographical sketch at the beginning of this chapter, Abdellah is known internationally for her contributions to nursing and to health policy.

STRENGTHS AND LIMITATIONS

A strength and a limitation are related to research. A major strength of Abdellah's work is that the 21 nursing problems were developed through extensive research— at least three separate research projects over a five-year period. A major limitation is the lack of continued research to link the effectiveness of use of the 21 nursing problems to successful outcomes of nursing care.

Another strength is the driving force behind the development of the 21 nursing problems. Abdellah wanted to move nursing care from a base in medical diagnosis and procedures to a patient-centered base. Interestingly, an approach taken to achieve this was to encourage the use of the 21 nursing problems in shaping the curricula of nursing education programs. In *Patient-centered approaches to nursing*, Matheny discusses application in an associate degree program, Martin discusses application in a diploma program, and Beland discusses application in a bachelor of science program. Abdellah also discusses application in nursing service (Abdellah, et al., 1960). While the use of the 21 nursing problems to structure nursing curricula has not been widely documented, the concept of patient-centered care and care of the total person has certainly evolved over the decades since the problems were initially identified.

Another strength can be seen in the emphasis placed on the importance of recognizing and correctly identifying both overt and covert problems. The link to Nightingale's emphasis on the value of careful observations only enhances the significance of this idea. Abdellah made a major contribution in reminding us to look below the surface—to seek out the covert problems since they are often the cause of the overt problems.

The label of "nursing problems" is a limitation. Labeling the list of 21 problems as nursing problems tends to lead the reader to the belief that Abdellah's work is nursing centered when she stated she was seeking to move nursing to being patient-centered. It would have been helpful had she used other terminology or explained more clearly how this label relates to patient-centered care.

Also, especially in care settings where a nurse has very limited time to spend with each patient, the use of the 21 nursing problems could further fractionalize care. This could happen if the focus is placed only on a problem or a series of problems, rather than on the total person. Abdellah's intention was for a total person approach. Having a list of discrete problems, and using this list in time-constrained circumstances, could easily lead to dealing with parts rather than the whole.

Overall, the strengths of this work outweigh the limitations. This is particularly true when the limitations are taken into careful consideration since overcoming the limitations is within the capacity of the individual nurse.

SUMMARY

Using Abdellah's concepts of health, nursing problems, and problem solving, the theoretical statement of nursing that can be derived is the use of the problem-solving approach with key nursing problems related to the health needs of people. From this framework, 21 nursing problems were developed. These problems may be compared to Henderson's 14 components of nursing and Maslow's hierarchy of needs. Ways to use the nursing problems in the nursing process are explored. Some modification of the nursing problems to more clearly promote a patient-centered orientation would encourage effective use of the theory in professional nursing practice.

REFERENCES

Abdellah, F. G. (1991a). The funding crisis in biomedical research, Part I—Addressing the issue. *Journal of Professional Nursing, 7,* 7.

Abdellah, F. G. (1991b). The funding crisis in biomedical research, Part II—Options for action. *Journal of Professional Nursing, 7,* 75.

Abdellah, F. G. (1991c). The human genome initiative—Implications for nurse researchers. *Journal of Professional Nursing, 7,* 332.

Abdellah, F. G. (1991d). Summary statements of the NIH Nursing Research Grant Applications. *Nursing Research, 40,* 346–351.

Abdellah, F. G. (1993). Doctoral preparation and research productivity. *Journal of Professional Nursing, 9,* 71.

Abdellah, F. G. (1995). Management perspectives. I'm the aspiring vice president of nursing at a university hospital and I'm wondering how to avoid hitting the "glass ceiling." *Nursing Spectrum, 5*(9), 7.

Abdellah, F. G. (1997). Managing the challenges of role diversification in an interdisciplinary environment. *Military Medicine, 162,* 453–458.

Abdellah, F. G. (1998). An interview with Faye G. Abdellah on nursing research and health policy. *Image: Journal of Nursing Scholarship, 301,* 215–219.

Abdellah, F. G., Beland, I. L., Martin, A., & Matheney, R. V. (1960). *Patient-centered approaches to nursing.* New York: Macmillan. (out of print)

Abdellah, F. G., Beland, I. L., Martin, A., & Matheney, R. V. (1973). *New directions in patient-centered nursing.* New York: Macmillan.

Abdellah, F. G., & Levine, E. (1965). *Better patient care through nursing research.* New York: Macmillan.

Abdellah, F. G., & Levine, E. (1986). *Better patient care through nursing research* (3rd ed.). New York: Macmillan.

American Nurses' Association. (1998). *Standards for clinical nursing practice.* Washington, DC: Author.

Bloch, D. (1977). Criteria, standards, norms—Crucial terms in quality assurance. *Journal of Nursing Administration, 7,* 22.

Carter, J. H., Hilliard, M., Castles, M. R., Stoll, L. D., & Cowan, A. (1976). *Standards of nursing care.* NY: Springer.

DeYoung, L. (1976). *The foundations of nursing.* St. Louis: Mosby.

Henderson, V. (1991). *The nature of nursing: A definition and its implications for practice, research, and education. Reflections after 25 years* (Pub. No. 15-2346). New York: National League for Nursing Press.

Maslow, A. (1954). *Motivation and personality.* New York: Harper & Row.

McFadden, W. (2000). Message from the Dean Graduate School of Nursing. Available: *www.usuhs.mil/gsn/msgdean.html*

Nicholls, M. E., & Wessells, V. G. (Eds.). (1977). *Nursing standards and nursing process.* Wakefield, Mass.: Contemporary Publishing.

Torres, G., & Stanton, M. (1982). *Curriculum process in nursing: A guide to curriculum development.* Upper Saddle River, NJ: Prentice Hall.

CHAPTER 10

NURSING PROCESS DISCIPLINE
IDA JEAN ORLANDO

Julia B. George

■ ■ ■

Ida Jean Orlando Pelletier (b. 1926) has had a varied career as a practitioner, educator, researcher, and consultant in nursing. During the early part of her career, she worked as a staff nurse in such areas as obstetrics, medicine, surgery, and the emergency room. She also held supervisory positions and the title of Second Assistant Director of Nurses. She received a diploma in nursing from New York Medical College, Flower Fifth Avenue Hospital School of Nursing in 1947, and a B.S. in Public Health Nursing from St. John's University in Brooklyn, New York, in 1951. In 1954, she received her M.A. in mental health consultation from Columbia University, New York. She then went to Yale University as a research associate and principal investigator on a project studying the integration of mental health concepts into the basic nursing curriculum. This led to the publication of her first book, The dynamic nurse–patient relationship: Function, process, and principles, *in 1961 (reprinted 1990). She also served as director of the graduate program in mental health and psychiatric nursing at Yale.*

In 1962, Orlando married Robert Pelletier and moved to Massachusetts. She became a clinical nursing consultant to a psychiatric hospital, McLean Hospital, and at a veterans' hospital. At McLean Hospital, she carried out the research that led to the publication in 1972 of her second book, The discipline and teaching of nursing process.

Since 1972, Orlando has been associated intermittently with Boston University School of Nursing, teaching nursing theory and supervising graduate students in the clinical area. She also served as a project consultant for The New England Board of Higher Education in their Mental Health Project for Associate Degree Faculties. She also served as a nurse educator at Metropolitan State Hospital in Waltham, Massachusetts.

Throughout her career, Orlando has been active in a variety of organizations, including the Massachusetts Nurses' Association and the Harvard Community Health Plan. She has also lectured and offered workshops and consultation to a wide variety of agencies.

Ida Jean Orlando Pelletier describes a nursing process based on the interaction between a patient and a nurse. Her nursing process discipline was developed through research and presented in two books. Her initial work, *The dynamic nurse–patient relationship: Function, process and principles*, was originally published in 1961 and reprinted in 1990. *The discipline and teaching of nursing process*, showing further testing and refinement of her work, appeared in 1972.

Orlando's educational background and the work that led to her publications provide insight into the content of her theory. Her advanced nursing preparation and area of teaching responsibility and practice were in mental health and psychiatric nursing. Although she applied her ideas to many nursing specialty areas, the focus of her work is interaction.

The dynamic nurse–patient relationship was written to report the results of a five-year project at Yale University in the mid-1950s. The purpose of this project, supported by a grant from the National Institute of Mental Health, was "to identify the factors which enhanced or impeded the integration of mental health principles in the basic nursing curriculum" (Orlando, 1961/1990, p. vii). This research resulted in the identification that a nurse's statement of her perception, thought, or feeling about the patient's behavior differentiated between effective and ineffective communication. The book describes the curriculum content developed from the study. Its stated purpose is "to offer the professional nursing student a theory of effective nursing practice" (p. viii). This book was completed in 1958 and was initially rejected for publication as not being marketable in nursing. Finally, in 1961, it was recognized as having an important contribution to make to the practice of nursing.

Orlando refined her ideas and put them into practice at a private psychiatric facility, McLean Hospital in Belmont, Massachusetts. Again with a National Institute of Mental Health grant, she studied an objective means to evaluate her process and training in its discipline. The discipline variable was found to make a statistically significant difference in patient outcomes. This work, done during the 1960s, led to *The discipline and teaching of nursing process* (1972), in which she was concerned with the specific definition of nursing function and with incorporating nursing activities beyond the nurse–patient relationship into a total nursing system. She also developed more readily measured criteria to guide the nurse in her reaction to patient behavior.*

Orlando's work spans a fertile period of nursing thinking. She was influenced by, as well as an influence on, other nursing theorists. For example, Orlando is similar to Nightingale when she states, "It is important for the nurse to concern herself with the patient's distress because the treatment and prevention of disease proceed best when conditions extraneous to the disease itself and its management do not cause the patient additional suffering" (Orlando, 1961/1990, pp. 22–23). Another nursing theorist, Peplau (1952/1988), published her highly interpersonal theory two years

---

*In this chapter, the feminine pronoun is used when referring to the nurse and the masculine pronoun when referring to the patient. This is consistent with Orlando's use of these pronouns and terms.

before Orlando began her first study. Henderson also was refining her definition of nursing during Orlando's first study. Henderson's 1955 definition is consistent with Orlando when she states, "Nursing is primarily assisting the individual . . . in the performance of those activities . . . that he would perform unaided if he had the necessary strength, will, or knowledge" (Harmer & Henderson, 1955, p. 4). Ernestine Wiedenbach's interest in the initial study led to an increased concentration of data collection about nursing practice in the maternal/newborn area (Trench, Wallace, & Coberg, 1987).

ORLANDO'S KEY CONCEPTS

Certain major concepts are evident in Orlando's theory of nursing. She believes that nursing is *unique* and *independent* because it concerns itself with an *individual's need for help*, real or potential, in an *immediate* situation. The process by which nursing resolves this helplessness is *interactive* and is pursued in a *disciplined* manner that requires *training*. She believes one's actions should be based on rationale, not protocols.

Throughout her career, Orlando has been concerned with identifying that which is *uniquely* nursing. In her first book, she presents principles to guide nursing practice (Orlando, 1961/1990). She believes that the use of general principles from other fields is not sufficient to help the nurse in her interaction with patients. She identifies nursing's role as follows, "It is the nurse's direct responsibility to see to it that the patient's needs for help are met either by her own activity or by calling in the help of others" (p. 22).

Orlando (1972) also suggests that nursing's failure to establish its uniqueness is a result of the lack of a clearly identifiable function, which leads to inadequate care and insufficient attention to the patient's reactions to his immediate experiences. Thus, she identifies nursing's function as being "concerned with providing direct assistance to individuals in whatever setting they are found for the purpose of avoiding, relieving, diminishing, or curing the individual's sense of helplessness" (p. 12). She also indicates that policies and practices developed for the purposes of institutional bureaucracy or the aims of medicine place nurses in a dependent position (Orlando, 1987).

It is the unique function of nursing and the license held by the individual nurse that gives nurses the authority to work *independently* (Orlando, 1987). Orlando recommends that "nurses . . . must radically shift their focus from assistance to physicians and institutions to assisting patients with what they cannot do alone" (Pelletier, 1967, p. 28). Physicians' orders are directed to patients, not to nurses. Moreover, at times nurses may even assist patients in *not* complying with medical orders when such orders are in conflict with the patient's need for help. Nurses must also resolve conflicts between the patient's need for help and institutional policies. Nursing's unique function allows nurses to work in any setting where persons experience a need for help that they cannot resolve themselves. Thus, nurses may practice with well or ill persons in an independent practice or in an institutional setting.

Orlando's theory focuses on the patient as an *individual*. Each person, in each situation, is different. To be appropriate, nursing actions for two patients with the same presenting behavior, or the same patient at different times, are to be individualized. Nurses cannot automatically act only on the basis of principles, past experience, or physicians' orders. They must first ascertain that their actions will meet the patient's specific need for help.

Nursing is concerned with "individuals who suffer or anticipate a sense of helplessness" (Orlando, 1961/1990, p. 12). Orlando (1972) defines need as "a requirement of the patient which, if supplied, relieves or diminishes his immediate distress or improves his immediate sense of adequacy or well-being" (p. 5). In many instances, people can meet their own needs, do so, and do not require the help of professional nurses. When they cannot do so, or do not clearly understand these needs, a *need for help* is present. The nurse's function is to correctly identify and relieve this need.

The *immediacy* of the nursing situation is a vital concept in Orlando's theory. Each patient's behavior must be assessed to determine whether it expresses a need for help. Furthermore, identical behaviors by the same patient may indicate different needs at different times. The nursing action must also be specifically designed for the immediate encounter. Long-term planning has no part in Orlando's theory except as it pertains to providing adequate staff coverage for a job setting.

Orlando describes a nursing process discipline that is totally *interactive*. It describes, step by step, what goes on between a nurse and a patient in a specific encounter. A patient behavior causes the process discipline to begin. The process discipline involves the nurse's reaction to this behavior and the nurse's consequent action. The nurse shares her reaction with the patient to identify the need for help and the appropriate action. The nurse also verifies that the action met the need for help. Orlando's principles are meant to guide the nurse at various stages of the interaction. She emphasizes the importance of interaction when she writes, "Learning how to understand what is happening between herself and the patient is the central core of the nurse's practice and comprises the basic framework for the help she gives to patients" (Orlando, 1961/1990, p. 4).

The actual *process* of a nurse–patient interaction may be the same as that of any interaction between two persons. When nurses use this process to communicate their reactions in caring for patients, Orlando calls it the "nursing process discipline." It is the tool that nurses use to fulfill their function to patients. In an attempt to extend her theory to encompass all nursing activities, Orlando (1972) broadens the use of the process discipline beyond the individual nurse–patient relationship in her book, *The discipline and teaching of nursing process*. She applies the process discipline to contacts between a nurse leader and those she supervises or directs. When it is used in this manner, she refers to the process discipline as the "directive or supervisory job process in nursing" (p. 29).

If the nursing process is the same as the interactive process between any two individuals, how can nursing call itself a profession? The key is *discipline* in use of the process. Orlando (1972) provides three criteria to evaluate this discipline. These criteria differentiate an "automatic personal response" from a "disciplined professional response" (p. 31). Only the latter leads to effective nursing care, that is, relief of the patient's sense of helplessness. Learning to employ the process discipline requires *training*. This justifies the need for specific education in nursing. Orlando's nursing process discipline and the criteria for its use are discussed in more detail.

ORLANDO'S NURSING PROCESS DISCIPLINE

Orlando's (1972) nursing process discipline is based on the "process by which any individual acts" (p. 24). The purpose of the process discipline, when it is used between a nurse and a patient, is to meet the patient's immediate need for help. Improvement in the patient's behavior that indicates resolution of the need is the desired result. The process discipline is also used with other persons working in a job setting. The purpose here is to understand how the professional and job responsibilities of each affect the other. This understanding allows each nurse to effectively fulfill her professional function for the patient within the organizational setting.

Patient Behavior

The nursing process discipline is set in motion by *patient behavior*. All patient behavior, no matter how insignificant, must be considered an expression of need for help until its meaning to a particular patient in the immediate situation is understood. Orlando (1961/1990) stresses this in her first principle: "The presenting behavior of the patient, regardless of the form in which it appears, may represent a plea for help" (p. 40).

Patient behavior may be verbal or nonverbal. Inconsistency between these two types of behavior may be the factor that alerts the nurse that the patient needs help. Verbal behavior encompasses all the patient's use of language. It may take the form of "complaints . . . , requests . . . , questions . . . , refusals . . . , demands . . . , and . . . comments or statements" (Orlando, 1961/1990, p. 11). Nonverbal behavior includes physiological manifestations such as heart rate, perspiration, edema, and urination, and motor activity such as smiling, walking, and avoiding eye contact. Nonverbal patient behavior may also be vocal, including such actions as sobbing, laughing, shouting, and sighing.

When the patient experiences a need that he cannot resolve, a sense of helplessness occurs. The patient's behavior reflects this distress. In *The dynamic nurse–patient relationship*, Orlando (1961/1990) describes some categories of patient distress: "physical limitations, . . . adverse reactions to the setting and . . . experiences which prevent the patient from communicating his needs" (p. 11). Feelings of helplessness caused by physical limitations may result from incomplete development, temporary or permanent disability, or restrictions of the environment, real or imagined. Adverse reactions to the setting, on the other hand, usually result from incorrect or inadequate understanding of an experience there. Patients may become distressed by a negative reaction to any aspect of the setting, despite its helpful or therapeutic intent. A need for help may also arise from the patient's inability to communicate effectively. This inability may be due to such factors as ambivalence concerning dependency brought on by illness, embarrassment related to the need, lack of trust in the nurse, and inability to state the need precisely.

Although all patient behavior may indicate a need for help, the behavior may not effectively communicate that need. When the behavior does not communicate the need, problems in the nurse–patient relationship can arise. Ineffective patient behavior "prevents the nurse from carrying out her concerns for the patient's care or from maintaining a satisfactory relationship to the patient" (Orlando, 1961/1990, p. 78). Ineffective patient behavior may also indicate difficulties in the initial establishment of the nurse–patient relationship, inaccurate identification of the patient's need by the nurse, or negative patient reaction to automatic nursing action. Resolution of ineffective patient behavior deserves high priority, for the behavior usually becomes worse over time if the need for help that it expresses remains unresolved. The nurse's reaction and action are designed to resolve ineffective patient behaviors as well as to meet the immediate need.

Nurse Reaction

The patient behavior stimulates a *nurse reaction*, which marks the beginning of the nursing process discipline. This reaction is comprised of three sequential parts (Orlando, 1972). First, the nurse perceives the behavior through any of her senses. Second, the perception leads to automatic thought. Finally, the thought produces an automatic feeling. For example, the nurse sees a patient grimace, thinks he is in pain, and feels concern. The nurse then shares her reaction with the patient to ascertain that she has correctly identified the need for help and to identify the nursing action appropriate to resolve it. Orlando (1961/1990) offers a principle to guide the nurse in her reaction to patient behavior. "The nurse does not assume that any aspect of her reaction to the patient is correct, helpful, or appropriate until she checks the validity of it in exploration with the patient" (p. 56).

Perception (sees the grimace), thought (thinks he is in pain), and feeling (feels concern) occur automatically and almost simultaneously. Therefore the nurse must learn to identify each part of her reaction. This helps her to analyze the reaction to determine why she responded as she did. The process becomes logical rather than intuitive and, thus, disciplined rather than automatic. The nurse is able to use her reaction for the purpose of helping the patient.

The discipline in the nursing process prescribes how the nurse shares her reaction with the patient. Orlando (1961/1990) offers a principle to explain the usefulness of this sharing: "Any observation shared and explored with the patient is immediately useful in ascertaining and meeting his need or finding out that he is not in need at that time" (pp. 35–36).

Orlando (1972) also provides three criteria to ensure that the nurse's exploration of her reaction with the patient is successful:

1. What the nurse says to the individual in the contact must match (*be consistent with*) any or all of the items contained in the immediate reaction, and what the nurse does nonverbally must be verbally expressed and the expression must match one or all of the items contained in the immediate reaction; 2. The nurse must clearly communicate to the indi-

vidual that the item being expressed belongs to herself; 3. The nurse must ask the individual about the item expressed in order to obtain correction or verification from that same individual (pp. 29–30).

Which aspect of her reaction the nurse shares with the patient is not as important as that it be shared in the manner described in the criteria. From a practical standpoint, it may be more expeditious to share a perception than a thought or feeling. "You are grimacing" contains less assumption than "Are you in pain?" In this way the patient can more easily express his need for help without having to correct the nurse's misconception.

Feelings can and should be shared even when they are negative. The nonverbal action of the nurse will usually show her feelings even if they are not verbally expressed. Thus, the nurse's verbal and nonverbal behavior may be inconsistent. Proper sharing of feelings can effectively help the patient to express his need for help. For example, a nurse may react to a patient's refusal of a medication with anger. If she says, "I am angry with your refusal of your medication. Could you explain to me why you have refused?" she invites the patient to explain the need for help that his refusal expressed. Her expression meets the three criteria, and the patient's need for help can be identified and resolved.

This example shows the importance of the nurse sharing her reaction as a fact about herself. She states, "I am angry," rather than, "You make me angry." This clear identification of the reaction as her own reduces the chance of misinterpretation by the patient. The sharing of the nurse's immediate reaction creates a climate in which the patient is more able to share his own reaction.

Adequate identification of the three aspects of the nurse's reaction helps to resolve extraneous feelings that may interfere with the patient's care. The nurse may find that her feelings come from her personal belief of how people should act or from stresses in the organizational setting or in her personal life. These feelings or stresses are unrelated to meeting the patient's need. If they are not resolved, the nurse's verbal and nonverbal behavior will again be inconsistent. This same process should be employed with nurses or other professionals in the job setting to resolve any conflicts that interfere with the nurse's fulfilling her professional function for the patient.

Orlando (1972) used her three criteria in the study described in *The discipline and teaching of nursing process* and found that use of the process discipline is positively related to improvement in patient behavior. The study also showed a positive relationship between the nurse's use of the process discipline and its use by the patient. Thus, use of the process discipline alone can help the patient communicate his need more effectively.

Orlando (1972) offers a diagram depicting open sharing of the nurse's reaction versus keeping the reaction secret (see Figs. 10–1 and 10–2). The nurse action that results from the reaction becomes a behavior that stimulates a reaction by the patient. Only openness in sharing of the nurse's reaction assures that the patient's need will be effectively resolved. This sharing, in the manner prescribed, differentiates professional nursing practice from automatic personal response.

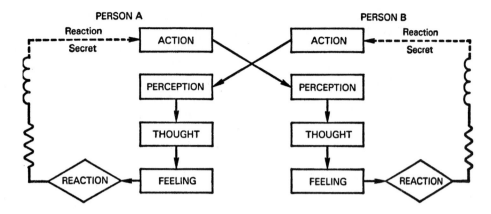

Figure 10–1. The action process in a person-to-person contact functioning in secret. The perceptions, thoughts, and feelings of each individual are not directly available to the perception of the other individual through the observable action. (*From Orlando, I. J. (1972). The discipline and teaching of nursing process, New York: G. P. Putnam's Sons, p. 26. Used with permission.*)

Nurse's Action

Once the nurse has validated or corrected her reaction to the patient's behavior through exploration with him, she can complete the nursing process discipline with the *nurse's action*. Orlando (1961/1990) includes "only what she [the nurse] says or does with or for the benefit of the patient" as professional nursing action (p. 60). The nurse must be certain that her action is appropriate to meet the patient's need for help. Orlando's principle for guiding nursing action states, "The nurse initiates a process of exploration to ascertain how the patient is affected by what she says or does" (p. 67).

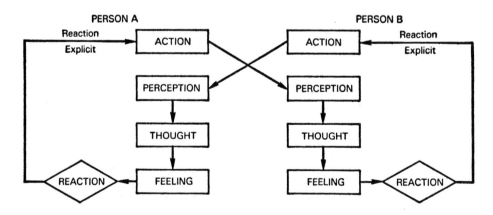

Figure 10–2. The action process in a person-to-person contact functioning by open disclosure. The perceptions, thoughts, and feelings of each individual are directly available to the perception of the other individual through the observable action. (*From Orlando, I. J. (1972). The discipline and teaching of nursing process, New York: G. P. Putnam's Sons, p. 26. Used with permission.*)

The nurse can act in two ways: automatic or deliberative. Only the second manner fulfills her professional function. Automatic actions are "those decided upon for reasons other than the patient's immediate need," whereas deliberative actions ascertain and meet this need (Orlando, 1961/1990, p. 60). There is a distinction between the purpose an action actually serves and its intention to help the patient. For example, a nurse administers a sleeping pill because the physician orders it. Carrying out the physician's order is the purpose of the action. However, the nurse has not determined that the patient is having trouble sleeping or that a pill is the most appropriate way to help him sleep. Thus, the action is automatic, not deliberative, and the patient's need for help is unlikely to be met. The following list identifies the criteria for deliberative actions:

1. Deliberative actions result from the correct identification of patient needs by validation of the nurse's reaction to patient behavior.
2. The nurse explores the meaning of the action with the patient and its relevance to meeting his need.
3. The nurse validates the action's effectiveness immediately after completing it.
4. The nurse is free of stimuli unrelated to the patient's need when she acts.

Automatic actions fail to meet one or more of these criteria. Automatic actions are most likely to be done by nurses primarily concerned with carrying out physicians' orders, routines of patient care, or general principles for protecting health or by nurses who do not validate their reactions to patient behaviors. Although any nursing action may be purported to have occurred with the intention of helping the patient, deliberation is needed to determine if the action achieved its purpose and to identify if the patient was helped.

Professional Function

Nurses often work within organizations with other professionals and are subject to the authority of the organization that employs them. It is inevitable, therefore, that at times conflicts will arise between the actions appropriate to the nurse's profession and those required by the job. Nonprofessional actions can prevent the nurse from carrying out her professional function, and this can lead to inadequate patient care. A well-defined function of the profession can help to prevent and resolve this conflict.

Ideally, nurses should not accept positions that do not allow them to meet their patients' needs for help. If a conflict does arise, the nurse must present data to show that nursing is unable to fulfill its professional function. Orlando (1972) believes that an employer is unlikely to continue to require job activities that interfere with a well-defined function of a profession. For an agency to do so "would be to completely abandon the whole point of having enlisted the services of that profession in the agency or institution" (p. 16).

Nurses must be constantly aware that their "activity is professional only when it deliberately achieves the purpose of helping the patient" (Orlando, 1961/1990,

p. 70). Some automatic activities may be necessary to the running of an institution. These should, however, be kept to a minimum and should be carried out as much as possible by support personnel. The nurse must attend to helping patients resolve any conflict between these routines and their needs for help.

In many health care institutions the potential demand for nursing skill and judgment exceeds the availability of such qualities. As a result, nursing care delivery systems may be evaluated and revised to enable the nurse to practice in those situations or areas where she is most needed. Some of these situations are reflected in the accreditation standards of the Joint Commission on Accreditation for Health Care Organizations. These include nursing assessment at the time of admission (identify the need for help); planning and delivery of patient education (deliberative action to meet the need); and preparation for discharge (verifying that the need has been met). In each of these situations, the use of Orlando's theory would guide the nurse in expeditiously meeting the patient's need. Nurses in acute care facilities are expected to use their professional skills and knowledge to recognize and resolve the patient's need for help. Some of this recognition of the nursing contribution may be related to the situational pressures arising out of the prospective payment reimbursement system in place in health care institutions. Under this system, emphasis is placed on the patient being treated and discharged within a predetermined number of days or cost of care. Nursing can capitalize on this situation and use it to the patient's and profession's best interests. Orlando's theory, although simple in nature, provides direction and focus for identifying, understanding, and meeting the patient's need in a potentially cost-effective manner. If the needs identified by the patient are met, then less nursing time should be involved than if the nurse uses primarily automatic actions and must provide additional care when the need has not been met.

Thus, the nursing process discipline is set in motion by a patient behavior that may indicate a need for help. The nurse reacts to this behavior with perceptions, thoughts, and feelings. She shares an aspect of her reaction with the patient, making sure that her verbal and nonverbal actions are consistent with her reaction, that she identifies the reaction as her own, and that she invites the patient to comment on the validity of her reaction. A properly shared reaction by the nurse helps the patient to use the same process to more effectively communicate his need. Next, an appropriate action to resolve the need is mutually decided on by the patient and nurse. After the nurse acts, she immediately asks the patient if the action has been effective. Throughout the interaction, the nurse makes sure that she is free of any extraneous stimuli that interfere with her reaction to the patient.

ORLANDO'S THEORY AND NURSING'S METAPARADIGM

Orlando includes material specific to three of the four major concepts: the human, health, and nursing. The fourth concept, society, is not included in her theory.

She uses the concept of *human* as she emphasizes individuality and the dynamic nature of the nurse–patient relationship. For Orlando, humans in need are the focus of nursing practice.

Although *health* is not specified by Orlando, it is implied. In her initial work, Orlando focused on illness. Later, she indicated that nursing deals with the individual whenever there is a need for help. Thus, a sense of helplessness replaces the concept of health or illness as the initiator of a need for nursing.

Orlando largely ignores *society*. She deals only with the interaction between a nurse and a patient in an immediate situation and speaks to the importance of individuality. She does discuss the overall nursing system in an institutional setting. However, she does not discuss how the patient is affected by the society in which he lives nor does she use society as a focus of nursing action. It is possible the immediate need could involve persons other than the patient. However, Orlando does not discuss nursing action with families or groups.

Nursing is, of course, the focus of Orlando's work. She speaks of nursing as unique and independent in its concerns for an individual's need for help in an immediate situation. The efforts to meet the individual's need for help are carried out in an interactive situation and in a disciplined manner that requires proper training.

COMPARISON OF ORLANDO'S PROCESS DISCIPLINE AND THE NURSING PROCESS

Orlando's nursing process discipline may be compared with the nursing process described in Chapter 2. Figure 10–3 helps to guide this comparison.

Certain overall characteristics are similar in both processes. For example, both are interpersonal in nature and require interaction between patient and nurse. The patient is asked for input throughout the process. Both processes also view the patient as a

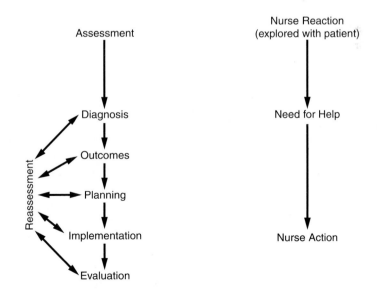

Figure 10–3. Comparison of Orlando's process with the nursing process.

total person. He is not merely a disease process or body part. Orlando does not use the term *holistic*, but she effectively describes a holistic approach. Both processes are also used as a method to provide nursing care and as a means to evaluate that care. Finally, both are deliberate intellectual processes.

The *assessment* phase of the nursing process corresponds to the sharing of the nurse reaction to the patient behavior in Orlando's process discipline. Patient behavior initiates the assessment. The collection of data includes only information relevant to identifying the patient's need for help. An ongoing database is not useful to the immediate situation of the patient. The nurse's reaction, however, is probably influenced by her past experiences with the patient and other patients.

Orlando (1961/1990) discusses data collection in her first book, *The dynamic nurse–patient relationship*. She defines observation as "any information pertaining to a patient which the nurse acquires while she is on duty" (p. 31). Direct data are comprised of "any perception, thought, or feeling the nurse has from her own experience of the patient's behavior at any or several moments in time" (p. 32). Indirect data come from sources other than the patient, such as records, other health team members, or the patient's significant others. Both types of data require exploration with the patient to determine their relevance to the specific situation. Both verbal and nonverbal patient behaviors are important. Their consistency or inconsistency is a data piece in itself. This corresponds somewhat with subjective and objective data in the nursing process.

The sharing of the nurse's reaction in Orlando's process discipline has components similar to the analysis in the nursing process. Although the nurse's reaction is automatic, her awareness of it and the way she shares it is a deliberate intellectual activity. Orlando's sharing of the reaction, however, is a process of exploration with the patient. The nursing process, on the other hand, makes use of nursing's theoretical base and principles from the physical and behavioral sciences.

The product of the analysis in the nursing process is the *nursing diagnosis*. Exploration of the nurse's reaction with the patient in Orlando's process discipline leads to identification of his need for help. The statement of the nursing diagnosis is a more formal process than that of need. Many nursing diagnoses may be made, given priority ratings, and resolved over time. Orlando deals with immediate nurse–patient interaction; only one need is dealt with at a time.

The *outcomes and planning* phases of the nursing process involve writing outcomes, goals, and objectives and deciding on appropriate nursing action. This corresponds to the nurse's action phase of Orlando's process discipline. Any outcome beyond the immediate situation is not likely in Orlando's process discipline. Her goal is always relief of the patient's need for help; the objective relates to improvement in the patient's behavior. The nursing process mandates a more formal action of writing and giving priority to goals and objectives.

Both processes require patient participation in determining the appropriate action. In the nursing process this participation occurs mostly in identification of outcomes and goal setting. Outcomes are based on mutual decision making of what the patient wants to change. This is similar in both processes and begins the nurse action phase. Orlando's process discipline sees the patient as an active participant in determining the actual nurse action. The nursing process, on the other hand, relies more heavily on scientific principles and nursing theories in deciding how the nurse will act.

Implementation involves the final selection and carrying out of the planned action and is also part of the nurse's action phase of Orlando's process discipline. Both processes mandate that the action be appropriate for the patient as a unique individual. The nursing process expects the nurse to consider all possible effects of the action on the patient. Orlando's process discipline is concerned only with the effectiveness of the action in resolving the immediate need for help.

Evaluation is inherent in Orlando's action phase of her process discipline. For an action to be deliberative, the nurse must evaluate its effectiveness when it is completed. Failure to evaluate can result in a series of ineffective actions including failure to meet the patient's need and an increase in the cost of nursing care and materials.

Evaluation in both processes is based on objective criteria. In the nursing process, evaluation asks whether the outcome was achieved. In Orlando's process discipline, the nurse observes patient behavior to see whether the patient has been helped. Thus, both processes evaluate in terms of outcomes of care.

Both the nursing process and Orlando's process discipline are described as a series of sequential steps. The steps do not actually occur discretely and in order in either process. As new information becomes available, earlier steps may be repeated. Thus, new assessment data may alter the nursing diagnosis or the plan. Orlando's process discipline is almost a continuous interchange in which patient behavior leads to nurse reaction, which leads to nurse behavior, which leads to patient reaction (see Figs. 10–2 and 10–3). Thus, both processes are dynamic and responsive to changes in the patient's situation.

The six-step nursing process used today and Orlando's process discipline have many similarities. They do, however, have important differences. The nursing process is far more formal and has more detailed phases than does Orlando's process discipline. The nursing process requires the nurse to use her knowledge of scientific principles and nursing theory to guide her behavior. Orlando demands only that the nurse follow the principles she lays down to guide nursing care. Long-term planning is part of the nursing process but is not relevant to Orlando's process discipline. Although both processes call for patient involvement in his care, Orlando's demands this participation more comprehensively.

An example of Orlando's process follows:

> **Case Situation**: One of your patients is Jeremy Isaac, a 20-year-old college senior. This is Jeremy's first postoperative day after exploratory abdominal surgery that resulted in a splenectomy. He is an athlete and has been having abdominal muscle spasms. These spasms have been well controlled with his pain medication and a muscle relaxant. His vital signs have been stable and he does not yet have bowel sounds. He has expressed a clear preference for the room temperature to be no greater than 72° F. He has been resting comfortably at this temperature. Within the last hour, a new admission has been placed in the other bed in Jeremy's room. This patient is an 80-year-old man who has noisily and frequently complained since his admission that the room is too cold. You have just entered the room.

Patient behavior: Jeremy is moving restlessly in his bed. Previously, he was sleeping.

Nurse's reaction: You perceive that Jeremy is now restless, think that this is a change in his behavior, and feel that he may be in pain. You say to him, "It appears to me that you are uncomfortable. Do you need pain medication?" His response is, "No, I'm not in pain. I just want to sleep." At this moment, the roommate once again yells out that the room is too cold. You quietly ask Jeremy if that is what is keeping him awake and Jeremy nods yes, thus validating your perception that the most recent dose of pain medication is still effective and the disturbance is the noisy roommate.

Nurse's action: You arrange for the roommate to be moved into another room with a patient closer to his age. Within 30 minutes of taking this deliberative action you note that Jeremy is once again resting quietly, thus validating that the action was effective.

CRITIQUE OF ORLANDO'S NURSING PROCESS DISCIPLINE

1. What is the historical context of the theory? Orlando's disciplined nursing process was developed from research conducted on nursing practice, as discussed earlier in this chapter. Orlando's research was being conducted during the same time that Henderson was developing her components and definition of nursing and Wiedenbach was developing her prescriptive theory of nursing. All of these theorists were at Yale. The observations from the original research were divided into "good" and "bad" nursing and the disciplined sharing of the nurse's reaction was identified as the primary difference between good and bad nursing. Orlando's nursing process discipline is easy to understand and is needs based.

2. What are the basic concepts and relationships presented by the theory? Nursing is presented as a unique, independent, and disciplined profession. Nursing functions to meet the immediate need that is demonstrated by the patient's behavior. The nurse's reaction to the patient's behavior (perception, thought, feeling) is shared with the patient in order to validate, or correct, the accuracy of that reaction. This disciplined nursing process leads to deliberative nursing actions taken to meet the patient's need. Automatic actions may be taken for reasons other than meeting the patient's immediate need. This interactive process requires training for the nurse to be effective.

3. What major phenomena of concern to nursing are presented? There phenomenon may include *but are not limited to*: human being, environment, health, interpersonal relations, caring, goal attainment, adaptation, and energy fields. The phenomena of concern to nursing presented in Orlando's theory include the human being, interactive communication, immediate need, validation, and deliberative actions. She also describes nursing as unique, independent, and disciplined. These have been discussed within this chapter.

4. To whom does it apply? In what situations? In what ways? This theory applies to anyone with an immediate need who is in contact with a nurse. The situations are limited only by the requirements of the presence of a nurse and a person with an immediate need. The requirement for the need to be immediate does limit the application for long-term needs, anticipatory guidance, or education when the need is not recognized by the person, and for most planning situations. This does not mean Orlando's work cannot be used in long-term care settings but that the focus would be on the patient's immediate need rather than on long-term goals. Rosenthal (1996) has described the beneficial use of this theory in the perioperative setting.

Other situations in which the theory may be used are those in which the nurse is functioning as a leader or manager. In these situations, another nurse or staff member will be the person in need. The effectiveness of this theory in nursing leadership has been supported by Schmeiding (1988, 1990a, 1990c, 1991), Sheafor (1991), and Laurent (2000).

5. By what method or methods can this theory be tested? This theory was derived from initial research that used a qualitative, observational methodology. Orlando's second research project was quantitative in nature as it used statistical analysis. However, this second study focused on the effects on nursing outcomes of teaching the disciplined process to nurses rather than on manipulating nurse–patient interactions. With the strong support received for the effectiveness of the disciplined nursing process, it would not be ethical to use a true experimental model in which one group of patients was assigned to receive only nursing care that has been delivered based solely on the nurse's reaction rather than on the validation of that reaction with the patient.

Research studies reported in the literature have used a variety of quasi- and non-experimental methods to study this theory. Potter and Bockenhauer (2000) used a quasi-experimental method to support positive outcomes in decreasing patients' levels of distress. Ellis (1999) used a quantitative survey to identify barriers experienced by registered nurses in the emergency department in relation to screening for domestic violence. Haggerty (1987), using videotaped patient situations, found that the type of patient distress was more predictive of the response of senior nursing students than was the type of educational program in which the students were enrolled (associate degree or baccalaureate). Ponte (1988) investigated the relationship between nurses' empathy skills and patient distress in adult cancer patients. Ponte found a positive relationship between empathy skills and use of Orlando's deliberative process. However, she also found that while nurses scored low in the use of empathy skills as well as in the use of the deliberative nursing process, the patients demonstrated low levels of distress.

The most common research methodology has been descriptive correlational. Olson (1993) and Olson and Hanchett (1997) investigated the relationships between nurse-expressed empathy and the outcomes of patient perception of empathy and patient distress. They found a statistically significant negative relationship between nurse-expressed empathy and patient distress as well as between patient-perceived empathy and patient distress. The relationship between nurse-expressed empathy

and patient perception of empathy was moderately positive and statistically significant. Schmieding (1987, 1988, 1990a, 1990b, 1990c, 1991) has proposed a model
for exploring the relationship between the responses of nurse administrators and the
actions of staff nurses and reported several descriptive correlational studies conducted using the model. She has found that administrators often respond in ways
that prevent staff participation in problem solving, which may limit the development of inquiry skills in staff nurses but that many staff nurses preferred not being
included in the identification of problems (Schmieding, 1990a, 1990c). In studying
the relationship between the responses of head nurses and staff responses to patients, she found a positive relationship with little influence from the characteristics
of the nurses or the size of the hospital (Schmieding, 1991). The primary mode of
response was the one termed nonexploratory by Schmieding. This response parallels Orlando's automatic actions.

6. Does this theory direct critical thinking in nursing practice? Critical thinking is absolutely necessary in using Orlando's disciplined nursing process. The
nurse must collect data (the patient's behavior), analyze it (the nurse's reaction),
and choose how to share the reaction while claiming ownership of that reaction.
Once the nurse and patient have validated the patient's need, they then must decide
what should be done to meet that need. The nurse takes the action they have decided
on (deliberative action) and then seeks to verify that the action taken has met the
need. Critical thinking is involved in each of these steps.

7. Does this theory direct therapeutic nursing interventions? The purpose of
the nursing process discipline is for deliberative nursing actions to be taken to meet
the patient's immediate need. If the need is met, the nursing interventions were therapeutic, the patient outcomes are positive. Potter and Bockenhauer (2000) and
Rosenthal (1996) speak to the positive effect of the use of the nursing process discipline on patient outcomes.

8. Does this theory direct communication in nursing practice? Communication is imperative for the success of the nursing process discipline. The discipline
described by Orlando is for the nurse to share the nurse reaction with the patient in
order to identify the match between the patient's behavior and the nurse's interpretation of that behavior. The interaction that evolves as this validation is occurring is
based in, and dependent on, communication. Orlando not only supports the importance of communication, but also indicates the content of the nurse's communication about the patient's behavior, along with guidelines for that content.

9. Does this theory direct nursing actions that lead to favorable outcomes? As
previously discussed, Potter and Bockenhauer (2000) supported that the use of the
disciplined nursing process leads to positive patient outcomes. Deliberative nursing
actions are taken for the purpose of meeting the patient's identified immediate need.
The outcomes of these actions must be favorable or the need has not been met and
new actions must be selected. Automatic nursing actions may or may not lead to favorable outcomes and do not require that the nurse validate the effectiveness of the

actions. Orlando's disciplined nursing process indicates that nursing actions should not be taken until the patient's need has been validated and the planned actions are agreed on between the nurse and the patient as being appropriate to meet the need.

10. How contagious is this theory? This use of this theory has been documented in clinical practice, nursing administration, and nursing education. It has been used primarily in the United States. An electronic search did locate two references from Japan (Ikeda, 1975; Kawakami, Kawashima, Hirao, Yamane, & Kosaka, 1972). Also, Olson and Hanchett (1977) have reported its use in Canada. Thus, the theory is contagious as to the areas of nursing in which it can be used, but the literature does not support that it has been widely contagious in any particular area of practice or throughout the world.

STRENGTHS AND LIMITATIONS

Orlando's theory has much to offer to nursing. The predominant strength of her work is its usefulness in nursing practice. It guides nurses through their interactions with patients. Use of her theory virtually assures that patients will be treated as individuals and that they will have an active and constant input into their own care. The nurse's focus must remain on the patient rather than on the demands of the work setting. Use of the process discipline helps the nurse deal with her personal reactions and leads her to value her own individuality as a thinking person.

The nurse can keep Orlando in mind while applying the nursing process. Use of her theory prevents inaccurate diagnosis or ineffective plans because the nurse has to constantly explore her reactions with the patient. No nurse, following Orlando's principles, could fail to evaluate the care she has given.

Another of Orlando's strengths is her assertion of nursing's independence as a profession and her belief that this independence must be based on a sound theoretical framework. She bases this belief on her definition of nursing function. She believes that this clearly defined function will assist nursing in establishing its independence and in structuring the work setting so that nurses can effectively meet their patients' needs for help. The function of finding and meeting the patient's immediate need for help is broad enough to encompass nurses practicing in all settings and in all specialty areas. It allows nursing to evolve over time by avoiding a rigid list of nursing activities.

Orlando guides the nurse to evaluate her care in terms of objectively observable patient outcomes. It is not the structure of the setting or the number of nurses on duty that determines effective care. Orlando and others have found a positive relationship between the use of her process and favorable outcomes of patient behavior. The immediate and interactive nature of her process does, however, make evaluation a time-consuming process.

As previously alluded to, the nursing profession's input into accreditation standards for health care organizations has placed great emphasis on the evaluation of interventions in terms of patient outcomes. Consistent use of Orlando's theory by nurses could make evaluation a less time-consuming and more deliberate function, the results of which would be documented in patient charts. Such documentation of patient needs, planned interventions, and evaluation of interventions would provide data for analysis that would contribute to the general body of knowledge within the field of nursing.

Orlando's testing of her theory in the practice setting lends further support to its usefulness. Her first study, published in *The dynamic nurse–patient relationship*, provided a basis for future work. For a second study, described in *The discipline and teaching of the nursing process*, she developed specific criteria amenable to statistical testing. Nursing can pursue Orlando's work by retesting and further developing her work.

Orlando's mental health background is probably responsible for the highly interactive nature of her theory. Although this interactive nature is one of the theory's strengths, it also provides limitation in her ideas. Nurses deal extensively with monitoring and controlling the physiological processes of patients to prevent illness and restore health. Orlando scarcely mentions this aspect of the nurse's role other than to question if monitoring machines is practicing nursing. The decidedly interactive nature of Orlando's theory makes it hard to include the highly technical and physical care that nurses give in certain settings, such as intensive care units. Her theory does, however, prevent the nurse from forgetting the patient in her efforts to fulfill the technical aspects of her job.

Orlando's theory is also limited by its focus on interaction with an individual, whereas the patient should be viewed as a member of a family and within a community. Often it is vital to deal with the family as a whole to help the patient. Orlando does not deal with these areas.

Long-term care and planning are not applicable to Orlando's focus on the immediate situation. She views long-term planning only as it is related to adequate staffing within an institution. Orlando herself recognizes this problem. In *The dynamic nurse–patient relationship* she speculated that "repeated experiences of having been helped undoubtedly culminate over periods of time in greater degrees of improvement" (p. 90). She also identified the cumulative effect of nursing as an area for further study.

In *The discipline and teaching of nursing process*, Orlando sought to define the entire nursing system. She described the system as the "regularly, interacting parts of a nursing service" (p. 18). This part of her theory attempts to incorporate nurses' relationships with other nurses and with members of different professions in the job setting. Her theory struggles with the authority derived from the function of the profession and that of the employing institution's commitment to the public. The same process is offered for dealing with others as for working with an individual patient.

When a nurse–manager deals with staff, Orlando's theory provides a framework for an interaction that leads to a positive result. As the nurse executive listens to the needs of the staff, she must decide if deliberate action is needed; such action may take the form of a policy or procedure change, staffing variation, or institutional policy change. The nurse executive may need to influence another department, group, or level within the organization to effect a positive intervention with staff. On the administrative level, Orlando's theory is used, but the time span needed to complete all components varies depending on the situations. An organization that consistently and methodically uses Orlando's theory can positively respond to all issues that need to be confronted. In such an environment, needs can be met and emphasis placed on the present rather than the past or the way it has always been done. Thus, the organization is able to maintain its competitive edge.

Orlando can be considered a nursing theorist who made a significant contribution to the advancement of nursing practice. She helped nurses to focus on the patient rather than on the disease or institutional demands. The nurse is firmly viewed as the handmaiden of the patient, not of the physician. Nurses must base their practice on logical thinking rather than on intuition. Orlando's nursing process discipline continues to be useful to nurses in their interactions with patients.

SUMMARY

Orlando's nursing process discipline is rooted in the interaction between a nurse and a patient at a specific time and place. A sequence of interchanges involving patient behavior and nurse reaction takes place until the patient's need for help, as he perceives it, is clarified. The nurse then decides on an appropriate action to resolve the need in cooperation with the patient. This action is evaluated after it is carried out. If the patient behavior improves, the action was successful, the desired outcomes were achieved, and the process is completed. If there is no change or the behavior gets worse, the process recycles with new efforts to clarify the patient's behavior or the appropriate nursing action. Orlando (1961/1990) summarizes her process as follows:

> A deliberative nursing process has elements of continuous reflection as the nurse tries to understand the meaning to the patient of the behavior she observes and what he needs from her in order to be helped. Responses comprising this process are stimulated by the nurse's unfolding awareness of the particulars of the individual situation. (p. 67)

REFERENCES

Ellis, J. M. (1999). Barriers to effective screening for domestic violence by registered nurses in the emergency department. *Critical Care Nursing Quarterly, 22*(1), 27–41.

Haggerty, L. A. (1987). An analysis of senior nursing students' immediate response to distressed patients. *Journal of Advanced Nursing, 12,* 451–461.

Harmer, B., & Henderson, V. (1955). *Textbook of the principles and practice of nursing* (5th ed.). New York: Macmillan.

Ikeda, S. (1975). [Ms. Ida Jean Orlando's nursing theory and my own concepts] (Japanese). *Kango (KUI), 27*(10), 30–35.

Kayakami, T., Kawashima, M., Hirao, H., Yamane, M., & Kosaka, F. (1972). [Nursing theory for nurses. 8. On Orlando's "Nursing Research"](Japanese). *Kangogaku Zasshi (KNM), 36,* 1018–1022.

Laurent, C. L. (2000). A nursing theory for nursing leadership. *Journal of Nursing Management, 8,* 83–87.

Olson, J. K. (1993). Relationships between nurse expressed empathy, patient perceived empathy and patient distress. *Dissertation Abstracts International, 55–02B*, 0369. (University Microfilms No. AAG9418218).

Olson, J., & Hanchett, E. (1997). Nurse-expressed empathy, patient outcomes, and development of a middle-range theory. *Image: Journal of Nursing Scholarship, 29*, 71–76.

Orlando, I. J. (1972). *The discipline and teaching of nursing process.* New York: G. P. Putnam's Sons. (out of print)

Orlando, I. J. (1987). Nursing in the 21st century: Alternate paths. *Journal of Advanced Nursing, 12*, 405–412.

Orlando, I. J. (1990). *The dynamic nurse–patient relationship: Function, process and principles.* New York: National League for Nursing. (Reprinted from 1961, New York: G. P. Putnam's Sons.)

Pelletier, I. O. (1967). The patient's predicament and nursing function. *Psychiatric Opinion, 4*, 25–30.

Peplau, H. E. (1988). *Interpersonal relations in nursing.* London: Macmillan Education. (Original work published 1952, New York: G. P. Putnam's Sons).

Ponte, P. A. R. (1988). The relationships among empathy and the use of Orlando's deliberative process by the primary nurse and the distress of the adult cancer patient. *Dissertation Abstracts International, 50–07B*, 2848. (University Microfilms No. AAG8916380).

Potter, M. L., & Bockenhauer, B. J. (2000). Implementing Orlando's nursing theory: A pilot study. *Journal of Psychosocial Nursing and Mental Health Services, 38*(3), 14–21.

Rosenthal, B. C. (1996). An interactionist's approach to perioperative nursing. *Association of Operating Room Nurses Journal, 64*, 254–260.

Schmieding, N. J. (1987). Analysing managerial responses in face-to-face contacts . . . Orlando's theory. *Journal of Advanced Nursing, 12*, 357–365.

Schmieding, N. J. (1988). Action process of nurse administrators to problematic situations based on Orlando's theory. *Journal of Advanced Nursing, 13*, 99–107.

Schmieding, N. J. (1990a). A model for assessing nurse administrators' actions. *Western Journal of Nursing Research, 12*, 293–306.

Schmieding, N. J. (1990b). An integrative nursing theoretical framework. *Journal of Advanced Nursing, 15*, 463–467.

Schmieding, N. J. (1990c). Do head nurses include staff nurses in problem-solving? *Nursing Management, 21*(3), 58–60.

Schmieding, N. J. (1991). Relationship between head nurses responses to staff nurses and staff nurse responses to patients. *Western Journal of Nursing Research, 13*, 746–760.

Sheafor, M. (1991). Productive work groups in complex hospital units: Proposed contributions of the nurse executive. *Journal of Nursing Administration, 21*(5), 25–30.

Trench, A. S. (Executive producer), Wallace, D. (Producer), & Coberg, T. (Director). (1987). *Ida Jean Orlando—The nurse theorists: Portraits of excellence* [Videotape]. Oakland, CA: Studio Three Production, Samuel Merritt College of Nursing.

CHAPTER 11

THE PRESCRIPTIVE THEORY OF NURSING
ERNESTINE WIEDENBACH*

Agnes M. Bennett
Peggy Coldwell Foster

■ ■ ■

Ernestine Wiedenbach was born in Germany in 1900 to an affluent family. Her family came to the United States during her early childhood. She graduated from Wellesley College, Wellesley, Massachusetts, in 1922 with a liberal arts degree. Her interest in nursing had been stimulated by the care given her ailing grandmother and the stories told by a medical student friend of her sister. Nickel, Gesse, and MacLaren (1992) reported that, much to the distress of her family, she enrolled in the Post Graduate Hospital School of Nursing. She was expelled from this program after she served as the spokesperson for student grievances. Adelaide Nutting arranged for Wiedenbach to continue her nursing preparation at the Johns Hopkins School of Nursing, Baltimore, Maryland, but only after she agreed that she would neither organize nor encourange any student dissent. She received her nursing diploma from Johns Hopkins in 1925. Since she held a bachelor's degree she was offered supervisory positions after graduation and worked at Johns Hopkins and at Bellevue in New York City. She attended night classes and received her master's degree and a certificate in public health nursing from Teachers College, Columbia University, New York, in 1934. For a time she worked with the Association for Improving Conditions of the Poor from the Henry Street Settlement. She then became a professional writer with the Nursing Information Bureau of the American Journal of Nursing *where she also worked to prepare nurses to enter World War II. She was unable to serve overseas due to a minor cardiac problem. Interested in returning to patient care, Wiedenbach obtained a certificate in nurse midwifery from the Maternity Center Association in New York in 1946. She practiced as a nurse midwife and a public health nurse, and taught in a number of schools of nursing. She was an Associate Professor Emeritus from Yale University School of Nursing where she had been director of the graduate program in maternal-newborn health nursing. She served as a visiting professor at*

---

*Wiedenbach consistently uses the term *patient* and refers to the nurse as *her* in her writings. This approach will be used in this chapter.

California State University, Los Angeles, and at the College of Nursing, University of Florida, Gainesville. In 1978, she received the Hattie Hemschemeyer award from the American College of Nurse Midwives for exceptional achievements in her professional life (Burst, 1979). Ernestine Wiedenbach died in April 1999 in Florida.

Ernestine Wiedenbach, a progressive nursing leader, began her nursing career in the 1920s. Wiedenbach first published *Family-centered maternity nursing* in 1958. It is of interest that in that book she recommended that babies be in hospital rooms with their mothers rather than in a central nursery. This innovative concept was not widely implemented until 20 years later. In 1964 she wrote *Clinical nursing—A helping art*, in which she described her ideas about nursing as a "concept and philosophy" derived from 40 years of nursing experience. She credited Patricia James, James Dickoff, and Ida Orlando Pelletier as great influences in her nursing writing and theory development. In collaboration with Dickoff and James, she presented the symposium and co-authored, "Theory in a practice discipline" (1968a, 1968b). In 1970 Wiedenbach defined the essentials of her prescriptive theory in "Nurses' wisdom in nursing theory."

According to Ernestine Wiedenbach (1964), nursing is nurturing and caring for someone in a motherly fashion. That care is given in the immediate present and can be given by any caring person. Nursing is a helping service that is rendered with compassion, skill, and understanding to those in need of care, counsel, and confidence in the area of health (Wiedenbach, 1977).

Nursing wisdom is acquired through meaningful experience (Wiedenbach, 1964). Sensitivity alerts the nurse to an awareness of inconsistencies in a situation that might signify a problem. It is a key factor in assisting the nurse to identify the patient's need for help (Wiedenbach, 1977).

The nurse's beliefs and values regarding reverence for the gift of life, the worth of the individual, and the aspirations of each human being determine the quality of the nursing care. The nurse's purpose in nursing represents a professional commitment (Wiedenbach, 1970).

Wiedenbach (1964) states the characteristics of a professional person that are essential for the professional nurse include the following [italics added]:

1. *Clarity* of purpose.
2. *Mastery* of skills and knowledge essential for fulfilling the purpose.
3. *Ability* to establish and sustain purposeful working relationships with others, both professional and nonprofessional individuals.
4. *Interest* in advancing knowledge in the area of interest and in creating new knowledge.
5. *Dedication* to furthering the good of mankind rather than to self-aggrandizement (p. 2).

The practice of nursing comprises a wide variety of services, each directed toward the attainment of one of its three components: (1) *identification* of the patient's need for help, (2) *ministration* of the help needed, and (3) *validation* that the help provided was indeed helpful to the patient (Wiedenbach, 1977). Within Wiedenbach's (1964) "identification of the patient's need for help," she presents three principles of helping: (1) the principle of inconsistency/consistency, (2) the principle of purposeful perseverance, and (3) the principle of self-extension. The *principle of inconsistency/consistency* refers to the assessment of the patient to determine some action, word, or appearance that is different from that expected—that is, something out of the ordinary for this patient. It is important for the nurse to observe the patient astutely and then critically analyze her observations. The *principle of purposeful perseverance* is based on the nurse's sincere desire to help the patient. The nurse needs to strive to continue her efforts to identify and meet the patient's need for help in spite of difficulties she encounters while seeking to use her resources and capabilities effectively and with sensitivity. The *principle of self-extension* recognizes that each nurse has limitations that are both personal and situational. It is important that she recognize when these limitations are reached and that she seek help from others, including through prayer.

WIEDENBACH'S PRESCRIPTIVE THEORY

Theory may be described as a system of conceptualizations invented to some purpose. Prescriptive theory (a situation-producing theory) may be described as one that conceptualizes both a desired situation and the prescription by which it is to be brought about. Thus, a prescriptive theory directs action toward an explicit goal. Wiedenbach's (1969) prescriptive theory is made up of three factors, or concepts, (see Fig. 11–1) [italics added]:

1. The *central purpose* which the practitioner recognizes as essential to the particular discipline.
2. The *prescription* for the fulfillment of the central purpose.
3. The *realities in the immediate situation* that influence the fulfillment of the central purpose (p. 2).

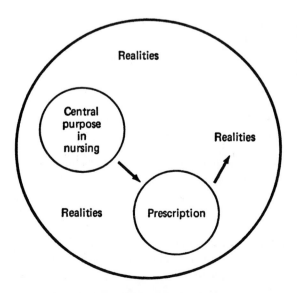

Figure 11–1. Wiedenbach's prescriptive theory. (*Adapted from Wiedenbach, E. (1969).* Meeting the realities in clinical teaching, *New York: Springer, p. x. Used with permission.*)

The Central Purpose

The nurse's central purpose defines the quality of health she desires to effect or sustain in her patient and specifies what she recognizes to be her special responsibility in caring for the patient (Wiedenbach, 1970). This central purpose (or commitment) is based on the individual nurse's philosophy. Wiedenbach (1964) states:

> Purpose and philosophy are, respectively, goal and guide of clinical nursing. . . . Purpose—that which the nurse wants to accomplish through what she does—is the overall goal toward which she is striving, and so is constant. It is her reason for being and doing. . . . Philosophy, an attitude toward life and reality that evolves from each nurse's beliefs and code of conduct, motivates the nurse to act, guides her thinking about what she is to do and influences her decisions. It stems from both her culture and subculture, and is an integral part of her. It is personal in character, unique to each nurse, and expressed in her *way* of nursing. Philosophy underlies purpose, and purpose reflects philosophy (p. 13).

Wiedenbach (1970) identifies three essential components for a nursing philosophy: (1) a reverence for the gift of life, (2) a respect for the dignity, worth, autonomy, and individuality of each human being, and (3) a resolution to act dynamically in relation to one's beliefs. Any of these concepts might be further developed. However, Wiedenbach (1964, 1970) emphasizes the second in her work, formulating the following beliefs about the individual:

1. Human beings are endowed with unique potential to develop within themselves the resources that enable them to maintain and sustain themselves.
2. Human beings basically strive toward self-direction and relative independence, and desire not only to make the best use of their capabilities and potentialities but also to fulfill their responsibilities.
3. Human beings need stimulation in order to make the best use of their capabilities and realize their self-worth.
4. Whatever individuals do represents their best judgment at the moment of doing it.
5. Self-awareness and self-acceptance are essential to the individual's sense of integrity and self-worth.

Thus, the central purpose is a concept the nurse has thought through—one she has put into words, believes in, and accepts as a standard against which to measure the value of her action to the patient. It is based on her philosophy and suggests the nurse's reason for being, the mission she believes is hers to accomplish (Wiedenbach, 1970).

The Prescription

Once the nurse has identified her own philosophy and recognizes that the patient has autonomy and individuality, she can work *with* the individual to develop a *prescription* or plan for his or her care.

A *prescription* is a directive to activity (Wiedenbach, 1969). It "specifies both the *nature of the action* that will most likely lead to fulfillment of the nurse's central purpose and the *thinking process* that determines it" (Wiedenbach, 1970, p. 1059). A prescription may indicate the broad general action appropriate to implementation of the basic concepts as well as suggest the kind of behavior needed to carry out these actions in accordance with the central purpose. These actions may be voluntary or involuntary. Voluntary action is an intended response, whereas involuntary action is an unintended response.

A prescription is a directive to at least three kinds of voluntary action: (1) *mutually understood and agreed upon* action ("the practitioner has . . . evidence that the recipient understands the implications of the intended action and is psychologically, physically and/or physiologically receptive to it."); (2) *recipient-directed* action ("the recipient of the action essentially directs the way it is to be carried out."); and (3) *practitioner-directed* action ("the practitioner carries out the action . . . .") (Wiedenbach, 1969, p. 3). Once the nurse has formulated a central purpose and has accepted it as a personal commitment, she not only has established the prescription for her nursing but also is ready to implement it (Wiedenbach, 1970).

The Realities

When the nurse has determined her central purpose and has developed the prescription, she must then consider the *realities* of the situation in which she is to provide nursing care. Realities consist of all factors—physical, physiological, psychological, emotional, and spiritual—that are at play in a situation in which nursing actions occur at any given moment. Wiedenbach (1970) defines the five realities as: (1) the agent, (2) the recipient, (3) the goal, (4) the means, and (5) the framework.

The *agent*, who is the practicing nurse or her delegate, is characterized by personal attributes, capacities, capabilities, and most importantly, commitment and competence in nursing. As the agent, the nurse is the propelling force that moves her practice toward its goal. In the course of this goal-directed movement, she may engage in innumerable acts called forth by her encounter with actual or discrepant factors and situations within the realities of which she herself is a part (Wiedenbach, 1967). The agent or nurse has the following four basic responsibilities:

1. To reconcile her assumptions about the realities . . . with her central purpose.
2. To specify the objectives of her practice in terms of behavioral outcomes that are realistically attainable.
3. To practice nursing in accordance with her objectives.
4. To engage in related activities which contribute to her self-realization and to the improvement of nursing practice (Wiedenbach, 1970, p. 1060).

The *recipient*, the patient, is characterized by personal attributes, problems, capacities, aspirations, and most important, the ability to cope with the concerns or problems being experienced (Wiedenbach, 1967). The patient is the recipient of the nurse's actions or the one on whose behalf the action is taken. The patient is vulnerable, dependent on others for help, and risks losing individuality, dignity, worth, and autonomy (Wiedenbach, 1970).

The *goal* is the desired outcome the nurse wishes to achieve. The goal is the end result to be attained by nursing action. The stipulation of an activity's goal gives focus to the nurse's action and implies her reason for taking it (Wiedenbach, 1970).

The *means* comprises the activities and devices through which the practitioner is enabled to attain her goal. The means includes skills, techniques, procedures, and devices that may be used to facilitate nursing practice. The nurse's way of giving treatments, of expressing concern, of using the means available is individual and is determined by her central purpose and the prescription (Wiedenbach, 1970).

The *framework* consists of the human, environmental, professional, and organizational facilities that not only make up the context within which nursing is practiced but also constitute its currently existing limits (Wiedenbach, 1967). The framework is composed of all the extraneous factors and facilities in the situation that affect the nurse's ability to obtain the desired results. It is a conglomerate of "objects, existing or missing, such as policies, setting, atmosphere, time of day, humans, and happenings that may be current, past, or anticipated" (Wiedenbach, 1970, p. 1061).

The realities offer uniqueness to every situation. The success of professional nursing practice is dependent on them. Unless the realities are recognized and dealt with, they may prevent the achievement of the goal.

The concepts of central purpose, prescription, and realities are interdependent in Wiedenbach's theory of nursing. The nurse develops a prescription for care that is based on her central purpose, which is implemented in the realities of the situation.

WIEDENBACH'S CONCEPTUALIZATION OF NURSING PRACTICE AND PROCESS

According to Wiedenbach (1967), nursing practice is an art in which the nursing action is based on the principles of helping. Nursing action may be thought of as consisting of the following four distinct kinds of actions:

- Reflex   (spontaneous)
- Conditioned   (automatic)
- Impulsive   (impulsive)
- Deliberate   (responsible)

Nursing as a practice discipline is goal-directed. The nature of the nursing act is based on thought. The nurse thinks through the kind of results she wants, gears her actions to obtain those results, then accepts responsibility for the acts and the outcome of those acts (Wiedenbach, 1970). Since nursing requires thought, it can be considered a deliberate responsible action.

Nursing practice has three components: (1) identification of the patient's need for help, (2) ministration of the help needed, and (3) validation that the action taken was helpful to the patient (Wiedenbach, 1977). Within the identification component, there are four distinct steps. First, the nurse observes the patient, looking for an inconsistency between the expected behavior of the patient and the apparent behavior. Second, she attempts to clarify what the inconsistency means. Third, she determines the cause of the inconsistency. Finally, she validates with the patient that her help is needed.

The second component is the ministration of the help needed. In ministering to her patient, the nurse may give advice or information, make a referral, apply a comfort measure, or carry out a therapeutic procedure. Should the patient become uncomfortable with what is being done, the nurse will need to identify the cause and, if necessary, make an adjustment in the plan of action.

The third component is validation. After help has been ministered, the nurse validates that the actions were indeed helpful. Evidence must come from the patient that the purpose of the nursing actions has been fulfilled (Wiedenbach, 1964).

Wiedenbach (1977) views the nursing process essentially as an internal personalized mechanism. As such, it is influenced by the nurse's culture, purpose in nursing, knowledge, wisdom, sensitivity, and concern.

In Wiedenbach's (1977) nursing process (see Fig. 11–2), she identifies seven levels of awareness: sensation, perception, assumption, realization, insight, design, and decision. Wiedenbach's nursing process begins with an activating situation. This situation exists among the realities and serves as a stimulus to arouse the nurse's consciousness. This consciousness arousal leads to a subjective interpretation of the first three levels, which are defined as: *sensation* (experienced sensory impression), *perception* (the interpretation of a sensory impression), and *assumption* (the meaning the nurse attaches to the perception). These three levels of awareness are obtained through the focus of the nurse's attention on the stimulus; they are intuitive rather than cognitive and may initiate an involuntary response. For example, a nurse enters a patient's room and states, "My, it's hot in here!" She immediately goes to the thermostat and sets it to a lower temperature. The *sensation* is the room temperature. The *perception* is "It feels hot." The *assumption* is "If I am hot, then the patient must be hot." The involuntary response is to adjust the thermostat.

Progressing from intuition to cognition, the nurse's actions become voluntary rather than involuntary. The next four levels of awareness occur in the voluntary phase: *realization* (in which the nurse begins to validate the assumption previously made about the patient's behavior); *insight* (which includes joint planning and additional knowledge about the cause of the problem); *design* (the plan of action decided on by the nurse and confirmed by the patient); and *decision* (the nurse's performance of a responsible action) (Wiedenbach, 1977).

To continue with the previous example: The nurse asks, "Are you too warm?" and the patient replies, "No, I'm not. I have felt cold since I washed my hair." The nurse responds, "I will readjust the thermostat and get you a blanket." The patient agrees, "That would be wonderful!" The nurse readjusts the thermostat and gets a blanket for the patient.

The *realization* is the validation of the patient's perception of temperature comfort. The *insight* is the additional information that the patient had washed his or her hair. The *design* is the plan to readjust the thermostat and get a blanket as confirmed by the patient. The *decision* is the nurse readjusts the thermostat and gets a blanket for the patient.

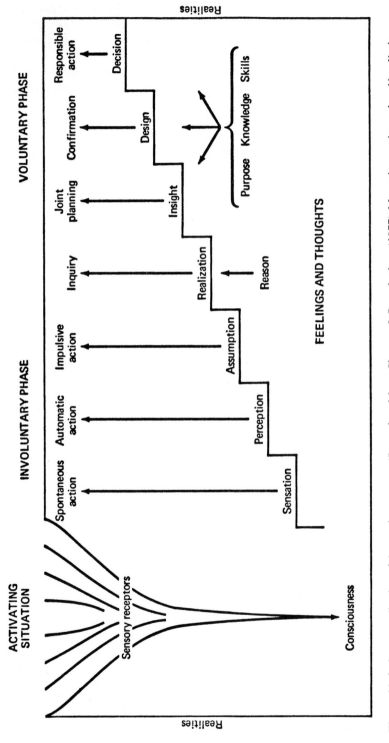

Figure 11–2. Conceptualization of the nursing process. *(Reproduced from Clausen, J. P. and others (1977). Maternity nursing today, New York: MacGraw-Hill, p. 43. Used with permission.)*

In summary, the comparison of Wiedenbach's prescriptive theory, the practice of nursing, and the nursing process as outlined in Chapter 2 of this book is as follows: In the practice of nursing, a nurse with her unique personality, philosophy, education, and life experiences (her central purpose), assesses the individual's health status and potential for development. She identifies the patient's need for help (makes a *nursing diagnosis*). She formulates a *plan* with the patient, identifying outcomes and setting goals that they will act on (*implement*). This plan or prescription and its implementation are affected by the realities, or the strengths and limitations of the situation (the *environment*). Their plan is implemented or the nurse provides the help needed. Validation is then obtained that the help provided was indeed helpful to the patient (*evaluation*).

WIEDENBACH'S THEORY AND NURSING'S METAPARADIGM

Wiedenbach (1964) emphasizes that the human or *individual* possesses unique potential, strives toward self-direction, and needs stimulation. Whatever the individual does represents his or her best judgment at the moment. Self-awareness and self-acceptance are essential to the individual's sense of integrity and self-worth. Wiedenbach believes these characteristics require respect from the nurse.

Wiedenbach (1977) does not define the concept of *health*. However, she supports the World Health Organization's definition of health as a state of complete physical, mental, and social well-being, and not merely the absence of disease and infirmity.

In Wiedenbach's work, she incorporates the *environment* within the realities—a major component of her theory. One element of the realities is the framework. According to Wiedenbach (1970), the framework is a complex of extraneous factors and circumstances that are present in every nursing situation. The framework may include objects "such as policies, setting, atmosphere, time of day, humans, and happenings" (p. 1061).

According to Wiedenbach (1969), *nursing*, a clinical discipline, is a practice discipline designed to produce explicit desired results. The art of nursing is a goal-directed activity requiring the application of knowledge and skill toward meeting a need for help experienced by a patient. Nursing is a helping process that will extend or restore the patient's ability to cope with demands implicit in the situation.

COMPARISON OF THE NURSING PROCESS WITH WIEDENBACH'S NURSING PROCESS AND NURSING PRACTICE

The comparison of the nursing process described in Chapter 2 and Wiedenbach's conceptualization of the nursing process and nursing practice yields some similarities and several significant differences (see Table 11–1). In Wiedenbach's nursing practice, the steps of (1) observation, (2) ministration of help, and (3) validation are comparable with the nursing process's phases of *assessment, implementation,* and *evaluation.*

TABLE 11–1. COMPARISON OF THE NURSING PROCESS WITH WIEDENBACH'S NURSING PROCESS AND NURSING PRACTICE

Nursing Process	Wiedenbach's Nursing Process	Wiedenbach's Nursing Practice
1. Nursing assessment	Stimulus	1. Observation
	Voluntary	
	Involuntary	
	1. Sensation	
	2. Perception	
	3. Assumption	
1.(a) Analysis and synthesis	2. Realization with reason—Inquiry	
2. Nursing Diagnosis	3. Insight—Joint planning	
3. Outcomes	4. Design—Confirmation	
4a. Goals and objectives	5. Spontaneous action	
4b. Plans	6. Automatic action	
	7. Impulsive action	2. Ministration of help
5. Implementation with scientific rationale	7 Decision with responsible action	
6. Nursing evaluation		3. Validation

Assessment, the first phase of the nursing process, considers the person holistically and requires extensive data collection. In Wiedenbach's (1977) model (see Fig. 11–3), there is a stimulus to which the nurse reacts. This stimulus produces a reaction at the level of sensation or perception. These levels are involuntary and intuitive. The nurse then makes an assumption about the situation and may act involuntarily. Such acts are spontaneous, automatic, or impulsive. They occur on the spur of the moment and are precipitated by unchecked, rampant thoughts and feelings. Occasionally in an emergency they may be lifesaving. However, these involuntary acts can frequently do more harm than good.

If the nurse makes an assumption, she might act impulsively. However, Wiedenbach (1964) points out that the nurse needs to willfully apply a strategy brake (see Fig. 11–3). This provides time for her to assemble the resources necessary for disciplined thought to control her action. This strategy brake then is applied just before Wiedenbach's realization level. At the realization level the process becomes voluntary, for the nurse uses reason and inquiry.

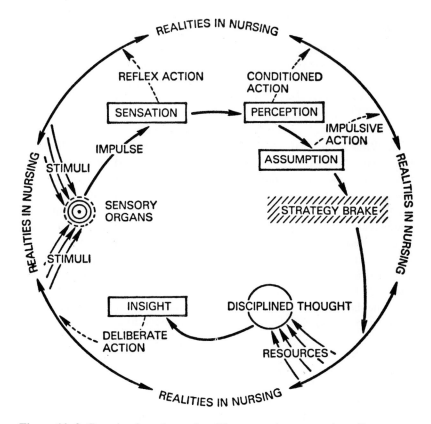

Figure 11–3. Genesis of nursing action. Diagrammatic presentation of how an impulse to act originates and how it is converted into action. Broken lines represent overt processes; solid lines represent covert processes. (*Reprinted by permission of G. P. Putnam's Sons from* Family-Centered Maternity Nursing *(2nd ed.) by Wiedenbach, E., 1967, G. P. Putnam's Sons.*)

Within the *assessment* phase of the nursing process the components of *analysis* and *synthesis* require much conscious thought and deliberation about the corrected data before the nurse can make a *nursing diagnosis*. Once the nursing diagnosis has been determined, the nurse identifies *outcomes,* sets goals and objectives, and *plans* the nursing care. This planning phase can be compared to Wiedenbach's levels of insight and design, which are part of her voluntary phase. The insight level of her nursing process model includes joint planning. This joint planning is between the nurse and the patient and does not necessarily involve other health care professionals.

Wiedenbach (1964) does not directly incorporate the concepts of outcomes or goals as part of the nursing process, although goals is one of her realities. However, the nurse's central purpose could be considered an outcome or a goal. On the design level the nurse plans a course of action. After the plan is decided on, the nurse confirms it with the patient. Once the plan has been decided on and confirmed, the nurse performs the responsible, deliberate nursing action. This level is comparable to the *implementation* phase of the nursing process.

In Wiedenbach's (1977) model of the nursing process, she does not identify *evaluation*. However, she does refer to evaluation in her discussion of nursing practice, emphasizing that the nurse needs "validation that the help provided was indeed helpful to the patient" (p. 39).

CRITIQUE OF WIEDENBACH'S PRESCRIPTIVE THEORY

1. What is the historical context of the theory? Ernestine Wiedenbach began her nursing career in the 1920s. She was one of the first nurses to develop a nursing theory and was strongly influenced by her work with Dickoff and James. Her theory was first published in 1964 in *Clinical nursing—A helping art*. It is a situation-producing theory that conceptualizes both a desired situation and the prescription by which that situation is to be brought about. Wiedenbach insists that every nursing act be examined in the light of its purpose. Each nurse's central purpose or commitment is based on that nurse's philosophy. It is assumed that the nurse is a well-intentioned, self-sacrificing individual who values human life. Florence Wald credited Wiedenbach with helping her recognize that purpose differentiates the theory of practitioners from the theory of basic scientists (Wiedenbach, 1964). That purpose and true commitment to nursing Wiedenbach derived from over 40 years of nursing practice.

2. What are the basic concepts and relationships presented by the theory? The basic concepts of Wiedenbach's theory include the nurse's central purpose, prescription, and the realities of the situation. She uses these concepts consistently throughout her work. The nurse is an agent, the patient a recipient. Nursing is provided with a goal and means within a framework. She recognizes that there are variables in every situation that may affect the patient, the nurse, and the outcome. She recommends the use of responsible, deliberative actions with validation that the actions met the patient's need for help. Her concepts are presented clearly to the reader.

3. What major phenomena of concern to nursing are presented? These phenomenon may include *but are not limited to*: human beings, environment, health, interpersonal relations, caring, goal attainment, adaptation, and energy fields. Wiedenbach's major phenomena include: human beings, environment (her framework and realities), interpersonal relationships, and nursing as a practice discipline in and among realities. The nurse is compassionate, caring, loving, nurturing, competent, knowledgeable, and altruistic. Wiedenbach does not specifically define the concept of health.

4. To whom does this theory apply? In what situations? In what ways? Wiedenbach's theory applies to individuals needing care and especially to the nurse who provides that care. It has a global philosophical blessing for nursing do-gooders. Wiedenbach does not discuss prevention and does not discuss the application of her prescriptive theory to groups needing care. This is a prescriptive predictive theory. Weidenbach (1969) applied her theory to the teaching of students of nursing in the clinical area in *Meeting the realities in clinical teaching*. VandeVusse (1997) also describes the use of Wiedenbach's work in educating nurse-midwives.

5. By what method or methods can this theory be tested? While little research has been reported, Weidenbach's theory has been tested using qualitative methods. Trefz (1999) addressed nurses' satisfaction in relation to patient teaching. Gustafson (1988) used naturalistic inquiry to identify behaviors of women during the first stage of labor that signaled a need-for-help. Thompson (1998) incorporated Wiedenbach's central purpose in her study of staff nurses' lived experiences in relating to student nurses in clinical practice and found that the expectations (central purpose) of both the staff and student nurses influenced the experience.

6. Does this theory direct critical thinking in nursitng practice? Wiedenbach believes nurses must have knowledge. In order to make knowledgeable decisions, the nurse must be educated, caring, competent, and committed. The application of Wiedenbach's strategy brake requires critical thinking as do the interactions expected during the voluntary phase of her nursing process.

7. Does this theory direct therapeutic nursing interventions? This theory directs therapeutic interventions because nursing interventions are aimed at a specific goal. The goal is determined in part by the nurse's central purpose and, if deliberative actions are taken, planned mutually with the patient in relation to the patient's need for help. Wiedenbach also specifies that the helpfulness of the nurse's actions must be validated.

8. Does this theory direct communication in nursing practice? Yes, Wiedenbach's theory directs communication because the nurse must validate her perceptions with the patient. If these perceptions are in error, then her actions must be redirected. The voluntary phase of her nursing process is based on communication.

9. Does this theory direct nursing actions that lead to favorable outcomes? Yes, nursing actions will lead to favorable outcomes in Wiedenbach's theory because the nurse works in collaboration with the patient. Together, they identify the common goal and then work together to achieve it. They also decide if the outcomes achieved are those that were desired.

10. How contagious is this theory? While it is one of the first nursing theories proposed as a theory rather than being developed with another primary purpose, Wiedenbach's prescriptive theory has not been very contagious. An electronic search of the literature identified a limited number of articles with very little recent discussion. A major aspect of the importance of Wiedenbach's theory historically is that it was intentionally developed as a framework for clinical nursing practice—both for the practitioner and for the teacher of practitioners.

STRENGTHS AND LIMITATIONS

Weidenbach describes nursing as a helping art. The nurse renders compassionate care to those in need of help. Nursing requires a professional commitment and is based on the individual nurse's philosophy. For Wiedenbach (1970) the concepts that epitomize the nurse's philosophy are the "reverence for the gift of life," "respect for the dignity, worth, autonomy, and individuality of each human being," and the "resolution to act dynamically in relation to one's beliefs" (p. 1058). The components of nursing practice are identification of the patient's need for help, ministration of help, and validation that the help given is beneficial.

Wiedenbach identifies seven levels within her nursing process: sensation, perception, assumption, realization, insight, design, and decision. Sensation through realization involves involuntary action, insight through design involves voluntary action. With increased purpose, knowledge, experience, and skill, the nurse moves from an involuntary response to voluntary action that focuses on meeting the patient's identified need for help.

The reader perceives that the nurse acts with a self-sacrificing commitment to nursing. If a nurse values the life and dignity of human beings, then she will provide quality nursing care. Wiedenbach (1964) states that "although recognized as a humanitarian service, nursing in its entirety is hard to describe, and the nurse's responsibilities are hard to delineate" (p. 1).

Wiedenbach's nursing process is different from the nursing process outlined in Chapter 2 in this text. She identifies the nursing process as being activated by a stimulus that may result in an involuntary response unless this reflexive action is halted by a strategy brake. This brake, or pause, allows the nurse to think, gather more data, analyze, and then plan before a voluntary deliberate action is taken. The nursing process in Chapter 2 more closely parallels Wiedenbach's definition of nursing practice, that is, observation, ministration of help, and validation.

This theory is useful with an individual patient but not with groups. With this theory, Wiedenbach recognizes that the "need for help" must be verified with the patient. This factor would require the patient to be coherent and responsive and limits the types of patients with whom the theory can be used.

Wiedenbach's work occurred early in the development of the theoretical nursing models. Her prescriptive theory defines her concepts of central purpose, prescription, and realities. However, these concepts are broad, vary with each nurse, each patient, each situation, and are difficult to use in research.

SUMMARY

Wiedenbach's theory for nursing, a prescriptive theory, contains three concepts: *central purpose, prescription,* and *realities.* The interrelationship of these three concepts is as follows: Within the realities, the nurse develops a prescription for nursing care based on her central purpose. The central purpose is the nurse's philosophy for care; the prescription is the directive to activity; the realities are the matrix in which the action occurs. These concepts are all interdependent. She also presents a three-phase nursing practice and seven-levels of nursing process.

Wiedenbach's theory presents a philosophical, altruistic approach to nursing. The nurse is viewed as a loving, caring individual. The nurse's philosophy about the value and worth of the individual directs her care. Wiedenbach (1967) states: "Nursing [is] a service which ideally exemplifies man's humanity to man" (p. 5).

Wiedenbach's work is innovative within the nursing profession. Her classic writings, including those written with Dickoff and James, serve as a basis for the development of nursing theory. Wiedenbach is a "mother" of nursing theory development.

REFERENCES

Burst, H. V. (1979). Presentation of the Hattie Hemschemeyer Award. *Journal of Nurse-Midwifery, 24*(5), 35–36.

Dickoff, J., James, P., & Wiedenbach, E. (1968a). Theory in a practice discipline I: Practice-orientated research. *Nursing Research, 17,* 415–435.

Dickoff, J., James, P., & Wiedenbach, E. (1968b). Theory in a practice discipline II: Practice-orientated research. *Nursing Research, 17,* 545–554.

Gustafson, D. C. (1988). Signaling behavior in stage I labor to elicit care: A clinical referent for Wiedenbach's need-for-help. *Dissertation Abstracts International, 49–10B,* 4230.

Nickel, S., Gesse, T., & MacLaren, A. (1992). Ernestine Wiedenbach: Her professional legacy. *Journal of Nurse-Midwifery, 37*(3), 161–167.

Thompson, J. M. (1998). The lived experience of the staff nurse relating to the student nurse during the clinical learning experience. *Dissertation Abstracts International, 58–12B,* 6493.

Trefz, L. M. (1999). *Nursing staff perceptions about breastfeeding: An education task force survey.* Unpublished master's thesis, University of Cincinnati, Ohio.

VandeVusse, L. (1997). Education exchange. Sculpting a nurse-midwifery philosophy: Ernestine Wiedenbach's influence. *Journal of Nurse-Midwifery, 42*(1), 43–48.

Wiedenbach, E. (1958). *Family-centered maternity nursing.* New York: G. P. Putnam's.

Wiedenbach, E. (1964). *Clinical nursing—A helping art.* New York: Springer.

Wiedenbach, E. (1967). *Family-centered maternity nursing* (2nd ed.). New York: G. P. Putnam's.

Wiedenbach, E. (1969). *Meeting the realities in clinical teaching.* New York: Springer.

Wiedenbach, E. (1970). Nurse's wisdom in nursing theory. *American Journal of Nursing, 70,* 1057–1062.

Wiedenbach, E. (1977). The nursing process in maternity nursing. In J. P. Clausen, M. H. Flook, & B. Ford. *Maternity nursing today* (2nd ed.) (pp. 39–51). New York: McGraw-Hill.

BIBLIOGRAPHY

Dickoff, J. J. (1968). Symposium in theory development in nursing: Researching research's role in theory development. *Nursing Research, 17,* 204–206.

Dickoff, J. J., & James, P. A. (1968). Symposium of theory development in nursing: A theory of theories: A position paper. *Nursing Research, 17,* 197–203.

Holland, M. A. (1989). *An examination of the propositions of James Dickoff, Patricia James: Implications for nursing research.* Unpublished doctoral dissertation, Temple University.

Wiedenbach, E. (1949). Childbirth as mothers say they like it. *Public Health Nursing, 51,* 417–421.

Wiedenbach, E. (1960). Nurse-midwifery, purpose, practice and opportunity. *Nursing Outlook, 8,* 256.

Wiedenbach, E. (1963). The helping art of nursing. *American Journal of Nursing, 63,* 54–57.

Wiedenbach, E. (1965). Family nurse practitioner for maternal and child care. *Nursing Outlook, 13,* 50.

Wiedenbach, E. (1968a). Genetics and the nurse. *Bulletin of the American College of Nurse Midwifery, 13,* 8–13.

Wiedenbach, E. (1968b). The nurse's role in family planning—A conceptual base for practice. *Nursing Clinics of North America, 3,* 355–365.

Wiedenbach, E. (1970). Comment on beliefs and values: Basis for curriculum design. *Nursing Research, 19,* 427.

Wiedenbach, E., & Falls, C. (1978). *Communication: Key to effective nursing.* New York: Tiresias Press.

CHAPTER 12

THE CONSERVATION PRINCIPLES: A MODEL FOR HEALTH
MYRA ESTRIN LEVINE

Julia B. George

■ ■ ■

Myra E. Levine (1920–1996) was born in Chicago, the first child in a family of three siblings. Her experiences during her father's frequent illnesses contributed to her interest in and dedication to nursing. She received a diploma from Cook County School of Nursing in 1944, a B.S. from the University of Chicago in 1949, and an M.S. in nursing from Wayne State University in 1962. Her career in nursing was varied. Clinically, she held positions as a private duty nurse, a civilian nurse for the U. S. Army, surgical supervisor, and director of nursing. She held faculty positions at Cook County School of Nursing, Loyola University, Rush University, and the University of Illinois, Chicago. She was Professor Emerita, Medical-Surgical Nursing, University of Illinois, Chicago. Levine filled visiting professorships at Tel-Aviv University and Recanati School of Nursing, Ben Gurion University of the Negev, both in Israel.

Levine was a charter fellow in the American Academy of Nursing and was honored by the Illinois Nurses Association. She was the first recipient of Sigma Theta Tau's Elizabeth Russell Belford Award for teaching excellence. She was granted an honorary doctorate by Loyola University, Chicago, in 1992.

Myra Levine said she had no intention of developing a theory when she first began putting her ideas about nursing into writing (Trench, Wallace, & Coberg, 1987). In fact, nearly two decades after the initial publication of *Introduction to clinical nursing* (Levine, 1969, 1973) she referred to her work as a theory but preferred to identify it as a conceptual model. She stated she was looking for a way to teach all the major concepts in medical-surgical nursing in three quarters and for a way to generalize the content, to move away from a procedurally oriented educational process. She was interested in helping nurses realize that every nurse–patient contact leads to a puzzle in relation to nursing care that needs to be solved in an individualized manner. Her work evolved over the years, with the most recent comprehensive update of the theory published in 1989 and additional discussions in 1990, 1991, and 1996.

Levine (1990) believed that entry into the health care system is associated with giving up some measure of personal independence. To designate the person who has entered the health care system a client reinforces the state of dependency, for a client is a follower. She supported the term *patient* because patient means sufferer, and dependency is associated with suffering.

> It is the condition of suffering that makes it possible to set independence aside and accept the services of another person. It is the challenge of the nurse to provide the individual with appropriate care without losing sight of the individual's integrity, to honor the trust that the patient has placed in the nurse, and to encourage the participation of the individual in his or her own welfare. The patient comes in trust and dependence only for as long as the services of the nurse are needed. The nurse's goal is always to impart knowledge and strength so that the individual can . . . walk away . . . as an independent individual (p. 199).

It was Levine's intent that such dependency be a very temporary state of affairs (Trench, Wallace, & Coberg, 1987). In accord with Levine's belief, the term *patient* is used throughout this chapter.

Levine (1989, 1990, 1991, 1996) was careful to credit the scientists' works upon which she built. She spoke to the importance of recognizing and building on these vital adjuncts to knowledge. This knowledge is not borrowed but, rather, is shared. In discussing physiological mechanisms, she drew on Cannon's (1939) description of the flight or fight response. Selye's (1956) stress theories provided further information about protection from the hazards of living. Gibson's (1966) perceptual systems about how people are actively involved in gathering information from their environments to aid them in moving safely through those environments were drawn on. Erikson's (1969, 1975) discussions of the influence of environment on development further expanded Levine's information about the person–environment interaction. Bates' (1967) description of three types of environment was also important. The works of Dubos (1965), Cohen (1968), and Goldstein (1963) contributed to Levine's concept of adaptation.

LEVINE'S THEORY

Levine discussed adaptation, conservation, and integrity. *Adaptation* is the process by which *conservation* is achieved, and the purpose for conservation is *integrity*. The core of Levine's theory are her four principles of conservation.

Adaptation

Adaptation is the life process by which, over time, people maintain their wholeness or integrity as they respond to environmental challenges; it is the consequence of interaction between the person and the environment (Trench, Wallace, & Coberg,

1987; Levine, 1989). Successful engagement with the environment depends on an adequate store of adaptations (Levine, 1990).

Both physiological and behavioral responses are different under different conditions—for example, responses to intensely quiet or extremely noisy environments will vary. It is possible to anticipate certain kinds of reactions, but the individuality of responses prevents accurate prediction. Adaptation is explanatory rather than predictive.

Adaptation includes the concepts of *historicity, specificity,* and *redundancy.* Adaptation is a historical process, responses are based on past experiences, both personal and genetic. Each individual's genetic pattern is unique. This uniqueness is further developed by the individual's experiences.

Adaptation is also specific. Each system has very specific responses. The physiological responses that "defend oxygen supply to the brain are distinct from those that maintain the appropriate blood glucose levels" (Levine, 1989, p. 328). Particular responses are called into action by a particular challenge; responses are task-specific. They are also synchronized. Although the changes that occur are sequential, they should not be viewed as linear. Rather, Levine (1989) describes them as occurring in "cascades" in which there is an interacting and evolving effect in which one sequence is not yet completed when the next begins.

"One of the most remarkable things about living species is the number of levels of response which permit them to confront the reality of their environment in ways that somehow maintain their well being" (Trench, Wallace, & Coberg, 1987). These redundant systems are both protective and adaptive. If one system does not adapt, another can take over. Levine (1989) indicated that redundant systems may function in a time frame; some are corrective whereas others permit a previously failed response to be re-established. Redundancy results in the most parsimonious use of energy (Levine, 1996).

Levine described adaptation as the best "fit of the person with his or her predicament of time and space" (Trench, Wallace, & Coberg, 1987). She differentiated between fit and congruence by using an example of shoes. Most of us have many pairs of shoes that are congruent with our feet. We also have certain pairs that we prefer to wear because they are the most comfortable—they are the best fit.

Conservation

The product of adaptation is conservation. Conservation is a universal concept, a natural law, that deals with defense of wholeness and system integrity (Levine, 1990, 1991, 1996). "Conservation defends the wholeness of living systems by ensuring their ability to confront change appropriately and retain their unique identity" (Levine, 1990, p. 192). Conservation describes how complex systems continue to function in the face of severe challenges; it provides not only for current survival but also for future vitality through facing challenges in the most economical way possible. An example Levine used to illustrate conservation is that of the thermostat. The thermostat is set at a selected temperature. As long as the temperature in the room is the same as the set temperature, nothing occurs. When the room temperature falls below the selected temperature, the thermostat activates the heating system—but only until the room temperature again reaches the thermostat setting. When the setting is reached, the thermostat turns the heating system off. Levine (1990) describes this as conserving energy—using it in "the most frugal, economic, and energy-sparing fashion" (p. 192). The essence of conservation is the successful use of responses that cost the least (Levine, 1989). "Conservation is clearly the consequence of the multiple, interacting, and synchronized negative feedback systems that provide for the stability of the living organism" (Levine, 1989, p. 329). As long as systems are physiologically stable, or in balance, negative feedback systems can function at minimal cost. Energy resources are conserved for use when needed to restore balance. Homeostasis is a state of conservation, a state of synchronized sparing of energy.

Levine (1989) stated that physiological and behavioral responses are essential components of the same activity. They are not parallel or simultaneous but part of the same whole. She also recognized that it is difficult to break down a body of knowledge and that often information must be gathered piece by piece (Trench, Wallace, & Coberg, 1987). Thus, physiological and behavioral responses are often identified and described as separate things. Since they represent the same whole, it is important to put the pieces together to represent that whole.

Levine (1989) described four levels of behavior. The first is Cannon's (1939) "fight or flight" response, the adrenocortical-sympathetic reactions that provide both physiological and behavioral readiness in the face of sudden and unexplained challenges in the environment. The second is the inflammatory-immune response, which we rely on for restoration of physical wholeness and healing. The third is Selye's (1956) stress response, described as an integrated defense that occurs over time and is "influenced by the accumulated experience of the individual" (p. 330). The fourth is Gibson's (1966) perceptual systems in which the senses not only provide access to environmental energy sources but also convert these sources into meaningful experiences; people not only see, they *look*; they not only hear, they *listen*. These levels of behavior support the individual as an active participant with the environment, not merely as a reactive being. The levels of responses are not sequential but rather redundant and integrated within the individual.

Nursing's role in conservation is to help the person with the process of "keeping together" the total person through the least expense of effort. Levine (1989) proposed the following four principles of conservation:

1. The conservation of energy of the individual.
2. The conservation of the structural integrity of the individual.
3. The conservation of the personal integrity of the individual.
4. The conservation of the social integrity of the individual. (p. 331)

The conservation of *energy* is basic to the natural, universal law of conservation. Levine (1989) stated that energy is not hidden; "it is eminently identifiable, measurable, and manageable" (p. 331). Within nursing practice, the measurement of vital signs is a daily measurement of energy parameters. For example, body temperature is an indication of the heat (energy) generated by living cells as they accomplish their work. Energy conservation is encouraged through the limitation of activities for coronary patients or the planned gradual resumption of activities postoperatively. It is important that, even at rest, energy costs are incurred through the activities necessary to support living. Levine (1989) identified these as those activities involved in growth, transport, and biochemical and bioelectrical change. She stated, "The conservation of energy is clearly evident in the very sick, whose lethargy, withdrawal, and self-concern are manifested while, in its wisdom, the body is spending its energy resources on the processes of healing" (p. 332). Levine (1996) also discussed conservation of energy as universal and increasingly justified through scientific data.

The second, third, and fourth principles continue the theme of conservation and include integrity—structural integrity, personal integrity, and social integrity. Levine (1990) also described the conservation of energy as protecting functional integrity. Levine presented the idea that "health" and "whole" are derived from the same root word and that another synonym for "whole" is "integrity." "Integrity means being in control of one's life . . . having the freedom to choose: to move without constraint . . . to exercise decisions on all matters . . . without apology, indebtedness, or guilt" (Levine, 1990, p. 193). We are concerned with the integrity of the whole person; the essence of wholeness is integrity.

Conservation of *structural integrity* focuses on the healing process (Levine, 1989). Through multiple experiences with scraped knees and such that heal with no scarring, humans develop a mind-set that expects perfect restoration of structural integrity throughout life. "Healing is the defense of wholeness" (p. 333). Nurses support structural integrity through efforts to limit injury and thus limit scarring, through proper positioning and range of motion to prevent skeletal deformity, pressure areas, or loss of muscle tone. To Levine the phantom limb phenomenon (Sacks, 1985) supports the idea that a sense of structural integrity is more than a physiological need.

Conservation of *personal integrity* focuses on a sense of self—"that intensely private, always unique and secret knowledge that we use to define ourselves" (Levine, 1996). Levine described Goldstein's (1963) identification of self-actualization as observed in efforts of severely brain injured persons to retain their personal identity. She pointed out that both Maslow (1968) and Rogers (1961) discussed self-actualization as a reaching beyond. Goldstein's concept, the one supported by Levine, is a reaching into the person rather than a reaching beyond. Humans have both a public and a very private self. At least some portion of the private self is not known even to those who are closest to the person. The self "is defined, defended, and described only by the soul that owns it. That private self is unique and whole. A person can share mere fragments of it with others" (Levine, 1990, p. 194). In this way a separation between self and other is maintained. Levine (1989) stated that efforts at collecting a complete psycho–social database may well violate this need to maintain separation, and therefore these efforts violate personal integrity. She stated, "the most generous psycho–social approach would be to limit the recording of confidences to only those generalizations that actually make a difference in the choice of treatment plans" (p. 334). She likened the awareness of self to independence.

Conservation of *social integrity* involves a definition of self that goes beyond the individual and includes the holiness of each person (Levine, 1989, 1996). Individuals use their relationships to define themselves. One's identity is connected to family, friends, community, workplace, school, culture, ethnicity, religion, vocation, education, and socioeconomic status. To function successfully in this wide variety of social environments requires a broad behavioral repertoire. The ultimate direction for social integrity is derived from the ethical values of the social system. "The health care system is a vast social order with its own rules, but it is an instrument of society and must guarantee privacy, personhood, and respect as moral imperatives" (Levine, 1989, p. 336). Levine (1990) pointed out that disease prevention is an issue of social integrity and discusses the need both to discuss and to fund studies and programs to deal with overwhelming health problems such as smoking, drug abuse, HIV, and cancer. She also stated, "It is difficult to foresee a time when conservation of social integrity is realistically possible" (Levine, 1996, p. 41).

> The conservation principles do not, of course, operate singly and in isolation from each other. They are joined within the individual as a cascade of life events, churning and changing as the environmental challenge is confronted and resolved in each individual's unique way. The nurse as caregiver becomes part of that environment, bringing to every nursing opportunity his or her own cascading repertoire of skill, knowledge, and compassion. It is a shared enterprise and each participant is rewarded (Levine, 1989, p. 336).

LEVINE'S THEORY AND NURSING'S METAPARADIGM

Levine skillfully wove her beliefs about human beings, environment, health, and nursing throughout her discussions of conservation and adaptation. They are fundamental to her work.

In relation to *human beings*, Levine (1990) stated that when a person is being studied, the focus should be on wholeness. She also maintained that a person cannot be understood outside the context of the place and time in which he or she is functioning, or separated from the influence of everything that is happening around him or her. Not only are human beings influenced by their current circumstances, they also are "burdened by a lifetime of experience," which has been recorded on the tissues of the body as well as on the mind and spirit (p. 197). Human beings are continually adapting in their interactions with their environment. The process of adaptation results in conservation. Human beings have need for nursing when they are suffering and can set aside independence and accept the services of another.

Levine (1984) indicated that *health* and disease are patterns of adaptive change. Some adaptations are more successful than others; all adaptations are seeking the best fit with the environment. The most successful adaptations are the ones that achieve the best fit in the most conserving manner. Health is the goal of conservation (Levine, 1990). She also discusses the words *health, whole,* and *integrity* as all being derived from the same root word and that, even with a multiplicity of definitions of health, each individual still defines health for him- or herself (Levine, 1991).

In defining *environment* Levine (1990) drew upon Bates's (1967) classifications of three aspects of environment. The *operational environment* consists of those undetected natural forces that impinge on the individual. The *perceptual environment* consists of information that is recorded by the sensory organs. The *conceptual environment* is influenced by language, culture, ideas, and cognition. Levine also said that even with definition, the environment is difficult to measure. However, because adaptation and conservation are based on the human being's interaction with the environment, efforts to understand the environment and the role it plays in an individual's predicament are vital. The *social context* is also important to consideration of the wholeness of an individual. Levine (1991) included the individual's "ethnic and cultural heritage, economic niche, the opportunities ignored or seized" in social context (p. 9). She said, "It is the social system that, in every place and in every generation, establishes the values that direct it and sets the rules by which its members are judged. The social integrity of the individual mirrors the community to which he or she belongs" (p. 9).

For Levine (1989) the purpose of *nursing* is to take care of others when they need to be taken care of. The dependency created by this need is a very temporary state. Nursing takes place wherever there is an individual who needs care to some degree. Levine discussed the fact that the person who provides nursing care has special burdens of concern since the "permission to enter into the life goals of another human being bears onerous debts of responsibility and choice" (p. 336). The nurse–patient relationship is based on the willful participation of both parties, and in such a relationship there cannot be "a substitute for honesty, fairness, and mutual respect" (p. 336). Nursing theory "is tested finally in the pragmatic, humble daily exchanges between nurse and patient . . . [its] success [is demonstrated in its ability to] equip individuals with renewed strength to pursue their lives in independence, fulfillment, hope, and promise" (pp. 336–337).

LEVINE'S THEORY AND THE NURSING PROCESS

Levine's concepts of adaptation, conservation, and integrity can be used to guide patient care within the nursing process.

In *assessment*, an understanding of the wholeness of the patient needs to be the end result. However, because we lack the mechanisms for assessing the whole as such, the principles of conservation can be used as a guide to structure the assessment. The assessment would not be initiated unless the person is suffering and willing to become to some degree dependent on the nurse. The overarching question could be, "What adaptation is needed, or has not been successful?" The history, specificity, and potential for redundancy in this area of adaptation need to be investigated. For example, with the cardiac patient it is important to gather information about the signs and symptoms that brought the person into the health care system. Is there a family or personal history of cardiac problems or of being at risk for such problems? Can the incident that initiated this problem be identified (e.g., response to sudden change in temperature would indicate a different specific response than to overexertion)? Have compensating efforts been made?

Under the first principle, conservation of energy, assessment data would relate to energy sources and expenditure. Data would include vital signs, laboratory values related to uptake and use of oxygen and nutrients, activities of daily living, nutrition, exercise, elimination, menstrual cycles . . . any aspect of living that requires energy. The primary focus would be on identifying the areas of energy expenditure that are related to the suffering that brought the patient into contact with the nurse. Information about the balance between energy input and output is also important.

Assessment data in relation to conservation of structural integrity would relate to information about injury and disease processes. Data would include laboratory values that reflect the immune/inflammatory response, direct observations of wounds, and any visible indications of disease (e.g., the "pox" in chicken pox), and information from the patient about symptoms that are not observable (e.g., nausea, pain).

Assessment data related to conservation of personal integrity need to be collected very carefully. Levine (1989) warns about the threat to the self of the patient that can be created if the nurse seeks a too thorough investigation of the self of that patient. Her guideline to use "only those generalizations that actually make a difference in the choice of treatment plans" is helpful (p. 334). For example, knowing that the person prefers to learn from reading material and receiving instruction individually rather than in a group setting would influence the choice of treatment plans. The patient will be comfortable in sharing his or her public self but reluctant to share the private self. To assist in maintaining independence, assessment needs to be limited to those portions of the self that the person is willing to share, and is capable of sharing.

Assessment data related to the conservation of social integrity includes information about others who have influenced the person's identification of self. Again, the kind and amount of data collected in this area need to be constructed carefully, with due sensitivity to the needs of the person to maintain privacy. Information may be obtained about family, the community in which the person lives and works, religious preferences, cultural and ethnic influences, and any other social information that the person deems important to share and that could influence the plan of care.

Assessment of the patient's nursing requirements leads to the development of *trophicognosis*. Trophicognosis is a nursing care judgment that is arrived at through the use of the scientific method (Trench, Wallace, & Coberg, 1987). Levine proposed the use of the term *trophicognosis* as an alternative to nursing diagnosis in 1966. In her more recent writings (1989, 1990) she does not include trophicognosis. She does state, "No diagnosis should be made that does not include the other persons whose lives are entwined with that of the individual (1989, p. 336). The *nursing diagnosis* focuses on the cause of the patient's suffering—what has put him or her in the predicament of need—and on the areas in which adaptation needs to be supported in order to achieve conservation and integrity.

Outcomes would center on Levine's goal of returning the patient to independence. In Levine's terms, an outcome might be that the patient can walk away from the nurse.

Planning focuses on what the nurse needs to do to aid the patient in again becoming independent. The goals that are set will reflect the patient's behavior and the planned activities will include both willing participants—the nurse and the patient. Levine has made no effort to be prescriptive about the kinds of actions that would be planned. She is very clear, however, that the intent is to return the patient to a state of independence as quickly and fully as possible.

Implementation is structured according to the four conservation principles. For conservation of energy, actions will seek to balance energy input with energy output. The actions may focus on increasing energy input through improved nutrition or in decreasing energy output through changes in activity. The classic example of decreasing energy output is full bed rest. However, it is important to remember, as Levine (1989) pointed out, even at purportedly complete rest, the body is still using energy. Levine reported that Winslow's research demonstrates that energy conservation can be *predicted* (personal communication, 1994). For structural integrity, nursing actions will be "based on limiting the amount of tissue involvement in infections and disease" (Trench, Wallace, & Coberg, 1987). Such actions could include appropriate positioning to prevent the formation of decubiti, dressing changes, and administration of antibiotics. For personal integrity, efforts will be "based on helping the person to preserve his or her identity and selfhood" (Trench, Wallace, & Coberg, 1987). These actions may begin in deciding to protect the private self by *not* collecting complete psycho–social data and continue through the design of treatment plans that take individual characteristics into account. Levine indicated it is important to observe a strict moral approach. For social integrity, nursing actions are "based on helping the patient to preserve his or her place in a family, community, and society" (Trench, Wallace, & Coberg, 1987). Such nursing actions may include teaching the family about the patient's care needs or teaching persons with new colostomies how to handle food and fluid intake and how to change the ostomy bag in a manner that helps to minimize its being evident to those they meet.

Evaluation is not specifically discussed by Levine but outcomes were discussed by Taylor (1974) for neurological patients. However, Levine's emphasis on the importance of assisting the person to return to independence as soon as possible supports the need for evaluation. It is important to know that the person's suffering has been relieved and that he or she is willing and capable of no longer being dependent. The evaluation data focus on the effectiveness of adaptation in achieving conservation and integrity in the four areas of energy, structural integrity, personal integrity, and social integrity. See Table 12–1 for an example of an application to clinical practice.

TABLE 12–1. APPLICATION OF CONSERVATION PRINCIPLES TO CLINICAL PRACTICE

Patient: Lester Douglas admitted with medical diagnoses of hypertension and peripheral vascular disease.

Assessment:

Conservation of energy:

> Mr. Douglas reports he cannot walk more than 1/2 block without resting due to pain in his legs. He must climb three steps to enter his house and can usually do so without difficulty. He lives in a two story house but has a bedroom on the first floor.
>
> Vital signs are within normal limits—Mr. Douglas says that as long as he takes his antihypertension medicine and limits the salt in his diet, his high blood pressure is controlled.
>
> Chest x-ray clear
>
> Lab values: Only abnormal level is cholesterol at 260
>
> Mr. Douglas reports he takes care of himself and hires someone to come in to clean his house and do his laundry once a week. He states he eats 2 meals a day and he cooks for himself.
>
> He has to get up at least once a night to void. His bowels are usually regular—sometimes he is constipated.

Conservation of Structural Integrity:

> Medical diagnosis of peripheral vascular disease is consistent with Mr. Douglas' description of difficulty walking and indicates impairment of his vascular system.
>
> Mr. Douglas reports that his left leg either hurts or "feels strange" most of the time. Pedal pulses on the left are diminished.
>
> History of smoking 1/2 pack per day for 40 years—stopped smoking 10 years ago and reports his breathing is better since then.
>
> Reports arthritis in both hands; physical examination indicates arthritic nodules distal joints of index fingers. Mr. Douglas reports pain in the proximal joints of both thumbs and that this has weakened his grip strength. He can fully close each hand.

Conservation of Personal Integrity:

> 89-year-old male

Conservation of Social Integrity:

> Widower, lives alone
>
> Believes in God but doesn't "get out to church much anymore. It's just too much effort."
>
> Has 3 living children—all are in their 60s and live out of state. Mr. Douglas states they call and write regularly and each visits once or twice a year.
>
> He has neighbors on either side of him who "keep an eye out." One of these neighbors likes to cook and regularly brings food over—"he can't seem to make a recipe small enough for just him so he shares with me. He's a pretty good cook, too!"

Nursing Diagnoses:

> Pain related to arthritis in hands and peripheral vascular disease in legs.
>
> Limited mobility associated with pain and peripheral vascular disease.

Desired Outcome: Able to continue to care for self and live in own home.

Planning:

> Pain control using prescribed medication and possible physical therapy to support continued function.
>
> Support for medical workup that could result in the recommendation of vascular surgery—provide appropriate education and opportunity for questions and discussion. Explain all tests in the level of detail he desires. Be sensitive to how much detail he really wants.

TABLE 12–1. (*CONT.*)

Implementation:
Conservation of energy:
  Increase the servings of fruits and vegetables to at least 5 daily to help assure regularity of his bowels.
  Arrange his bath and other care activities to allow rest before and after his physical therapy.
  Conservation of structural integrity:
  Work with physician and patient to establish an effective plan of analgesia to decrease his pain—help him accept that the pain will not totally disappear.
  Conservation of Personal and Social Integrity:
  Encourage him to keep up the good work!
Evaluation:
  Can he walk with more comfort?
  Can he use his hands for activities of daily living and desired recreation?
  Is he ready to resume independence?

CRITIQUE OF LEVINE'S CONSERVATION PRINCIPLES

1. What is the historical context of the theory? Levine developed her work to teach nursing students the practice of medical-surgical nursing. She had a practice-oriented focus in doing so and only began to discuss the work in terms of a theory about two decades after the initial publication. She was attuned to the origin of words and took care in her use of words and how they relate to one another.

Levine clearly identified those ideas from adjunctive disciplines that she used in her work. These include Cannon's (1939) flight or fight response, Selye's (1956) stress theories, Gibson's (1966) perceptual systems, Erikson's (1969, 1975) discussions of the influence of environment on development, Bates's (1967) three types of environment, and the works of Dubos (1965), Cohen (1968), and Goldstein (1963) in relation to adaptation. She clearly and carefully includes information about how she used these ideas. Her work is consistent with these works but builds on them in a way that creates questions to be answered. Such questions could include: Does change in one type of environment have a greater effect on adaptation than changes in the other two types? Why are some people more (or less) effective than others in adapting, conserving, and thus maintaining integrity? What are the most effective ways of conserving social integrity through disease prevention activities?

Levine's work is most consistent with the totality paradigm. She supported holism and stressed the importance of the whole person. However, she indicated that we must look at the parts to understand the whole.

2. What are the basic concepts and relationships presented by the theory? The basic concepts are adaptation, conservation, and integrity. The relationships are presented in the theory statement, a*daptation* is the process by which *conservation* is achieved, and the purpose for conservation is *integrity*.

3. What major phenomena of concern to nursing are presented? These phenomenon may include *but are not limited to***: human being, environment, health, interpersonal relations, caring, goal attainment, adaptation, and energy fields.** The major phenomena begin with the basic concepts of adaptation, conservation, and integrity. In addition, the conservation principles include the phenomena of energy, structural integrity, personal intergrity, and social integrity. The human being who needs nursing is seen as a person who is in a predicament of illness, who is willing to enter a dependent state, and who needs to return to independence as soon as possible. Levine emphasized that the person who is receiving nursing should be identified as a patient.

4. To whom does this theory apply? In what situations? In what ways? Because Levine's three concepts apply to all living human beings and, according to Levine, nursing is not setting specific, the theory is generalizable. It can be used in any setting with any human being who is suffering and willing to seek assistance from a nurse.

5. By what method or methods can this theory be tested? Hypotheses have been developed from Levine's theory, and research has been conducted to test these hypotheses. The results of these research studies have contributed to the general body of knowledge in nursing. Levine (1989) discusses the studies conducted by Wong (1968) and Winslow, Lane, and Gaffney (1985) that support the importance of energy conservation for patients with myocardial infarctions. Research has also been conducted in using Levine's theory with confused patients over age 60 and caring for neonates and for women in labor (Foreman, 1989; 1991; Newport, 1984; Yeates & Roberts, 1984). Pappas (1990) investigated the relationship between nursing care and anxiety in patients with sexually transmitted diseases and found significant relationships between constructs of nursing and components of anxiety. MacLean (1987) used the principles of conservation of energy and conservation of structural integrity in identifying cues that nurses use to diagnose activity intolerance. Foreman (1987) found that variables that represented the four conservation principles were more important in combination than separately when used to diagnose confusion in hospitalized elderly patients. Nagley (1984) did not find significant differences in groups of hospitalized elderly in relation to confusion between those treated with nursing measures derived from the four principles of conservation and those who did not receive such treatment. However, she questioned the accuracy of the initial diagnosis of confusion for these patients.

Other studies have also been conducted. A number of these are included in Schaefer and Pond (1991). Others are unpublished master's theses or doctoral dissertations, and thus are less accessible than published materials, especially when they are not included in either *Masters Abstracts International* or *Dissertation Abstracts International*.

The studies reported in the literature have been primarily descriptive correlational studies. Many have both quantitative and qualitative aspects.

6. Does this theory direct critical thinking in nursing practice? Critical thinking is required for effective use of the principles of conservation. Critical thinking is particularly important in the conservation of personal integrity since the nurse must be sensitive to what data is imperative to identifying appropriate therapeutic measures and which is best left to the person rather than filling in the blanks in a standardized assessment form.

7. Does this theory direct therapeutic nursing interventions? The desired outcome of nursing interventions is to return a person who has become dependent due to the predicament of an illness to a state of independence as quickly as possible. Levine's work certainly provides a guide to practice and if used consistently can improve practice. Areas of nursing practice that have been reported in the literature as using Levine's work include the homeless; patients with burns, cervical cancer, chronic pain, congestive heart failure, and epilepsy; and clinical settings that include critical care, emergency room, intensive care nursery, long-term care, pediatrics, perioperative nursing, and smoking cessation (Bayley, 1991; Brunner, 1985; Cox, 1991; Crawford-Gamble, 1986; Dever, 1991; Erwin & Biordi, 1991; Fawcett, et al., 1987; Langer, 1990; Lynn-McHale & Smith, 1991; McCall, 1991; Neswick, 1997; O'Laughlin, 1986; Pasco & Halupa, 1991; Pond, 1991; Pond & Taney, 1991; Savage & Culbert, 1989; Schaefer, 1991). Levine's work has also been used in both undergraduate and graduate education (Grindley & Paradowski, 1991; Schaefer, 1991).

8. Does this theory direct communication in nursing practice? Communication is required to help a person in a predicament of illness to accept temporary dependence and to conserve, adapt, and regain or maintain integrity. Specific directions for communication skills are not included.

9. Does this theory direct nursing actions that lead to favorable outcomes? The purpose of the nursing actions is to help the person return to a state of health, a state of independence. This favorable outcome is clearly included as part of the theory.

10. How contagious is this theory? Unfortunately, a search of the literature does not clearly reflect the full use of Levine's work. The literature does support its use in a variety of clinical settings and some research has been conducted using the theory as a framework for the study or as a guide in assessing the data. There is also documentation of its use in Brazil (Fagundes, 1983).

STRENGTHS AND LIMITATIONS

A major strength of Levine's work is its universality. Her concepts apply to all human beings wherever they may be. She also indicates when nursing is needed—it is needed by the person in a predicament of illness who is willing to become dependent in relation to that predicament. Thus, the use of this work is not limited to any given setting but may be used wherever there is a nurse and a patient.

Levine's careful use of words is also a strength. Her careful selection of terminology provides clarity to the reader. She provides clear connections to the works of others (the adjunctive disciplines) and certainly helps the reader understand how these works can be used in a way that is specific to nursing.

Her stress on the wholeness of the person, the importance of integrity, is very useful. Also, her statement that adaptation is a process, not a value, helps us understand that adaptation is what is, rather than a positive or negative state. She describes adaptation as a bridge between environments (Levine, 1996).

A limitation could be considered to be the need for each nurse to create his or her own assessment tool to use Levine's conservation principles. This could also be viewed as providing flexibility and allowing each nurse to create a personal fit with the principles.

SUMMARY

Myra Levine's theory has evolved from a publication whose initial intention was the organization of medical-surgical nursing content to facilitate student learning. Her theory interrelates the concepts of adaptation, conservation, and integrity. Adaptation is the process by which conservation occurs. Human beings are constantly in interaction with their environments. It is this interaction that creates the need for adaptation. As the environment changes, the human must adapt. Successful adaptation will achieve the best fit with the environment and will do so in a manner that conserves energy, structural integrity, personal integrity, and social integrity. The purpose of conservation is health, or integrity—the wholeness of the individual. This theory has been tested through research and its usefulness demonstrated in clinical practice and education.

REFERENCES

Bates, M. (1967). A naturalist at large. *Natural history, 76*(6), 8–16.

Bayley, E. W. (1991). Care of the burn patient. In K. M. Schaefer & J. B. Pond (Eds.), *Levine's conservation model: A framework for nursing practice* (pp. 91–99). Philadelphia: Davis.

Brunner, M. (1985). A conceptual approach to critical care nursing using Levine's model. *Focus on Critical Care, 12*(2), 39–44.

Cannon, W. B. (1939). *The wisdom of the body.* New York: Norton.

Cohen, Y. (1968). *Man in adaptation: The biosocial background.* Chicago: Aldine.

Cox, S. R. A. (1991). A tradition of caring: Use of Levine's model in long-term care. In K. M. Schaefer & J. B. Pond (Eds.), *Levine's conservation model: A framework for nursing practice* (pp. 179–197). Philadelphia: Davis.

Crawford-Gamble, P. E. (1986). An application of Levine's conceptual model. *Perioperative Nursing Quarterly, 2*(1), 64–70.

Dever, M. (1991). Care of children. In K. M. Schaefer & J. B. Pond (Eds.), *Levine's conservation model: A framework for nursing practice* (pp. 71–82). Philadelphia: Davis.

Dubos, R. (1965). *Man adapting.* New Haven, CT: Yale University Press.

Erikson, E. (1969). *Ghandi's truth.* New York: Norton.

Erikson, E. (1975). *Life history and the historical moment.* New York: Norton.

Erwin, S., & Biordi, D. (1991). A smoke-free environment: Psychiatric nurses respond. *Journal of Psychosocial Nursing and Mental Health Services, 29*(5), 12–18.

Fagundes, N. C. (1983). O processo de enfermagem em saude comunitaria a partir de teoria de Myra Levine (The nursing process in community health as derived from Myra Levine's theory). *Rev Bras Enferm, 38,* 265–273.

Fawcett, J., Cariello, F. P., Davis, D. A., Farley, J., Zimmaro, D. M., & Watts, R. J. (1987). Conceptual models of nursing: Application to critical care nursing practice. *Dimensions of Critical Care Nursing, 6*, 202–213.

Foreman, M. D. (1987). The development of confusion in the hospitalized elderly. *Dissertation Abstracts International, 48-08B*, 2261.

Foreman, M. D. (1989). Confusion in the hospitalized elderly: Incidence, onset, and associated factors. *Research in Nursing and Health, 12*, 21–29.

Foreman, M. D. (1991). Conserving cognitive integrity of the hospitalized elderly. In K. M. Schaefer & J. B. Pond (Eds.), *Levine's conservation model: A framework for nursing practice* (pp. 133–149). Philadelphia: Davis.

Gibson, J. E. (1966). *The senses considered as perceptual systems*. Boston: Houghton-Mifflin.

Goldstein, K. (1963). *Human nature*. New York: Schocken.

Grindley, J., & Paradowski, M. (1991). Developing an undergraduate program using Levine's model. In K. M. Schaefer & J. B. Pond (Eds.), *Levine's conservation model: A framework for nursing practice* (pp. 199–208). Philadelphia: Davis.

Langer, V. S. (1990). Minimal handling protocol for the intensive care nursery. *Neonatal Network, 9*(3), 23–27.

Levine, M. E. (1966). Trophicognosis: An alternative to nursing diagnosis. In *American Nurses' Association Regional Clinical Conference Vol. 23* (pp. 55–70). New York: American Nurses' Association.

Levine, M. E. (1969). *Introduction to clinical nursing*. Philadelphia: Davis. (out of print)

Levine, M. E. (1973). *Introduction to clinical nursing* (2nd ed.). Philadelphia: Davis. (out of print)

Levine, M. E. (1989). The conservation principles of nursing: Twenty years later. In J. Riehl-Sisca (Ed.), *Conceptual models for nursing practice* (3rd ed.) (pp. 325–337). Norwalk, CT: Appleton & Lange.

Levine, M. E. (1990). Conservation and integrity. In M. E. Parker (Ed.), *Nursing theories in practice* (pp. 189–201) (Pub. No. 15-2350). New York: National League for Nursing.

Levine, M. E. (1991). The conservation principles: A model for health. In K. M. Schaefer & J. B. Pond (Eds.), *Levine's conservation model: A framework for nursing practice* (pp. 1–11). Philadelphia: Davis.

Levine, M. E. (1996). The conservation principles: A retrospective. *Nursing Science Quarterly, 9*, 38–41.

Lynn-McHale, D. J., & Smith, A. (1991). Comprehensive assessment of families of the critically ill. *AACN Clinical Issues in Critical Care Nursing, 2*, 195–209.

MacLean, S. L. (1987). Description of cues nurses use for diagnosing activity intolerance. *Dissertation Abstracts International, 48–08B*, 2264.

Maslow, A. (1968). *Toward a psychology of being* (2nd ed.). Princeton, NJ: VanNostrand.

McCall, B. H. (1991). Neurological intensive monitoring system: Unit assessment tool. In K. M. Schaefer & J. B. Pond (Eds.), *Levine's conservation model: A framework for nursing practice* (pp. 83–90). Philadelphia: Davis.

Nagley, S. J. (1984). Prevention of confusion in hospitalized elderly persons. *Dissertation Abstracts International, 45–06B*, 1732.

Neswick, R. S. (1997). Myra E. Levine: A theoretic basis for ET nursing. *Journal of WOCN, 21*(1), 6–9.

Newport, M. A. (1984). Conserving thermal energy and social integrity in the newborn. *Western Journal of Nursing Research, 6*, 176–197.

O'Laughlin, K. M. (1986). Changes in bladder function in the woman undergoing radical hysterectomy for cervical cancer. *JOGNN: Journal of Obstetric, Gynecologic, and Neonatal Nursing, 15*, 380–385.

Pappas, W. S. (1990). The sexually transmitted disease patient's satisfaction with nursing care and impact on anxiety level. *Masters Abstracts International, 29–01*, 97.

Pasco, A., & Halupa, D. (1991). Chronic pain management. In K. M. Schaefer & J. B. Pond (Eds.), *Levine's conservation model: A framework for nursing practice* (pp. 101–117). Philadelphia: Davis.

Pond, J. B. (1991). Ambulatory care of the homeless. In K. M. Schaefer & J. B. Pond (Eds.), *Levine's conservation model: A framework for nursing practice* (pp. 167–178). Philadelphia: Davis.

Pond, J. B., & Taney, S. G. (1991). Emergency care in a large university emergency department. In K. M. Schaefer & J. B. Pond (Eds.), *Levine's conservation model: A framework for nursing practice* (pp. 151–166). Philadelphia: Davis.

Rogers, C. R. (1961). *On becoming a person.* Boston: Houghton Mifflin.

Sacks, O. (1985). *The man who mistook his wife for a hat.* New York: Summit.

Savage, T. A., & Culbert, C. (1989). Early intervention: The unique role of nursing. *Journal of Pediatric Nursing, 4*, 339–345.

Schaefer, K. M. (1991). Developing a graduate program in nursing: Integrating Levine's philosophy. In K. M. Schaefer & J. B. Pond (Eds.), *Levine's conservation model: A framework for nursing practice* (pp. 209–217). Philadelphia: Davis.

Schaefer, K. M., & Pond, J. B. (Eds.). (1991). *Levine's conservation model: A framework for nursing practice.* Philadelphia: Davis.

Selye, H. (1956). *The stress of life.* New York: McGraw-Hill.

Taylor, J. W. (1974). Measuring the outcomes of nursing care. *Nursing Clinics of North America, 9*, 337–349.

Trench, A. S. (Executive producer), Wallace, D. (Producer), & Coberg, T. (Director). (1987). *Myra E. Levine—The nurse theorists: Portraits of excellence* [Videotape]. Oakland, CA: Studio Three Production, Samuel Merritt College of Nursing.

Winslow, E., Lane, L. D., & Gaffney, F. A. (1985). Oxygen consumption and cardiovascular response in control adults and acute myocardial infarction patients during bathing. *Nursing Research, 34*, 164–169.

Wong, S. (1968). *Rehabilitation of a patient following myocardial in/out.* Unpublished master's thesis, Loyola University of Chicago School of Nursing.

Yeates, D. A., & Roberts, J. E. (1984). A comparison of two bearing-down techniques during the second stage of labor. *Journal of Nurse-Midwifery, 29*, 3–11.

BIBLIOGRAPHY

Levine, M. E. (1967). The four conservation principles of nursing. *Nursing Forum, 6*, 45–59.

Levine, M. E. (1969). The pursuit of wholeness. *American Journal of Nursing, 69*, 93–98.

Levine, M. E. (1970). The intransgient patient. *American Journal of Nursing, 70*, 2106–2111.

Levine, M. E. (1971). Holistic nursing. *Nursing Clinics of North America, 6*, 253–264.

Levine, M. E. (1988). Antecedents from adjunctive disciplines: Creation of nursing theory. *Nursing Science Quarterly, 1*, 16–21.

ANNOTATED BIBLIOGRAPHY

Blasage, M. C. (1987). Toward a general understanding of nursing education: A critical analysis of the work of Myra Estrin Levine. *Dissertation Abstracts International, 47-11B*, 4467.

 The purpose of this research was to review and identify trends in the writings of Myra Estrin Levine. In addition, the study compared and contrasted Levine's model with those of Imogene King and Dorothea Orem. Levine's model was identified as one of her greatest contributions to nursing. Four trends were identified in her writings. These trends included holistic patient care, communication, nursing education, and ethics in nursing practice.

CHAPTER 13

SYSTEMS FRAMEWORK AND THEORY OF GOAL ATTAINMENT
IMOGENE M. KING

Julia B. George

Imogene M. King was born in 1923, the youngest of three children. She received her basic nursing education from St. John's Hospital School of Nursing in St. Louis, Missouri, graduating in 1945. Her B.S. in nursing and education with minors in philosophy and chemistry (1948) and M.S. in nursing (1957) are from St. Louis University and her Ed.D. (1961) is from Teachers College, Columbia University, New York. She has done postdoctoral study in research design, statistics, and computers (King, 1986b).

King has had experience in nursing as an administrator, an educator, and a practitioner. Her area of clinical practice is adult medical-surgical nursing. She has been a faculty member at St. John's Hospital School of Nursing, St. Louis; Loyola University, Chicago; and the University of South Florida. She served as director of the School of Nursing at The Ohio State University, Columbus. She was an Assistant Chief of the Research Grants Branch, Division of Nursing, Department of Health, Education, and Welfare in the mid-1960s and on the Defense Advisory Committee on Women in the Services for the Department of Defense in the early 1970s. She is professor emeritus from the University of South Florida and continues to consult and work on the further application of her theory. She has been actively involved in the establishment of the King International Nursing Group, headquartered at Oakland University's School of Nursing (www.snaou.nursing.oakland.edu/king/index.htm).

From the early 1960s the rapidity of knowledge development in many arenas has had as great an impact on the profession of nursing as on the rest of society. In the 1960s, as emerging professionals, nurses were identifying the knowledge base specific to nursing practice and to an expanding role for nurses. In this environment, Imogene M. King (1971) sought to answer several questions:

1. What are some of the social and educational changes in the United States that have influenced changes in nursing?
2. What basic elements are continuous throughout these changes in nursing?
3. What is the scope of the practice of nursing, and in what kind of settings do nurses perform their functions?
4. Are the current goals of nursing similar to those of the past half century?
5. What are the dimensions of practice that have given the field of nursing unifying focus over time? (p. 19).

In exploring the literature on systems analysis and general system theory, King (1971) developed additional questions:

1. What kind of decisions are nurses required to make in the course of their roles and responsibilities?
2. What kind of information is essential for them to make decisions?
3. What are the alternatives in nursing situations?
4. What alternative courses of action do nurses have in making critical decisions about another individual's care, recovery, and health?
5. What skills do nurses now perform and what knowledge is essential for nurses to make decisions about alternatives? (pp. 19–20).

King's *Toward a theory for nursing: General concepts of human behavior* was published in 1971 and *A theory for nursing: Systems, concepts, process* in 1981 (reprinted in 1990). These publications grew from King's thoughts about the vast amount of knowledge available to nurses and the difficulty this presents to the individual nurse in choosing the facts and concepts relevant to a given situation. In the preface to *Toward a theory for nursing* (1971), King clearly states she was proposing a conceptual framework for nursing and not a nursing theory. As she denoted in the title, her purpose was to help move *toward* a theory for nursing. In contrast, in the preface to *A theory for nursing* (1981/1990a), she indicates that she has expanded and built on the original framework. In this second publication, she again presents her system based conceptual framework and discusses the relationship of the concepts she identifies as fundamental to comprehending nursing as a system in the health care systems. In this text she also discusses concept development and knowledge application in nursing and, through explication of her Theory of Goal Attainment, derived from the open systems framework, shows one way of constructing a theory.

King (1997, 2001) now identifies her framework as a conceptual system. The function of a conceptual system is to give support for arranging ideas or concepts into a grouping that provides meaning. As her extensive documentation indicates, she has drawn from a wide variety of sources in developing the conceptual system and deriving the theory from that conceptual system. Because the Theory of Goal Attainment is derived from the conceptual system, the conceptual system and its assumptions and concepts are presented first, and then the goal attainment theory is discussed.

KING'S CONCEPTUAL SYSTEM

The purposes of the conceptual system are to 1) name concepts necessary to nursing as a discipline, 2) provide for the derivation of theories that are tested through research as part of the development of the scientific base for nursing knowledge, 3) provide an organizing structure for nursing curricula and 4) lead to nursing practice, based in theory, that supports quality care in all settings in which nursing occurs (King, 1990c, 1997). Concepts and knowledge may be similar across disciplines, but the way each profession uses them will differ (King, 1989). The conceptual system includes goal, structure, functions, resources, and decision making, which King (1990c, 1997) says are essential elements. The conceptual system has health as the *goal* for nursing. *Structure* is represented by three open systems. *Functions* are demonstrated in reciprocal relations of individuals in interaction and transactions. *Resources* include both people (health professionals and their clients) and money, goods, and services for items needed to carry out specific activities. *Decision making* occurs when choices are made in resource allocation to support attaining system goals.

King (1989) presents several assumptions that are basic to her conceptual system. These include the assumptions that human beings are open systems in constant interaction with their environment, that nursing's focus is human beings interacting with their environment, and that nursing's goal is to help individuals and groups maintain health.

The conceptual system is composed of three interacting systems: the personal systems, the interpersonal systems, and the social systems. Figure 13–1 presents a schematic diagram of these interacting systems. King (1995) summarizes the conceptual system as focusing on human behavior. Each personal system represents an individual. When individuals interact with others, they form interpersonal systems that may range in size from two people to a large group. Groups interact with one another and form social systems that in turn are part of a community; communities reside in societies.

The unit of analysis for the conceptual system is the behavior of humans in various social environments (King, 1995). King identifies several concepts as relevant for each of these systems. However, she also states that the placement of concepts with each system is arbitrary because all the concepts are interrelated in the human–environment interaction and that knowledge of all the concepts is used by the nurse in most situations. King (1981/1990a) has defined most of these concepts and refers back to these definitions in her later publications.

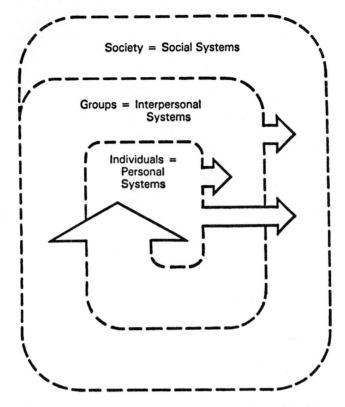

Figure 13–1. Dynamic interacting systems. (*Adapted from King, I. M. (1971). Toward a theory for nursing, New York: Wiley, p. 20. Copyright (c) 1971, by John Wiley & Sons, Inc. Used with permission.*)

Personal Systems

Each individual is a personal system. For a personal system the relevant concepts are perception, self, growth and development, body image, space, and time (King, 1986a 1988). *Perception* is presented as the major concept of a personal system, the concept that influences all behaviors or to which all other concepts are related. The characteristics of perception are that it is universal, or experienced by all; subjective or personal; and selective for each person, meaning that any given situation will be experienced in a unique manner by each individual involved. Perception is focused on activity in the present that is based on the available information. Also, perception is transactions; that is, individuals are active participants in situations and their identities are affected by their participation (King, 1981/1990a). King further discusses perception as a process in which data obtained through the senses and from memory are organized, interpreted, and transformed. This process of human interaction with the environment influences behavior, provides meaning to experience, represents the individual's image of reality and includes learning.

The characteristics of *self* are the dynamic person who is an open system, and whose actions are oriented toward achieving goals. King (1981/1990a) accepts Jersild's (1952) definition of self that includes self as made up of those thoughts and feelings related to one's awareness of being a person separate from others and influencing one's view of who and what he or she is. Included are attitudes, ideas, values, and commitments. Also, self differentiates one's inner world from the outer world in which other people and objects exist.

The characteristics of *growth and development* include changes in behavior at the cellular and molecular levels in individuals. These changes usually occur in an orderly manner, one that is predictable but has individual variations. They are influenced by genetic makeup; life experiences, especially those that have meaning and lead to satisfaction; and by an environment that supports movement toward maturity (King, 1981/1990a). Growth and development can be defined as the processes in people's lives through which they move from a potential for achievement to actualization of self. Theorists mentioned are Freud (1966), Erikson (1950), Piaget (Inhelder & Piaget, 1964), Gesell (1952), and Havinghurst (1953), but no particular model, theory, or framework of growth and development is specifically selected.

Body image is characterized as very personal and subjective, acquired or learned, dynamic and changing as the person redefines self. Body image is part of each stage of growth and development. King (1981/1990a) indicates body image includes both the way one perceives one's body and others' reactions to one's appearance.

Space is characterized as universal because everyone has some concept of it. It may be personal and subjective; situational and dependent on the relationships in the situation; dimensional as a function of volume, area, distance, and time; and transactional or based on the individual's perception of the situation. King (1981/1990a) states that space occurs in every direction, is universally the same, and is defined by the physical area known as territory and by the behaviors of those who occupy it. Individual definitions of space are influenced by culture.

Time is characterized as universal and inherent in life processes; relational or dependent on distance and the amount of information occurring; unidirectional or irreversible as it moves from past to future with a continuous flow of events; measurable; and subjective because it is based on perception. King (1981/1990a) defines time as an interval between the two events that is experienced differently by each person.

In 1986, King (1986a) added *learning* as a concept in the personal system. She did not further define learning as a concept. Learning is included in 1995, but is not discussed as a separate concept in later publications.

Perception, self, growth and development, body image, space, and time are the concepts of the personal system. The focus of nursing in the personal system is the person (King, 1986a). When personal systems come in contact with one another, they form interpersonal systems.

Interpersonal Systems

Interpersonal systems are formed by human beings interacting. Two interacting individuals form a dyad, three form a triad, and four or more form small or large groups. The complexity of the interactions increases as the number of people interacting increases. The relevant concepts for interpersonal systems are interaction, communication, transaction, role, and stress (King, 1981/1990a, 1995). The concepts from the personal system are also used in understanding interactions (King, 1989). In 1992, King included interpersonal relationships as a concept of interpersonal systems. She did not define this concept and it has not been included in later works.

Interaction is characterized by values; mechanisms for establishing human relationships; being universally experienced; being influenced by perceptions; reciprocity; being mutual or interdependent; containing verbal and nonverbal communication; learning occurring when communication is effective; unidirectionality; irreversibility; dynamism; and existing in time and space (King, 1981/1990a). Interactions are defined as the observable behaviors of two or more persons in mutual presence.

Characteristics of *communication* are that it is verbal and nonverbal situational; perceptual; transactional; irreversible, or moving forward in time; personal; and dynamic (King, 1981/1990a). Symbols for verbal communications are provided by language, for such communication includes the spoken and written language that conveys ideas from one person or group to another. An important aspect of nonverbal behavior is touch. Other aspects of nonverbal behavior are distance, posture, facial expression, physical appearance, and body movements. Communication involves the exchange of information between persons. This may occur face-to-face, through electronic media, and through the written word. Communication as a fundamental social process develops and maintains human relations and facilitates the ordered functioning of human groups and societies. As the information component of human interactions, communication occurs in all behaviors. King also discusses communication as intrapersonal or occurring within the person. She includes genetics, metabolic changes, hormonal fluctuations, neurological signals as well as psychological processes and indicates that intrapersonal communication can affect the person's social exchanges.

Transactions, for this conceptual system, are derived from cognition and perceptions and not from transactional analysis. The characteristics of transactions are that they are unique because each person has a distinctive view of the world based on that person's perceptions; they occur in space and time; and they are experience—a series of events in time. King (1981/1990a) defines transactions as a series of exchanges between human beings and the environment that include observable behaviors that seek to reach goals of worth to the participants.

The characteristics of *role* include reciprocity in that a person may be a giver at one time and a taker at another time, with a relationship between two or more individuals who are functioning in two or more roles that are learned, social, complex, and situational (King, 1981/1990a). There are three major elements of role. The first is that role consists of a set of expected behaviors of those who occupy an identified position in a social system. The second is a set of procedures or rules that define the obligations and rights associated with a position in an organization. The third is a relationship of two or more persons who are interacting for a purpose in a particular situation. The nurse's role can be defined as interacting with one or more others in a nursing situation in which the nurse as a professional uses the skills, knowledge, and values identified as belonging to nursing to identify goals with others and help them achieve the goals.

The characteristics of *stress* are that it is universal dynamic as a result of open systems being in continuous exchange with the environment; the intensity varies; there is a temporal-spatial dimension that is influenced by past experiences; it is individual, personal, and subjective—a response to life events that is uniquely personal. King (1981/1990a) defines stress as an ever changing condition in which an individual, through environmental interaction, seeks to keep equilibrium to support growth and development and activity. This environmental interaction is based on an open system process of exchange of information and energy with the purpose of regulating and controlling stressors. In addition, stress involves objects, persons, and events as stressors that evoke an energy response from the person. Stress may be positive or negative, and may simultaneously help an individual to a peak of achievement and wear the individual down.

The defined concepts of interpersonal systems are interaction, communication, transaction, role, and stress. The focus of nursing in the interpersonal system is the environment (King, 1986a). Interpersonal systems join together to form larger systems known as social systems.

Social Systems

A social system is a structured large group in a system that includes the roles, behaviors, and practices defined by the system for the purposes of sustaining desirable attributes and for creating methods to maintain the practices and rules of the system (King, 1981/1990a). Examples of social systems include peers, families, community groups, religious groups, educational organizations, governments, and work systems. The concepts relevant to social systems are organization, authority, power, status, decision making, and control plus all the concepts from the personal and interpersonal systems (King, 1989). In 1992, 1995, and 2001 control is not included as a concept of social systems and control has not been defined.

King (1981/1990a) proposes four parameters for *organization*. The first is those values held by human beings as well as the patterns of behavior and the expectations, needs, and desired outcomes of the individuals in the system. The second is the environment in which the system exists and which influences the availability of resources, both material and human. The third is the humans in the system—family members, administration and staff, officers and members. The fourth involves the technology used to reach the goals of the organization.

An *organization* is characterized by a structure that orders positions and activities and includes formal and informal arrangements of people to gain both personal and organizational goals; has functions that describe the roles and positions of people as well as the activities to be performed; goals or outcomes to be achieved; and resources. King defines organization as being made up of individuals who have prescribed roles and positions and who make use of resources to meet goals—both personal and organizational.

The characteristics of *authority* include that it is observable through the regularity, direction, and responsibility for actions it provides; universal; necessary to formal organizations; reciprocal because it requires cooperation; resides in a holder who must be perceived as legitimate; situational; essential to goal achievement; and associated with power (King, 1981/1990a). Assumptions about authority include that it can be discerned by human beings and seen as legitimate; it can be associated with a position in which the position holder distributes rewards and sanctions; it can be held by professionals through their competence in using special knowledge and skills; and it can be exercised through group leadership by those with human relations skills. King defines authority as an active, reciprocal process of transaction in which the actors' experience, understanding, and values influence the meaning, legitimacy, and acceptance of those in organizational positions associated with authority.

Power is characterized as universal, situational (i.e., not a personal attribute but existing in the situation), necessary in the organization, influenced by resources in a situation, dynamic, and goal directed (King, 1981/1990a). Premises about power are that energy that is potential rather than actual, is necessary to avoid chaos in society, increases group integration, is related to organizational position, has a direct association with authority, is a function of the communication of human beings, and is associated with decision making. King defines power in a variety of ways including organizational capacity to use resources to meet goals, one person influencing others, capability to attain goals, existing in every area of life with all having potential for power, and a social force.

Status is characterized as situational, position dependent, and reversible. King (1981/1990a) defines status as the relationship of one's place in a group to others in the group or of a group to other groups. She also identifies that status is accompanied by advantages, accountabilities, and requirements.

Decision making is characterized as necessary to provide order in an individual's or group's living and working, universal, individual, personal, subjective, situational, a continuous process, and goal directed. Decision making in organizations is defined as a changing and orderly process through which choices related to goals are made among identified possible activities and individual or group actions are taken to move toward the goal (King, 1981/1990a).

The major theses of King's (1981/1990a) conceptual system are that every individual views the world as a whole as goals are identified and sought with other people and with objects in the environment. Also, the establishment of and movement toward goals occur in life situations characterized by the interaction of the perceiver and the perceived (person or object) with each person being an active participant and each participant changed by the activities and exchanges the occur.

Theories may be derived from conceptual frameworks. King has derived a Theory of Goal Attainment from the concepts and systems of her conceptual system.

KING'S THEORY OF GOAL ATTAINMENT

The major elements of King's middle range Theory of Goal Attainment are seen "in the interpersonal systems in which two people, who are usually strangers, come together in a health care organization to help and be helped to maintain a state of health that permits functioning in roles" (King, 1981/1990a, p. 142). The theory's focus on interpersonal systems reflects King's belief that the practice of nursing is differentiated from that of other health professions by what nurses do with and for individuals. The concepts of the theory are interaction, perception, communication, transaction, self, role, stress, growth and development, time, and personal space (King, 1990c 1995, 1999). In her 2001 overview, King added decision making and omitted growth and development, stress, time, and space without discussion of a rationale for change. The most frequently identified concepts will be used in the following discussion.

These concepts of the theory are interrelated in every nursing situation (King, 1989, 1995). Although these terms have already been defined in the conceptual system discussion, they are defined again here as part of the Theory of Goal Attainment. King states that although all have been conceptually defined, only transaction has been operationally defined. However, the operational definition given for transaction is also used for interaction in another publication (King, 1990c).

Interaction is the observable verbal and nonverbal goal directed behaviors of two or more people in mutual presence and includes perception and communication (King, 1981/1990a). King diagrams interaction as seen in Figure 13–2. This is also known as the transaction process model. Each of the individuals involved in an interaction brings different ideas, attitudes, and perceptions to the exchange. The individuals come together for a purpose and perceive each other; each makes a judgment and takes mental action or decides to act. Then each reacts to the other and the situation (perception, judgment, action, reaction). King indicates that only the interaction and transaction are directly observable. Her law of nurse-patient interaction is "nurses and patients in mutual presence, interacting purposefully, make transactions in nursing situations based on each individual's perceptions, purposeful communication and valued goals" (King, 1997, p. 184).

Perception is reality as seen by each individual (King, 1981/1990a) The elements of perception are the importing of energy from the environment and organizing it by information, transforming energy, processing information, storing information, and exporting information in the form of observable behaviors.

Communication is the exchange of information between people that may occur during a face-to-face meeting, through electronic media, and through the written word (King, 1981/1990a). Communication represents, and is part of, the information aspect of interaction and may occur within a person as well as between people.

Transaction is a series of exchanges between human beings and their environment that include observable behaviors that seek to reach goals of worth to the participants (King, 1981/1990a). Transactions represent the aspect of human interactions in which values are apparent and involve compromising, conferring, and social exchange. When transactions occur between nurses and clients, goals are attained.

Role is defined as a set of expected behaviors (King, 1981/1990a). Related to role is the position held by the person, the rights and responsibilities associated with that position, and the relationship between the interacting individuals. It is important that roles be understood and interpreted clearly by all persons involved in defining the expected behaviors to avoid conflict and confusion.

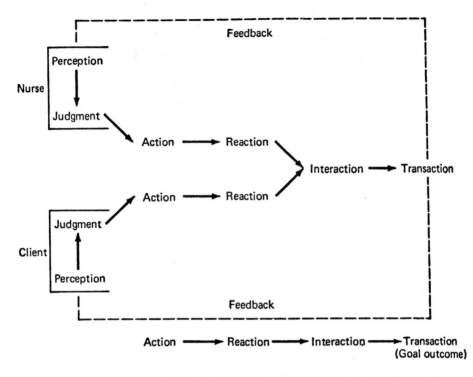

Figure 13–2. Interaction. (*Adapted from King, I. M. (1971). Toward a theory for nursing: General concepts of human behavior, New York: Wiley, pp. 26, 92. Copyright (c) 1971, by John Wiley & Sons, Inc. Used with permission.*)

Stress is an ever changing condition in which an individual, through environmental interaction, seeks to keep equilibrium to support growth and development and activity. This environmental interaction is based on an open system process of exchange of information and energy with the purpose of regulating and controlling stressors (King, 1981/1990a). Although stress may be positive or negative, too high a level of stress may decrease an individual's ability to interact and to attain goals. It may be the level of stress rather than the positive or negative nature of the stress that is most important.

Growth and development can be defined as the ever occurring changes in behavior and at the cellular and molecular levels in individuals. These changes serve to move the person from potential to achievement (King, 1981/1990a).

Time is an interval between two events that is experienced differently by each person. Time is also involved in relating one event to another (King, 1981/1990a).

Space exists in every direction and is the same in all directions. Space includes that physical area named territory. Space is defined by the behaviors of those individuals who occupy it (King, 1981/1990a).

Health is not stated as a concept in the theory but is identified as the goal for nursing (King, 1990b). King (1986a) indicates the outcome is an individual's state of health or ability to function in social roles.

King's (1981/1990a, 1989, 1990c) operational definition of transaction has been used to identify the elements in interactions, at other times called a model of transactions. These elements are *action, reaction, disturbance (problem), mutual goal setting, exploration of means to achieve the goal, agreement on means to achieve the goal, transaction,* and *goal attainment.* The model essentially describes an interpersonal dyad (nurse and client) in interactions, using mutual goal setting or decision making as a process that leads to goal attainment.

From the Theory of Goal Attainment, King (1990c) has developed predictive propositions that 1) Perceptual accuracy, role congruence, and communication in a nurse–client interaction leads to transactions; 2) Transactions lead to goal attainment and growth and development; and 3) Goal attainment leads to satisfaction and to effective nursing care (pp. 80–81). She suggests that additional propositions may be generated.

Originally, King (1981/1990a) specified internal and external boundary-determining criteria. Internal boundary criteria were derived from the characteristics of the concepts of the theory and spoke to the theory itself. External boundary criteria spoke to the domain of the theory. King (personal communication, 2001) no longer supports boundary criteria as she states open systems do not have boundaries. However, these former boundary criteria do point out some important aspects of the Theory of Goal Attainment that are still pertinent.

- The nurse is a licensed practitioner of professional nursing.
- The client had a need for services provided by nursing.
- Generally, the nurse and client initially meet as strangers.
- The nurse and client meet in mutual presence and interact with the purpose of meeting goals.
- The nurse-client relationship is one of reciprocity
   ○ The nurse brings specialized knowledge and skills and can communicate information that is helpful in setting goals.
   ○ The client has information and knowledge about self and can communicate concerns and viewpoints to help in mutual goal setting.
- Interactions occur in a dyad (this is the original statement. More recently King has spoken to working with families, groups, and communities and identified the work of others in relation to interactions beyond the dyad).
- Interactions occur between the professional nurse and the client in need of nursing.
- The environment for interactions is a natural one.

In 1995, King includes these ideas in her discussion of the transaction process model and adds that nurses may interact with family members when the client in not verbal. In 1987, King discussed the idea of client locus of control and stated that it is difficult to achieve mutual goal setting with a client who has an external locus of control.

Thus, King is saying that a professional nurse, with special knowledge and skills, and a client in need of nursing, with knowledge of self and perceptions of personal problems, meet as strangers in a natural environment. They interact mutually to identify problems and to establish and achieve goals. The personal system of the nurse and the personal system of the client meet in interaction with the interpersonal system of their dyad. Their interpersonal system is influenced by the social systems that surround them as well as by each of their personal systems.

KING'S THEORY AND NURSING'S METAPARADIGM

In discussing her conceptual system as an introduction to the presentation of her Theory of Goal Attainment, King (1981/1990a) indicates that the abstract concepts of the conceptual system are human beings, health, environment, and society. Because the theory is presented as a theory for nursing, King also defines nursing. Thus, the four major concepts of human beings, health, environment/society, and nursing are discussed by King.

King (1981/1990a) identifies several assumptions about *human beings*. She describes human beings as social, sentient, rational, reacting, perceiving, controlling, purposeful, action-oriented, and time-oriented. From these beliefs about human beings, she has derived the following assumptions that are specific to nurse–client interaction:

- Perceptions of nurse and of client influence the interaction process.
- Goals, needs, and values of nurse and client influence the interaction process.
- Individuals have a right to knowledge about themselves.
- Individuals have a right to participate in decisions that influence their life, their health, and community services.
- Health professionals have a responsibility to share information that helps individuals make informed decisions about their health care.
- Individuals have a right to accept or to reject health care.
- Goals of health professionals and goals of recipients of health care may be incongruent (pp. 143–144).

King (1981/1990a) further states that a concern for nursing is helping people interact with their environment in a manner that will support health maintenance and growth toward self fulfillment. Human beings have three fundamental health needs: (1) the need for health information that is usable at the time when it is needed and can be used, (2) the need for care that seeks to prevent illness, and (3) the need for care when human beings are unable to help themselves. King indicates that nurses have the opportunity to find out what health information the client has, how the client views his or her own health, and what actions the client takes for health maintenance.

King defines *health* as "dynamic life experiences of a human being, which implies continuous adjustment to stressors in the internal and external environment through optimum use of one's resources to achieve maximum potential for daily living" (King, 1989, p. 152) and as "a dynamic state of an individual in which change is constant and ongoing and may be viewed as the individual's ability to function in his or her usual roles (King, 1990b, p. 76). King (1990b) affirms that health is not a continuum but a holistic state and identifies the characteristics of health as "genetic, subjective, relative, dynamic, environmental, functional, cultural, and perceptual" (p. 124). She discusses health as a functional state and illness as an interference with that functional state. She defines illness as a deviation from or imbalance in the person's normal functioning. This deviation may be related to biological structure, psychological make up, or social relationships (King, 1981/1990a).

Environment and *society* are indicated as major concepts in King's conceptual system but are not specifically defined in her work. Society may be viewed as the social systems portion of her conceptual system. In 1983, King extended the ability to interact in goal setting and selection of means to achieve the goal to include mutual goal setting with family members in relation to clients and families. Although her definition of health mentions both internal and external environment, and she has stated, "environment is a function of balance between internal and external interactions" (1990b, p. 127), the usual implication of the use of environment in *A theory for nursing* is that of external environment. Because she presents her material as based on open systems, it is assumed that a definition of external environment may be drawn from general system theory. Systems are considered to have semipermeable boundaries that help differentiate their internal components from the rest of the world. The external environment for a system is the portion of the world that exists outside of the system. Of particular interest as a system's external environment is the part of the world that is in direct exchange of energy and information with the system. King (1981/1990a) does say that the three systems form the environments that influence individuals.

Nursing is defined as the nurse and client using action, reaction, and interaction in a health care situation to share information about their perception of each other and the situation; this communication enables them to set goals and choose the methods for meeting the goals (King, 1981/1990a). *Action* is defined as a sequence of behaviors involving mental and physical activity. The sequence is first mental action to recognize the presenting conditions; then physical action to begin activities related to those conditions; and finally, mental action in an effort to exert control over the situation, combined with physical action seeking to achieve goals. *Reaction* is not specifically defined but might be considered to be included in the sequence of behaviors described in action. *Interaction* has been discussed previously. Although King has altered her definition of nursing from that published in 1971, she has continued to refer to nursing as that which is done by nurses. "Lawyer" and "legal situation," "physical therapist" and "therapy situation," or any other practitioner who interacts with clientele could be substituted for "nurse" and "healthcare situation" in her definitions of nursing. Such substitution would create definitions that could be applied to these other practices. This weakens her definition.

In addition to the foregoing definition of nursing, King (1981/1990a) discusses the goal, domain, and function of the professional nurse. The goal of the nurse is "to help individuals maintain health or regain health" (King, 1990b, pp. 3–4). Nursing's domain includes promoting, maintaining, and restoring health, and caring for the sick, injured, and dying. The function of the professional nurse is to interpret information in what is known as the nursing process to plan, implement, and evaluate nursing care for individuals, families, groups, and communities.

THEORY OF GOAL ATTAINMENT AND THE NURSING PROCESS

The basic assumption of the Theory of Goal Attainment—that nurses and clients communicate information, set goals mutually, and then act to attain those goals—is also the basic assumption of the nursing process. King (1990c, 1997) describes the steps of the nursing process as a system of interrelated actions and identifies concepts from her work that provide the theoretical basis for the nursing process as method.

According to King (1981/1990a, 1997), *assessment* occurs during the interaction of the nurse and client, who are likely to meet as strangers. Assessment may be viewed as paralleling action and reaction. The concepts King identifies are the perception, communication, and interaction of nurse and client. The nurse brings to this meeting special knowledge and skills, whereas the client brings knowledge of self and perceptions of the problems that are of concern. Assessment, interviewing, and communication skills are needed by the nurse as is the ability to integrate knowledge of natural and behavioral sciences for application to a concrete situation.

All concepts of the theory apply to assessment. Growth and development, knowledge of self and role, and the amount of stress influence perception and in turn influence communication, interaction, and transaction. In assessment, the nurse needs to collect data about the client's level of growth and development, view of self, perception of current health status, communication patterns, and role socialization, among other things. Factors influencing the client's perception include the functioning of the client's sensory system, age, development, sex, education, drug and diet history, and understanding of why contact with the health care system is occurring. The perceptions of the nurse are influenced by the cultural and socio-economic background and age of the nurse and the diagnosis of the client (King, 1981/1990a). Perception is the basis for gathering and interpreting data, thus the basis for assessment. Communication is necessary to verify the accuracy of perceptions. Without communication, interaction and transaction cannot occur.

For example, the nurse is meeting for the first time with Kelly Jenkins and gathers the following assessment data. She perceives Mrs. Jenkins as a well-groomed pregnant female who appears to be comfortable in the examination room and who makes eye contact with the nurse. As they interact, the nurse finds out that Kelly is 25 years old, married, about six months pregnant, and has gained 12 pounds so far during the pregnancy (growth and development); Kelly views herself as essentially healthy (self); she has a B.S. in English and taught high school English before the family's recent move to the area; she plans to look for a teaching position after the baby is born (role); the family's recent move has been a bit stressful since they must change health care providers in the middle of her first pregnancy, but also exciting because they have moved into their first house. Kelly indicates she is using e-mail more than she ever did before because it helps her keep in touch with friends and family "back home." She asks questions about Lamaze classes, and how she might locate a good dentist and pediatrician. She also reports she is very glad the nausea and vomiting she experienced during the first three months of her pregnancy are no longer bothering her. Her pregnancy appears to be progressing normally and without complications.

The information shared during assessment is used to derive a *nursing diagnosis*, defined by King (1981/1990a) as a statement that recognizes the distresses, difficulties, or worries identified by the client and for which help is sought. The implication is that the nurse makes the nursing diagnosis as a result of the mutual sharing with the client during assessment. Stress may be a particularly important concept in relation to nursing diagnosis because stress, distress, difficulty, and worry may be closely connected.

The nursing diagnoses for Kelly Jenkins would include "healthy primipara progressing normally through pregnancy" and "knowledge deficit about local resources for health care and childbirth related to recent move to the area." These are derived from the interactions that occurred during assessment.

After the nursing diagnosis is made, *outcomes* are identified and *planning* occurs. King (1997, 2001) indicates that goal attainment equates to outcomes. King (1997) says that the concepts involved are *decision making* about goals and *agreeing to means* to attain goals. King describes planning as setting goals and making decisions about how to achieve these goals. This is part of transaction and again involves mutual exchange with the client. She specifies that clients are requested to participate in decision making about how the goals are to be met. Although King assumes that in nurse–client interactions clients have the right to participate in decisions about their care, she does not say they have the responsibility. Thus, clients are requested to participate, not expected to do so. Carter and Dufour (1994) discuss that this ability of the client to decide not to decide enhances the cultural flexibility of King's work.

Implementation occurs in the activities that seek to meet the goals. Implementation is a continuation of transaction in King's theory. She states that the concept involved is the making of *transactions*.

With Kelly Jenkins, the mutually established desired outcome (or goal, in King's terminology) would be a healthy mother, father, and baby. The transactions would involve establishing and keeping a schedule of regular prenatal visits and the nurse providing referrals and information about community resources for the family to identify appropriate health care providers and childbirth education.

Evaluation involves descriptions of how the outcomes identified as goals are attained. In King's (1981/1990a) description, evaluation not only speaks to the attainment of the client's goals but also to the effectiveness of nursing care. She also indicates that the involved concept is goal attainment or, if not, why not (King, 1997).

Evaluation data would include the vaginal delivery of a 9 pound 2 ounce boy. Father is beaming and making plans for baseball and football games. The pediatrician selected by the family has seen the baby and pronounced him healthy. Mother and baby have had a successful initial experience with breastfeeding, with support of the nursing staff.

Although all the theory concepts apply throughout the nursing process, communication with perception, interaction, and transaction are vital for goal attainment and need to be apparent in each phase. King emphasizes the importance of mutual participation in interaction that focuses on the needs and welfare of the client and of verifying perceptions while planning and activities to achieve goals are carried out together. Although King emphasizes mutuality, she does not limit it to verbal communication, nor does she require the client's active physical participation in actions to achieve goal attainment. In situations where the nurse cannot interact directly with the client, Carter and Dufour (1994) support interaction with the family or other members of the client's interpersonal and social systems.

King (2001) has developed a documentation system, known as the goal oriented nursing record, to facilitate the implementation of the transaction process model and the attainment of goals. She has also developed the Goal Attainment Scale for use in measuring goal attainment.

CRITIQUE OF KING'S THEORY OF GOAL ATTAINMENT

1. What is the historical context of the theory? King began her study of the literature to answer her questions about the influence of changes on nursing as the rapid expansion of knowledge was being recognized. She supported her ideas from the literature and applied that information to the practice of nursing. She identifies an overall assumption for the Theory of Goal Attainment as including "that the focus of nursing is human beings interacting with their environment, leading to health for individuals, which is the ability to function in social roles" (King, 1992, p. 21). Assumptions about nurse–client interactions include that

> perceptions of nurse and client influence the interaction process. Individuals and families have a right to knowledge about their health. They have a right to accept or reject health care. They have a right to participate in decisions that influence their life, their health and community services. Health professionals have a responsibility to share information that helps individuals make informed decisions about their health. Health professionals have a responsibility to gather relevant information about the perceptions of the client so that their goals and the goals of the client are congruent (p. 21).

These latter assumptions were first presented for individuals in King's 1981 publication and include families in 1992. These assumptions are easily understood.

King derived a Theory of Goal Attainment from her conceptual system of personal, interpersonal, and social systems. This middle range theory was developed in the middle of the surge of nursing theory development in the latter part of the twentieth century. With the emphasis on holistic systems and perceptions, this theory fits best with the simultaneity paradigm.

2. What are the basic concepts and relationships presented by the theory? King used the concepts of interaction, perception, communication, transaction, self, role, stress, growth and development, time, and space for the Theory of Goal Attainment. Her theory deals with a nurse–client dyad, a relationship to which each brings perceptions of self, role, and levels of growth and development. The nurse and client communicate, first in interaction and then in transaction, to attain mutually set goals. The relationship takes place in space identified by their behaviors and occurs in forward-moving time. The specification of transaction as dealing with mutual goal attainment is a unique way of looking at the phenomenon of nurse–client relationships.

3. What major phenomena of concern to nursing are presented? These phenomenon may include *but are not limited to*: human being, environment, health, interpersonal relations, caring, goal attainment, adaptation, and energy fields. In addition to the four major concepts of human being, environment, health, and nursing, King has included the personal, interpersonal, and social systems. She also emphasizes the importance of interaction for transaction and of transaction for goal attainment. Health is identified as a goal.

4. To whom does it apply? In what situations? In what ways? Even though King indicates that many of her concepts are situation dependent, they are not situation specific; that is, they are influenced by the situation but may occur in many different situations. The Theory of Goal Attainment is limited in setting only in regard to "natural environments" and, with growth and development as a major concept, is certainly not limited in age. The Theory of Goal Attainment is generalizable to any dyadic nursing situation with a possible limitation relating to difficulties associated with seeking mutual goal setting with a client who has an external locus of control. The emphasis on mutuality would initially appear to limit the theory to dealing with those clients who can verbally interact with the nurse and physically participate in implementations to meet goals. However, King points to observable behaviors and to both verbal and nonverbal communication. Indeed, even the comatose individual has observable behaviors in the form of vital signs and does communicate nonverbally. Also, family members may be involved in transactions for the nonverbal individual. King predicts that with transactions and mutual goal setting the goals will be attained.

5. By what method or methods can this theory be tested? The research related to King's theory and conceptual system that has been reported in the literature has primarily used qualitative or descriptive methods of research (Bryant-Lukosius, 1993; Desruisseaux, 1991; Kirkpatrick, 1992; Lockhart, 1992; Lott, 1996; Rhodes, 1995; Talosi, 1993). Exceptions include Froman's (1995) factor relating research, Frey's (1988) and Doornbos' (1995) theory development studies, Bagby's (1994) use of Q-sort and three quasi-experimental studies (Cox, 1995; Fredenburgh, 1993; Harman, 1998). Those studies that have investigated transactions or goal attainment have supported that mutual goal setting and transactions increase goal attainment, or conversely, the lack of transactions is associated with lower levels of goal attainment (Ford, 1992; Froman, 1995; Hanna, 1993; Kameoka, 1995; Quirk, 1995). A number of studies have indicated the use of King as a guide or framework for studies involving perceptions (Harrity, 1992; Kirkpatrick, 1992; Lockhart, 1992; Lott, 1996; McGeein, 1992; Monti, 1992; Theobald, 1992; Villaneuva-Noble, 1998). In some of these studies the purpose of the study was to describe the perceptions of a group of people, such as nurses in a particular setting, rather than to investigate the effect of the nurse's perceptions and the client's perceptions on the ability of the nurse and client to interact and transact. It is questionable that these studies are testing relationships within the theory.

King (1990c) presents the following hypotheses that she states are being tested:

- Mutual goal setting will increase ability to perform activities of daily living.
- Mutual goal setting by nurse and patient leads to goal attainment.
- Goal attainment will be greater in patients who participate in goal setting than those who do not participate in goal setting.
- Mutual goal setting will increase elderly patients' morale.
- Perceptual congruence in nurse–patient interactions increases mutual goal setting.
- Goal attainment decreases stress and anxiety in nursing situations.
- Congruence in role expectations and role performance increases transactions in nurse–patient interactions (pp. 81–82).

King (1981/1990a) reports the results of a descriptive study conducted to test the theory of goal attainment. The study resulted in a classification system to analyze nurse–patient interactions and found that goal attainment is facilitated when the nurse and patient have congruent perceptions, adequate communication, and set goals mutually. She also states that data about interactions from two separate studies have confirmed the presence of transactions (King, 1990c).

6. Does this theory direct critical thinking in nursing practice? The activities involved in being aware of one's own perceptions and judgments, as well as those of the other and deciding how these influence the nurse-client interaction require critical thinking. The process of transactions to achieve goal attainment is also dependent on the exercise of critical thinking skills.

7. Does this theory direct therapeutic nursing interventions? Goal attainment requires therapeutic nursing interventions in the nurse–client relationship. Health is defined as involving the ability to function in social roles. The nurse–client relationship of interaction and transaction occurs because the client's interactions with the environment in some way requires support, information, or intervention. King does not define or specify therapeutic nursing interventions but indicates that the nurse and client bring knowledge and information to the relationship that will support the identification and development of such interventions.

8. Does this theory direct communication in nursing practice? Absolutely!! Interaction and transaction are dependent on communication. It is important to remember that communication occurs on many levels and through many mechanisms. King emphasizes the importance of both verbal and nonverbal forms of communication.

9. Does this theory direct nursing actions that lead to favorable outcomes? The focus of the theory is the attainment of goals. King (1981/1990a) has developed the goal-oriented nursing record in an effort to document the implementation of the transaction process model and goal attainment. She has also developed a criterion-referenced tool for measuring attainment of health goals (King, 1988, 2001). The theory predicts that the use of mutually set goals will lead to favorable outcomes.

10. How contagious is this theory? King's conceptual system and Theory of Goal Attainment are widely used, as evidenced by a growing body of literature about the conceptual system and theory. Studies reported in the literature include using King's conceptual system and/or Theory of Goal Attainment to investigate nurses' attitudes/characteristics/perceptions/knowledge (Brower, 1981; Kaminski, 1999; Keyworth, 1998; Lockhart, 1992; Lott, 1996; Mann, 1997; McGeein, 1992; Monna, 1989; Oates, 1994; Quirk, 1995; Ventresca, 1994); the effects of nursing actions (Duffy, 1990; Rosendahl & Ross, 1982); client's perceptions (Allan, 1995; Cox, 1995; Desruisseaux, 1991; Glasgow, 1998; Harrity, 1992; Hobdell, 1995; Monti, 1992; Morris, 1996; Rhodes, 1995; Rooke, 1995a); organizational structure or social systems (Dawson, 1996; Winker, 1996); and care in a variety of clinical areas or topics including children and adolescents, cardiac rehabilitation, chemical addiction, chronic illness, community mental health, diabetic care, families, health behavior change, menopause, parenting, postpartum and newborn care, and self-care (Binder, 1992; Campbell-Begg, 1998; Church, 1997; Fredenburgh, 1993; Frey, 1988, 1989, 1995; Hanucharunkui & Vinya-nguag, 1991; Kirkpatrick, 1992; Konkle-Parker, 1996; Laben, Dodd, & Sneed, 1991; Lincoln, 1997; Marasco, 1990; McGirr, Rukholm, Salmoni, O'Sullivan, & Koren, 1990; Meighan, 1998; Norris & Hoyer, 1993; Parsons & Ricker, 1993; Sharts-Engel, 1984; Sharts-Hopko, 1995; Skariah, 1999; Talosi, 1993; Villaneuva-Noble, 1998; White-Linn, 1994; Wicks, 1992).

Articles relating to the use of King's conceptual system or Theory of Goal Attainment in practice include such clinical areas and topics as carpal tunnel syndrome, case management, cultural diversity, diabetic care, discharge planning, documentation, the elderly, emergency care, genetics, HIV, managed care, neonates, oncology, orthopedics, organizational structure, parenting, practice framework, pregnancy, psychotherapy, tertiary care, and quality care (Alligood, 1995; Bauer, 1998, 1999; Benedict & Frey, 1995; Byrne & Schreiber, 1989; Coker, et al, 1995; DeHowitt, 1992; Fawcett, Vaillancourt, & Watson, 1995; Gill, et al, 1995; Hampton, 1994; Husband, 1988; Husting, 1997; Jolly & Winker, 1995; Jonas, 1987; Jones, Clark, Merker, & Palau, 1995; Kemppainen, 1990; Laben, Sneed, & Seidel, 1995; Messmer, 1995; Messner & Smith, 1986; Norgan, Ettipio, & Lasome, 1995;

Norris & Hoyer, 1993; Omar, 1989; Porter, 1991; Rooda, 1992; Shea, et al, 1989; Smith, 1988; Sowell & Lowenstein, 1994; Temple & Fawdry, 1992; Tritsch, 1998; West, 1991; Woods, 1994). Publications in relation to education have included preparation of certified nursing assistants, curriculum development, teaching methods, and student perceptions (Brown, 1999; Daubenmire, 1989; Dougal & Gonterman, 1999; Gold, Haas, & King, 2000; Gulitz & King, 1988; Harman, 1998).

Internationally, King's work has been used in relation to practice in Canada and Germany (Bauer, 1998, 1999; Fawcett, et al, 1995; Gill, et al, 1995; Porter, 1991; Shea, et al, 1989; West, 1991; Woods, 1994). In addition, it has been extended and tested in Sweden and Japan as well as used for education in Sweden (Frey, et al, 1995; Kameoka, 1995; Rooke, 1995b).

King's conceptual system and theory have demonstrated contagiousness. Further research is needed to establish the relationships among the concepts in the theory.

STRENGTHS AND LIMITATIONS

It is apparent from the use of the conceptual system and theory across multiple cultures, that King's work is not limited to use in the United States. This is a major strength in a time when communication can be instantaneous and multicultural situations are becoming the norm. Husting (1997) speaks to the importance of the cultural facets in each of the interacting systems in the conceptual system.

Although the presentation appears to be complex, King's Theory of Goal Attainment is relatively simple. Ten concepts are identified, defined, and their relationships considered; two concepts are identified only. King's Theory of Goal Attainment describes a logical sequence of events and, for the most part, concepts are clearly defined. However, a major inconsistency within her writing is the lack of a clear definition of environment, which is identified as a basic concept for the conceptual system from which she derives her theory. In addition, she indicates that nurses are concerned about the health care of groups and commiunities but concentrates her discussion on nursing as occurring in a dyadic relationship. Thus, the theory essentially draws on only two of the three systems described in the conceptual system. The social systems portion of the conceptual system is less clearly connected to the Theory of Goal Attainment than are the personal and interpersonal systems. This may help explain Carter and Dufour's (1994) concern that critiques of King's work have not always differentiated between the conceptual system and the theory.

The definition of stress indicates that it is both negative and positive, but discussion of stress always implies that it is negative. Finally, King says that the nurse and client are strangers, yet she speaks of their working together for goal attainment and of the importance of health maintenance. Attainment of long-term goals, such as those concerning health maintenance, is not consistent with not knowing each other.

A limitation is the effort required of the reader to sift through the presentation of a conceptual system and a theory with repeated definitions to find the basic concepts. Another limitation relates to the lack of development of application of the theory in providing nursing care to groups, families, or communities.

SUMMARY

Imogene King has presented a conceptual system from which she derived a Theory of Goal Attainment. The conceptual system consists of three systems—personal, interpersonal, and social—all of which are in continuous exchange with their environments. The concepts of the personal systems are perception, self, body image, growth and development, time, and space. The concepts of the interpersonal systems are role, interaction, communication, transaction, and stress. Social systems concepts are organization, power, authority, status, decision making, control, and role.

From these systems and their abstract concepts of human beings, health, environment, and society, King derives a Theory of Goal Attainment. The major concepts of the Theory of Goal Attainment are interaction, perception, communication, transaction, role, stress, and growth and development. Each of these is defined, and overall propositions and criteria for determining internal and external boundaries of the theory are presented.

Imogene King has developed a Theory of Goal Attainment that is based on a philosophy of human beings and a conceptual system. She presents the results of some of the research conducted to test the theory and proposes a goal-oriented nursing record to document, and a Goal Attainment Scale to measure, goal attainment.

The theory is useful, testable, and applicable to nursing practice. Although it is not the "perfect theory," it is widely generalizable and not situation specific. Dr. King's work is solidly based in the literature and provides the reader with a rich set of resources for further study.

REFERENCES

Allan, N. J. (1995). Goal attainment and life satisfaction among frail elderly. *Masters Abstracts International, 33–05*, 1486.

Alligood, M. R. (1995). Theory of Goal Attainment: Application to adult orthopedic nursing. In M. A. Frey & C. L. Sieloff (Eds.). *Advancing King's systems framework and theory of nursing* (pp. 209–222). Thousand Oaks, CA: Sage.

Bagby, A. M. (1994). Nurse caring behaviors: The perceptions of potential health care consumers in a community setting. *Masters Abstracts International, 33–03*, 864.

Bauer, R. (1998). A dialectical study of the psychotherapeutic effectives of nursing interventions [German]. *Pflege, 11*, 305–311.

Bauer, R. (1999). A dialectical perspective of the psychotherapeutic effectiveness of nursing therapeutics [German]. *Pfege, 12*, 5–10.

Benedict, M., & Frey, M. A. (1995). Theory-based practice in the emergency department. In M. A. Frey & C. L. Sieloff (Eds.), *Advancing King's systems framework and theory of nursing* (pp. 317–324). Thousand Oaks, CA: Sage.

Binder, B. K. (1992). King's transaction elements indentified in adolescents' interactions with health care providers. *Dissertation Abstracts International, 54–01B, 163*.

Brower, H. T. (1981). Social organization and nurses' attitudes toward older persons. *Journal of Gerontological Nursing, 7*, 293–298.

Brown, S. J. (1999). Student nurses' perceptions of elderly care. *Journal of National Black Nurses' Assocation, 10*(2), 29–36.

Bryant-Lukosius, D. E. (1993). Patient and nurse perceptions of the needs of patients with non-Hodgkin's lymphoma: A qualitative study. *Masters Abstracts International, 31–04*, 1730.

Byrne, E., & Schreiber, R. (1989). Concept of the month: Implementing King's conceptual framework at the bedside. *Journal of Nursing Administration, 19*(2), 28–32.

Campbell-Begg, T. (1998). Promotion of transactions during animal-assisted, group therapy with individuals who are recovering from chemical addictions. *Masters Abstracts International, 37–04*, 1175.

Carter, K. F., & Dufour, L. T. (1994). King's theory: A critique of the critiques. *Nursing Science Quarterly, 7*(3), 128–133.

Church, C. J. (1997). The relationship of interaction between peer counselors and low-income women and duration of breastfeeding. *Masters Abstracts International, 36–04*, 1061.

Coker, E., Fradley, T., Harris, J., Tomarchio, D., Chan, V., & Caron, C. (1995). Implementing nursing diagnosis within the context of King's conceptual framework. In M. A. Frey & C. L. Sieloff (Eds.), *Advancing King's systems framework and theory of nursing* (pp. 161–175). Thousand Oaks, CA: Sage.

Cox, M. A. C. (1995). Exercise adherence: Testing a goal attainment intervention program. *Dissertation Abstracts International, 56–09B*, 4813.

Daubenmire, M. J. (1989). A baccalaureate nursing curriculum based on King's conceptual framework. In J. Riehl-Sisca (Ed.), *Conceptual models for nursing practice* (3rd ed.) (pp. 167–178). Norwalk, CT: Appleton & Lange.

Dawson, B. W. (1996). The relationship between functional social support, social network and the adequacy of prenatal care. *Masters Abstracts International, 35–01*, 361.

DeHowitt, M. C. (1992). King's conceptual model and individual psychotherapy. *Perspectives in Psychiatric Care, 28*(4), 11–14.

Desruisseaux, B. (1991). A qualitative study: Goal attainment is the path to mastery—A factor contributing to patients' learning following ostomy surgery. *Masters Abstracts International, 30–02*, 296.

Doornbos, M. M. (1995). Using King's systems framework to explore family health in the families of the young chronically mentally ill. In M. A. Frey & C. L.Sieloff (Eds.), *Advancing King's systems framework and theory of nursing* (pp. 192–205). Thousand Oaks, CA: Sage.

Dougal, J., & Gonterman, R. (1999). A comparison of three teaching methods on learning and retention. *Journal for Nurses in Staff Development, 15*, 205–209.

Duffy, J. R. (1990). An analysis of the relationships among nurse caring behaviors and selected outcomes of care in hospitalized medical and/or surgical patients. *Dissertation Abstracts International, 51–08B*, 3777.

Erikson, E. (1950). *Childhood and society*. New York: Norton. (out of print)

Fawcett, J. M., Vaillancourt, V. M., & Watson, C. A. (1995). Integration of King's framework into nursing practice. In M. A. Frey & C. L. Sieloff (Eds.), *Advancing King's systems framework and theory of nursing* (pp. 176–191). Thousand Oaks, CA: Sage.

Ford, W. A. (1992). A study of productivity and quality on a pilot unit for patient centered care. *Masters Abstracts International, 30–04*, 1290.

Fredenburgh, L. (1993). The effect of mutual goal setting on stress reduction in the community mental health client. *Masters Abstracts International, 32–03*, 934.

Freud, S. (1966). *Introductory lectures on psychoanalysis*. (J. Strachey, trans.) New York: Norton. (out of print)

Frey, M. A. (1988). Health and social support in families with children with diabetes mellitus. *Dissertation Abstracts International, 48*, 4A.

Frey, M. A. (1989). Social support and health: A theoretical formulation derived from King's conceptual framework. *Nursing Science Quarterly, 2*, 138–148.

Frey, M. A. (1995). Toward a theory of families, children, and chronic illness. In M. A. Frey & C. L. Sieloff (Eds.), *Advancing King's systems framework and theory of nursing* (pp. 109–125). Thousand Oaks, CA: Sage.

Frey, M. A., Rooke, L., Sieloff, C., Messmer, P. R., & Kameoka, T. (1995). King's framework and theory in Japan, Sweden, and the United States. *Image: Journal of Nursing Scholarship, 27,* 127–130.

Froman, D. (1995). Perceptual congruency between clients and nurses: Testing King's Theory of Goal Attainment. In M. A. Frey & C. L.Sieloff (Eds.), *Advancing King's systems framework and theory of nursing* (pp. 223–238). Thousand Oaks, CA: Sage.

Gesell, A. (1952). *Infant development.* New York: Harper & Row. (out of print)

Gill, J., Hopwood-Jones, L., Tyndall, J., Gregoroff, S., LeBlanc, P., Lovett, C., Rasco, L., & Ross, A. (1995). Incorporating nursing diagnosis and King's theory in O.R. documentation. *Canadian Operating Room Nursing Journal, 13*(1), 10–14.

Glasgow, V. M. (1998). Preconceptual health and its effect on pregnancy outcomes in African-Canadian Women and their partners. *Masters Abstracts International, 36–06,* 1585.

Gold, C., Haas, S., & King, I. (2000). Conceptual frameworks: Putting the nursing focus into core curricula. *Nurse Educator, 25*(2), 95–98.

Gulitz, E. A., & King, I. M. (1988). King's general systems model: Application to curriculum development. *Nursing Science Quarterly, 1,* 128–132.

Hampton, D. C. (1994). King's theory of goal attainment as a framework for managed care implementation in a hospital setting. *Nursing Science Quarterly, 7,* 170–173.

Hanna, K. (1993). Effect of nurse–client transaction on female adolescents' oral contraceptive use. *Image, 25,* 285–290.

Hanucharunkui, S., & Vinya-nguag, P. (1991). Effects of promoting patient's participation in self-care on postoperative recovery and satisfaction with care. *Nursing Science Quarterly, 4,* 14–20.

Harman, B. J. (1998). The effects of a paraprofessional preceptor program for certified nursing assistants in dementia special care units. *Dissertation Abstracts International, 59–11B,* 5786.

Harrity, M. C. (1992). The characteristics of the military retirees who volunteered as civilians for a U. S. Army family support system during Operation Desert Shield/Storm. *Masters Abstracts International, 31–01,* 273.

Havinghurst, R. (1953). *Human development and education.* New York: McKay. (out of print)

Hobdell, E. F. (1995). Using King's interacting systems framework for research on parents of children with neural tube defect. In M. A. Frey & C. L. Sieloff (Eds.), *Advancing King's systems framework and theory of nursing* (pp. 126–136). Thousand Oaks, CA: Sage.

Husband, A. (1988). Application of King's theory of nursing to the care of the adult with diabetes. *Journal of Advanced Nursing, 13,* 484–488.

Husting, P. M. (1997). A transcultural critique of Imogene King's theory of goal attainment. *Journal of Multicultural Nursing & Health, 3*(3), 15–20.

Inhelder, B. F., & Piaget, J. (1964). *The early growth of logic in the child.* New York: Norton. (out of print)

Jersild, A. T. (1952). *In search of self.* New York: Columbia University Teachers College Press. (out of print)

Jolly, M. L., & Winker, C. K. (1995). Theory of Goal Attainment in the context of organizational structure. In M. A. Frey & C. L. Sieloff (Eds.), *Advancing King's systems framework and theory of nursing* (pp. 305–316). Thousand Oaks, CA: Sage.

Jonas, C. M. (1987). King's goal attainment theory: Use in gerontological nursing practice. *Perspectives, 11*(4), 9–12.

Jones, S., Clark, V. B., Merker, A., & Palau, D. (1995). Changing behaviors: Nurse educators and clinical nurse specialists design a discharge planning program. *Journal of Nursing Staff Development, 11,* 291–295.

Kameoka, T. (1995). Analyzing nurse–patient interactions in Japan. In M. A. Frey & C. L. Sieloff (Eds.), *Advancing King's systems framework and theory of nursing* (pp. 251–260). Thousand Oaks, CA: Sage.

Kaminski, L. A. (1999). Perceptions of homecare nurses as facilitators of discussions and advance directives. *Masters Abstracts International, 37–04*, 1179.

Kemppainen, J. K. (1990). Imogene King's theory: A nursing case study of a psychotic client with human immunodeficiency virus infection. *Archives of Psychiatric Nursing, 4*, 384–388.

Keyworth, C. A. (1998). Responses of visiting nurses to sexual harassment by clients. *Masters Abstracts International, 36–03*, 782.

King, I. M. (1971). *Toward a theory for nursing: General concepts of human behavior.* New York: Wiley. (out of print)

King, I. M. (1983). King's theory of nursing. In I. W. Clements & F. B. Roberts (Eds.), *Family health: A theoretical approach to nursing care.* New York: Wiley. (out of print)

King, I. M. (1986a). *Curriculum and instruction in nursing.* East Norwalk, CT: Appleton-Century-Crofts. (out of print)

King, I. M. (1986b). King's Theory of Goal Attainment. In P. Winstead-Fry (Ed.), *Case studies in nursing theory* (pp. 197-213) (Pub. No. 15-2152). New York: National League for Nursing.

King, I. M. (1987). *King's theory.* Paper presented at Nurse Theorist Conference, Pittsburgh, PA. (cassette recording).

King, I. M. (1988). Measuring health goal attainment in patients. In C. Waltz & O. Strickland (Eds.), *Measurement of nursing outcomes* (Vol I) (pp. 109–17). New York: Springer.

King, I. M. (1989). King's general systems framework and theory. In J. Riehl-Sisca (Ed.), *Conceptual models for nursing practice* (3rd ed.) (pp. 149–58). Norwalk, CT: Appleton & Lange.

King, I. M. (1990a). *A theory for nursing: Systems, concepts, process.* Albany, NY: Delmar. (Originally published 1981, NY:Wiley.)

King, I. M. (1990b). Health as a goal for nursing. *Nursing Science Quarterly, 3*, 123–128.

King, I. M. (1990c). King's conceptual framework and Theory of Goal of Attainment. In M. E. Parker (Ed.), *Nursing theories in practice* (pp. 73–84) (Pub. No. 15-2350). New York: National League for Nursing.

King, I. M. (1992). King's Theory of Goal Attainment. *Nursing Science Quarterly, 5*, 19–26.

King, I. M. (1995). A systems framework for nursing. In M. A. Frey & C. L. Sieloff (Eds.), *Advancing King's systems framework and theory of nursing* (pp. 14–22). Thousand Oaks, CA: Sage.

King, I. M. (1997). King's Theory of Goal Attainment in practice. *Nursing Science Quarterly, 10*, 180–185.

King, I. M. (1999). A Theory of Goal Attainment: Philosophical and ethical implications. *Nursing Science Quarterly*, 12, 292–296.

King, I. M. (2001). Theory of Goal Attainment. In M. Parker (Ed.), *Nursing theories and nursing practice* (pp. 275–286). Philadelphia: Davis.

Kirkpatrick, N. C. (1992). A phenomenological study of adolescent females' perceptions of death and dying in light of the AIDS epidemic. *Masters Abstracts International, 31–02*, 765.

Konkle-Parker, D. J. (1996). Survey of nurse practitioners' health counseling strategies. *Masters Abstracts International, 35–04*, 1000.

Laben, J. K., Dodd, D., & Sneed, L. (1991). King's theory of goal attainment applied in group therapy for inpatient juvenile sexual offenders, maximum security state offenders, and community parolees, using visual aids. *Issues in Mental Health Nursing, 12*(1), 51–64.

Laben, J. K., Sneed, L. D., & Seidel, S. L. (1995). Goal attainment in short-term group psychotherapy settings: Clinical implications for practice. In M. A. Frey & C. L. Sieloff (eds.). *Advancing King's systems framework and theory of nursing* (pp. 261–277). Thousand Oaks, CA: Sage.

Lincoln, K. E. (1997). A comparison of postpartum clients' and nurses' perceptions of priority information needs for early discharge. *Masters Abstracts International, 36–05*, 1330.

Lockhart, J. S. (1992). Female nurses' perceptions regarding the severity of facial disfigurement in patients following surgery for head and neck cancer: A comparison based on experience in head and neck oncology. *Dissertation Abstracts International, 54–02B*, 745.

Lott, C. E. (1996). Perceptions of acceptance and recognition among professional Black nurses. *Masters Abstracts International, 34–04*, 1551.

Mann, C. M. (1997). Home care nurses' perceptions of continuing their education. *Masters Abstracts International, 35–04*, 1000.

Marasco, G. (1990). Parents' perceptions of the effects of early postpartum discharge on family adjustment. *Masters Abstracts International, 29–01*, 95.

McGeein, M. L. S. (1992). A descriptive study of community health nurses' perceptions of elder maltreatment. *Masters Abstracts International, 31–01*, 278.

McGirr, M., Rukholm, E., Salmoni, A., O'Sullivan, P., & Koren, I. (1990). Perceived mood and exercise behaviors of cardiac rehabilitation program referras. *Canadian Journal of Cardiovascular Nursing, 1*(4), 14–19.

Meighan, M. M. (1998). Testing a nursing intervention to enhance paternal–infant interaction and promote paternal role assumption. *Dissertation Abstracts International, 60–07B*, 3204.

Messmer, P. R. (1995). Implementation of theory-based nursing practice. In M. A. Frey & C. L. Sieloff (Eds.), *Advancing King's systems framework and theory of nursing* (pp. 294–304). Thousand Oaks, CA: Sage.

Messner, R., & Smith, M. N. (1986). Neurofibromatosis: Relinquishing the masks; a quest for quality of life. *Journal of Advanced Nursing, 11*, 459–464.

Monna, K. A. (1989). The perception of job satisfaction of baccalaureate-prepared and diploma-prepared community health nurses. *Masters Abstracts International, 28–04*, 579.

Monti, A. (1992). Members' perceptions of the transactions within their psychosocial club. *Masters Abstracts International, 30–04*, 1296.

Morris, G. L. (1996). Client satisfaction with nursing care in the home. *Masters Abstracts International, 34–06*, 2348.

Norgan, G. H., Ettipio, A. M., & Lasome, C. E. M. (1995). A program plan addressing carpal tunnel syndrome: The utility of King's goal attainment theory. *AAOHN Journal, 43*, 407–411.

Norris, D. M., & Hoyer, P. J. (1993). Dynamism in practice: Parenting within King's framework. *Nursing Science Quarterly, 6*, 79–85.

Oates, S. J. (1994). Nurses' perceptions of participation in shaping the workplace. *Masters Abstracts International, 33–03*, 874.

Omar, M. A. (1989). Relationship of family processes to family life satisfaction in stepfamilies and biological families during pregnancy. *Dissertation Abstracts International, 51–03B*, 1196.

Parsons, A. E., & Ricker, V. J. (1993). Critique of practices used by Massachusetts nurse practitioners to promote breastfeeding. *Nursing Scan in Research, 6*(5), 4–5.

Porter, H. B. (1991). A theory of goal attainment and ambulatory care oncology nursing: An introduction. *Canadian Oncology Nursing Journal, 1*(4), 124–126.

Quirk, S. E. (1995). A study to determine if working on self-directed teams increases job satisfaction among home health registered nurses. *Masters Abstracts International, 34–01*, 283.

Rhodes, E. R. (1995). Perceptions of health among low-income African-Americans and utilization of health services. *Masters Abstracts International, 34–03*, 1153.

Rooda, L. A. (1992). The development of a conceptual model for multicultural nursing. *Journal of Holistic Nursing, 10*, 337–347.

Rooke, L. (1995a). The concept of space in King's systems framework: Its implications for nursing. In M. A. Frey & C. L. Sieloff (Eds.), *Advancing King's systems framework and theory of nursing* (pp. 79–96). Thousand Oaks, CA: Sage.

Rooke, L. (1995b). Focusing on King's theory and systems framework in education by using an experiential learning model: A challenge to improve the quality of nursing care. In M. A. Frey & C. L. Sieloff (Eds.), *Advancing King's systems framework and theory of nursing* (pp. 278–93). Thousand Oaks, CA: Sage.

Rosendahl, P. B., & Ross, V. (1982). Does your behavior affect your patient's response? *Journal of Gerontological Nursing, 8*, 572–575.

Sharts-Engel, N. C. (1984). On the vicissitudes of health appraisal. *Advances in Nursing Science, 7,* 12–23.

Sharts-Hopko, N. C. (1995). Using health, personal, and interpersonal system concepts within the King's systems framework to explore perceived health status during the menopause transition. In M. A. Frey & C. L. Sieloff (Eds.), *Advancing King's systems framework and theory of nursing* (pp. 147–160). Thousand Oaks, CA: Sage.

Shea, H., Rogers, M., Ross, E., Tucker, D., Fitch, M., & Smith, I. (1989). Implementation of nursing conceptual models: Observations of a multi-site research team. *Canadian Journal of Nursing Administration, 2*(1), 15–20.

Skariah, R. A. (1999). Analysis of first nation children's drawings of their perceptions of health. *Masters Abstracts International, 37–04,* 1184.

Smith, M. C. (1988). King's theory in practice. *Nursing Science Quarterly, 1,* 145–146.

Sowell, R. L., & Lowenstein, A. (1994). King's theory as a framework for quality: Linking theory to practice. *NursingConnections, 7*(2), 19–31.

Talosi, R. (1993). Puppetry simulation: The health education vehicle to goal attainment in children with asthma. *Masters Abstracts International, 32–04,* 1172.

Temple, A., & Fawdry, K. (1992). King's theory of goal attainment: Resolving filial caregiver role strain. *Journal of Gerontological Nursing, 18*(3), 11–15.

Theobald, S. K. (1992). Clinical teaching characteristics of baccalaureate and associate degree nursing faculty: A comparative study. *Masters Abstracts International, 31–01,* 284.

Tritsch, J. M. (1998). Application of King's theory of goal attainment and the Carondelet St. Mary's case management model. *Nursing Science Quarterly, 11,* 69–73.

Ventresca, A. R. (1994). Job satisfaction: Goal attainment of community health nurses. *Masters Abstracts International, 33–04,* 1232.

Villanueva-Noble, N. S. (1998). Cross-cultural analysis of perceptions of health in children's drawings: A replicate study. *Masters Abstracts International, 36–04,* 1070.

West, P. (1991). Theory implementation: A challenging journey. *Canadian Journal of Nursing Administration, 4*(1), 29–30.

White-Linn, V. M. (1994). Perceived quality of life of adults aged 30 to 50 years with Type I and II diabetes. *Masters Abstracts International, 33–05,* 1496.

Wicks, M. L. N. (1992). Family health in chronic illness. *Dissertation Abstracts International, 53–12B,* 6228.

Winker, C. K. (1996). A descriptive study of the relationship of interaction disturbance to the organizational health of a metropolitan general hospital. *Dissertation Abstracts International, 57–07B,* 4306.

Woods, E. C. (1994). King's theory in practice with elders. *Nursing Science Quarterly, 7,* 65–69.

ANNOTATED BIBLIOGRAPHY

Alligood, M. R., & May, B. A. (2000). A nursing theory of personal system empathy: Interpreting a conceptualization of empathy in King's interacting systems. *Nursing Science Quarterly, 13,* 243–247.

Through rational hermeneutic interpretation within King's personal system, and the personal system concepts, a theory of intrapersonal empathy was developed. This theory proposes that perceptions are organized by empathy; awareness of self and others is facilitated, sensitivity is increased, shared respect is promoted as are mutual goals and social awareness, understanding of individuals within both historical and social contexts is encouraged and learning is affected.

Glasgow, V. M. (1998). Preconceptual health and its effect on pregnancy outcomes in African-Canadian women and their partners. *Masters Abstracts International, 36–06*, 1585.

A sample of 30 African-Canadian women and their partners completed questionnaires about their perceptions of preconceptual health and these perceptions were related to pregnancy outcomes. Overall, the data supported a strong relationship between the perceptions of both partners and improved pregnancy outcomes.

Harman, B. J. (1999). The effects of a paraprofessional preceptor program for certified nursing assistants in dementia special care units. *Dissertation Abstracts International, 59–11B*, 5786.

This study utilized a multisite, repeated measures, quasi-experimental design to investigate the outcomes of a newly instituted paraprofessional mentor program for certified nursing assistants (CNAs) in dementia special care units. Participating CNAs attended a six-hour educational program to prepare them to serve as preceptors. Sixteen new CNAs were enrolled in the study with 11 completing the data collection. Of these 11, six had preceptors and five participated in the usual program, or served as the control group. Due to the sample size, statistical significance was not found. However, 100% of the experimental group continued employment as compared to 56% in the control group.

Quirk, S. E. (1995). A study to determine if working on self-directed teams increases job satisfaction among home health registered nurses. *Masters Abstracts International, 34–01*, 283.

This descriptive study investigated job satisfaction in 30 home health registered nurses in two agencies. In one agency, nurses participated in self-directed teams while in the other nurses did not have access to self-directed teams. Those who worked on self-directed teams exhibited higher levels of job satisfaction.

West, P. (1991). Theory implementation: A challenging journey. *Canadian Journal of Nursing Administration, 4*(1), 29–30.

Describes the implementation of King's conceptual system for theory-based practice in a large metropolitan hospital. Identifies that more time spent in educating the staff about the framework would have helped the staff understand and accept the value of theory-based practice.

CHAPTER 14

SCIENCE OF UNITARY HUMAN BEINGS
MARTHA E. ROGERS

Maryanne Garon

■ ■ ■

    Martha Rogers (1914–1994) was an influential and visionary nurse theorist, an innovative thinker, and an articulate spokesperson for professional nursing education. Her conceptual system has had a profound impact on practice, theory development, and research in the profession. But, in addition to all that, Martha Rogers was a warmly regarded and honored human being. She had a rich family life, and was much loved by her family members—from her sisters and brother to innumerable nieces, nephews, and grandnieces, as well as by her many friends and colleagues in nursing. Some of this respect and affection is reflected in her recognition as a fellow in the American Academy of Nursing and her induction into the American Nurses' Association Hall of Fame.

    Martha Rogers was born in Dallas, Texas, on May 12, 1914. She attended the University of Tennessee, Knoxville, from 1931–1933. Her broad academic and scientific interests were manifested early, as she took a science-med course, which she characterized as more substantial than pre-med, including French, zoology, genetics, embryology, and many other courses (Hektor, 1989). However, at some point during this period, she and her parents concluded that medicine was an inappropriate career for a woman (Garon, 1992). She decided to enter the Knoxville General Hospital School of Nursing, because one of her friends was planning to attend there. Being an independent and intelligent young woman, Martha Rogers found the routines of the hospital school to be restrictive. At one point she even left the school briefly, but returned to complete her nurses' training with her class (personal interview with M. Rogers, 1991). She received her nursing diploma in 1936. Rogers continued her education at George Peabody College in Nashville, receiving a Bachelor of Science Degree in Public Health. After receiving her B.S. degree, Rogers' first position was as a public health nurse in rural Michigan. She remained there for two years, until she returned to study for her first master's degree, an M.A. in Public Health Supervision from Teacher's College, Columbia University, in 1945 (Hektor, 1989). Rogers also worked as a staff nurse, supervisor, and education director for a visiting nurse agency in Hartford, Connecticut. After advancing to the position of acting Director of Education, she moved to Phoenix, Arizona, where she established and became the Executive

Director of the first Visiting Nursing Service in Phoenix (online source: archive.uwcm.ac.uk/uwcm/ns/martha/Biography.htm). *She later returned to the East Coast to continue her education. She earned a masters in public health in 1952 and a doctor of science degree in 1954, both from Johns Hopkins University. Rogers' career in academia began when she was appointed chairperson of the Department of Nursing Education at New York University in 1954. She officially retired in 1979, but continued as Professor Emerita. After retiring, she moved back to Phoenix where she lived until her death in 1994.*

"Ahead of her time, in and out of this world" (Ireland, 2000, p. 59)

Rogers' view of nursing as a separate and essential discipline and a unique field of study was influential in her life's work. She focused much of her writing, particularly prior to 1970, on working for the establishment of nursing in higher education. She believed that there was a unique body of knowledge in nursing that had not yet been identified or written about. In her books and articles that argued the need for higher education for nurses, Rogers developed and wrote about this unique body of knowledge that would eventually become her conceptual system (Garon, 1992).

Rogers' first book, published in 1961, *Educational revolution in nursing*, was a call for a broad liberal university education for nurses. It also contained the beginnings of her conceptual system. Further evidence of the development of the conceptual system is found in her second book, *Reveille in nursing*, published in 1964, in which she proposed a professional curriculum for nursing. As a focus of the curriculum, Rogers developed several assumptions that later became central to her conceptual system. Meleis (1985) credited these writings as the first comments on the theoretic basis of the nursing process. Rogers continued to refine her thinking about her conceptual system, and published *An introduction to the theoretical basis of nursing* in 1970. This book contains the basis for her conceptual system. There have been a number of updates and refinements to the conceptual system since 1970.

The concepts and principles presented in this section will include the later explications presented by Rogers, as well as references to the original work. While reading the 1970 book is necessary to better understand Rogers' conceptual system, knowledge of Rogers would be incomplete without including the revisions presented in her later publications.

Throughout her life Rogers was adamant that nursing is a science with a unique body of knowledge (Meleis, 1997). Nursing focuses on unitary human beings and their world. Rogers used the word *unitary* to connote human beings as unified wholes, greater than the sum of their parts; in fact, as not even being composed of parts. Rogers abandoned the word *holism*, because of its widespread and often inaccurate use, to describe everything from dietary regimens to massages to the use of colonics (Malinski, 1994, p. 203). Unitary human beings and their environments cannot be understood or studied by looking at their parts. Gathering information about physiological indices or a person's social context may be helpful for nurses in some of their collaborative functions, but this information would not lead to an understanding of the unitary human being.

Rogers (1990b/1994) argued that every discipline has many theories and that she was presenting an abstract or conceptual system, an abstract worldview from which theories could be derived. She emphasized that this is a new product, rooted in a different paradigm. The word *paradigm* has been noted to have many different meanings (Guba, 1990, p. 17). A paradigm may be defined as the way that scientists or persons in a given field approach the problems or areas of interest in their field (Briggs & Peat, 1984). It is a particular perspective of reality, and has been likened to a worldview. Thomas Kuhn (1970) wrote about scientific paradigms and how they change. He believed that knowledge advances through revolutions, or leaps in knowledge—what he called paradigm shifts. However, it is difficult for someone who has been rooted in one paradigm to shift to viewing things in the new paradigm. The shift is said to take place all at once—the old information is suddenly seen differently, as though the person were wearing a different shade of lenses. One example that has been used to demonstrate this shift in paradigm view is illustrated in the sketch shown in Figure 14–1.

Viewed from one perspective, the drawing appears to be a rabbit. But, by shifting the view—by rotating the page—one can suddenly see the duck. Once you make the shift, you can easily see both. It is now difficult to go back to where you were before, when you could see only one animal. This is likened to a paradigm shift. At first, you only see things from the old paradigm, but once you have made the shift, it is difficult to go backwards and not view things from the new paradigm while still including the old one.

Many nurses are accustomed to viewing people and the practice of nursing from a biomedical perspective that is based on reductionism. Nurses who practice from a

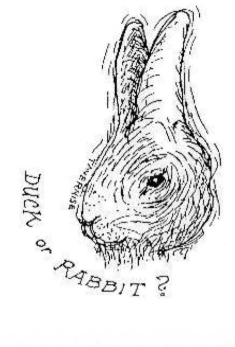

Figure 14–1

Drawing by Cindy Tavernise. Used with permission.

reductionistic perspective, or the biomedical model, need to make a paradigm shift to begin to understand the Science of Unitary Human Beings. The words and concepts are very different from those that most nurses use in everyday practice.

The conceptual system developed by Martha Rogers requires a paradigm shift similar to that illustrated in Figure 14–1. Initially, it is hard to "see," as the old views are paramount. After reading her conceptual system and applying it to practice, the paradigm shift may occur. Suddenly, the "duck" appears. The new views make sense—and it is difficult to ever go back to the old, or previous, view of reality. This does not mean that the old views are discarded; rather, they are now incorporated within the newer worldview.

ROGERS' CONCEPTUAL SYSTEM

In her 1970 book, *An introduction to the theoretical basis of nursing science*, Rogers outlined five assumptions that provide the foundation for the discipline of nursing. They were:

1. Man [Roger's used "Man" in place of person or human being in 1970] is a unified whole, possessing his own integrity and manifesting characteristics that are more than and different from the sum of his parts (p. 47).
2. Man [as an open system] and environment are continuously exchanging matter and energy with one another (p. 54).
3. The life process evolves irreversibly and unidirectionally along the space–time continuum (p. 59).
4. Pattern and organization identify man and reflect his innovative wholeness (p. 65).
5. Man is characterized by the capacity for abstraction and imagery, language and thought, sensation and emotion (p. 73).

Rogers drew on her readings from the arts, the sciences, and philosophy, as well as her scientific education, to develop this conceptual system for nursing. In deducing her conceptual system, she used terminology from the general system theory of Von Bertalanffy to support her conceptions of a universe of open systems and the continuous interaction of human and environmental fields (Meleis, 1997). She also drew on both physics and electrodynamic theory as underpinnings for some of her concepts. Other influences included early Greek philosophers, Lewin's field theory, and the works of theologian Teilhard de Chardin and of Polanyi (Garon, 1992). In later writings, Rogers refined and condensed the assumptions, finally settling on the five building blocks of the conceptual system (Rogers, 1992): *energy fields, pandimensionality, pattern, unitary persons,* and *environment.*

The first concept is that of *energy field*. An energy field is defined as "the fundamental unit of the living and the non-living" (Rogers, 1990b, p. 109;1994, p. 252). Understanding Rogers' view of energy fields is essential to understanding her conceptual system. *Energy* signifies the dynamic nature of the field; a *field* is in continuous motion and is infinite (Rogers, 1990b, 1994). Both human beings and their environment are conceptualized as energy fields in this system. Because both are infinite, their boundaries do not end at the physical body.

The concept of energy field seems to be particularly difficult for many nurses to understand. Because of this difficulty, they may either dismiss Rogers as "too abstract" or question how they can see, touch, or identify an energy field. Reeder (1999) acknowledged the questions that many nurses have, and raised the possibility of energy field in the Rogerian system as metaphor. Rogers constantly referred to human beings and their environments as energy fields, but gave little elaboration. Her few explanations revolved around the nature of energy fields as dynamic and unified. "Field is a unifying concept. Energy signifies the dynamic nature of the field; a field is in continuous motion and is infinite" (Rogers, 1990b, p. 109;1994, p. 252). Reeder wrote that it is possible that "Rogers deliberately chose the metaphor *energy field* as a figure of speech to evoke the imagination and wonderment of possibilities . . . to represent the revolutionary, fully pandimensional human being rather than . . . a literal entity connoting Newtonian three dimensionality" (1999, p. 7). Understanding the concept of energy fields becomes easier when it is viewed as a metaphor. While it may be difficult for some nurses to look at a person and see him or her as something like a Kirlian field photograph or a Star Trek version of an evolved alien, most every nurse can agree that people are incredibly dynamic, yet integral beings. Because it is difficult to measure or visualize energy fields, this perspective can be a good starting point for making the switch to viewing things in the Rogerian conceptual system.

Pattern, the next concept, received increasing importance in Rogers' writings in later years (Sarter, 1987, p. 54). This concept arises both from systems thinking and views from quantum physics. *Pattern* is defined as "the distinguishing characteristic of an energy field perceived as a single wave" (Rogers, 1990b, p. 109;1994, p. 252). Rogers used the concept of pattern to emphasize that unitary human beings cannot be understood by studying or summing their parts. Each human being instead has a unique identifiable pattern. Pattern is the unique configuration of relationships characteristic of a particular system. Capra, in *The web of life*, emphasized that the "study of pattern is essential to the understanding of living systems" (1996, p. 81). In systems thinking, it is not the structure or the physical parts that are important, but the pattern of relationships. Systemic properties *are* properties of a pattern. The irreducible, nonmaterial aspect of life is the pattern. One of the difficulties in operationalizing Rogers' model has been deciding on means to assess the pattern of the human energy field. Several nurse researchers have attempted to develop means to better identify and measure human field patterns. Examples of such research includes that by Bays, 1995, 2001; Bernardo, 1993, 1996; Brown, 1992; Butcher, 1994a, 1996; Matas, 1997; Rapacz, 1991; Yarcheski & Mahon, 1995 and others included in Malinski's (1986) *Explorations on Martha Rogers' Science of Unitary Human Beings*, Barrett's (1990) *Visions of Rogers' science-based nursing*, and Madrid and Barrett's (1994) *Rogers' scientific art of nursing practice*. Areas of human field patterns that have been explored include adolescents, chronic pain, hope, injury-associated behaviors and life events, repatterning, and time and creativity.

The next concept is *pandimensionality*. In her earliest writings, Rogers referred to this concept as space–time. Later, she refined it to four-dimensionality, then multidimensionality. In 1992 she finally settled on pandimensionality. Pandimensionality refers to an infinite domain without limit. Rogers drew on changes in knowledge from twentieth-century physics that theorized space–time dimensions beyond three dimensions. Human and environmental fields, and all reality, are believed to be pandimensional (Rogers, 1992). This is a way of perceiving reality, of moving beyond the standard view of the world as three-dimensional. When we move beyond the three-dimensional view of the world as one that we can experience with our five senses, there is no limit on the realm of possibility. The pandimensional nature of reality can explain a number of phenomena thought to be paranormal, such as déjà vu, precognition, and clairvoyance. A standard way to help with understanding these concepts can be found in Abbott's (1992) *Flatland*. In that book a resident of a two-dimensional world finds his way into a three-dimensional world. He had never imagined a reality beyond his two dimensions, and is both overwhelmed and enlightened by the idea of another dimension. Just as the protagonist of *Flatland* has difficulty in conceptualizing a third dimension, so do we have difficulty imaging a reality *beyond* three dimensions. Yet, theories from modern physics lend support to Rogers' conceptualization of multiple dimensions (Capra, 1983, p. 89). Our words and understandings lag behind reality in this case.

The *unitary human being* is defined by Rogers as "an irreducible, indivisible, pandimensional energy field identified by pattern and manifesting characteristics that are specific to the whole and which cannot be predicted from knowledge of the parts" (Rogers, 1992, p. 29). Unitary human beings and their environments are the focus of nursing science and give nursing its unique perspective and area of practice.

The *environment* or *environmental energy field* is defined as "an irreducible, pandimensional energy field identified by pattern and integral with the human field" (Rogers, 1992, p. 29).

In addition to these basic building blocks or concepts, Rogers (1992) proposed three principles. These principles express the nature of change in human and environmental fields. Like other aspects of her conceptual system, these have evolved and been refined over the years. Rogers was very concerned with language and the precise meanings of words. When she found that a particular word was not appropriate to the meaning of a concept or principle, she clarified it by refining, revising, or replacing the term. In regards to the principles, earlier writings will have different names for them. In the most current conceptualizations, the principles are: *Principle of Resonancy, Principle of Helicy*, and *Principle of Integrality*.

The *Principle of Resonancy* is defined as the "continuous change from lower to higher frequency wave patterns in human and environmental fields" (Rogers, 1992, p. 31). Human beings are perceived as wave patterns and a variety of life rhythms can be likened to wave patterns. These include things such as sleep–wake rhythms, hormone levels, and fluctuating emotional states (waves of joy or pain or loneliness). The changes that occur to these patterns of human beings are from lower to higher frequency patterns. Some examples of these changes are seen in Table 14–1, which illustrates the principle of resonancy. These changes are postulated to express the continuous creative change in the flow of human/environmental field patterning.

TABLE 14–1. MANIFESTATION OF FIELD PATTERNING IN UNITARY HUMAN BEINGS

Lower frequency	Higher frequency	Highest frequency
Pragmatic	Imaginative	Visionary
Time experienced as slower	Time experienced as faster	Timelessness
Lesser diversity		Greater diversity
Longer sleeping	Longer waking	Beyond waking
Longer rhythms	Shorter rhythms	Seems continuous
Slower motion	Faster motion	Seems continuous

Source: Rogers, M. (1992). Nursing science and the space age. *Nursing Science Quarterly, 5*, 27–34. Reprinted by permission of Sage Publications.

The *Principle of Helicy* is defined as "continuous, innovative, unpredictable, increasing diversity of human and environmental field patterns" (Rogers, 1992, p. 31). Rogers saw helicy as "an ordering of man's evolutionary emergence" (1970, p. 100). This principle underlies the fact that humans do not regress but become increasingly diverse and complex. Rogers frequently used the Slinky toy to illustrate the nature of human change as spiral-like, continually progressing towards increased diversity (see Fig. 14–2). She emphasized that this eliminates the idea of homeostasis. Human development is not static and humans do not ever return to exactly the same place that they were at before. Following a path along the Slinky, the person may have spiraled to a place that is similar to where he or she was before, but is just one circuit or turn on the Slinky from that original place. Unitary persons, in their development, do not go backward. This view of human development places a positive light on aging. Humans are becoming more diverse and complex as they age.

The *Principle of Integrality* is defined as "continuous mutual human field and environmental field process" (Rogers, 1992, p. 31). Integrality is derived from the word *integral* to explain the essential relationship between the human and environmental fields. Rogers emphasized the continuous mutual nature of the human–environmental field relationship by the deliberate use of the word *process*, instead of *interaction*. Interaction implies an episodic or even causal relationship. To illustrate this, imagine a child playing outside in the sun on a bright summer day. The child gets a sunburn. This might be perceived as an interaction between the child and the sun. However, consider the mutual process between the child and the sun as occurring simultaneously and continuously over a lifetime. Included in the process is everything from the necessity of the sun for life on this planet to Vitamin D absorption by the child to ongoing effects of radiation on the skin to the child's impact on the ozone layer. This ongoing mutual *process* is the nature of human beings and their environment.

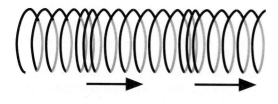

Figure 14–2. Slinky toy—Representation of Helicy (*From* http://www.messiah.edu/hpages/facstaff/barrett/slinky/home.htm/)

ROGERS' WORK AND THE FOUR MAJOR CONCEPTS

Rogers does address each of the four major concepts in her writings. Rogers defines and describes *human beings* as unitary persons, being irreducible, pandimensional energy fields identified by pattern and integral with the environment (Rogers, 1992). *Environment* is also defined as an irreducible, pandimensional energy field that is identified by pattern and is integral with the human field. Rogers repeatedly emphasized that *nursing* is a noun that referred to the body of knowledge and area of study that is unique to this profession. However, she also emphasized that nursing is both a science and an art. She wrote eloquently and passionately of the role of nursing in society.

> Nursing's story is a magnificent epic of service to mankind. It is about people: How they are born, and live and die; in health and in sickness; in joy and in sorrow. Its mission is the translation of knowledge into human service.
>
> Nursing is compassionate concern for human beings. It is the heart that understands and the hand that soothes. It is the intellect that synthesizes many learnings into meaningful ministrations (Rogers, 1966, cited in Barrett, 1990b, p. 31).

Furthermore, Rogers defined the purpose of nursing as promoting "symphonic interaction between man and environment, to strengthen the coherence and integrity of the human field, and to direct and redirect patterning of the human and environmental fields for realization of maximum health potential" (1970, p. 122) and "to promote human betterment wherever people are, on planet earth or in outer space" (Rogers, 1992, p. 33).

Rogers viewed *health* as a value term. She stated "unitary human health signifies an irreducible human field manifestation" (1990a, p. 10; 1994, p. 248) and "disease and pathology are value terms applied when the human field manifests characteristics that may be deemed undesirable" (1992, p. 33). Rogers believed that health is relative and infinite. She did not view health and illness as dichotomous, but as expressions of the life process. Nurses participate in the process of helping people to achieve their maximum health or well being, according to each person's own definitions and potentials. The concept of health is not as important in the Rogerian conceptual system as the concepts of unitary human beings and their mutual process with the environment.

Rogerian Practice Methodology

Rogers described nursing practice as "the process by which the body of scientific knowledge, (nursing science) is used for the purpose of assisting human beings to move in the direction of maximum well-being" (Rogers, 1994, p. 64). She described this process as subsumed under two categories: (1) evaluative and diagnostic, and (2) interventive. The evaluative/diagnostic phase is "the process of determining the position of an individual, family or group on the continuum of minimum to maximum well-being" (Rogers, 1994, p. 64). The interventive category is "the process of determining and initiating . . . processes characterized by ongoing modification, alteration, revision, and change" (p. 64). Rogers herself never specifically addressed whether the nursing process or nursing diagnosis fit well with her model. However, Rogers did participate in early conferences of the North American Nursing Diagnosis Association.

Barrett (1990a) developed a practice methodology consistent with the Science of Unitary Human Beings. She named this practice methodology, the health-patterning practice method. Barrett derived the method from Rogers' descriptions of health and nursing's role, as well as from her own experience in working with clients and developing a health-patterning practice.

In the health-patterning practice method there are two major processes: *pattern manifestation knowing* (originally pattern manifestation appraisal), and *voluntary mutual patterning* (originally deliberative mutual patterning). The processes are neither sequential nor separable. In the first, knowing includes to come to know, to recognize the nature of, and to discern. Barrett (1998) changed the term from *appraisal* to *knowing*, because she believed that appraisal implied an inequality between the nurse and client, as well as a suggestion of measurement, while knowing implies a more egalitarian view.

The second process, voluntary mutual patterning, acknowledges the client's free choice in making decisions about health. However, the nurse does have the obligation to encourage "the client to discover whether he/she is making choices without being fully aware or feeling free" (Barrett, 1998, p. 137). Barrett emphasized that clients are full participants in these processes. She suggested posing questions to clients such as "What do you want?" "What choices are open to you now?" . . .

Use in Actual Practice Situations

Roger's Science of Unitary Human Beings has appealed to many groups of nurses because of its emphasis on viewing human beings and environments as integral wholes. Both individuals and institutions have adopted it as their basis for nursing practice. An experience with an individual client will be presented followed by a discussion of use in nursing leadership.

Use in Clinical Practice

The first is an example of the use of Rogers' in clinical practice with an individual client.

The home health nurse, Ms. X., receives a referral from the Orthopedic Clinic physicians to make a home visit to Mr. S., an 82-year-old Caucasian male for whom hip surgery has been recommended. Mr. S. has missed several appointments, does not have a phone, and has not responded to letters requesting that he call for an appointment.

As the nurse drives into Mr. S.'s neighborhood, she observes and assesses the environmental energy field. Mr. S. lives in an impoverished area of a large western U.S. city. His neighborhood is just outside of the recently redeveloped downtown.

Many of the displaced homeless and less affluent are now living in this neighbor-hood. There are no new restaurants or stylish shops in this part of town. As the nurse pulls her car over to the curb, looking for the address, she can see a dry cleaner and liquor store storefronts. It is mid-day, yet a group of men lounge on the street corner, smoking cigarettes and passing time. Unable to find the address that she has for Mr. S., Ms. X. gets out of her car and ventures into the cleaners. "Oh, 1257 Apt E? Just go up those stairs over there," says the man behind the counter. As she exits the cleaners, she sees that one of the doors in the storefront hides a flight of stairs leading to some apartments. Nurse X. follows the staircase and finds a hallway of doors, apparently single-occupancy apartments. There are no numbers or letters on the rooms, but another resident peeks out of his room and directs Ms. X. to Mr. S.'s room.

Mr. S. answers the knock on his door tentatively, cracking the door open and peering through at Nurse X. After Ms. X. explains who she is and the reason for her visit, she is able to convince Mr. S. to fully open his door. An incredible sight con-fronts the nurse—an entire room filled, top to bottom, with books. Every inch of the floor is enveloped in piles of books. There is a small hollow near the door—evidently where Mr. S. sleeps. Other than that, it is a room of books.

At first, Ms. X.'s mind leaps to safety issues—fire hazard, building safety hazard, what should she do? But, she also senses that there is more to the whole of Mr. S. than this small roomful of books. She begins to talk to him. This amiable 82 year old has a twinkle in his eye and a lilt in his voice, as he answers Nurse X.'s standard questions. He is surprised to hear of the physicians' concerns and has some interest in the proposed hip surgery. As they speak he conveys to the nurse his love for read-ing and walking. He confides that he has had a long and fulfilling life. He even has a storage garage full of more books! For his daily routine, he awakens early every morning and walks downtown for coffee, breakfast, and newspapers. Then, he often spends the day walking around town, at times sitting and watching people. He does not perceive himself as ill or disabled. Health to him is being able to continue his current lifestyle. He would only be interested in surgery if it would not interfere with his life, and if he would be hospitalized for a minimum time. He does not want to leave his little room, or to change it. He is well aware that others view his room of books as a problem and a safety hazard—but he is not convinced of that or con-cerned about the potential hazards. He just wants to continue his walks and his reading.

With his consent, the nurse makes Mr. S. an appointment in the Orthopedic Clinic. She gives him information about the surgery and potential hospitalization time. Mr. S. keeps the appointment but later declines the surgery.

Several months later, a small earthquake shakes the city, and Mr. S.'s books fall on him. He is found in his room over 24 hours after the quake, and hospitalized for injuries and pneumonia. He never recovers and dies while hospitalized. Ms. X. is greatly saddened by Mr. S.'s death and reviews her actions carefully, still wonder-ing if she did the right thing by letting him continue his life as he desired.

Using Barrett's practice methodology, the nurse first uses *pattern manifestation knowing.* She needs to understand Mr. S. as a whole human being—what is his pat-tern? What is important to him in life? What is the meaning of health for him? In the other phase (which may actually occur simultaneously), *voluntary mutual patterning*, the nurse discusses Mr. S.'s health needs from his perspective. She determines what his values and knowledge levels are. Mr. S. is very knowledgeable about his need to continue to exercise his body and mind. He knows that his living situation might be viewed as unsafe, but he freely chooses to continue to live a life that he values. He is willing to listen to the physicians' view of his need for surgery and to assess how that fits within his view of life. He freely and knowledgeably chooses not to follow their advice. Mr. S.'s choices may not have been those of the nurse or of the physician, but he chose what made sense for him.

Use in Nursing Leadership

Rogers' conceptual model can also be used in administration and in education. Her conceptual system requires a view of human beings as "sentient and creative and held in high regard" (Gueldner, 1989, p. 114). Using the conceptualization of power that Barrett (1989) derived from Rogers, people may choose to knowingly create change. The nurse leader (whether administrator or educator) utilizes knowledge to create evolutionary change. Leaders must both practice and role model within the Rogerian conceptual system by being open in communication patterns and appreciating the unique and unitary nature of each individual with whom they interact. Nurse leaders also understand that the nursing and health care systems (or educational systems) are highly complex and continuously evolving toward higher-frequency diversifying wholeness. When the nurse leader helps to create environments characterized by acceptance for openness, creativity, and diversity, nurses and others are able to grow, evolve, improve, and shape their practices or educational experiences in ways that benefit them, their institutions, and their clients. The experience of implementing Rogers' model in practice at the San Diego Veterans Administration Medical Center has been described in Heggie, Schoenmehl, Greico, and Chang (1989) and Heggie, Garon, Kodiath, and Kelly (1994). These authors clearly demonstrate that the paradigm shift required to use Rogers' approach does not occur quickly and they describe the change process they employed, including modeling the use of Rogers' ideas. Administrative modeling resulted in the staff nominating their manager for a nursing service award for caring. The staff identified her Rogerian approach as having created a major, positive difference for them.

CRITIQUE OF ROGERS' SCIENCE OF UNITARY HUMAN BEINGS

1. What is the historical context of the theory? Rogers began to conceptualize her view of nursing in the mid-1950s and continued to develop her thinking until her death in 1994. She had studied sciences before becoming a nurse and earned a doctorate in science. She was very interested in the changes in science and approaches to knowledge development in the twentieth century. She drew on knowledge from fields as diverse as physics to theology (Garon, 1992). Rogers was one of the first nurses to think and write about the conceptual bases for nursing

(Meleis, 1985). Among other areas, the content of her work has been found to be consistent with Tao Te Ching and Buddhist thought (Hanchett, 1992; Overman, 1994).

The Science of Unitary Human Beings (SUHB) is not in itself a theory, but a number of theories have been derived from the SUHB. Examples of derived theories include enfolding health-as-wholeness-and-harmony (Carboni, 1995b), power (Barrett, 1984, 1989; Caroselli-Dervan, 1991, 1995; Caroselli & Barrett, 1998), and spirituality (Smith, D. W., 1994). Concept analyses include integrated awareness (Phillips & Bramlett, 1994), healing (Wendler, 1996), and beyond-waking experience (Watson, 1998).

2. What are the basic concepts and relationships presented by the theory? The basic concepts are energy field, pandimensionality, pattern, unitary human beings, and environment. The relationships are defined in the principles of resonancy, helicy, and integrality. The concepts of the theory are defined and used in a consistent fashion. Rogers was meticulous about use of language, and would refine word usage to appropriately present her meanings. The relationships among concepts are logical, and are based on the stated assumptions. However, the concepts and the relationship are stated in language that is not familiar to most nurses and is difficult to read and understand without substantial background information.

3. What major phenomena of concern to nursing are presented? These phenomena *may include but are not limited to*: **human being, environment, health, interpersonal relations, caring, goal attainment, adaptation, and energy fields.** Rogers wrote that the major phenomena of interest to nursing were unitary human beings and their environment. Her definition of unitary human beings and their environments is that they are unitary, indivisible energy fields. She also wrote of nursing as a compassionate concern for human beings, and that its purpose is to promote human health and well-being (Rogers, 1988).

4. To whom does the theory apply? In what situations? In what ways? Since humans are integral with their environment, Rogers' work is applicable whenever humans are located—including outer space. The Science of Unitary Human Beings (SUHB) has been applied in all aspects of nursing. It has been labeled a "grand" theory. Any limitations to the use of SUHB lie more within the practitioner than within the SUHB.

5. By what method or methods can the theory be tested? Rogers' conceptual system has been utilized as the underlying framework for multiple nursing studies. These research studies have used multiple modes of inquiry, but have remained consistent to Roger's epistemological holism (Barrett, 1990a). Rawnsley (1977) is credited with being the first nurse researcher to frame her study solely within the Science of Unitary Human Beings (Ference, 1986a). A number of nursing dissertations emerged from NYU framed within the Rogerian system, developing particular aspects into theory. Ference (1979) studied time experience, creativity traits, differentiation, and human field motion. From her study, she developed the Human Field Motion tool. Barrett (1990a) studied human field motion and power. From her study, she developed a theory of power as knowing participation in change.

From these studies and others, there has been some support for a number of Rogers' propositions. The continual mutual process of human and environmental fields has been supported in some of the studies (Meleis, 1997). However, there are also methodological difficulties in finding ways to do research that remain consistent with the Rogerian framework. Other approaches to knowledge generation, including philosophical explorations, have also added to the growth of knowledge within this conceptual system.

Both qualitative and quantitative methods have been used to test theories derived from the SUHB. Examples of descriptive research include Abu-Realh, Magwood, Narayan, Rupprecht, and Suraci (1996), Allen (1988), Alligood (1991), Alligood and McGuire (2000), Bray (1989), Donahue and Alligood (1995), Doyle (1995, 1998), Ireland (1996), MacNeil (1996), McNiff (1995a, 1995b), Morris (1991), Moulton (1994), Orshan (1996), Richard (1993), Rush (1997), Sherman (1993, 1996), Smith, D. W. (1992, 1995); phenomenological research include Dominguez (1996), Kells (1995), Klebanoff (1994), Smith, C. T. (1989), Sullivan (1994), and Thomas (1993). Examples of quasi-experimental studies include Biley (1996a), Bramlett and Gueldner (1993), Krause (1991), and Meehan (1993). Experimental studies include Butcher and Parker (1988), Girardin (1990), Mersmann (1993), Samarel, Fawcett, Ryan, and Davis (1998), Straneva (1992), Thornton (1996a, 1996b), and Wall (2000). Daingerfield (1993) used ethnography and Halkitis and Kirton (1999) used focus groups. Grounded theory methodology has been used by Krause (1991), Quinn (1988), and Schneider (1995a, 1995b). Pohl (1992) reports using both quantitative and qualitative methods in her study.

Obviously, no one methodology is identified as the "best" for studying and testing Rogers' conceptual system and the theories derived from that system. Alligood and Fawcett (1999) argue that rational interpretive hermeneutics methodology is compatible with the SUHB. Butcher (1994a, 1994b, 1998) has developed the Unitary Field Pattern Portrait Research Method (a phenomenological-hermeneutical method) and Carboni (1995a) describes a qualitative methodology called the Rogerian process of inquiry. Cowling (1998) argues for the use of case studies (unitary case inquiry), while Sherman (1997) supports the use of quantitative research methods and M. C. Smith and Reeder (1998) discuss how clinical outcomes research can be reconciled with the SUHB. One review of Rogerian research can be found in Dykeman and Loukissa (1993).

A number of tools have been developed for the SUHB. These include:

Power as Knowing Participation in Change Tool (Barrett & Caroselli, 1998)
Human Field Image Metaphor Scale (Johnston, 1993, 1994)
Person-Environment Participation Scale (Leddy, 1999)
Human Field Motion Tool (Ference, 1979, 1986b)
McCanse Readiness for Death Instrument (McCanse, 1995)

Mutual Exploration of the Healing Human Field-Environmental Field Relationship (Carboni, 1992)

Diversity of Human Field Pattern Scale (Hastings-Tolsma, 1992)

Temporal Experiences Scale (Paletta, 1990)

Assessment of Dream Experiences (Watson, 1999)

Time Metaphor Test (Allen, 1988; Hastings-Tolsma, 1992; Watson, Sloyan, & Robalino, 2000)

6. Does the theory direct critical thinking in nursing practice? Use of the Science of Unitary Human Beings in nursing practice requires both critical thinking and the ability to take a systems approach to knowledge. The nurse who utilizes Rogers in practice needs to be able to suspend judgment and accurately assess human beings from their own perspective as well as support them in making decisions.

7. Does the theory direct therapeutic nursing interventions? and **8. Does this theory direct communication in nursing practice?** Using Rogers' conceptual system directs nurses to consider a wide variety of interventions in their work with unitary human beings. Rogers (1970) emphasized that nursing interventions are not focused on disease states, but on wholeness. Interventions focusing on wholeness would include guided imagery, relaxation and stress reduction techniques, therapeutic touch, motion therapy, meditation and aromatherapy, among others. Communication is inherent in these interventions.

9. Does this theory direct nursing actions that lead to favorable outcomes? Rogers would view this question as value laden—it would depend on whose outcomes are being questioned and who defines favorable. As shown in the clinical example, the outcomes desired by the physician or the nurse may not be the same ones that the client perceives as favorable. For Mr. S., being able to live his life in the way that he desires, free to make his own choices, are more favorable outcomes for him than a longer life of lesser quality. The emphasis in health care has definitely been on outcomes recently, but in Rogers' practice model the person would provide the leadership in deciding which favorable outcomes to seek. While Barrett (1998) indicates the Rogerian practice model, health-patterning practice method, does not seek to identify or anticipate consequences, Smith and Reeder (1998) argue that clinical outcomes research can be reconciled with Rogerian science.

10. How contagious is this theory? Rogers' Science of Unitary Human Beings has definitely been contagious. There is a Society for Rogerian Scholars, a Rogerian newsletter, and an annual conference. Numerous graduates of NYU and other universities continue to research, write about, and apply the Rogerian conceptual system. Furthermore, it has served as the starting point for the development of other nursing theories, such as those of Fitzpatrick, Parse, and Margaret Newman. Sarter (1988) wrote that the profession would be at a very different point if not for Martha Rogers. Her ideas have brought a paradigm change to nursing and opened the door for ideas on alternative means of healing, Eastern philosophy, and philosophical explorations. Furthermore, her views of unitary human beings as irreducible wholes probably helped bring consensus to the profession about its holistic focus as the basis for practice (Garon, 1992).

Multiple areas of study have investigated specific principles. Research in relation to the principle of integrality includes studies of guided imagery and parent–fetal attachment (Kim, 1990); hardiness, uncertainty, power, and environment in adults waiting for kidney transplants (Stoeckle, 1993); health choices in older women (Johnson, 1996); human field pattern, risk-taking, and time experience (Hastings-Tolsma, 1992); leadership styles (Kilker, 1994); life satisfaction, purpose in life, power in those over 65 years of age (Rizzo, 1990); lightwave frequency and sleep–wakefulness frequency (Girardin, 1990); music and dyspnea (McBride, Graydon, Sidani, and Hall, 1999); music and human field motion (Edwards, 1991); music and perception of environment (Biley, 1996a); parent–fetus attachment and couvade (Schodt, 1989); rest and harmonics (Smith, M. J., 1986); sleep patterns and environment change (Dixon, 1994); temporal experience and musical sequence complexity (de Sevo, 1991); and unitary field practice modalities through use of complementary therapies by people with cancer (Abu-Realh, et al., 1996). Research in relation to the principle of resonancy includes studies of guided imagery (Butcher & Parker, 1988), and tension headache (MacNeil, 1996). Research in relation to helicy includes studies of creativity, time experience, and mystical experience (Bray, 1989); the theory of aging including time, sleep patterns, and activity (Alligood & McGuire, 2000); the theory of accelerating change (Alligood, 1991; Biley, 1992a); and time experience, human field motion, and creativity (Allen, 1988). Therapeutic touch is one of the most widely known interventions associated with the Science of Unitary Human Beings. Research on therapeutic touch includes studies on the experience of receiving therapeutic touch (Samarel, 1992); in vitro erythropoiesis (Straneva, 1992); milk letdown (Mersmann, 1993); pain and anxiety in burn patients (Turner, Clark, Williams, and Gauthier, 1998); pain in elders with degenerative arthritis (Peck, 1997, 1998); postoperative pain (Meehan, 1993); and stress reduction and immune function (Garrard, 1995).

Use of the Science of Unitary Human Beings has been discussed in multiple areas of practice. These areas include addiction/drug abuse (Compton, 1989; Conti-O'Hare, 1998); cardiac care (Contrades, 1987); care of the terminally ill (Buczny, Speirs, & Howard, 1989); caring (Smith, M. C., 1999); community health (Ruka, Brown, & Procope, 1997); family nursing (Winsted-Fry, 2000); home health (Heggie et al., 1994); innovative imagery as a health patterning modality (Barrett, 1992); menopause (Novak, 1999); oncology (Feber, 1996); postpartum assessment tool (Tettero, Jackson, & Wilson, 1993); preventing teen pregnancy (Porter, 1998); postmastectomy care (Biley, 1993); psychiatric care (Thompson, 1990); spirituality (Malinski, 1991); therapeutic touch (Benor, 1996; Biley 1996b; Green, 1998; Griffin, Moore, Ruge, and Weiter-Crespo, 1996; Kenosian, 1995; Mills, 1996; Samarel, 1997); unitary pattern appreciation (Cowling 2000); use in the future (Barrett, 2000); and use of the Personalized Nursing LIGHT model (Andersen & Smereck, 1989).

The Science of Unitary Human Beings has also been used in education. Batra (1995, 1996) discusses its use in baccalaureate and graduate nursing education. Hellwig and Ferrante (1993) describe the use of SUHB as a framework for an associate degree nursing education program. Klemm and Stashinko (1997) describe a method for teaching Rogers' work, and Patty (1999) presents a use of SUHB in teaching surgical technologists.

In addition to the widespread use of the Science of Unitary Human Beings in the United States, it has influenced nursing in many other countries. These include Australia (Powell, 1997); Canada (Chapman, Mitchell, & Forchuk, 1994); China (Sheu, Shiau, & Hung, 1997); Germany (Ammende, 1996a, 1996b; Madrid, 1996; Richter, 1998); Spain (Tejero, 1998); and the United Kingdom and Ireland (Benor, 1996; Biley, 1992a, 1992b, 1993, 1996a, 1996b, 1998, 1999; Feber, 1996; Green, 1998; Mills, 1996; Mills & Biley, 1994; Tettero, Jackson, & Wilson, 1993; Wendler, 1996).

STRENGTHS AND LIMITATIONS

Rogers presented us with an optimistic conceptual system that views human beings as unique, developing, "becoming" systems rather than compilations of mechanistic parts subject to breakdown. She gave us a view of nurses and the people for whom they provide care as partners in care, equal participants in ever-changing life processes. She has helped nurses refocus on the importance of the ever-developing environment, in continual process with human beings (Garon, 1992, p. 71).

Rogers' conceptual system is most often criticized for its abstractness and difficulty in application. Rogers herself recognized that she was oft criticized and stated, "people either think I'm great or that I should have died a long time ago!" (Safier, 1977). Cerilli and Burd (1989) critiqued the abstractness and difficulty in application to practice, and contended that the terminology is difficult to understand and apply. The experience of the nursing service at the San Diego Veterans Affairs Health Care System lends some support to these critiques. While individual nurses were enthusiastic and supportive, others were frustrated with the model's abstractness and difficulty of application. It was time consuming to continuously educate nurses to this way of thinking. In the end, it may not be Rogers' conceptual model that is the problem, but the readiness of nurses and health care systems for this innovative thinking.

SUMMARY

Rogers' conceptual system is acknowledged as being broad in scope and applicable in all nursing practice settings. The Rogerian conceptual system has been applied in education and practice settings. It has led to the growth of nursing research and the development of further theoretical knowledge. Her emphasis on viewing human beings and their environment as irreducible wholes has brought some consensus to nursing in regards to a focus on holism (Meleis, 1985). Her writings have given rise to explorations in nursing of new paradigm views consistent with the received view of science, feminist theory, and Eastern cultures and philosophy (Garon, 1992). Despite some difficulty in operationalizing some of her concepts, nurses will undoubtedly continue to explore her ideas and utilize them in practice.

REFERENCES

Abbott, E. (1992). *Flatland*. New York: Dover.

Abu-Realh, M. H., Magwood, G., Narayan, M. C., Rupprecht, C., & Suraci, M. (1996). The use of complementary therapies by cancer patients. *Nursing Connections, 9*(4), 3–12.

Allen, V. L. R. (1988). The relationship of time experience, human field motion, and clairvoyance: An investigation in the Rogerian conceptual framework. *Dissertation Abstracts International, 50*(1B), 121.

Alligood, M. R. (1991). Testing Roger's theory of accelerating change: The relationships among creativity, actualization, and empathy in persons 18 to 92 years of age. *Western Journal of Nursing Research, 13*(1), 84–96.

Alligood, M. R., & Fawcett, J. (1999). Acceptance of the invitation to dialogue: Examination of an interpretive approach for the Science of Unitary Human Beings. *Visions: The Journal of Rogerian Nursing Science, 7*(1), 5–13.

Alligood, M. R., & McGuire, S. L. (2000). Perception of time, sleep patterns, and activity in senior citizens: A test of a Rogerian theory of aging. *Visions: The Journal of Rogerian Nursing Science, 8*(1), 6–14.

Ammende, M. (1996a). Changes of paradigm in nursing. Part 1: Theory of Martha Rogers [German]. *Pflege, 9*, 5–11.

Ammende, M. (1996b). Change of paradigm in nursing: Part 2: Elizabeth Barrett's "Theory of power" [German]. *Pflege, 9*, 98–104.

Andersen, M. D., & Smereck, G. A. D. (1989). Personalized Nursing LIGHT model. *Nursing Science Quarterly, 2*, 120–130.

Barrett, E. A. M. (1984). An empirical investigation of Martha E. Rogers' principle of helicy: The relationship of human field motion and power. *Dissertation Abstracts International, 45*(2A), 615.

Barrett, E. A. M. (1989). A nursing theory of power for nursing practice: Derivation from Rogers' paradigm. In J. Riehl-Sisca (Ed.), *Conceptual models for nursing practice* (3rd ed.) (pp. 207–217). Norwalk, CT: Appleton & Lange.

Barrett, E. A. M. (1990a). Rogers' science-based nursing practice. In E. A. M. Barrett (Ed.), *Visions of Rogers' science based nursing* (pp. 31–44) (Pub. No. 15-2285). New York: National League for Nursing.

Barrett, E. A. M. (Ed.). (1990b). *Visions of Rogers' science based nursing* (Pub. No. 15-2285). New York: National League for Nursing.

Barrett, E. A. M. (1992). Innovative imagery: A health-patterning modality for nursing practice. *Journal of Holistic Nursing, 10*, 154–166.

Barrett, E. A. M. (1998). A Rogerian practice methodology for health patterning. *Nursing Science Quarterly, 11*, 136–138.

Barrett, E. A. M. (2000). Speculations on the unpredictable future of the Science of Unitary Human Beings. *Visions: The Journal of Rogerian Nursing Science, 8*, 15–25.

Barrett, E. A. M., & Caroselli, C. (1998). Methodological ponderings related to the Power as Knowing Participation in Change Tool. *Nursing Science Quarterly, 11*, 17–22.

Batra, C. (1995). Theory based curricula and utilization of Martha Rogers framework in undergraduate and graduate programs. *Rogerian Nursing Science News, 8*(2), 8–9.

Batra, C. (1996). Developing a baccalaureate curriculum based on Martha Rogers' framework. *Rogerian Nursing Science News, 9*(1), 10–11.

Bays, C. L. (1995). Older adults' descriptions of hope after a stroke. *Dissertation Abstracts International, 56*(10B), 5412.

Bays, C. L. (2001). Older adults' descriptions of hope after a stroke. *Rehabilitation Nursing, 26*(1), 18–20, 23–27.

Benor, R. (1996). Innovations in practice. Therapeutic touch. *British Journal of Community Health Nursing, 1*, 203–208.

Bernardo, L. M. (1993). Parent-reported injury-associated behaviors and life events among injured, ill, and well preschool children. *Dissertation Abstracts International, 54*(7B), 3548.

Bernardo, L. M. (1996). Parent-reported injury-associated behaviors and life events among injured, ill, and well preschool children. *Journal of Pediatric Nursing: Nursing Care of Children and Families, 11*, 100–110.

Biley, F. C. (1992a). The perception of time as a factor in Rogers' Science of Unitary Human Beings: A literature review. *Journal of Advanced Nursing, 17*, 1141–1145.

Biley, F. (1992b). The Science of Unitary Human Beings: A contemporary literature review. *Nursing Practice, 5*(4), 23–26.

Biley, F. C. (1993). Energy fields nursing: A brief encounter of a unitary kind. *International Journal of Nursing Studies, 30*, 519–525.

Biley, F. C. (1996a). An exploration of the Science of Unitary Human Beings and the principle of integrality: The effects of background music on patients and their perception of the environment. Unpublished Ph.D. thesis. *Rogerian Nursing Science News, 9*, 9.

Biley, F. C. (1996b). Rogerian science, phantoms, and therapeutic touch: Exploring potentials. *Nursing Science Quarterly, 9*, 165–169.

Biley, F. C. (1998). The Beat Generation and beyond: Popular culture and the development of the Science of Unitary Human Beings. *Visions: The Journal of Rogerian Nursing Science, 6*, 5–12.

Biley, F. (1999). The impact of the beat generation and popular culture on the development of Martha Rogers's Theory of the Science of Unitary Human Beings. *International History of Nursing Journal, 5*(1), 33–39.

Bramlett, M. H., & Gueldner, S. H. (1993). Reminiscence: A viable option to enhance power in elders. *Clinical Nurse Specialist, 7*(2), 68–74.

Bray, J. D. (1989). The relationships of creativity, time experience and mystical experience. *Dissertation Abstracts International, 50*(8B), 3394.

Briggs, J. P., & Peat, F. D. (1984). *The looking glass universe: The emerging science of wholeness.* New York: Cornerstone.

Brown, P. W. (1992). Sibling relationship qualities following the crisis of divorce. *Dissertation Abstracts International, 53*(11B), 5639.

Buczny, B., Speirs, J., & Howard, J. R. (1989). Nursing care of a terminally ill client: Applying Martha Rogers' conceptual framework. *Home Healthcare Nurse, 7*(4), 13–18.

Butcher, H. K. (1994a). A unitary field pattern portrait of dispiritedness in later life. *Dissertation Abstracts International, 55*(11B), 4784.

Butcher, H. K. (1994b). The unitary field pattern portrait method: Development of research method within Rogers' scientific art of nursing practice. In M. Madrid, & E. A. M. Barrett (Eds.), *Rogers' scientific art of nursing practice* (pp. 397-429) (Pub. No. 15-2610). New York: National League for Nursing Press.

Butcher, H. K. (1996). A unitary field pattern portrait of dispiritedness in later life. *Visions: the Journal of Rogerian Nursing Science, 4*, 41–58.

Butcher, H. K. (1998). Crystallizing the processes of the Unitary Field Pattern Portrait research method. *Visions: The Journal of Rogerian Nursing Science, 6*, 13–26.

Butcher, H. K., & Parker, N. I. (1988). Guided imagery within Rogers' Science of Unitary Human Beings: An experimental study. *Nursing Science Quarterly, 1*, 103–110.

Capra, F. (1983). *The turning point.* Toronto: Bantam Books.

Capra, F. (1996). *Web of life: A new scientific understanding of living systems.* New York: Anchor Books, Doubleday.

Carboni, J. T. (1992). Instrument development and the measurement of unitary constructs. *Nursing Science Quarterly, 5*, 134–142.

Carboni, J. T. (1995a). The Rogerian process of inquiry. *Nursing Science Quarterly, 8*, 22–37.

Carboni, J. T. (1995b). Enfolding health-as-wholeness-and-harmony: A theory of Rogerian nursing practice. *Nursing Science Quarterly, 8*, 71–78.

Caroselli-Dervan, C. (1991). The relationship of power and feminism in female nurse executives in acute care hospitals. *Dissertation Abstracts International, 52*(6B), 2990.

Caroselli, C. (1995). Power and feminism: A nursing science perspective. *Nursing Science Quarterly, 8*, 115–119.

Caroselli, C., & Barrett, E. A. M. (1998). A review of the power as knowing participation in change literature. *Nursing Science Quarterly, 11*, 9–16.

Cerilli, K., & Burd, S. (1989). An analysis of Martha Rogers' nursing as a Science of Unitary Human Beings. In J. Riehl-Sisca (Ed.), *Conceptual models for nursing practice* (3rd ed., pp. 189–95). Norwalk, CT: Appleton & Lange.

Chapman, J. S., Mitchell, G. J., & Forchuk, C. (1994). A glimpse of nursing theory-based practice in Canada. *Nursing Science Quarterly, 7*, 104–112.

Compton, M. A. (1989). A Rogerian view of drug abuse: Implications for nursing. *Nursing Science Quarterly, 2*, 98–105.

Conti-O'Hare, M. (1998). Examining the wounded healer archetype: A case study in expert addictions nursing practice. *Journal of the American Psychiatric Nurses Association, 4*(3), 71–76.

Contrades, S. (1987). Altered cardiac output: An assessment tool. *DCCN: Dimensions of Critical Care Nursing, 6*, 274–282.

Cowling, W. R. (1998). Unitary case inquiry. *Nursing Science Quarterly, 12*, 139–141.

Cowling, W. R. (2000). Healing as appreciating wholeness. *Advances in Nursing Science, 22*(3), 16–32.

Daingerfield, M. A. F. (1993). Communication patterns of critical care nurses. *Dissertation Abstracts International, 54*(4B), 1888.

de Sevo, M. R. (1991). Temporal experience and the preference for musical sequence complexity: A study based on Martha Rogers' conceptual system. *Dissertation Abstracts International, 52*(6B), 2991.

Dixon, D. S. (1994). An exploration of the sleep patterns of individuals when their environment changes from home to the hospital. *Dissertation Abstracts International, 55*(11B), 4785.

Dominguez, L. M. (1996). The lived experience of women of Mexican heritage with HIV/AIDS. *Dissertation Abstracts International, 57*(4B), 2475.

Donahue, L., & Alligood, M. R. (1995). A description of the elderly from self-selected attributes. *Visions: The Journal of Rogerian Nursing Science, 3*, 12–19.

Doyle, M. B. (1995). Mental health nurses' imagination, power, and empathy: A descriptive study using Rogerian nursing science. *Dissertation Abstracts International, 56*(11B), 6033.

Doyle, M. B. (1998). Mental health nurses' imagination, power, and empathy: A descriptive study using Rogerian nursing science. *Rogerian Nursing Science News, 10*(4), 8.

Dykeman, M. C., & Loukissa, D. (1993). The Science of Unitary Human Beings: An integrative review. *Nursing Science Quarterly, 6*, 179–188.

Edwards, J. V. (1991). The relationship of contrasting selections of music and human field motion. *Dissertation Abstracts International, 52*(6B), 2992.

Feber, T. (1996). Promoting self-esteem after laryngectomy. *Nursing Times, 92*(30), 37–39.

Ference, H. M. (1979). The relationship of time experience, creativity traits, differentiation, and human field motion: An empirical investigation of Rogers' correlates of synergistic human development. *Dissertation Abstracts International, 40*(11B), 5206.

Ference, H. (1986a). Foundations of a nursing science and its evolution: A perspective. In V. M. Malinski (Ed.), *Explorations on Martha Rogers' Science of Unitary Human Beings* (pp. 35–44). Norwalk, CT: Appleton-Century-Crofts.

Ference, H. M. (1986b). The relationship of time experience, creativity traits, differentiation, and human field motion. In V. M. Malinski (Ed.), *Explorations on Martha Rogers' Science of Unitary Human Beings* (pp. 95–106). Norwalk, CT: Appleton-Century-Crofts.

Garon, M. (1992). Contributions of Martha Rogers to the development of nursing science. *Nursing Outlook, 40*(2), 67–72.

Garrard, C. T. (1995). The effect of therapeutic touch on stress reduction and immune function in persons with AIDS. *Dissertation Abstracts International, 56*(7B), 3692.

Girardin, B. W. (1990). The relationship of lightwave frequency to sleepwakefulness frequency in well, full-term, Hispanic neonates. *Dissertation Abstracts International, 52*(2B), 748.

Green C. A. (1998). Critically exploring the use of Rogers' nursing theory of Unitary Human Beings as a framework to underpin therapeutic touch practice. *European Nurse, 3*, 158–169.

Griffin, W. M., Moore, P., Ruge, C., & Weiler-Crespo, W. (1996). Martha E. Rogers' nursing science: Application to Therapeutic Touch. *Rogerian Nursing Science News, 8*, 9–12.

Guba, E.G. (Ed.) (1990). *The paradigm dialogue.* Newbury Park, CA: Sage.

Gueldner, S. H. (1989). Applying Rogers' model to nursing administration: Emphasis on client and nursing. In B. Henry, C. Arndt, M. DiVincenti, & A. Marriner-Tomey (Eds.), *Dimensions of nursing administration* (pp. 113–119). Boston: Blackwell Scientific.

Halkitis, P. N., & Kirton, C. (1999). Self-strategies as means of enhancing adherence to HIV antiretroviral therapies: A Rogerian approach. *Journal of the New York State Nurses Association, 30*, 22–27.

Hanchett, E. S. (1992). Concepts from Eastern philosophy and Rogers' Science of Unitary Human Beings. *Nursing Science Quarterly, 5*, 164–170.

Hastings-Tolsma, M. T. (1992). The relationship of diversity of human field pattern to risk-taking and time experience: An investigation of Rogers' principles of homeodynamics. *Dissertation Abstracts International, 53*(8B), 4029.

Heggie, J., Garon, M., Kodiath, M., & Kelly, A. (1994). Implementing the Science of Unitary Human Beings at the San Diego VA Medical Center. In Madrid, M. & Barrett, E. A. M. (Eds.), *Rogers' scientific art of nursing practice* (pp. 285-304) (Pub. No. 15-2610). New York: National League for Nursing Press.

Heggie, J. R., Schoenmehl, P. A., Grieco, C., & Chang, M. K. (1989). Selection and implementation of Dr. Martha Rogers' nursing conceptual model in an acute care setting. *Clinical Nurse Specialist, 3*, 143–147.

Hektor, L. M. (1989). Martha E. Rogers: A life history. *Nursing Science Quarterly, 2*, 63–73.

Hellwig, S. D., & Ferrante, S. (1993). Martha Rogers' model in associate degree education. *Nurse Educator, 18*(5), 25–27.

Ireland, M. (1996). Death anxiety and self-esteem in children four, five and six years of age: A comparison of minority children who have AIDS with minority children who are healthy. *Rogerian Nursing Science News, 8*(4), 16.

Ireland, M. (2000). Martha Rogers' odyssey. *American Journal of Nursing, 100*(10), 59.

Johnson, E. E. (1996). Health choice-making: The experience, perception, expression of older women. *Dissertation Abstracts International, 57*(11B), 6851.

Johnston, L. W. (1993). The development of the Human Field Image Metaphor Scale. *Dissertation Abstracts International, 54*(4B), 1890.

Johnston, L. W. (1994). Psychometric analysis of Johnston's Human Field Image Metaphor Scale. *Visions: The Journal of Rogerian Nursing Science, 2*, 7–11.

Kells, K. J. (1995). Sensing presence as open or closed space: A phenomenological inquiry on blind individuals' experiences of obstacle detection. *Dissertation Abstracts International, 57*(1B), 239.

Kenosian, C. V. (1995). Wound healing with noncontact therapeutic touch used as an adjunct therapy. *Journal of WOCN, 22*, 95–99.

Kilker, M. J. (1994). Transformational and transactional leadership styles: An empirical investigation of Rogers' principle of integrality—dissertation abstract. *Rogerian Nursing Science News, 7*(2), 1.

Kim, H. (1990). Patterning of parent-fetal attachment during the experience of guided imagery: An experimental investigation of Martha Rogers human-environment integrality. *Dissertation Abstracts International, 51*(10B), 4778.

Klebanoff, N. A. (1994). Menstrual synchronization. *Dissertation Abstracts International, 56*(2B), 742.

Klemm, P. R., & Stashinko, E. E. (1997). Martha Rogers' Science of Unitary Human Beings: A participative teaching-learning approach. *Journal of Nursing Education, 36*, 341–345.

Krause, D. A. B. (1991). The impact of an individually tailored nursing intervention on human field patterning in clients who experience dyspnea. *Dissertation Abstracts International, 53*(3B), 1293.

Kuhn, T. (1970). *The structure of scientific revolutions* (2nd ed.). Chicago: The University of Chicago.

Leddy, S. K. (1999). Further exploration of the psychometric properties of the Person–Environment Participation Scale: Differentiating instrument reliability and construct stability. *Visions: The Journal of Rogerian Nursing Science, 7*, 55–57.

MacNeil, M. (1996). Therapeutic Touch and pain in tension headache. *Rogerian Nursing Science News, 8*(3), 13.

Madrid, M. (1996). The participating process of human field patterning in an acute-care environment [German]. *Pflege, 9*, 246–254.

Madrid, M., & Barrett, E. A. M. (Eds.) (1994). *Rogers' scientific art of nursing practice.* (Pub. No. 15-2610). New York: National League for Nursing Press.

Malinski, V. M. (1986). *Explorations on Martha Rogers' Science of Unitary Human Beings.* Norwalk, CT: Appleton-Century-Crofts.

Malinski, V. M. (1991). Spirituality as integrality: A Rogerian perspective on the path of healing. *Journal of Holistic Healing, 9*(1), 54–64.

Malinski, V.M. (1994). Highlights in the evolution of nursing science: Emergence of the Science of Unitary Human Beings. In V. M. Malinski & E. A. M.Barrett (Eds), *Martha E. Rogers: Her life and her work* (pp. 197–204). Philadelphia: Davis.

Matas, K. E. (1997). Human patterning and chronic pain. *Nursing Science Quarterly, 10*, 88–96.

McBride, S., Graydon, J., Sidani, S., & Hall, L. (1999). The therapeutic use of music for dyspnea and anxiety in patients with COPD who live at home. *Journal of Holistic Nursing, 17*, 229–250.

McCanse, R. P. (1995). The McCanse Readiness for Death Instrument (MRDI): A reliable and valid measure for hospice care. *Hospice Journal: Physical, Psychosocial, and Pastoral Care of the Dying, 10*(1), 15–26.

McNiff, M. A. (1995a). A study of the relationship of power, perceived health, and life satisfaction in adults with long-term care needs based on Martha E. Rogers' Science of Unitary Human Beings. *Dissertation Abstracts International, 56*(11B), 6037.

McNiff, M. A. (1995b). A study of the relationship of power, perceived health, and life satisfaction in adults with long-term care needs based on Martha E. Rogers' Science of Unitary Human Beings. *Rogerian Nursing Science News 8*(2), 1–2.

Meehan, T. C. (1993). Therapeutic touch and postoperative pain: A Rogerian research study. *Nursing Science Quarterly, 6*, 69–78.

Meleis, A. (1985). *Theoretical nursing: Development and progress.* Philadelphia: Lippincott.

Meleis, A. (1997). *Theoretical nursing: Development and progress* (3rd ed.). Philadelphia: Lippincott.

Mersmann, C. A. (1993). Therapeutic touch and milk letdown in mothers of non-nursing preterm infants. *Dissertation Abstracts International, 54*(4B), 4602.

Mills, A. (1996). Nursing. Therapeutic touch—Case study: The application, documentation and outcome. *Complementary Therapies in Medicine, 4*, 127–132.

Mills, A., & Biley, F. C. (1994). A case study in Rogerian nursing. *Nursing Standard, 9*(7), 31–34.

Morris, D. L. (1991). An exploration of elders' perceptions of power and well-being. *Dissertation Abstracts International, 52*(8B), 4125.

Moulton, P. J. (1994). An investigation of the relationship of power and empathy in nurse executives. *Dissertation Abstracts International, 55*(4B), 1379.

Novak, D. M. (1999). Perception of menopause and its application to Rogers' Science of Unitary Human Beings. *Visions: The Journal of Rogerian Nursing Science, 7*, 24–29.

Orshan, S. A. (1996). The relationships among perceived social support, self-esteem, and acculturation in pregnant and non-pregnant Puerto Rican teenagers. Abstract of doctoral dissertation. *Rogerian Nursing Science News,9*(1), 9–10.

Overman, B. (1994). Lessons from the Tao for birthing practice. *Journal of Holistic Nursing, 12*, 142–147.

Paletta, J. L. (1990). The relationship of temporal experience to human time. In E. A. M. Barrett (Ed.), *Visions of Rogers' Science Based Nursing* (pp. 239–253) (Pub. No. 15-2285). New York: National League for Nursing.

Patty, C. M. (1999). Teaching affective competencies to surgical technologists. *AORN Journal, 70*, 776, 778–781.

Peck, S. D. E. (1997). The effectiveness of therapeutic touch for decreasing pain in elders with degenerative arthritis. *Journal of Holistic Nursing, 15*, 176–198.

Peck, S. D. (1998). The efficacy of therapeutic touch for improving functional ability in elders with degenerative arthritis. *Nursing Science Quarterly, 11*, 123–132.

Phillips, B. B., & Bramlett, M. H. (1994). Integrated awareness: A key to the pattern of mutual process. *Visions: The Journal of Rogerian Nursing Science, 2*, 19–34.

Pohl, J. M. (1992). Mother–daughter relationships and adult daughters' commitment to caregiving to their aging disabled mothers. *Dissertation Abstract International, 53*(12B), 6225.

Porter, L. S. (1998). Reducing teenage and unintended pregnancies through client-centered and family-focused school-based family planning programs. *Journal of Pediatric Nursing: Nursing Care of Children and Families, 13*, 158–163.

Powell, G. M. (1997). The new physics: Health and nursing. *Australian Journal of Holistic Nursing, 4*(1), 17–23.

Quinn, A. A. (1988). Integrating a changing me: A grounded theory of the process of menopause for perimenopausal women. *Dissertation Abstracts International, 50*(1B), 126.

Rapacz, K. E. (1991). Human patterning and chronic pain. *Dissertation Abstracts International, 52*(9B), 4670.

Rawnsley, M. (1977). Relationships between the perception of the speed of time and the process of dying: An empirical investigation of the holistic theory of nursing proposed by Martha Rogers. Unpublished doctoral dissertation, Boston University.

Reeder, F. (1999). Energy: Its distinctive meanings. *Nursing Science Quarterly, 12*, 6–7.

Richard, M. A. (1993). Staff nurses' perception of power as a function of organizational factors. *Dissertation Abstracts International, 54*(2A), 466.

Richter, D. (1998). Holistic nursing—do nurses take on too much? [German]. *Pflege, 11*, 255–262.

Rizzo, J. A. (1990). An investigation of the relationships of life satisfaction, purpose in life, and power in individuals sixty-five years and older. *Dissertation Abstracts International, 51*(9B), 4280.

Rogers, M. E. (1961). *Education revolution in nursing*. New York: Macmillan.

Rogers, M. E. (1964). *Reveille in nursing*. Philadelphia: Davis.

Rogers, M. E. (1970). *An introduction to the theoretical basis of nursing*. Philadelphia: Davis.

Rogers, M. E. (1988). Nursing science and art: A prospective. *Nursing Science Quarterly, 1*, 99–102.

Rogers, M. E. (1990a). Nursing: Science of Unitary, Irreducible, Human Beings: Update 1990. In E. A. M. Barrett (Ed), *Visions of Rogers' science-based nursing* (pp. 5–11) (Pub. No. 15-2385). New York: National League for Nursing. Reprinted in 1994 in V. M. Malinski & E. A. M. Barrett (Eds), *Martha E. Rogers: Her life and her work* (pp. 244–249). Philadelphia: Davis.

Rogers, M. E. (1990b). Space-age paradigm for new frontiers in nursing. In M. E. Parker (Ed), *Nursing theories in practice* (pp. 105–113) (Pub. No. 12-2350). New York: National League for Nursing. Reprinted in 1994 in V.M. Malinski & E. A. M. Barrett (Eds), *Martha E. Rogers: Her life and her work* (pp. 250–255). Philadelphia: Davis.

Rogers, M. E. (1992). Nursing science and the space age. *Nursing Science Quarterly, 5*, 27–34.

Rogers, M. E. (1994). Educating the nurse for the future. In V.M. Malinski & E. A. M. Barrett (Eds). *Martha E. Rogers: Her life and her work* (pp. 61–68). Philadelphia: Davis.

Ruka, S. M., Brown, J. A., & Procope, B. (1997). Clinical exemplar. A blending of health strategies in a community-based nursing center. *Clinical Nurse Specialist, 11*, 179–187.

Rush, M. M. (1997). A study of the relations among perceived social support, spirituality, and power as knowing participation in change among sober female alcoholics within the Science of Unitary Human Beings. *Journal of Addictions Nursing, 9*, 146–155.

Safier, G. (1977). *Contemporary American leaders in nursing: An oral history.* New York: McGraw-Hill.

Samarel, N. (1992). The experience of receiving therapeutic touch. *Journal of Advanced Nursing, 17*, 651–657.

Samarel, N. (1997). Therapeutic touch, dialogue, and women's experiences in breast cancer surgery. *Holistic Nursing Practice, 12*(1), 62–70.

Samarel, N., Fawcett, J., Ryan, F. M., & Davis, M. M. (1998). Effects of dialogue and therapeutic touch on preoperative and postoperative experiences of breast cancer surgery: An exploratory study. *Oncology Nursing Forum, 25*, 1369–1376.

Sarter, B. (1987). Philosophical sources of nursing theory. *Nursing Science Quarterly, 1*, 52–57.

Sarter, B. (1988). *The stream of becoming: A study of Martha Rogers's theory* (Pub. No. 15-2205). New York: National League for Nursing.

Schneider, P. E. (1995a). Focusing awareness: The process of extraordinary healing from a Rogerian perspective. *Visions: The Journal of Rogerian Nursing Science, 3*, 32–43.

Schneider, P. E. (1995b). A model of alternative healing: A comparative case analysis. *Dissertation Abstracts International, 56*(4B), 1938.

Schodt, C. M. (1989). Patterns of parent-fetus attachment and the couvade syndrome: An application of human-environment integrality as postulated in the Science of Unitary Human Beings. *Dissertation Abstracts International, 50*(10B), 4455.

Sherman, D. W. (1993). An investigation of the relationships among spirituality, perceived social support, death anxiety, and nurses' willingness to care for AIDS patients. *Dissertation Abstracts International, 55*(5B), 1808.

Sherman, D. W. (1996). Nurses' willingness to care for AIDS patients and spirituality, social support, and death anxiety. *Image: Journal of Nursing Scholarship, 28*, 205–213.

Sherman, D. W. (1997). Rogerian science: Opening new frontiers of nursing knowledge through its application in quantitative research. *Nursing Science Quarterly, 10*, 131–135.

Sheu, S. L., Shiau, S. J., & Hung, C. H. (1997). The application of Rogers' Science of Unitary Human Beings to an adolescent with mental illness [Chinese]. *Journal of Nursing (China), 44*(2), 51–57.

Smith, C. T. (1989). The lived experience of staying healthy in rural Black families. *Dissertation Abstracts International, 50*(9B), 3925.

Smith, D. W. (1992). A study of power and spirituality in polio survivors using the nursing model of Martha E. Rogers. *Dissertation Abstracts International, 53*(4B), 1791.

Smith, D. W. (1994). Toward developing a theory of spirituality. *Visions: The Journal of Rogerian Nursing Science, 2*, 35–43.

Smith, D. W. (1995). Power and spirituality in polio survivors: A study based on Rogers' science. *Nursing Science Quarterly, 8*, 133–139.

Smith, M. C. (1999). Caring and the Science of Unitary Human Beings. *Advances in Nursing Science, 21*(4), 14–28.

Smith, M. C., & Reeder, F. (1998). Clinical outcomes research and Rogerian science: Strange or emergent bedfellows? *Visions: The Journal of Rogerian Nursing Science, 6*, 27–38.

Smith, M. J. (1986). Human-environment process: A test of Rogers' principle of integrality. *Advances in Nursing Science, 9*(1), 21–28.

Stoeckle, M. L. (1993). Waiting for a second chance at life: An examination of health-related hardiness, uncertainty, power, and the environment in adults on the kidney transplant waiting list. *Dissertation Abstracts International, 54*(6B), 3000.

Straneva, J. A. E. (1992). Therapeutic touch and in vitro erythropoiesis. *Dissertation Abstracts International, 54*(3B), 1338.

Sullivan, L. M. (1994). The meaning and significance of homelessness to a child: A phenomenological inquiry. *Dissertation Abstracts International, 56*(2B), 746.

Tejero, M. C. (1998). Reflections on Martha E. Rogers' theory [Spanish]. *Revista Rol de Enfermeria, 21*(238), 43–46.

Tettero, I., Jackson, S., & Wilson, S. (1993). Theory to practice: Developing a Rogerian based assessment tool. *Journal of Advanced Nursing, 18*, 776–782.

Thomas, D. J. (1993). The lived experience of people with liver transplants. *Dissertation Abstracts International, 54*(2B), 747.

Thompson, J. E. (1990). Finding the borderline's border: Can Martha Rogers help? *Perspectives in Psychiatric Care, 26*(4), 7–10.

Thornton, L. M. (1996a). A study of Reiki, an energy field treatment, using Rogers' science. *Rogerian Nursing Science News, 8*(3), 14–15.

Thornton, L. M. (1996b). A study of Reiki using Rogers' science, part II. *Rogerian Nursing Science News, 8*(4), 13–14.

Turner, J. G., Clark, A. J., Williams, M., & Gautheir, D. K. (1998). The effect of therapeutic touch on pain and anxiety in burn patients. *Journal of Advanced Nursing, 28*(1), 10–20.

Wall, L. M. (2000). Changes in hope and power in lung cancer patients who exercise. *Nursing Science Quarterly, 13*, 234–242.

Watson, J. (1998). Exploring the concept of beyond waking experience. *Visions: The Journal of Rogerian Nursing Science, 6*, 39–46.

Watson, J. (1999). Measuring dreaming as a beyond waking experience in Rogers' conceptual model. *Nursing Science Quarterly, 12*, 245–250.

Watson, J., Sloyan, C. M., & Robalino, J. E. (2000). The Time Metaphor Test re-visited: Implications for Rogerian research. *Visions: The Journal of Rogerian Nursing Science, 8*, 32–45.

Wendler, M. C. (1996). Understanding healing: A conceptual analysis. *Journal of Advanced Nursing, 24*, 836–842.

Winsted-Fry, P. (2000). Rogers' conceptual system and family nursing. *Nursing Science Quarterly, 13*, 278–280.

Yarcheski, A., & Mahon, N. E. (1995). Rogers' pattern manifestations and health in adolescents. *Western Journal of Nursing Research, 17*, 383–397.

On line source: *archive.uwcm.ac.uk/uwcm/ns/martha/Biography.htm*

ANNOTATED BIBLIOGRAPHY—NURSING

Barrett, E. A. M. (Ed.). (1990). *Visions of Rogers' science-based nursing* (Pub. No. 15-2285). New York: National League for Nursing.

A compilation of materials from scholars and clinicians who have worked with Rogerian science. One of the noteworthy contributions of this book is Rogers' 1990 update. In addition, it is divided into sections on practice, research, and education.

Bray, J. D. (1989). The relationships of creativity, time experience and mystical experience. *Dissertation Abstracts International, 50*(8B), 3394.

This study hypothesized a positive relationship between creativity and mystical experience, timelessness and mystical experience, and creativity and timelessness. A nonrandom sample of 193 college students provided the data. In the overall data analysis, no significant correlations were found. However, significant correlations between timelessness and mystical experience in males and between mystical experience and timelessness as well as creativity for participants who practiced mediation, prayer, or relaxation techniques were found.

Johnson, E. E. (1996). Health choice-making: The experience, perception, expression of older women. *Dissertation Abstracts International, 57*(11B), 6851.

This hermeneutic phenomenologic study conceptualized health choice-making as a pattern manifestation of the human/environment process. Commonalties found in the descriptions of 15 women, aged 75 or older, were combined to construct a unitary field pattern portrait of health choice-making. This pattern includes health choice-making as an awareness of an unsettled state of affairs, active participation in changing this state of affairs, hoping for the best, and taking a chance since change is unpredictable.

Madrid, M. (Ed.). (1997). *Patterns of Rogerian knowing.* New York: National League for Nursing.

The most recent compilations of writings from scholars and clinicians who share their applications of the Science of Unitary Human Beings.

Malinski, V. M., & Barrett, E. A. M. (1994). *Martha E. Rogers: Her life and her work.* Philadelphia: Davis.

One of the most comprehensive reviews of Martha Roger's life and her writings. In addition to chapters devoted to Rogers' work, it also includes a comprehensive bibliography of citations about Rogers and the Science of Unitary Human Beings, a review of her life history, and even her family genealogy provided by her sister. The publishers received word of Martha Roger's death, just as the book was being prepared for press and included the following tribute as a publisher's note:

> I climbed aboard her spacecraft a long time ago.
> It wasn't made of metal or plastic, and it had no
> rigid form. It was the web of the mind that carries
> us beyond our expectations. She brought a Slinky
> along to demonstrate "The Spiral of Life."

> I cannot visualize Martha at rest. She is out there
> somewhere discovering, developing, and nurturing ideas
> to challenge us when next we meet.
> Robert H. Craven, Sr. (p. iv)

Matas, K. E. (1997). Human patterning and chronic pain. *Nursing Science Quarterly, 10,* 88–96.

This study investigated pattern manifestations of chronic pain through comparing adults in chronic pain management programs and adults living in the community who did not report chronic pain. Findings included lower scores on human field motion and power as knowing participation measurements for the chronic pain group as compared to those without such pain, showing continued support for Rogers' abstract conceptual system. The author speculates that chronic pain may slow movement to higher frequency patterns.

Morris, D. L. (1991). An exploration of elders' perceptions of power and well-being. *Dissertation Abstracts International, 52*(8B), 4125.

This exploratory descriptive study involved interviews of 61 elders (31 living in the community and 30 nursing home residents), aged 61 to 97. The emerging power categories were mastery, resources, influence, values, personal attributes, interpersonal, and independence/dependence. The well-being categories were mastery, health, self-attitude, valued behavior, relationships, independence/dependence, spirituality, and security. Those living in the community had significantly higher scores for power and well-being and lower locus of control scores, indicating patterns of higher frequency.

Peck, S. D. (1998). The efficacy of therapeutic touch for improving functional ability in elders with degenerative arthritis. *Nursing Science Quarterly, 11,* 123–132.

In this study, 82 community living elders were randomly assigned to therapeutic touch or progressive muscle relaxation treatments. Both treatments resulted in improvements in pain, tension, mood, and satisfaction. Therapeutic touch improved hand function while progressive muscle relaxation improved walking and bending.

Phillips, B. B., & Bramlett, M. H. (1994). Integrated awareness: A key to the pattern of mutual process. *Visions: The Journal of Rogerian Nursing Science, 2,* 19–34.

This theoretical exploration sought to analyze the concept, integrated awareness, in its relationship with the Science of Unitary Human Beings. Integrated awareness has direct relevance to the nature of human to human mutual process, involves creating a matrix recognizing cognition of a greater awareness of self and environment, implies an abstract sense of connection in the evolution of the human and environmental fields, and may be seen as a unifying schema of inner peace, serenity, well-being, and power.

Sarter, B. (1987). Philosophical sources of nursing theory. *Nursing Science Quarterly, 1,* 52–59.

Sarter's thoughtful and well-written article helps to explain some of the philosophical underpinnings of Rogers' writings (and of others).

Sherman, D. W. (1996). Nurses' willingness to care for AIDS patients and spirituality, social support, and death anxiety. *Image: Journal of Nursing Scholarship, 28,* 205–213.

This descriptive correlational study collected data from 220 female RNs who cared for AIDS patients in the New York City Metropolitan area. Findings included that willingness to care for AIDS patients was positively correlated with spirituality and perceived social support and negatively correlated with death anxiety.

Smith, M. C. (1999). Caring and the Science of Unitary Human Beings. *Advances in Nursing Science, 21*(4), 14–28.

This concept clarification sought to elucidate ambiguity about the concept of caring. By examining points of congruence between the literature on caring and the Science of Unitary Human Beings five constitutive meanings of caring were identified. These are manifesting intentions, appreciating pattern, attuning to dynamic flow, experiencing the infinite, and inviting creative emergence. The article includes narratives to ground the abstract in concrete human experiences.

Web site: *archive.uwcm.ac.uk/uwcm/ns/martha/homepage.html*

Useful information about the conceptual system, research, conferences, and links.

ANNOTATED BIBLIOGRAPHY—NON-NURSING

Abbott, E. (1992). *Flatland.* New York: Dover.

This book, actually written at least a century ago, is an account of an intelligent creature from a two-dimensional world who finds his way to a three dimensional world. It is an easy and quick read, and is considered one of the best things of its kind that has ever been written. It is also a good introduction to the idea of dimensions beyond three.

Briggs, J. P., & Peat, F. D. (1984). *The looking glass universe: The emerging science of wholeness.* New York: Cornerstone.

A book about the science of wholeness, written for the general public. Dr. John Briggs is a science writer and Dr. David Peat a physicist. Together they produced an entertaining and enlightening book that helps explain many of the concepts underlying the Rogerian conceptual system.

Capra, F. (1996). *Web of life: A new scientific understanding of living systems.* New York: Anchor Books, Doubleday.

The most recent book by Fritjof Capra (*The Tao of physics, The turning point*). Capra is a theoretical physicist who is able to write about new conceptions of science for the general public. His writings are quite consistent with the Rogerian conceptual system, and provide both support and explanation for some of her views. His two earlier books are also helpful in understanding Rogers' conceptual system.

CHAPTER 15

ROY ADAPTATION MODEL
SISTER CALLISTA ROY

Julia Gallagher Galbreath

■ ■ ■

Sister Callista Roy, R.N., Ph.D. (b. 1939) is a nurse theorist at Boston College, Massachusetts. Before this appointment, Roy was a Post-Doctoral Fellow and Robert Wood Johnson Clinical Nurse Scholar at the University of California, San Francisco. Sr. Roy has served in many positions, including Chair of the Department of Nursing, Mount Saint Mary's College, Los Angeles; Adjunct Professor, Graduate Program, School of Nursing, University of Portland; and Acting Director and Nurse Consultant, Saint Mary's Hospital, Tucson, Arizona. Sr. Roy earned her B.S. in nursing in 1963 from Mount Saint Mary's College, Los Angeles, her M.S. in nursing in 1966, and doctorate in sociology in 1977 from the University of California, Los Angeles. She is a Fellow of the American Academy of Nursing and active in many nursing organizations including Sigma Theta Tau, the North American Nursing Diagnosis Association (1973–1983), and the Boston-Based Adaptation Research in Nursing Society (BBARNS). She is the author or co-author of a number of works including Introduction to nursing: An adaptation model *(Roy, 1976, 1984);* Essentials of the Roy Adaptation Model *(Andrews & Roy, 1986);* Theory construction in nursing: An adaptation model *(Roy & Roberts, 1981);* The Roy Adaptation Model *(Roy & Andrews, 1991, 1999).*

The Roy Adaptation Model has evoked much interest and respect since its 1964 inception by Sister Roy as part of her graduate work under the guidance of Dorothy E. Johnson at the University of California, Los Angeles. In 1970, the faculty of Mount Saint Mary's College in Los Angeles adopted the Roy Adaptation Model as the conceptual framework of the undergraduate nursing curriculum. That same year Roy first published her ideas about adaptation (Roy, 1970).

A text, written by Sr. Roy and fellow faculty, described the Roy Adaptation Model and presented nursing assessment and intervention reflective of the distinctive focus of the model (Roy, 1976). In 1991 Roy and Andrews presented *The Roy Adaptation Model: The definitive statement*, which included the collective experiences of several contributing authors who taught and practiced using the Roy model for over two decades. Based on four earlier books, this text included the diagrammatic conceptualizations of the model developed at the Royal Alexandra Hospital's School of Nursing, Edmonton, Alberta, Canada. In her recent book, *The Roy Adaptation Model*, Roy redefines elements in the Roy Adaptation Model (RAM) in preparation for nursing in the twenty-first century (Roy & Andrews, 1999).

Further, Roy and Roberts (1981) wrote *Theory construction in nursing: An adaptation model* to discuss the use of the Roy model to construct nursing theory. Interested readers can search for the *Roy Adaptation Model* in databanks such as CINAHL and Dissertation Abstracts International and find many matches for books, articles, and research discussing the model.

In 1989, a group of researchers who had been using the RAM to guide their individual studies began working together. They formed a society, now named the Boston-Based Adaptation Research in Nursing Society (BBARNS), whose purposes include

1. advancing nursing practice by developing nursing knowledge based on the RAM;
2. providing scholarly colleagueship needed for knowledge and research;
3. enhancing networks for dissemination and utilization of research for nursing practice; and
4. promoting the development of expert nurse scientists (Pollock, Frederickson, Carson, Massey, & Roy, 1994, p. 362).

THE ROY ADAPTATION MODEL

Roy credits the works of von Bertalanffy's (1968) general system theory and Helson's (1964) adaptation theory as forming the original basis of the scientific assumptions underlying the Roy model. Table 15–1 identifies the assumptions flowing from the initial philosophical and scientific perspectives. The philosophic assumptions flow, according to Roy, from humanism and veritivity. The term *veritivity* was coined by Roy to identify the common purposefulness of human existence (Roy, 1988).

In response to the 25th anniversary of the model's publication, Roy restated the assumptions that form the basis of the model and redefined adaptation. Adaptation is defined as, "the process and outcome whereby thinking and feeling persons, as individuals or in groups, use conscious awareness and choice to create human and environmental integration" (Roy & Andrews, 1999, p. 30). The most recent scientific and philosophic assumptions are presented in Table 15–2.

In expanding her philosophic statements in 1997, Roy drew on the richness found in a diversity of cultures. The philosophic premise is stated as "nursing sees persons as co-extensive with their physical and social environments. Nurse scholars

TABLE 15–1. ASSUMPTIONS UNDERLYING THE ROY ADAPTATION MODEL

Scientific	
Systems Theory	Adaptation-Level Theory
Holism	Behavior as adaptive
Interdependence	Adaptation as a function of stimuli and adaptation level
Control processes	Individual, dynamic adaptation levels
Information feedback	Positive and active processes of responding
Complexity of living systems	

Philosophic	
Humanism	Veritivity
Creativity	Purposefulness of human existence
Purposefulness	Unity of purpose
Holism	Activity, creativity
Interpersonal process	Value and meaning of life

Source: Originally from Roy, C., & Andrews, H. A. (Eds.). (1991). *The Roy Adaptation Model: The definitive statement* (p. 5). Norwalk, CT: Appleton & Lange. Used with permission. Also found in Roy & Andrews, (1999), p. 33.

TABLE 15–2. VISION BASIC TO CONCEPTS FOR THE 21st Century

Scientific Assumptions

Systems of matter and energy progress to higher levels of complex self-organization.

Consciousness and meaning are constitutive of person and environment integration.

Awareness of self and environment is rooted in thinking and feeling.

Humans by their decisions are accountable for the integration of creative processes.

Thinking and feeling mediate human action.

System relationships include acceptance, protection, and fostering of interdependence.

Persons and the earth have common patterns and integral relationships.

Persons and environment transformations are created in human consciousness.

Integration of human and environment meanings results in adaptation.

Philosophic Assumptions

Persons have mutual relationships with the world and God.

Human meaning is rooted in an omega point convergence of the universe.

God is intimately revealed in the diversity of creation and is the common destiny of creation.

Persons use human creative abilities of awareness, enlightenment, and faith.

Persons are accountable for the process of deriving, sustaining, and transforming the universe.

Source: Roy, Sr. C., & Andrews, H. A. (1999). *The Roy Adaptation Model* (2nd ed., p. 35). Stamford, CT: Appleton & Lange. Used with permission.

take a value-based stance. Rooted in beliefs and hopes about the nature of the human person, they fashion a discipline that participates in the well-being of persons" (Roy, 1997a, p. 42). Roy drew on the characteristics of creation spirituality (Swimme & Berry, 1992) as she redefined the philosophical assumptions of the model. Within this framework there is:

- A focus on awareness and the notion of eliminating false consciousness.
- Enlightenment to reach self-control, balance, and quietude.
- The reclamation of earthly creation as the core of faith (Roy & Andrews, 1999, p. 35).

Roy continued her development of philosophic assumptions to include a focus on people's mutuality with others, the world, and God (Roy & Andrews, 1999). A more complete discussion of the philosophic and scientific assumptions related to the model can be found in the publications *Future of the Roy model: Challenge to redefine adaptation* and *Knowledge as universal cosmic imperative* (Roy, 1997a, 1997b).

The four major concepts of the Roy Adaptation Model (RAM) are the following:

1. Humans as adaptive systems as both individuals and groups
2. The environment
3. Health
4. The goal of nursing (Roy & Andrews, 1999, p. 35).

The model presents concepts related to these four areas, clarifying each and defining their interrelationships.

Humans as Adaptive Systems

The first area of focus is humans as adaptive systems, both as individuals and in groups. The model offers a point of view or paradigm for shaping nursing activities. The focus of nursing relationships and interactions can be at the level of the individual, groups, organizations, communities, and societies in which they are included (Roy & Andrews, 1999, p. 35). Any of these may be considered a human system and each is considered by the nurse as a holistic adaptive system. The idea of an adaptive system combines the concepts of system and adaptation.

Human adaptive system. Roy conceptualizes the human system in a holistic perspective as holism stems from the underlying philosophic assumption of the model. Holism is the aspect of unified meaningfulness of human behavior in which the human system is greater than the sum of individual parts (Roy & Andrews, 1999, p. 35). As living systems, persons are in constant interaction with their environments. Between the system and the environment occurs an exchange of information, matter, and energy. Characteristics of a system include inputs, outputs, controls, and feedback.

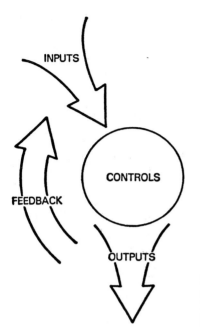

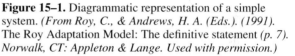

Figure 15–1. Diagrammatic representation of a simple system. *(From Roy, C., & Andrews, H. A. (Eds.). (1991). The Roy Adaptation Model: The definitive statement (p. 7). Norwalk, CT: Appleton & Lange. Used with permission.)*

Dunn (1971), a system theorist, calls our attention to the smallest unit of life, the cell. The cell is a living open system. The cell has its inner and outer worlds. From its outer world, it must draw forth the substances it needs to survive; within itself, the cell must maintain order over its vast number of molecules. System openness, therefore, implies the constant exchange of information, matter, and energy between the system and the environment. These system qualities are held by the individual as well as by groups or aggregates of humans. Figure 15–1 illustrates a simple system.

Adaptation. Figure 15–2 is used by Roy to represent humans as adaptive systems. The human adaptive system has inputs of stimuli and adaptation level, outputs as behavioral responses that serve as feedback, and control processes known as coping mechanisms. The human adaptive system has input coming from the external environment as well as from within the system. Roy identifies inputs as *stimuli* and *adaptation level* (a particular internal pooling of stimuli). Stimuli are conceptualized as falling into three classifications: focal, contextual, and residual. The stimulus most immediately confronting the human system is the *focal stimulus*. The focal stimulus demands the highest awareness from the human system. It is the center of the system's consciousness. *Contextual stimuli* are all other stimuli of the human system's internal and external worlds that can be identified as having a positive or negative influence on the situation. *Residual stimuli* are those internal or external factors whose current effects are unclear. In nursing practice, the nurse considers general knowledge related to the event or situation that has possible but unknown influences as residual stimuli. Along with stimuli, the adaptation level of the human

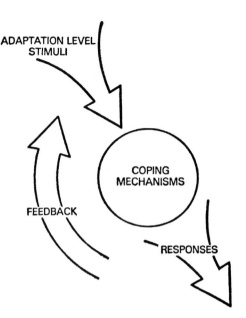

Figure 15–2. The person as a system. *(From Roy, C., & Andrews, H. A. (Eds.). (1991). The Roy Adaptation Model: The definitive statement (p. 8). Norwalk, CT: Appleton & Lange. Used with permission.)*

system acts as an important internal input to that system as an adaptive system. *Adaptation level* is the combining of stimuli that represents the condition of life processes for the human adaptive system. The three levels defined by Roy are: integrated, compensatory, and compromised life processes. *Integrated* processes are present when the adaptation level is working as a whole to meet the needs of the human system. *Compensatory* processes occur when the human's response systems have been activated and *compromised* processes occur when the compensatory and integrated processes are not providing for adaptation. Integrated life process can change to compromised processes, which activates the system's compensatory processes (Roy & Andrews, 1999, pp. 36–43).

Outputs of the human adaptive system are behavioral responses (see Fig. 15–2). Output responses can be both external and internal; thus, these responses are the system's behaviors. They can be observed, intuitively perceived by the nurse, measured, and subjectively reported by the human system. Output responses become feedback to the system and to the environment. Roy categorizes outputs of the system as either adaptive responses or ineffective responses. *Adaptive responses* are those that promote the integrity of the human system. The system's integrity, or wholeness, is behaviorally demonstrated when the system is able to meet the goals in terms of survival, growth, reproduction, mastery, and transformations of the system and the environment (Roy & Andrews, 1999, p. 44). In turn, the groups, communities, and society of which the individual is a member must sense and respond to changes in the person. An example of group consciousness and adaptation would include a citizen's planning meeting. In the Miami Valley region of Ohio, one such group is called "Communities Alive." This open citizens' group looks at areas of concerns and needs for change and growth. Strategies have included "Hidden Hero Awards" to recognize people who quietly work for the good of a person, family, or subgroup in the community. In another example, high school counselors came to a local industry to increase understanding of modern manufacturing job opportunities.

Ineffective responses, on the other hand, do not support the goals of humans as adaptive systems. Ineffective responses can immediately or gradually threaten the system's survival, growth, reproduction, mastery, or transformations (Roy & Andrews, 1999, p. 44). Ineffective responses can occur at the higher system level such as in the family or in a group. A business, for example, is a team of persons who must adapt to the constantly changing demands of the marketplace. These changes might include the impact of government regulations, competition with other providers, cost changes, or computer system changes. Business people speak of being in a "downward spiral," keenly aware of their inability to effectively respond to change.

For the human adaptive system, complex internal dynamics act as control processes. Roy has used the term *coping mechanisms* to describe the control processes of the human as an adaptive system. Some coping mechanisms are inherited or genetic, such as the white blood cell defense system against bacteria that seek to invade the body. Other mechanisms are learned, such as the use of antiseptics to cleanse a wound. Roy presents a unique nursing science concept of control mechanisms: the *regulator* and the *cognator*. Roy's model considers the regulator and cognator coping mechanisms to be subsystems of the person as an adaptive system and the *innovator* and *stabilizer* as control mechanisms inherent to the functioning of groups (Roy & Anway, 1989).

The *regulator subsystem* has the components of input, internal process, and output. Input stimuli may originate externally or internally to the person. The transmitters of the regulator system are chemical, neural, or endocrine in nature. Autonomic reflexes, which are neural responses originating in the brain stem and spinal cord, are generated as output responses of the regulator subsystem. Target organs and tissues under endocrine control also produce regulator output responses. Finally, Roy presents psychomotor responses originating from the central nervous system as regulator subsystem responses (Roy & Roberts, 1981). Many physiological processes can be viewed as regulator subsystem responses. For example, several regulatory feedback mechanisms of respiration have been identified. One of these is increased carbon dioxide, the end product of metabolism, which stimulates chemoreceptors in the medulla to increase the respiratory rate. Strong stimulation of these centers can increase ventilation six- to sevenfold (Guyton, 1971). An example of a regulator process is when a noxious external stimulus is visualized and transmitted via the optic nerve to higher brain centers and then to lower brain autonomic centers. The sympathetic neurons from these origins have multiple visceral effects, including increased blood pressure and increased heart rate. Roy's schematic representation of the regulator processes is seen in Figure 15–3.

When considering the individual, the other control subsystem original to the Roy model is the *cognator subsystem* (Roy & Andrews, 1999). Stimuli to the cognator subsystem are also both external and internal in origin. Output responses of the regulator subsystem can be feedback stimuli to the cognator subsystem.

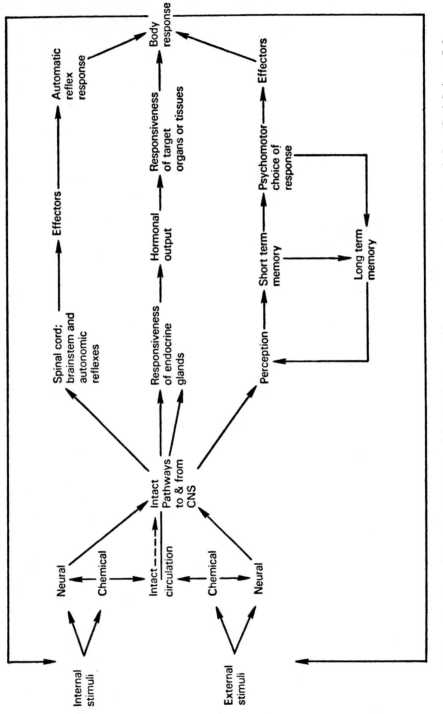

Figure 15–3. The Regulator (*From Roy, C., & McLeod, D. (1984). Theory of the person as an adaptive system. In Roy, C., & Roberts, S. L. Theory construction in nursing: An adaptation model (p. 61). Upper Saddle River, NJ: Prentice-Hall. Used with permission.*)

Cognator control processes are related to the higher brain functions of perception or information processing, learning, judgment, and emotion. Perception, or information processing, is related to the internal processes of selective attention, coding, and memory. Learning is correlated to the processes of imitation, reinforcement, and insight. Problem solving and decision making are examples of the internal processes related to judgment; and finally, emotion has the processes of defense to seek relief, affective appraisal, and attachment. A schematic presentation by Roy of the cognator subsystem is presented in Figure 15–4. In maintaining the integrity of the person, the regulator and cognator are postulated as interrelated and acting together.

Individual Situation. A decrease in the oxygen supply to Albert Smith's heart muscle stimulates pain receptors that transmit the message of pain along sympathetic afferent nerve fibers to his central nervous system. The autonomic centers of his lower brain then stimulate the sympathetic efferent nerve fibers, and there is an increase in heart and respiratory rates. The result is an increase in the oxygen supply to the heart muscle. This increase can be viewed as regulator subsystem action.

The cognator subsystem also receives the internal pain stimuli as input. Mr. Smith has learned from past experiences that the left chest and arm pain are related to his heart. His judgment is activated in deciding what action to take. He decides to go inside to air conditioning, to sit with his legs elevated, and to take slow, deep breaths. He also decides not to call for emergency help. Certainly, he believes an adaptive response secondary to these actions will occur. However, he may be increasingly alert for further regulator subsystem output responses that might cause him to question his decision. This represents the cognator process of selective attention and coding. Following the episode of pain, Mr. Smith may attempt to gain further insight into the cause of the episode. He may decide that the 90°F weather was causal and remember to limit his activities during extreme heat. In this example, Mr. Smith used the cognator subsystem processes of perception, learning, and judgment.

Control mechanisms are proposed by the RAM as inherent to the functioning of groups. Roy categorizes family, group, and collective system control mechanisms as the stabilizer and the innovator subsystems (Roy & Andrews, 1999, pp. 47–48). This conceptualization suggests that groups have two goals: stabilization and change. *Stabilizer* processes are those of established structure, values, and daily activities where the work of the group is done and the group contributes to the general well-being of society. The *innovator* subsystem is the second of the group control mechanisms and identifies structures and processes that promote change and growth.

Group Situation. A town counsel's set of by-laws and budget could be considered stabilizer control mechanisms. These structures aid in the work of the counsel by clarifying the order and process of the work. Examples of innovator control mechanisms would be a needs survey or an open town meeting. Both have the potential of promoting new thinking or awareness in the community and can lead to change.

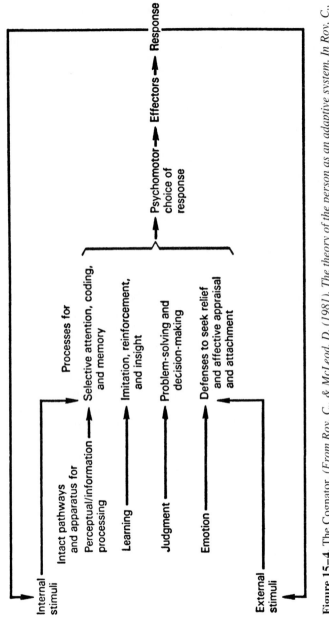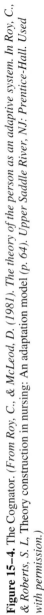

Figure 15–4. The Cognator. *(From Roy, C., & McLeod, D. (1981). The theory of the person as an adaptive system. In Roy, C., & Roberts, S. L, Theory construction in nursing: An adaptation model (p. 64). Upper Saddle River, NJ: Prentice-Hall. Used with permission.)*

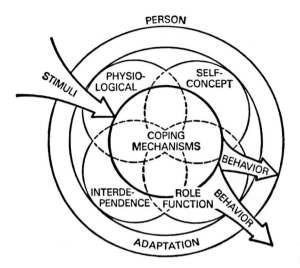

Figure 15–5. The person as an adaptive system. *(From Roy, C., & Andrews, H. A. (Eds.). (1991). The Roy Adaptation Model: The definitive statement (p. 17). Norwalk, CT: Appleton & Lange. Used with permission.)*

The Four Adaptive Modes

The coping processes, cognator-regulator and stabilizer-innovator, promote adaptation in human adaptive systems. However, the coping processes are not directly observable. Only the responses of the person or group can be observed, measured, or subjectively reported. Roy has identified four adaptive modes as categories for assessment of behavior resulting from regulator-cognator coping mechanism in persons or stabilizer-innovator coping processes in groups. These adaptive modes are the *physiological-physical, self-concept-group identity, role function,* and *interdependence* modes. By observing behavior in relation to the adaptive modes, the nurse can identify adaptive or ineffective responses in situations of health and illness. Figure 15–5 diagrammatically conceptualizes the human system as an adaptive system that includes the four adaptive modes for assessment. Further explanation of the four adaptive modes follows.

Physiological-physical Mode. The physiological mode represents the human system's physical responses and interactions with the environment (Roy & Andrews, 1999). For the individual, the underlying need of this mode is physiologic integrity, which is composed of the basic needs associated with oxygenation, nutrition, elimination, activity and rest, and protection. The complex processes of this mode are associated with the senses; fluid, electrolyte, and acid-base balance; neurological function; and endocrine function. These needs and processes may be defined as follows:

> • Oxygenation   The processes (ventilation, gas exchange, and transport of gases) by which cellular oxygen supply is maintained by the body (p. 126)

• Nutrition	The series of processes by which a person takes in nutrients, then assimilates and uses them to maintain body tissue, promote growth, and provide energy (p. 149)
• Elimination	Expulsion from the body of undigested substances, fluid wastes, and excess ions (p. 171)
• Activity and rest	Body movement that serves various purposes and changes in such movement so energy requirements are minimal (pp. 192–193)
• Protection	Nonspecific (surface membrane barriers and chemical and cellular defenses) and specific (immune system) defense processes to protect the body from foreign substances (p. 233)
• Senses	The processes by which energy (light, sound, heat, mechanical vibration, and pressure) changes to neural activity and becomes perception (p. 259)
• Fluid, electrolyte, and acid-base balance	The complex process of maintaining a stable internal environment of the body (p. 295)
• Neurological function	Key neural processes and the complex relationship of neural function to regulator and cognator coping mechanisms (p. 313)
• Endocrine function	Patterns of endocrine control and regulation that act in conjunction with the autonomic nervous system to maintain control of all physiologic processes (p. 355)

The *physical* is the focus of assessment in the first adaptive mode for a family, group, or collective human adaptive system. The need underlying this mode is resource adequacy or wholeness. For groups, the mode relates to basic operating resources such as participants, physical facilities, and fiscal resources (Roy & Andrews, 1999, p. 49).

Self-Concept-Group Identity Mode. For individuals, the self-concept mode relates to the basic need for psychic and spiritual integrity or a need to know the self with a sense of unity. Self-concept is central to the person's behavior because it consists of a person's beliefs or feelings about himself or herself at any given time (Roy & Andrews, 1999, p. 49). Self-concept has the components of physical self and personal self. The physical self includes body sensation and body image; the personal self includes self-consistency, self-ideal, and the moral-ethical-spiritual self. Body sensation is how the person experiences the physical self, and body image is how the person views the physical self. Self-consistency represents the person's efforts to maintain self-organization and avoid disequilibrium; self-ideal represents what the person expects to be and do; and the moral-ethical-spiritual self represents the person's belief system and self-evaluator (pp. 379–382). The need underlying the group identity mode for a family, group, or a collective is identity integrity. In collectives, "the mode consists of interpersonal relationships, group self-image, social milieu, and culture" (p. 49).

Role Function Mode. Role function mode is a category of behavior for both individuals and groups. A role consists of a set of expectations of how a person in a particular position will behave in relation to a person who holds another position. The need underlying this mode is social integrity. More specifically, Roy states that social integrity is knowing who one is in relation to others so that one can act appropriately. For the individual this mode focuses on the roles of the individual in society. Role behavior in groups is the means through which the social system achieves goals and functions. The need underlying the role function mode in groups is termed *role clarity*. The mode includes functions of members of the administration and staff, information management, decision-making systems, systems to maintain order, or the need for group members to understand and commit to fulfilling expected responsibilities (Roy & Andrews, 1999, pp. 49–50).

Interdependence Mode. The interdependence mode applies to adaptive behavior for both individuals and groups. Behavior is assessed as it relates to interdependent relationships of individuals and groups. For individuals, the underlying need of this mode is relational integrity or security in nurturing relationships. The mode focuses on the giving and receiving of love, respect, and value with significant others and support systems. Significant others are those persons who are of greatest importance to the person. Support systems are identified as those who help the person meet the needs for love, respect, and value. For groups, interdependence relates to social context, including both public and private contacts within and outside the group. The components are context, infrastructure, and resources (Roy & Andrews, 1999, p. 50).

Environment

Stimuli from within the human adaptive system and stimuli from around the system represent the element of environment, according to Roy. Roy specifically defines environment as "all conditions, circumstances, and influences that surround and affect the development and behavior of humans as adaptive systems, with particular consideration of person and earth resources" (Roy & Andrews, 1999, p. 52).

Health

Roy defines health as "a state and a process of being and becoming an integrated and whole human being" (Roy & Andrews, 1999, p. 54). The integrity of the person is expressed as the ability to meet the goals of survival, growth, reproduction, mastery, and person and environment transformation. Roy states that the term *integrity* is used to mean "soundness or an unimpaired condition leading to wholeness" (p. 54). One's sense of purpose in life and the meaning of life, according to Roy, are significant factors relating to integration and wholeness. This view of health transcends a simple absence of disease. In fact health, as viewed in this perspective, can exist for persons with physical, emotional, or other changes. More important than the existence of a condition, illness, or change is the response of the person. Health in the RAM is a state and a process of integration that indicates successful adaptation. The aim of the nurse practicing under the RAM is to promote the health of the human by promoting adaptive responses in all life processes, including dying with dignity.

Goal of Nursing

Roy defines the *goal of nursing* as the promotion of adaptive responses in relation to the four adaptive modes: physiological-physical, self-concept-group identity, role function, and interdependence. *Adaptive responses* are those that positively affect health, that is, support the integrity of the human adaptive system. In the perspective of the RAM, human responses include not only problems, needs, and deficiencies, but also capacities, assets, knowledge, skills, abilities, and commitments (Roy & Andrews, 1999). All responses are *behavior. Nursing activities* support adaptive responses and seek to reduce ineffective responses. The nurse may anticipate that the human system has a potential for ineffective responses secondary to stimuli likely to be present in a particular situation. The nurse acts to prepare the human system through anticipatory guidance. Nursing actions suggested by the model include approaches aimed at maintaining adaptive responses.

> In the example of the person experiencing chest pain, the stimulus immediately confronting Albert Smith (the focal stimulus) is the deficit of oxygen supply to his heart muscle. The contextual stimuli include the 90°F temperature, the sensation of pain, and Mr. Smith's age, weight, blood sugar level, and degree of coronary artery patency. The residual stimuli include his history of cigarette smoking and work-related stress.

> For Mr. Smith, the stimuli, adaptation level, and coping processes have resulted in an ineffective response. The deficit of oxygen to his heart is a threat to his physiologic integrity and will not maintain his survival. This response became feedback to the system and a focal stimulus. Mr. Smith used the cognator mechanism to adjust the total stimuli by going indoors to a cooler room and decreasing his oxygen needs by sitting down and elevating his legs. After the adjustment of the stimuli, the oxygen needs of his heart muscle were met, and the pain stopped.

THE NURSING PROCESS

The *nursing process* is a vehicle or decision-making method compatible with the practice of nursing using the RAM. After making a behavioral assessment and a nursing judgment, nurses assess stimuli affecting responses, make a nursing diagnosis, set goals, and implement interventions to promote adaptation (Roy & Andrews, 1999, p. 55). Roy offers the following broad aims for nursing in response to the assumptions written for the twenty-first century: "nurses aim to enhance system relationships through acceptance, protection, and fostering of interdependence and to promote personal and environmental transformations" (p. 55).

The RAM offers guidelines to the nurse in application of the *nursing process*. The elements of the Roy nursing process include assessment of behavior, assessment of stimuli, nursing diagnosis, goal setting, intervention, and evaluation (Roy & Andrews, 1999).

Assessment of Behavior

Assessment of behavior is considered to be the gathering of responses or output behaviors of the human system as an adaptive system in relation to each of the four adaptive modes: physiological-physical, self-concept-group identity, role function, and interdependence. Roy defines behavior as "actions or reactions under specified circumstances. It can be observable or nonobservable" (Roy & Andrews, 1999, p. 67). The nurse, through the processes of observation, careful measurement, and skilled interview techniques, gathers the specific data.

Assessment of the client in each of the four adaptive modes enhances a systematic and holistic approach. Such assessment clarifies the focus that the nurse or nursing team will use in caring for the client. Ideally, thoroughly conducted and recorded nursing assessment in the four adaptive modes sets the tone for understanding of the particular situation of a client for an entire health care team. Proficiency in the practice of nursing requires skilled assessment of behaviors and the knowledge to compare the person to specific criteria to evaluate behavioral responses as adaptive or ineffective. Figure 15–6 shows a Nursing History/Assessment developed by the nurses at Upper Valley Medical Center in Troy, Ohio. This form uses the four adaptive modes of the Roy model. Guide questions related to each adaptive mode can be developed to reflect the age or acuity of the client population being assessed. Information collected includes subjective, objective, and measurement data. Extensive discussion of assessment of behavior related to the four adaptive modes can be found in *The Roy Adaptation Model* (Roy & Andrews, 1999) and *Nursing Manual: Assessment tool according to the Roy Adaptation Model* (Cho, 1998).

Assessment of Stimuli

After gathering behavioral assessment data, the nurse analyzes the emerging themes and patterns of client behavior to identify ineffective responses or adaptive responses requiring nurse support with continual involvement of the human system receiving

UPPER VALLEY MEDICAL CENTERS
PMMC   STOUDER
ADMISSION NURSING ASSESSMENT

INSTRUCTIONS: Check all boxes that apply. For Surgical Admissions: complete white area at P.A.T. and grey area day of admission. *See Care Plan / 24 HR Nursing Assessment & Care Record.   N/A-Not Applicable

Date	Time	Received From: ☐ ER ☐		VIA ☐ w/c	Room	Family Physician		☐ male	Age
		☐ admitting ☐ doctor's office		☐ ambulatory ☐ cart				☐ female	

Temp.			☐ Regular ☐ Irregular	Resp.		BP (LA)	BP (RA)	Height	Weight
	Pulse		☐ Regular ☐ Irregular						

Informant: ☐ patient ☐ family member ☐ friend ☐ transfer form ☐ prior medical record / date: _____ ☐ interview per phone
☐ current ER record ☐ other _____

History and present status of chief complaint: _____

Pain Present: ☐ no ☐ yes / location | **Intensity Scale** 1 (mild) – 10 (severe) | **When did pain start?** | **How was pain managed at home?**

Allergies: (describe reaction) ☐ Medications ☐ food ☐ environment ☐ None   Allergy band on? ☐ yes ☐ N/A

PATIENT HISTORY:

No Yes
☐ ☐ Heart disease (MI, angina, CHF, arrhythmia, murmur, mitral valve, prolapse, pacemaker)
☐ ☐ High Blood Pressure
☐ ☐ Stroke
☐ ☐ Respiratory (asthma, emphysema, bronchitis)
☐ ☐ Kidney (stones, infection, hemodialysis)
☐ ☐ Liver (hepatitis, mono, jaundice)
☐ ☐ Cancer
☐ ☐ Blood Disorder (bleeding, clots, anemia, phlebitis)

No Yes
☐ ☐ Blood Transfusion
☐ ☐ Diabetes
☐ ☐ Thyroid Disease
☐ ☐ Seizures/Fainting
☐ ☐ Muscle Disease
☐ ☐ Neck/Back Disorder, Arthritis
☐ ☐ Depression, Mental Illness
☐ ☐ Alcohol/Drug Abuse
☐ ☐ Communicable disease (TB, STD, ...)
☐ ☐ Other _____

Past Surgeries: ☐ none   Pt/Family Reactions to anesthesia: ☐ N/A   ☐ no   ☐ yes _____

Past Medical Hospitalizations: ☐ none   Recent xrays: ☐ no ☐ yes _____   Recent lab: ☐ no ☐ yes

FAMILY HEALTH HISTORY: (Check conditions that apply)   ☐ none
☐ cancer ☐ diabetes ☐ stroke ☐ high blood pressure ☐ heart disease ☐ muscle disease ☐ other _____

Medications: (prescription, O.T.C., recreational) Include dose and frequency.   Admission Nurse, note time last dose taken.
☐ None

Are medications taken as prescribed: ☐ yes ☐ no ☐ N/A

Home Situation: (marital status, children, significant others, living environment – stairs, etc.)

(vertical left margin) **INTERDEPENDENCE – ROLE FUNCTION – SELF-CONCEPT**

NSG-001   **Admission Nursing Assessment** (page 1)   UVMC 3/88
                                                                     Rev. 3/92

Figure 15–6. Upper Valley Medical Center Admission Nursing Assessment. *C. Mikolajewski, J. Frantz, C. Garber, J. Snyder, J. Boles, S. Deslich, L. Enz, R. A. Kuntz, C. Strawser, M. Langenkamp. Used with permission.*

INTERDEPENDENCE ROLE-SELF CONCEPT (cont.)

Occupation:

Social History: (education, special learning needs, religion, hobbies)

Utilization of community resources: ☐ no ☐ home care ☐ hospice ☐ Meals on Wheels ☐ church group ☐ support groups ☐ other _____
Personal Concerns: _____
Do you have any religious special requests? ☐ no ☐ yes _____
Emotional Status: ☐ calm ☐ anxious ☐ angry ☐ quiet ☐ talkative ☐ sad ☐ agitated ☐ other _____
Life changes in past 1-2 years? ☐ none ☐ change in health ☐ new baby ☐ marriage / divorce ☐ death someone close
☐ job / business related change ☐ other _____
Do you feel you deal successfully with stress? ☐ yes ☐ no ☐ depends on circumstance Describe:

NEUROLOGICAL

Mental Status: ☐ alert ☐ oriented ☐ disoriented ☐ restless ☐ drowsy ☐ unresponsive ☐ memory loss
☐ other _____

Speech: ☐ clear ☐ slurred ☐ garbled ☐ aphasic ☐ hoarse ☐ barriers/ foreign language _____

2	3	4	5	6	7	8	9	+ Reactive

− Nonreactive
± Sluggish

Ability to Move Extremities to Command
0 (no movement)   1 (weak)   2 (strong)
RA: LA: RL: LL:

Right Eye: ___ mm   Left Eye: ___ mm

SENSES

Vision Impairment: ☐ no ☐ yes   ☐ glasses / contacts   ☐ artificial eye   ☐ cataracts   ☐ glaucoma ☐ blind ☐ R ☐ L

Hearing Impairment: ☐ no ☐ yes   partial deaf ☐ R ☐ L   total deaf ☐ R ☐ L   hearing aid ☐ R ☐ L

ACTIVITY / REST

Sleep: (Usual time of day and hours) _____
Sleep problems: ☐ none ☐ unrested after sleep ☐ insomnia ☐ nightmares ☐ other _____

SELF-CARE ABILITY (Check appropriate column)

ACTIVITY	0	1	2	3	4	5
Eating / Drinking						
Bathing						
Dressing / Grooming						
Toileting						
Bed mobility						
Transferring						
Ambulating						
Stair Climbing						
Shopping						
Cooking						
Home Maintenance						

0 - Independent
1 - Assistive Device
2 - Assistance from person
3 - Assistance from person & equipment
4 - Dependent/ unable
5 - Change in last week

FALL RISK EVALUATION

Age <3 or >75	10 points
Confused and disoriented, hallucinating, senile	15 points
History of falls	15 points
Recent history of loss of consciousness, seizure disorder	15 points
Unsteady on feet / amputation	10 points
Poor eyesight	5 points
Poor hearing	5 points
Drug / alcohol problem, sedatives	5 points
Postop condition / sedated	5 points
Language barrier	5 points
Attitude (resistant, belligerent, combative, fearful)	10 points
Postural hypotension	5 points
15 or more indicates risk. Fall precautions started:	TOTAL POINTS

Fall Band on ☐

Assistive Devices: ☐ none ☐ crutches ☐ bedside commode ☐ walker ☐ cane ☐ splint / brace ☐ wheelchair ☐ prosthesis
☐ other _____
Activity Tolerance: ☐ no problem ☐ weakness ☐ vertigo ☐ unsteady gait ☐ angina ☐ dyspnea ☐ dyspnea at rest
☐ other _____

Admission Nursing Assessment (page 2)

Figure 15–6. (Continued)

OXYGENATION - SKIN INTEGRITY		
Skin: ☐ Warm ☐ Hot ☐ Cool ☐ Dry ☐ Diaphoretic ☐ Clammy	**Skin Color** ☐ Normal ☐ Pale ☐ Cyanotic ☐ Jaundiced ☐ Mottled ☐ Flushed	

Edema: ☐ none ☐ yes / location: _____

Pedal Pulses: ☐ Present ☐ Abnormal / Explain: _____

Skin Lesions: (mark location of skin lesions by number on diagram)
☐ none ☐ scar (1) ☐ rash (2) ☐ wound or open area (3) ☐ bruise (4) ☐ incision (5) ☐ sutures / staples (6)
☐ abrasions (7) ☐ discolorations (8) ☐ other (9)
Describe _____

Dressings: ☐ no ☐ yes / location: _____

Monitor pattern: ☐ N/A

Respirations: ☐ nonlabored ☐ labored ☐ rapid ☐ shallow

Heart sounds: ☐ audible ☐ abnormal

Cough: ☐ no ☐ yes ☐ non-productive
☐ productive / color: _____

Oxygen: ☐ no ☐ yes - method / amt.: _____

Tobacco Use: ☐ no ☐ yes / type: _____
_____ pkg/day x _____ years

Breath Sounds: ☐ clear ☐ abnormal / describe: _____

RISK PREDICTORS FOR SKIN BREAKDOWN*

BRADEN SCALE

SENSORY PERCEPTION	1. COMPLETELY LIMITED	2. VERY LIMITED	3. SLIGHTLY LIMITED	4. NO IMPAIRMENT
MOISTURE	1. CONSTANTLY MOIST	2. VERY MOIST	3. OCCASIONALLY MOIST	4. RARELY MOIST
ACTIVITY	1. BEDFAST	2. CHAIRFAST	3. WALKS OCCASIONALLY	4. WALKS FREQUENTLY
MOBILITY	1. COMPLETELY IMMOBILE	2. VERY LIMITED	3. SLIGHTLY LIMITED	4. NO LIMITATIONS
NUTRITION	1. VERY POOR	2. PROBABLY INADEQUATE	3. ADEQUATE	4. EXCELLENT
SHEAR & FRICTION	1. PROBLEM	2. POTENTIAL PROBLEM	3. NO APPARENT PROBLEM	

* Refer to Braden Scale for description of each subscale category
Score of 15 or less indicates that patient is a risk. Refer to SKIN CARE DECISION TREE. **TOTAL**

ELIMINATION	
Abdomen ☐ soft ☐ firm ☐ distended / girth _____ ☐ non-distended ☐ tender / location: _____	
Bowel Sounds: ☐ present ☐ absent	**Last BM** / color / character: _____

Bowel Pattern: ☐ diarrhea ☐ constipation ☐ blood in stool ☐ hemorrhoids
☐ no problem ☐ incontinence ☐ laxative / enema Use/List: _____

Bladder Pattern: ☐ burning ☐ nocturia (No. times/night) ☐ difficulty starting flow ☐ frequency
☐ no problem ☐ incontinence - ☐ total ☐ daytime ☐ night time ☐ occasional ☐ urgency ☐ hematuria

Drainage Tubes: ☐ none ☐ indwelling catheter (1) ☐ intermittant catheterization (2) _____ ☐ N/G (3) ☐ G-tube (4)
☐ chest tube (5) ☐ T-tube (6) ☐ penrose (7) ☐ ostomy (8) type: _____
☐ other (9) _____
Describe Drainage: _____

LYTES - NUTRITION			
Current Diet/Restrictions: ☐ Regular	Is diet followed: ☐ yes ☐ no	Last fluid / food intake	**Appetite:** ☐ good ☐ fair ☐ poor

Recent weight change last 6 months: ☐ no ☐ yes / describe: _____

Fluid Intake: ☐ restricted ☐ 0 - 5 glasses / day ☐ 5 - 10 glasses / day ☐ > 10 glasses / day

☐ Caffeine use: Amt. _____ ☐ Alcohol use: Type/Amt. _____

Eating disorders: ☐ none ☐ nausea ☐ emesis ☐ chewing / swallowing difficulty ☐ sore mouth ☐ taste alterations ☐ mouth ulcers
☐ indigestion ☐ ulcer ☐ mouth-white patches ☐ erythema ☐ other

Dentures: ☐ no ☐ yes/ ☐ upper: ☐ full ☐ partial ☐ lower: ☐ full ☐ partial ☐ caps ☐ bridges ☐ loose teeth ☐ retainer ☐ crowns

IV ☐ no ☐ yes - solution - rate - site - cath no.	☐ IML	☐ vascular access device

Admission Nursing Assessment (page 3)

Figure 15–6. (Continued) Braden Scale © *Braden, B. J., & Bergstrom, N. Used with permission.*

ADMISSION NURSING ASSESSMENT

ENDOCRINE	□ N/A	Last Menstrual Period Problems: □ none □ abnormal bleeding □ breast lump history	Breast self-exam done: □ no □ yes
		□ vaginal drainage □ other □ breast feeding	Frequency
		Pap smear requested during hospitalization: □ no □ yes* *See sticker on front of chart	Last Pap Exam:
	□ N/A	Last Rectal Exam Rectal exam requested during hospitalization □ no □ yes* *see sticker on front chart	

Concerns about current or future effects of illness / surgery / treatment on:
□ appearance   □ male / female roles   □ other _____

NOTES: _____

_____

_____

_____

_____

Admission Nursing Assessment (page 4)

Figure 15–6. (Continued)

TABLE 15–3. INDICATIONS OF ADAPTATION DIFFICULTY

Signs of pronounced regulator activity:

1. Increase in heart rate or blood pressure
2. Tension
3. Excitement
4. Loss of appetite
5. Increase in serum cortisol

Signs of cognator ineffectiveness include:

1. Faulty perception and information processing
2. Ineffective learning
3. Poor judgment
4. Inappropriate affect

Source: Adapted from Roy, C., & Andrews, H. A. (eds.). (1999). *The Roy Adaptation Model* (2nd ed., p. 70). Stamford, CT: Appleton & Lange. Used with permission.

care. Behavior that varies from expectations, norms, and guidelines frequently represents ineffective responses. Roy has identified frequently occurring signs of pronounced regulator activity and cognator ineffectiveness (see Table 15–3). The presence of these behaviors also suggests ineffective responses. When ineffective behaviors or adaptive behaviors requiring support are present, the nurse assesses internal and external stimuli that may be affecting behavior. In this phase of assessment, the nurse collects data about the focal, contextual, and residual stimuli challenging the person's coping. For groups, ineffective responses may be indicated by increased stabilizer activity associated with innovator ineffectiveness. For example, the death of the wage earner in a family could result in frenzied housecleaning by the rest of the family in preparation for the return of that member to the house (increased stabilizer activity) along with refusal to arrange the funeral (innovator ineffectiveness). Adaptive responses requiring nursing support include behaviors related to promoting, maintaining, or improving adaptive responses that will not continue to be effective with the occurrence of anticipated future changes. They may also include behaviors that are adaptive but that could be strengthened through education or anticipatory guidance.

The assessment of stimuli uses the same skills as assessment of behavior and clarifies the nature of the focal stimulus; that is, the focal stimulus makes the greatest demand on the human system or provides the most immediate cause of the behavior. In identifying the focal stimulus, it should be remembered that behavior in one mode can serve as a focal stimulus for another mode, and that a given focal stimulus may influence more than one mode. The first priority is given to behaviors that indicate a threat to the integrity of the system (ineffective responses). The nurse identifies significant contextual and residual stimuli. Common influencing stimuli have been identified by Roy and her colleagues and are listed in Table 15–4.

The nurse assesses the *adaptation level* (a pooling of internal stimuli), a significant internal stimulus, to assess *life processes* as integrated, compensated, or compromised. In *The Roy Adaptation Model*, the life processes and indicators of integration, compromise, and compensation are discussed in detail by chapter authors (Roy & Andrews, 1999). Other areas of stimuli to be considered include the acquired coping processes of the cognator and innovator mechanisms and changes in the environment.

TABLE 15–4. COMMON STIMULI AFFECTING ADAPTATION

Culture. Socioeconomic status, ethnicity, belief system.

Family/aggregate participants. Structure and tasks.

Developmental stage. Age, sex, tasks, heredity, genetic factors, longevity of aggregate, vision.

Integrity of adaptive modes. Physiologic (including disease pathology): physical (including basic operating resources); self-concept-group identity; role function; interdependence modes.

Cognator–Innovator effectiveness. Perception, knowledge, skill.

Environmental considerations. Change in internal or external environment; medical management; use of drugs, alcohol, tobacco; political or economic stability.

Source: Roy, C., & Andrews, H. A. (1999). *The Roy Adaptation Model* (2nd ed., p. 72). Stamford, CT: Appleton & Lange. Used with permission.

Nursing Diagnosis

A *nursing diagnosis* is an interpretative statement that represents a judgment that the nurse makes in relation to the adaptation status of the human adaptive system (Roy & Andrews, 1999, p. 77). The method suggested by Roy is stating the observed behavior along with the most influential stimuli. Using this method, a diagnosis for Mr. Smith could be stated as: "Chest pain caused by a deficit of oxygen to the heart muscle associated with an overexposure to hot weather." A nursing diagnosis can also be a statement of adaptive responses that the nurse wishes to support. For example, if Mr. Smith is seeking help through vocational counseling to adapt to his physical limitation, the nurse may diagnose a need to support this behavior. In this case, an appropriate diagnosis would be: "Adaptation to role failure by seeking an alternative career." Roy and others also have developed a typology of indicators of positive adaptation (see Table 15–5). Roy indicates that the NANDA diagnostic categories may be related to adaptation problems and refers to these categories as clinical classifications (Roy & Andrews, 1999) (see Table 15–6).

Goal Setting

The goal of nursing intervention is to maintain and enhance adaptation, and to change ineffective behavior to adaptive behavior. Goal setting involves making clear statements of the desired behavioral outcomes of nursing care. These outcomes will reflect adaptation. Roy suggests that goal statements be in terms of the desired *behavior* of the human system. A complete statement is described as one that includes the *behavior* desired, the *change* expected, and a *time frame* (Roy & Andrews, 1999, p. 85). Goals may be short term or long term relative to the situation.

In the case of Mr. Smith presented in this chapter, the short-term goal would read: Mr. Smith will proceed with daily activities (*behavior*) with no chest pain (*change*) after 30 minutes of rest (*time frame*). The long-term goal statement would read: Mr. Smith will be able to resume work (*behavior*) in a new field (*change*) in six months (*time frame*).

TABLE 15–5. TYPOLOGY OF INDICATORS OF POSITIVE ADAPTATION

Physiologic-Physical Mode

Individuals	Groups
Oxygenation	
Stable processes of ventilation	Adequate fiscal resources
Stable pattern of gas exchange	Member capability
Adequate transport of gases	Availability of physical facilities
Adequate processes of compensation	

Nutrition
Stable digestive processes
Adequate nutritional pattern for body requirements
Metabolic and other nutritive needs met during
   altered means of ingestion

Elimination
Effective homeostatic bowel processes
Stable pattern of bowel elimination
Effective processes of urine formation
Stable pattern of urine elimination
Effective coping strategies for altered elimination

Activity and Rest
Integrated processes of mobility
Adequate recruitment of compensatory
   movement processes during inactivity
Effective pattern of activity and rest
Effective sleep pattern
Effective environmental changes for altered
   sleep conditions

Protection
Intact skin
Effective healing response
Adequate secondary protection for changes
   in integrity and immune status
Effective processes of immunity
Effective temperature regulation

Senses
Effective processes of sensation
Effective integration of sensory input into
   information
Stable patterns of perception, interpretation,
   and appreciation of input
Effective coping strategies for altered sensation

Fluid, Electrolyte, and Acid-Base Balance
Stable processes of water balance
Stability of electrolytes in body fluids
Balance of acid-base system
Effective chemical buffer regulation

Neurologic Function
Effective processes of arousal and attention;
   sensation and perception; coding, concept
   formation, memory, language; planning,
   motor response
Integrated thinking and feeling processes
Plasticity and functional effectiveness of
   developing, aging, and altered nervous system

316

TABLE 15–5. (CONT.)

Physiologic-Physical Mode

Individuals	Groups

Endocrine Function
  Effective hormonal regulation of metabolic
    and body processes
  Effective hormonal regulation of
    reproductive development
  Stable patterns of closed loop negative
    feedback hormone systems
  Effective coping strategies for stress

Self-Concept-Group Identity Mode

Individuals	Groups

Physical Self
  Positive body image
  Effective sexual function
  Psychic integrity with physical growth
  Adequate compensation for bodily changes
  Effective coping strategies for loss
  Effective process of life closure

Personal Self
  Stable pattern of self-consistency
  Effective integration of self-ideal
  Effective processes of moral-ethical-spiritual growth
  Functional self-esteem
  Effective coping strategies for threats to self

Groups column:
  Effective interpersonal relationships
  Supportive culture
  Positive morale
  Group acceptance
  Principle-based relationships
  Value-driven relationships

Role Function Mode for Individuals and Groups

Role clarity
Effective processes of role transition
Integration of instrumental and expressive role behaviors
Integration of primary, secondary, and tertiary roles
Effective pattern of role performance
Effective processes for coping with role changes
Role performance accountability
Effective group role integration
Stable pattern or role mastery

Interdependence Mode for Individuals and Groups

Affectional adequacy
Stable pattern of giving and receiving
Effective pattern of dependency and independency
Effective coping strategies for separation and loneliness
Developmental adequacy
Resource adequacy

Source: Roy, Sr. C., & Andrews, H. A. (1999). *The Roy Adaptation Model* (2nd ed., pp. 79–81). Stamford, CT: Appleton & Lange. Used with permission.

TABLE 15–6. TYPOLOGY OF COMMONLY RECURRING PROBLEMS

Physiologic-Physical Mode

Individuals	Groups
Oxygenation	
Hypoxia	Inadequate fiscal resources
Shock	Capability deficits
Ventilatory impairment	Inadequate physical facilities
Inadequate gas exchange	
Inadequate gas transport	
Altered tissue perfusion	
Poor recruitment of compensatory process for changing oxygen need	
Nutrition	
Weight 20–25% above or below average	
Nutrition more or less than body requirements	
Anorexia	
Nausea and vomiting	
Ineffective coping strategies for altered means of ingestion	
Elimination	
Diarrhea	
Bowel incontinence	
Constipation	
Urinary incontinence	
Urinary retention	
Flatulence	
Ineffective coping strategies for altered elimination	
Activity and Rest	
Immobility	
Activity intolerance	
Inadequate pattern of activity and rest	
Restricted mobility, gait, and/or coordination	
Disuse syndrome	
Sleep deprivation	
Potential for sleep pattern disturbance	
Protection	
Disrupted skin integrity	
Pressure sores	
Itching	
Delayed wound healing	
Infection	
Potential for ineffective coping with allergic reaction	
Ineffective coping with changes in immune status	
Ineffective temperature regulation	
Fever	
Hypothermia	
Senses	
Impairment of a primary sense	
Potential for injury	
Loss of self-care abilities	
Sensory monotony or distortion	
Sensory overload or deprivation	
Potential for distorted communication	
Acute pain	
Chronic pain	
Perceptual impairment	
Ineffective coping strategies for sensory impairment	

TABLE 15–6. (*CONT.*)

Physiologic-Physical Mode

Individuals	Groups

Fluid and Electrolytes
    Dehydration
    Edema
    Intracellular water retention
    Shock
    Hyper- or hypo-calcemia, kalemia, or natremia
    Acid-base imbalance
    Ineffective buffer regulation for changing pH

Neurologic Function
    Decreased level of consciousness
    Defective cognitive processing
    Memory deficits
    Instability of behavior and mood
    Ineffective compensation for cognitive deficit
    Potential for secondary brain damage

Endocrine Function
    Ineffective hormone regulation
    Ineffective reproductive development
    Instability of hormone system loops
    Instability of internal cyclical rhythms
    Stress

Self-Concept-Group Identity Mode

Individuals	Groups
Physical Self	
Body image disturbance	Ineffective interpersonal relationships
Sexual dysfunction	Oppressive culture
Rape trauma syndrome	Low morale
Unresolved loss	Stigma
Personal Self	
Anxiety	Abusive relationships
Powerlessness	Valueless relationships
Guilt	
Low self-esteem	

Role Function Mode for Individuals and Groups

Ineffective role transitions
Prolonged role distance
Role conflict—intrarole and interrole
Role failure
Role ambiguity
Outgroup stereotyping

Interdependent Mode for Individuals and Groups

Ineffective pattern of giving
Ineffective pattern of dependency and independency
Separation anxiety
Loneliness
Ineffective development of relationships
Inadequate resources

Source: Roy, Sr. C., & Andrews, H. A. (1999). *The Roy Adaptation Model* (2nd ed., pp. 82–84). Stamford, CT: Appleton & Lange. Used with permission.

Intervention

Nursing interventions are planned with the purpose of altering stimuli or strengthening adaptive processes. The nurse plans specific activities to alter the selected stimuli appropriately (Roy & Andrews, 1999). Nursing activities manage stimuli by "altering, increasing, decreasing, removing, or maintaining them" as most appropriate to the situation (p. 86). By using these strategies, the nurse adjusts stimuli so that the total stimuli fall within that person's ability to cope. The coping processes of the person are the usual means of adaptation for the human adaptive system. It is when the coping processes are unable to respond effectively that the integrity of the person is compromised.

> Consider Mr. Smith, previously discussed, who has chest pain. The nurse might identify a need for information related to heart disease, a need for low-fat diet information, a need for cooking classes, as well as a need for a program of cardiac rehabilitation exercises to increase cardiac strength and endurance. These plans of care alter the contextual stimuli and assist the patient in reaching the long-term goal of resuming productive work.

Because many alternatives may be available to the nurse to alter the focal and contextual stimuli in any situation, Roy suggests the use of a nursing judgment method developed by McDonald and Harms in 1966. First, relevant stimuli and coping processes are identified. Then, nursing intervention alternatives are considered in terms of the anticipated *consequences* of changing each stimulus, the *probability* of the occurrence of the consequences (high, moderate, or low), and the *value* of the change (desirable or undesirable). The use of this judgment method includes collaboration with the members of the human adaptive system (Roy & Andrews, 1999, p. 87).

> In the case of Mr. Smith, the nurse judges the consequences of taking a cooking class as increasing the likelihood of maintaining a low-fat diet. The probability of success is rated high. This rating is based on a class being available at no cost at a community agency close to the client's home. In addition, the value is seen as desirable. The nurse and Mr. Smith select this intervention strategy along with others for implementation. The implementation requires that the nurse work with the patient, the family, the doctor, and the community agency. On the other hand, the nurse may find that the community does not have such a program to help Mr. Smith. While exploring the alternatives with Mr. Smith, the nurse may also identify a community need to enhance the health of community members. The nurse then works with community agencies and groups, using the nursing judgment method to change this ineffective community response. In either situation, the identified actions must be initiated.

Evaluation

Evaluation occurs to establish the effectiveness of the actions taken. The nurse and the involved individual(s) look collaboratively at the behaviors to see if the behavioral goals have been reached. Goal behaviors are compared to the client's output responses, and movement toward or away from goal achievement is determined. If the goals have not been achieved, the nursing process begins again with additional questions relating to the accuracy and completeness of the assessment data, the match between identified goals and the client system's wishes, and the ways in which interventions were carried out. Readjustments to goals and interventions are made on the basis of evaluation data (Roy & Andrews, 1999).

The Roy Nursing Process Applied to Nursing Practice

Individual Situation. In a recovery room, the RAM can be applied to nursing assessment and interventions in various clinical situations. In the following case study, the Roy model is applied to a person during the period of immediate recovery from surgery and anesthesia.

Assessment of behavior focuses on the physiologic mode responses during the first hour of recovery time after a person experiences surgery and general anesthesia. By applying the RAM, significant behaviors can be conceptualized as regulator output responses. Increased sympathetic or parasympathetic system activity can signal regulator system activity. Regulator output responses that vary from baseline values determined for the person may be the first warning of an ineffective response to postoperative stimuli. Key baseline values are the person's presurgery measures of heart rate, blood pressure, and respiratory rate. Immediately upon observation of changes from the baseline, assessment of stimuli is done. Goals are set with the basic survival of the person as a priority. Interventions are taken so that focal and contextual stimuli are altered and adaptation is promoted. The evaluation of goal achievement is made, and further actions are taken as necessary.

Mrs. Reed is received from surgery after a major abdominal operation. Before surgery, her baseline vital signs were: heart rate, 80 beats per minute; blood pressure, 120/80 mm Hg; and respiratory rate, 16 per minute. After 45 minutes in recovery, her vital signs are: heart rate, 150 beats per minute; blood pressure, 90/60 mm Hg; respiratory rate, 32 per minute. Increased regulator output response is signaled by sympathetic nervous system stimulation of the heart in response to decreased blood pressure. The nurse decides that Mrs. Reed is showing an ineffective response. Therefore, assessment of stimuli is done.

The focal stimulus is a decrease in arterial blood pressure secondary to an unknown underlying cause. The contextual stimuli are: age 45 years, cool extremities, poor nail blanching, no food or drink for 12 hours, and intravenous infusion (IV) of dextrose 5 percent in water with lactated Ringer's solution at 100 cc per hour. Also, contextual stimuli include 200 cc of IV fluids infused during surgery, 10 cc of urine excreted during the first 45 minutes in recovery, 1.5 hours of general anesthesia, estimated blood loss of 500 cc during surgery, no operative site bleeding, and level of consciousness slow to respond to tactile stimuli after 45 minutes in recovery. The residual stimuli include history of renal infections.

The nursing diagnosis of a decreased arterial blood pressure secondary to fluid volume deficit is made. A fluid volume loss is suggested both by the contextual data and by the changes in the baseline heart rate, blood pressure, and urine output. The nurse then intervenes by altering contextual stimuli so that an adaptive response is promoted. The goal of a circulatory volume adequate to maintain a blood pressure of plus or minus 20 mm Hg of baseline levels within 15 minutes is set. The nurse plans and then takes the following intervention steps. The IV rate is increased to 300 cc per hour. The foot of the bed is elevated to increase venous return. Forty-percent oxygen is given by mask. Mrs. Reed is verbally and tactilely stimulated and told to take slow deep breaths. The nurse prepares vasopressor medications for immediate use and applies an external continuous blood pressure cuff for constant blood pressure monitoring. The nurse also consults with other team members as to Mrs. Reed's clinical presentation.

A constant evaluation of the effectiveness of the nursing actions is made. The nurse holds Mrs. Reed in recovery until the goal of adequate circulation volume is met. Evaluation criteria include urine output greater than 30 cc per hour, mental alertness, rapid nail bed blanching, blood pressure plus or minus 20 mm Hg of presurgery levels, pulse plus or minus 20 beats per minute of baseline, and respirations plus or minus 5 per minute of presurgery levels.

Group Situation. A school nurse surveys the members of the tenth grade in her school about personal substance use and finds that 30 percent of the teens are smoking more than two cigarettes a day. The students state that smoking is "cool," gives them a "buzz," is a way to "break away from control by parents," and that the health risk is "almost none." Stimuli are assessed as: lack of positive role modeling in advertisements that present smoking as "cool," lack of adaptive coping by students to control developmental anxieties, lack of involvement by parents in building parent–teen communication, and lack of knowledge related to the health risk of smoking. The nursing diagnoses include: ineffective use of substance to create sense of self-worth and -esteem, ineffective use of substance to control developmental anxieties, ineffective use of substance in separation issues with the family, and inadequate knowledge of health risks of smoking. The nurse sets the following goals: Within three months, the students will state the myths related to the image of smoking created by advertising. Within four months, the tenth grade students will state the health risks of cigarette smoking. Within six months, the rate of cigarette use by tenth graders will decrease by 50 percent. Within one year, students will identify positive coping strategies to deal with developmental anxieties, and parents will increase involvement in teen activities. The nurse creates a core group of concerned teens, parents, and teachers to plan strategies. The team decides to alter stimuli related to lack of positive role modeling in advertising that presents smoking as "cool." Plans include use of posters that show a "different" image of the smoker, and talks by nonsmoking college nursing students about setting life goals and building self-esteem without use of substance. The group members secure resources including funding, space, and scheduling assistance. The team that the nurse has assembled develops many other strategies. One year later, smoking has decreased to 17 percent of the teens.

CRITIQUE OF THE ROY ADAPTATION MODEL

1. What is the historical context of the theory? The Roy Adaptation Model has been a phenomena in nursing since the mid-1960s and continues to grow in use in educational, practice, and research settings. The underlying assumptions are well detailed and have been recently expanded to meet the challenges of nursing in the next millennium. The scientific assumptions initially were drawn from von Bertalanffy's (1968) general system theory, Helson's (1964) view of adaptation as a pooled effect with three categories of stimuli, Davies' (1988) discussion of the ability to self-organize, and Swimme and Berry's (1992) concepts to accept, protect, and foster. Roy has added unity and meaningfulness of the created universe. The philosophical assumptions originated from humanism with emphasis on mutuality with others, the work, and God. Roy considers the place of the human system in creation and the meaning of human existence. She indicates human decisions are accountable for the integration of the creative processes and draws on Fox (1983) and deChardin (1966, 1969) in relation to creation spirituality. Roy states "new knowledge can be developed related to higher levels of complex self-organization; consciousness and meaning; integration of creative processes; common person and earth patterns; diversity and destiny; convergence and transformation of the universe; and human creative abilities of awareness, enlightenment, and faith" (Roy & Andrews, 1999, p. 44). This tremendously potent sentence provides direction for the future of nursing.

2. What are the basic concepts and relationships presented by the theory? The RAM offers a conceptual path to aid in the understanding of human behavior that is of interest to nursing and the identification of interventions that promote the well being of people and society. The concepts are presented in Figure 15–7. The

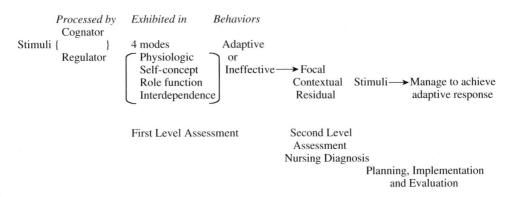

Figure 15–7. Relationship of concepts in the Roy Adaptation Model. *From Julia B. George, California State University, Fullerton, 1997. Used with permission.*

sequence of concepts in the Roy model follows logically. In the presentation of each of the key concepts there is the recurring idea of adaptation to maintain integrity. The definition of health is based on the idea of integrity, which in turn is operationalized to mean responses that meet the person's goals of survival, growth, reproduction, mastery, and person and environment transformations. Promoting adaptive responses is the goal of nursing.

3. What major phenomena of concern to nursing are presented? These phenomena may include *but are not limited to*: **human being, environment, health, interpersonal relations, caring, goal attainment, adaptation, and energy fields.** The Roy Adaptation Model considers the phenomena of individuals and of groups. It concerns itself with the control processes of individual coping, the regulator and cognator mechanisms; and of groups, the stabilizer and innovator coping processes. It concerns itself with the behavioral focus of nursing assessment and develops extensive guidelines for each area of assessment. It suggests a scientific and philosophic perspective for nursing interaction with human systems based on the concepts of wholeness, veritivity, and cosmic openness. It presents adaptation of the human adaptive system as the reflection of health and the concept of wholeness as the system's process of meeting the goals of survival, growth, reproduction, mastery, and person–environment transformation. It concerns itself with the integration of the human system and the universe.

4. To whom does the theory apply? In what situations? In what ways? The Roy Adaptation Model has broad implications for the practice of nursing. The concepts of the model have application for individuals across the life span and for families, groups, and other collective human adaptive systems. No age or situation is particularly outside the scope of the model. Portions of the model may be of greater concern to the nurse at different times. For example, if a child has been hit by an automobile, the physiological integrity is assessed and survival is the most important goal. As priorities shift in a given situation, the model continues to give the practicing nurse direction and guidance. As the nurse cares for the injured child, the nurse begins to care for the family. The group-identity of the family is now affected by having an injured child and the nurse assesses the contextual stimuli related to this change. The model helps the nurse organize and apply the vast body of knowledge of nursing science and related sciences and arts to promote adaptation of individuals and groups.

5. By what method or methods can this theory be tested? While both quantitative and qualitative methods have been used to observe and test the concepts and relationships of the RAM, the preponderance of the studies reviewed were quantitative in nature and many of these were descriptive correlational studies. Areas of study using quantitative methods include *adolescents* (Modrcin-Talbott, Pullen, Ehrenberger, Zandstra, & Muenchen, 1998; Modrcin-Talbott, Pullen, Zandstra, Ehrenberger, & Muenchen, 1998); *arthritis* (Newman, A. M., 1991); *battered women* (Woods, 1997); *cardiac* (Rees, 1995); *caregivers* (Ellison, 1993; Jensen,

1996; Sirapo-Ngam, 1994; Smith, Mayer, Parkhurst, Perkins, & Pingleton, 1991); *childbearing* (Corbett, 1995; Fawcett, Tulman, & Spedden, 1994; Khanobdee, 1994); *children and families* (Bournaki, 1997; Bufe, 1996; Hamid, 1993); *diabetes* (LeMone, 1995; Willoughby, 1995); *gerontology* (Collins, 1992; McGill & Paul, 1993; Murphy, 1993; Ryan, 1996; Taylor, 1997; Zhan, 2000); *grieving* (Robinson, 1995); *gynecology* (Sheppard & Cunnie, 1996); *HIV/AIDS* (Jarczewski, 1995; Orsi, Grandy, Tax, & McCorkle, 1997; Phillips, K. D., 1994; Vicenzi & Thiel, 1992); *nursing administration* (Lutjens, 1994); *nursing home care* (Toye, Percival, & Blackmore, 1996); *occupational health* (Phillips, J. A., 1991); *oncology* (Chen, Ma, Kuo, & Shyr, 1999; Fredrickson, Jackson, Strauman, & Strauman, 1991; Grimes, 1997; Nuamah, Cooley, Fawcett, & McCorkle, 1999; Samarel, & Fawcett, 1992; Samarel, Fawcett, Krippendorf, et al., 1998; Samarel, Fawcett, & Tulman, 1997; Shuler, 1990; Wright, 1993); *pain* (Calvillo & Flaskerud, 1993); *perception of control* (Hamner, 1996); *psychosocial determinants of adaptation* (Ducharme, Ricard, Duquette, Levesque, & Lachance, 1998; Levesque, Ricard, Ducharme, Duquette, & Bonin, 1998); *spousal presence* (Baker, 1993); *theory-based practice* (Tolson & McIntosh, 1996); *theory development* (Burns, 1997; Ciambelli, 1996); *tool development* (Burgess & Fawcett, 1996; Modrcin-McCarthy, McCue, & Walker, 1997; Newman, D. M. L., 1997a); *urinary incontinence* (Gallagher, 1998; Johnson, 1997). Qualitative methods have been used in the study of *adolescents* (McLeod-Fletcher, 1996); *gerontology* (Lee & Ellenbecker, 1998); *multiple sclerosis* (Fawcett, Sidney, Riley-Lawless, & Hanson, 1996); *neonatal intensive care units* (Nyqvist & Sjoden, 1993; Raeside, 1997, 2000); *oncology* (Phuphaibul & Muensa, 1999); *parenting* (Niska, 1999; Niska, Lia-Hoagberg, & Snyder, 1997; Niska, Snyder, & Lia-Hoagberg, 1999); *practice framework* (Weiss, Hastings, Holly, & Craig, 1994); *pregnancy* (Martin, 1995; Reichert, Baron, & Fawcett, 1993); and *urinary incontinence* (Patterson, 1995).

The BBARNS study reported by Pollock, et al., (1994) provides an example of research findings reported in the literature. Pollock et al., presented a synthesis of findings across selected studies that used Roy's model. Commonalities between studies existed in the conceptualization of input stimuli with focal and contextual stimuli as subcategories. The studies analyzed were by Carson, 1991; Fredrickson, Jackson, Strauman, & Strauman, 1991; Massey, 1990; Pollock, 1993; and Roy & Andrews, 1991. The focal stimulus was viewed as health-related stressors defined as either an actual or potential health problem. The focal stimuli were operationalized in three studies as having lived with a specific health problem for a designated time. In one study the focal stimulus was a physiologic stressor in healthy adults.

Pollock et al. (1994) found that all investigators conceptualized contextual stimuli to include general social and demographic characteristics such as age, gender, marital status, and social status. Other contextual stimuli identified by investigators included "health-related hardiness" (Pollock, et al., 1994, p. 366) and anxiety-level (Carson, 1991). Instruments used by investigators to measure contextual stimuli included the Health-Related Hardiness Scale (Pollock & Duffy, 1990) and the State-Trait Anxiety Inventory (Spielberger, Gorsuch, Lushen, Vagg, & Jacobs, 1983).

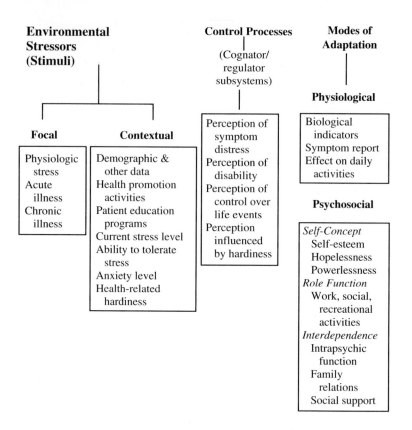

Figure 15–8. Classification of study variables according to the Roy Adaptation Model. From Pollock, S. E., Frederickson, K., Carson, M. A., Massey, V. H., & Roy, C. (1994). *Contributions to nursing science: Synthesis of findings from adaptation model research.* Scholarly Inquiry for Nursing Practice, 8, *365. Used by permission of Springer Publishing Company, Inc., New York 10012.*

Figure 15–8 is a classification of study variables according to the Roy Adaptation Model as developed by Pollack et al.

Because Roy presents her work as a model, subtheorizing is present when application of the model is made for predictive understanding in a clinical situation. The model must be able to clearly identify the connecting relationships between underlying theories. Testable hypotheses are thus generated. Hill and Roberts (1981) discuss "relevant theory derivations" in their study of nursing interventions to promote the health of children with birth defects who are in need of habilitation. Developmental and social learning concepts related to the Roy premises and hypotheses for testing are proposed (see Table 15–7). Multiple examples of hypotheses for testing are generated by Roy and Roberts (1981). Because the model is an umbrella that can link theories, its contributions in the future to the body of nursing knowledge may be considerable.

TABLE 15–7. RELEVANT THEORY DERIVATIONS

Roy's Premises	Developmental Unit–Child Habilitation	Social Learning Unit—Maternal Locus of Control
Man is an adaptive being.	Habilitation is an adaptation problem.	Generalized expectancy of control is directional towards internality or externality.
If man is an adaptive being, he has an adaptation level. The adaptation level is a function of the interaction between adaptation mechanisms and the environment.	The greater the adaptation level, the greater the habilitation level. The habilitation level is a function of the interaction between adaptation mechanisms and the environment	
	The greater the deficits in habilitation, the greater the impairment of adaptation level.	
	The greater the impairment of adaptation level, the greater the impairment of activities of daily living.	
	The greater the impairment of adaptation level, the greater the significance of the environment.	A significant stimulus in a child's environment is the mother.
		The greater the maternal internal locus of control, the greater the parenting patterns fostering independence of a child.
		The greater the maternal external locus of control, the less the parenting patterns fostering the independence of a child.
Nursing intervention is directed towards manipulation of the environment.	The less the habilitation level of the child, the greater the need for nursing intervention.	The less the parenting patterns fostering independence of a child, the less the habilitation level of the child.

Source: Roy, C., & Roberts, S. L. (1981). *Theory construction in nursing: An adaptation model* (pp. 36–37). Upper Saddle River, NJ: Prentice Hall. Used with permission.

6. Does this theory direct critical thinking in nursing practice? The Roy model describes a systematic approach to nursing care. Critical thinking skills are required for success in each of the steps of the RAM nursing process. Assessment of behavior and of stimuli requires the organized collection, synthesis, and analysis of data. Decisions must be made to establish priorities. Nursing diagnoses are identified using the critical thinking skills involved in decision making. Planning includes the use of perception, inference, and short- and long-range projections to establish goals and select appropriate actions. Nursing interventions are carried out while continuing to collect assessment data—what are the behavioral responses to the altering of stimuli? Evaluation requires the use of all the previously employed critical thinking skills as each of the aspects of assessment, diagnosis, goal setting, and intervention are reviewed and decisions made about their adequacy and accuracy.

7. Does this theory direct therapeutic nursing interventions? Perhaps the most important question that one can consider is the usefulness of the RAM in directing therapeutic nursing interventions. The model suggests that nurses alter, increase, decrease, remove, or maintain the focal stimulus or, if that is not possible, manage the contextual stimuli to promote adaptation. The search for nursing knowledge lies in greater understanding of the relative impact of contextual stimuli and the coping mechanisms in human adaptive systems. For example, should the nurse *teach* (contextual stimuli being lack of information) teens about the physiologic risks of smoking or guide a group discussion on the *perception* (cognator coping mechanism) advertisers create to make smoking look "cool"?

Pollock, et al. (1994) together formed the society known as the Boston-Based Adaptation Research in Nursing Society (BBARNS). Among other purposes, BBARNS proposes the advancement of nursing practice by developing nursing knowledge based on the RAM. Pollack et al. presented a set of middle-range theo-

TABLE 15–8. MIDDLE-RANGE THEORIES DERIVED FROM QUALITATIVE SYNTHESIS OF RESEARCH BASED ON ROY ADAPTATION MODEL (RAM)

Component of RAM	Middle-Range Theories
Focal Stimuli	1. In both healthy adults and those with health problems, actual physiological status and functioning in psychosocial areas such as interpersonal relationships and attitudes about self are not related. 2. In adults with health problems, severity of physical illness and functioning in psychosocial areas such as interpersonal relationships and attitudes about self are not related.
Contextual Stimuli	1. In healthy adults and those with health problems, current stress level and anxiety level and functioning in psychosocial areas such as interpersonal relationships and attitudes about self are not related. 2. In adults with chronic illnesses, presence of health-related hardiness and involvement in health promotion exercises positively affects functioning in psychosocial areas such as interpersonal relationships and attitudes about self.
Control Processes	1. In adults with chronic illnesses, perception of disability is related to functioning in psychosocial areas such as work, family relation, and self-esteem. 2. In healthy adults and adults with health problems, perception of physical status, disability, or well being are not related to actual physical status.
Adaptive Modes	1. In adults with chronic illnesses, actual physiological status and functioning in psychosocial areas such as work, family relations, and self-esteem are not related.

Source: Pollock S. E., Frederickson K., Carson M. A., Massey, V. H., & Roy, C. (1994). Contributions to nursing science: Synthesis of findings from Adaptation Model Research. *Scholarly Inquiry for Nursing Practice 8*(4), 361–374. Used by permission of Springer Publishing Company, Inc. New York 10012.

ries derived from the qualitative synthesis of selected studies using the RAM. The interventions that flow from the middle-range theory are identified in Table 15–8. The authors strongly insist that repeated testing should be done before implementation in practice is instituted.

8. Does this theory direct communication in nursing practice? The RAM does direct communication in nursing practice. The nurse may be able to identify a focal stimulus strictly though observation, but verification of the impact of stimuli to move them from residual to contextual requires communication. In addition, much of the content of the psychosocial modes requires communication. Also, communication is needed to establish goals that are acceptable to the patient and to implement effective management of stimuli to support goal attainment. While the RAM calls for and relies on communication, it does not specify the manner in which that communication should occur.

9. Does this theory direct nursing actions that lead to favorable outcomes? The model sets the goal of promoting adaptation for human adaptive systems—a favorable outcome. Consider again the philosophical assumptions for the twenty-first century (Table 15–2). When the nurse promotes survival, growth, reproduction, mastery, and person and environment transformation, the well being of the individual and the society of which he or she is a member is enhanced. The role of the person in creating and driving his or her life decisions is strongly respected.

10. How contagious in this theory? In the process of teaching, the Roy model has been used to organize curriculum by the faculty at Mount Saint Mary's College in Los Angeles. Similarly, extensive use of the model, as well as pictorial representations of it, has been made by the faculty and students of the Royal Alexandra Hospital's School of Nursing (Andrews & Roy, 1986).

Few can fail to be excited by the explosive use of the Roy Adaptation Model in clinical practice, nursing administration, nursing education, and scholarly research. In addition to widespread use in the United States in practice, administration, research, and education (Curl, Hoehn, & Theile, 1988; De Villers, 1998; Dixon, 1999; Dunn & Dunn, 1997; Duquette, 1997; Frederickson, 2000; Frederickson, Williams, et al., 1997; Gless, 1995; Harding-Okimoto, 1997; Haunt, Peddicord, & O'Brien, 1994; Hennessey-Harstad, 1999; Higgins, 1996; Janelli, Kanski, Jones, & Kennedy, 1995; Keen, et al., 1998; Lutjens, 1992; Morales-Mann & Logan, 1990; Morgan, 1997; Newman, D.M.L., 1997b; Samarel, Fawcett, Tulman, Rothman, et al., 1999), publications support the use of the RAM in research in Australia, Indonesia, Taiwan, and Thailand (Chen, et al., 1999; Hamid, 1993; Khanobdee, 1994; Phuphaibul & Muensa, 1999; Toye, et al., 1996); in practice, research, and education in Canada (de Montigny, 1995; Ducharme, et al., 1998; Laschinger & Duffy, 1991; Levesque, et al., 1998; Morales-Mann & Logan, 1990; Thelot & Guimond-Papai, 2000); in education in India (Kurian, 1992); in practice in Pakistan (Zindani, 1996); and in practice and research in the Untied Kingdom and Sweden (Cook, 1999; Dawson, 1998; Ingram, 1995; Lankester & Sheldon, 1999; Nyqvist & Karlsson, 1997; Nyqvist & Sjoden, 1993; Raeside, 1997, 2000; Tolson & McIntosh, 1996).

STRENGTHS AND WEAKNESSES OF THE ROY ADAPTATION MODEL

The RAM offers a variety of strengths for all areas of nursing. First, is the focus on, and inclusion of, the whole person or group. The four modes provide an opportunity for consideration of multiple aspects of the human adaptive system and support gaining an understanding of the whole system. The importance of the spiritual aspects of the human adaptive system, often omitted from nursing assessment, is included in a manner that allows for incorporation of spirituality without imposition of the nurse's beliefs. It is evident from the amount of research using the RAM reported in the literature, and through the formation of BBARNS, that research is supported. Due to this research connection, the RAM is evolving rather than static. It is logically organized and draws on the nurse's observational and interviewing skills.

Weaknesses have been identified in relation to research and to practice. One is the need for consistent definitions of the concepts and terms within the RAM, as well as for more research based on such consistent definitions. Also, in a practice arena that is increasingly challenged with time constraints, the amount of time required to fully implement the two areas of RAM assessment may be viewed as insurmountable. This is particularly true as one begins to use the RAM; a nurse more experienced in the use of the RAM may find the time constraints less compelling.

SUMMARY

The Roy Adaptation Model identifies the essential concepts relevant to nursing as the human adaptive system, the environment, health, and nursing. The human adaptive system is viewed as constantly interacting with internal and external environmental stimuli. The human adaptive system is active and reactive to these stimuli. Stimuli are defined as focal, contextual, and residual. The *focal stimulus* is that most immediately confronting the human system and demanding the greatest awareness or consciousness of the system. *Contextual stimuli* are internal and/or external factors that can be identified as having a positive or negative effect. *Residual stimuli* are those factors in the internal or external environment whose affect on the present situation is not known. The model suggest that nurses seek to identify influencing stimuli and intervention strategies center around the changing stimuli or strengthening adaptive responses. For example, if the contextual stimulus of *lack of transportation to prenatal care* is identified by the nurse through community assessment, then community-based strategies to address the concern can be developed. The internal coping processes of regulator and cognator for the individual and stabilizer and innovation for collective human adaptive systems are phenomena of concern to nursing. Support of coping processes may be the focus of nursing intervention. The four adaptive modes—physiological-physical, self-concept-group identity, role function, and interdependence—are areas for *behavioral* assessment. The four adaptive modes may be the first aspect of the model that the student or nurse is able to assimilate. Based on nursing tradition, assessment of behavior related to fluid and electrolytes, elimination, oxygenation, self-concept, role, and such evoke familiar images. Roy and colleagues offer extensive direction to behavioral assessment in *The Roy Adaptation Model* (Roy & Andrews, 1999). By observing behavior in relation to the adaptive modes, the nurse can identify adaptive or ineffective responses in life situations. *Nursing diagnoses* are judgments that the nurse makes in relation to the adaptation status of the human adaptive system. The goal of nursing is to promote adaptation in each of the adaptive modes. The nurse changes stimuli or strengthens adaptive responses to promote the integrity of wholeness in the human adaptive system. The model suggest that nurses alter, increase, decrease, remove, or maintain the focal stimulus or, if that is not possible, change the contextual stimuli so that adaptation is promoted. Health is defined as being or becoming an integrated whole person (Roy & Andrews, 1999).

REFERENCES

Andrews, H. A., & Roy, C. (1986). *Essentials of the Roy Adaptation Model.* Norwalk, CT: Appleton-Century-Crofts.

Baker, A. C. (1993). The spouse's positive effect on the stroke patient's recovery. *Rehabilitation Nursing, 18*(1), 30–33, 67–68.

Bournaki, M. (1997). Correlates of pain-related responses to venipunctures in school-age children. *Nursing Research, 46,* 147–154.

Bufe, G. M. (1996). *A study of opinions of children about mental illness and associated predictor variables.* (On-line) Dissertation abstract from: CINAHL Accession No: 2000006208.

Burgess, A. W., & Fawcett, J. (1996). The Comprehensive Sexual Assault Assessment Tool. *Nurse Practitioner: American Journal of Primary Health Care, 21*(4), 66, 71–72, 74–76.

Burns, D. P. (1997). *Coping with hemodialysis: A mid-range theory deduced from the Roy Adaptation Model.* (On-line) Dissertation abstract from: CINAHL Accession No: 2000013715.

Calvillo, E. R., & Flaskerud, J. H. (1993). The adequacy and scope of Roy's Adaptation Model to guide cross-cultural pain research. *Nursing Science Quarterly, 6,* 118–129.

Carson, M. A. (1991). *The effect of discrete muscle activity on stress response.* Doctoral dissertation, Boston College School of Nursing. University Microfilm, Inc.

Chen, H., Ma, F., Kuo, B., & Shyr, Y. (1999). Physical and psychological adjustment in women with mastectomy: Based on Roy's Adaptation Model [Chinese]. *Nursing Research (China), 7,* 321–332.

Cho, J. (1998). *Nursing manual: Assessment tool according to Roy Adaptation Model.* Glendale, CA: Polaris.

Ciambelli, M. M. (1996). *Adaptation in marital partners with fertility problems: Testing a midrange theory derived from Roy's Adaptation Model.* (On-line) Dissertation abstract from: CINAHL Accession NO: 2000006126.

Collins, J. M. (1992). *Functional health, social support, and morale of older women living alone in Appalachia.* (On-line) Dissertation abstract from: CINAHL Accession No: 1994089996.

Cook, N. F. (1999). Clinical. Self-concept and cancer: Understanding the nursing role. *British Journal of Nursing, 8,* 318–324.

Corbett, R. W. (1995). *The relationship among trace elements, pica, social support and infant birthweight.* (On-line) Dissertation abstract from: CINAHL Accession No. 1999006484.

Curl, L., Hoehn, J., & Theile, J. R. (1988). Computer applications in nursing: A new course in the curriculum. *Computers in Nursing, 6,* 263–268.

Davies, P. (1988). *The cosmic blueprint*. New York: Simon and Schuster.

Dawson, S. (1998). Adult/elderly care nursing. Pre-amputation assessment using Roy's Adaptation Model. *British Journal of Nursing 7*, 536, 538–542.

deChardin, P. T. (1966). *Man's place in nature*. New York: Harper & Row.

deChardin, P. T. (1969). *Human energy*. New York: Harcourt Brace Jovanovich.

de Montigny, R. (1995). Family nursing interventions during hospitalization [French]. *Canadian Nurse, 91*(10), 38–42.

De Villers, M. J. (1998). The clinical nurse specialist as expert practitioner in the obstetrical/gynecological setting. *Clinical Nurse Specialist, 12*(5), 193–199.

Dixon, E. L. (1999). Community health nursing practice and the Roy Adaptation Model. *Public Health Nursing, 16*, 290–300.

Ducharme, F., Ricard, N., Duquette, A., Levesque, L., & Lachance, L. (1998). Empirical testing of a longitudinal model derived from the Roy Adaptation Model. *Nursing Science Quarterly, 11*, 149–159.

Dunn, H. C., & Dunn, D. G. (1977). The Roy Adaptation Model and its application to clinical nursing practice. *Journal of Ophthalmic Nursing & Technology, 16*, 74–78.

Dunn, H. L. (1971). *High level wellness*. Arlington, VA: Beatty.

Duquette, A. M. (1997). Adaptation: A concept analysis. *Journal of School Nursing, 13*(3), 30–33.

Ellison, K. J. (1993). *Focal and contextual stimuli influencing caregiving in spouses of older adults with diabetes*. (On-line) Dissertation abstract from: CINAHL Accession No: 1998018590.

Fawcett, J., Sidney, J. S., Riley-Lawless, K., & Hanson, M. J. S. (1996). An exploratory study of the relationship between alternative therapies, functional status, and symptom severity among people with multiple sclerosis. *Journal of Holistic Nursing, 14*, 115–129.

Fawcett, J., Tulman, L., & Spedden, J. P. (1994). Responses to vaginal birth after cesarean section. *JOGNN: Journal of Obstetric, Gynecologic, and Neonatal Nursing, 23*(3), 253–259.

Fox, M. (1983). *Original blessing: A primer in creation spirituality*. Santa Fe: Bear & Co.

Fredrickson, K. (2000). Research issues. Nursing knowledge development through research: Using the Roy Adaptation Model. *Nursing Science Quarterly, 13*, 12–17.

Fredrickson, K., Jackson, B. S., Strauman, T., & Strauman, J. (1991). Testing hypotheses derived from the Roy Adaptation Model. *Nursing Science Quarterly, 4*, 168–174.

Frederickson, K., Williams, J. K., Mitchell, G. J., Bernardo, A., Bournes, D., & Smith M. C. (1997). Nursing theory—guided practice. *Nursing Science Quarterly, 10*, 53–58.

Gallagher, M. S. (1998). Urogenital distress and the psychosocial impact of urinary incontinence on elderly women . . . including commentary by Baggerly, J. *Rehabilitation Nursing, 23*(4), 192–197.

Gless, P. A. (1995). Applying the Roy Adaptation Model to the care of clients with quadriplegia. *Rehabilitation Nursing 20*(1), 11–16.

Grimes, C. E. (1997). *The relationship of daily hassles, life change events, and pain to hopelessness in the ambulatory cancer patient*. (On-line) Dissertation abstract from: CINAHL Accession No: 2000013802.

Guyton, A. C. (1971). *Basic human physiology: Normal function and mechanisms of disease*. Philadelphia: Saunders.

Hamid, A.Y.S. (1993). *Child-family characteristics and coping patterns of Indonesian families with a mentally retarded child*. (On-line) Dissertation abstract from: CINAHL Accession No: 1996002845.

Hamner, J. B. (1996). Preliminary testing of a proposition from the Roy Adaption [sic] Model. *Image: Journal of Nursing Scholarship, 28*, 215–220.

Harding-Okimoto, M. B. (1997). Pressure ulcers, self-concept and body image in spinal cord injury patients. *SCI Nursing, 14*(4), 111–117.

Haunt, C., Peddicord, K., & O'Brien, E. (1994). Supporting parental bonding in the NICU: A care plan for nurses. *Neonatal Network: Journal of Neonatal Nursing, 13*(8), 19–25.

Helson, H. (1964). *Adaptation level theory.* New York: Harper & Row.

Hennessey-Harstad, E. B. (1999). Empowering adolescents with asthma to take control through adaptation. *Jorunal of Pediatric Health, 13,* 273–277.

Higgins, K.M. (1996). *The entrepreneurial nurse-midwife: A profile of successful business practice.* (On-line) Dissertation abstract from: CINAHL Accession No: 2000013738.

Hill, B. J., & Roberts, C. S. (1981). Formal theory construction: An-example of the process. In C. Roy & S. L. Roberts, *Theory construction in nursing: An adaptation model* (pp. 30–39). Upper Saddle River, NJ: Prentice-Hall.

Ingram, L. (1995). Roy's Adaptation Model and accident and emergency nursing. *Accident and Emergency Nursing, 3*(3), 150–153.

Janelli, L. M., Kanski, G. W., Jones, H. M., & Kennedy, M. C. (1995). Exploring music intervention with restrained patients. *Nursing Forum, 30*(4), 12–18.

Jarczewski, P.A.H. (1995). *Social support, self-esteem, symptom distress, and anxiety of adults with acquired immune deficiency syndrome.* (On-line) Dissertation abstract from: CINAHL Accession No: 1998079907.

Jensen, K. A. (1996). *Stress and coping of caregivers to individuals with dementia.* (On-line) Dissertation abstract from: CINAHL Accession No: 1999064041.

Johnson, V. Y. (1997). *Effects of a submaximal exercise protocol to recondition the circumvaginal musculature in women with genuine stress urinary incontinence.* (On-line) Dissertation abstract from: CINAHL Accession No: 2000013731.

Keen, M., Breckenridge, D., Frauman, A. C., Hartigan, M. F., Smith, L., Butera, E., Hooper, S. T., Mapes, D., Neff, M., & Fawcett, J. (1998). Nursing assessment and intervention for adult hemodialysis patients: Application of Roy's Adaptation Model. *ANNA Journal, 25,* 311–319.

Khanobdee, C. (1994). *Hope and social support of Thai women experiencing a miscarriage.* (On-line) Dissertation abstract from: CINAHL Accession No: 1998051367.

Kurian, A. (1992). Effective teaching and its application in nursing: Problem solving method of teaching in nursing. *Nursing Journal of India, 83,* 251–254.

Lankester, K., & Sheldon, L. M. (1999). Health visiting with Roy's model: A case study. *Journal of Child Health Care, 3*(1), 28–34.

Laschinger, H. K., & Duffy, V. (1991). Attitudes of practicing nurses toward theory-based nursing practice. *Canadian Journal of Nursing Administration, 4*(1), 6–10.

Lee, A. A., & Ellenbecker, C. H. (1998). The perceived life stressors among elderly Chinese immigrants: Are they different from those of other elderly Americans? *Clinical Excellence for Nurse Practitioners, 2*(2), 96–101.

LeMone, P. (1995). Assessing psychosexual concerns in adults with diabetes: Pilot project using Roy's modes of adaptation. *Issues in Mental Health Nursing, 16*(1), 67–78.

Levesque, L., Ricard, N., Ducharme, F., Duquette, A., & Bonin, J. (1998). Empirial verification of a theoretical model derived from the Roy Adaptation Model: Findings from five studies. *Nursing Science Quarterly, 11,* 31–39.

Lutjens, L. R. J. (1992). Derivation and testing of tenets of a theory of social organizations as adaptive systems. *Nursing Science Quarterly, 5,* 62–71.

Lutjens, L. R. J. (1994). Hospital payment source and length-of-stay. *Nursing Science Quarterly, 7,* 174–179.

Martin, B. P. (1995). *An analysis of common postpartum problems and adaptation strategies used by women during the first two to eight weeks following delivery of a full-term healthy newborn.* (On-line) Dissertation abstract from: CINAHL Accession No: 1999014948.

Massey, V. H. (1990). *Psychosocial adaptation in acute and chronic health problems during hospitalizations.* Unpublished manuscript.

McGill, J. S., & Paul, P. B. (1993). Functional status and hope in elderly people with and without cancer. *Oncology Nursing Forum, 20,* 1207–1213.

McLeod-Fletcher, C. (1996). *Appraisal and coping with vaso-occlusive crisis in adolescents with sickle cell disease.* (On-line) Dissertation abstract from: CINAHL Accession No: 1999084234.

Modrcin-McCarthy, M. A., McCue, S., & Walker, J. (1997). Preterm infants and STRESS: A tool for the neonatal nurse. *Journal of Perinatal and Neonatal Nursing, 10*(4), 62–71.

Modrcin-Talbott, M. A., Pullen, L., Ehrenberger, H., Zandstra, K., & Muenchen, B. (1998). Self-esteem in adolescents treated in an outpatient mental health setting. *Issues in Comprehensive Pediatric Nursing, 21*, 159–171.

Modrcin-Talbott, M. A., Pullen, L., Zandstra, K., Ehrenberger, H., & Muenchen, B. (1998). A study of self-esteem among well adolescents: Seeking a new direction. *Issues in Comprehensive Pediatric Nursing, 21*, 229–241.

Morales-Mann, E. T., & Logan, M. (1990). Implementing the Roy model: Challenges for nurse educators. *Journal of Advanced Nursing, 15*, 142–147.

Morgan, M. G. (1997). The Roy Adaptation Theory and multicultural nursing. *Journal of Multicultural Nursing & Health, 3*(3), 10–14.

Murphy, K. P. (1993). *Relationships between biopsychosocial characteristics and adaptive health patterns in elder women.* (On-line) Dissertation abstract from: CINAHL Accession No: 1998038215.

Newman, A. M. (1991). *The effect of the arthritis self-help course on arthritis self-efficacy, perceived social support, purpose and meaning in life, an arthritis impact in people with arthritis.* (On-line) Dissertation abstract from: CINAHL Accession No: 1993157036.

Newman, D. M. L. (1997a). The Inventory of Functional Status—Caregiver of a Child in a Body Cast. *Journal of Pediatric Nursing: Nursing Care of Children and Families, 12*(3), 142–147.

Newman, D. M. L. (1997b). Responses to caregiving: A reconceptualization using the Roy Adaptation Model. *Holistic Nursing Practice, 12*(1), 80–88.

Niska, K. J. (1999). Family nursing interventions: Mexican American early family formation . . . third part of a three-part study. *Nursing Science Quarterly, 12*, 335–340.

Niska, K. J., Lia-Hoagberg, B., & Snyder, M. (1997). Parental concerns of Mexican American first-time mothers and fathers. *Public Health Nursing, 14*, 111–117.

Niska, K. J., Snyder, M., & Lia-Hoagberg, B. (1999). The meaning of family health among Mexican American first-time mothers and fathers. *Journal of Family Nursing, 5*, 218–233.

Nuamah, I. F., Cooley, M. E., Fawcett, J., & McCorkle, R. (1999). Testing a theory for health-related quality of life in cancer patients: A structural equation approach. *Research in Nursing & Health, 22*, 231–242.

Nyqvist, K. H., & Karlsson, K. H. (1997). A philosophy of care for a neonatal intensive care unit: Operationalization of a nursing model. *Scandinavian Journal of Caring Sciences*, 11(2), 91–96.

Nyqvist, K. H., & Sjoden, P. (1993). Advice concerning breastfeeding from mothers of infants admitted to a neonatal intensive care unit: The Roy Adaptation Model as a conceptual structure. *Jouranl of Advanced Nursing, 8*(1), 54–63.

Orsi, A. J., Grandy, C., Tax, A., & McCorkle, R. (1997). Nutritional adaptation of women living with HIV: A pilot study. *Holistic Nursing Practice, 12*(1), 71–79.

Patterson, J. E. (1995). *Responses of institutionalized older adults to urinary incontinence: Managing the flow.* (On-line) Dissertation abstract from: CINAHL Accession No: 1999006488.

Phillips, J. A. (1991). *Adaptation and injury status of industrial workers on a rotating shift pattern.* (On-line) Dissertation abstract from: CINAHL Accession No: 1993152180.

Phillips, K. D. (1994). *Testing biobehavioral adaptation in persons living with AIDS using Roy's theory of the person as an adaptive system.* (On-line) Dissertation abstract from: CINAHL Accession No: 1998065077.

Phuphaibul, R., & Muensa, W. (1999). International pediatric nursing. Negative and positive adaptive behaviors of Thai school-aged children who have a sibling with cancer. *Journal of Pediatric Nursing: Nursing Care of Children and Families, 14*, 342–348.

Pollock, S. E. (1993). Adaptation to chronic illness: A program of research for testing nursing theory. *Nursing Science Quarterly, 6,* 86–92.

Pollock, S. E., & Duffy, M. E. (1990). The health-related hardiness scale: Development and psychometric evaluation. *Nursing Research, 39,* 218–222.

Pollock, S. E., Frederickson, K., Carson, M. A., Massey, V. H., & Roy C. (1994). Contributions to nursing science: Synthesis of findings from adaptation model research. *Scholarly Inquiry for Nursing Practice, 8,* 361–374.

Raeside, L. (1997). Clinical. Perceptions of environmental stressors in the neonatal unit. *British Journal of Nursing, 6,* 914–916.

Raeside, L. (2000). Caring for dying babies: Perceptions of neonatal nurses. *Journal of Neonatal Nursing, 6*(3), 93–99.

Rees, B. S. (1995). *Influences of coronary artery disease knowledge, anxiety, social support, and self-efficacy on adaptive health behaviors of patients treated with a percutaneous transluminal coronary angioplasty.* (On-line) Dissertation abstract from: CINAHL Accession No: 1999015007.

Reichert, J.A., Baron, M., & Fawcett, J. (1993). Changes in attitudes toward cesarean birth. *JOGNN: Journal of Obstetric, Gynecologic, and Neonatal Nursing, 22,* 159–167.

Robinson, J. H. (1995). Grief responses, coping processes, and social support of widows: Research with Roy's model. *Nursing Science Quarterly, 8,* 158–164.

Roy, C. (1970). Adaptation: A conceptual framework for nursing. *Nursing Outlook, 18,* 43–45.

Roy, C. (1976). *Introduction to nursing: An adaptation model.* Upper Saddle River, NJ: Prentice Hall. (out of print)

Roy, C. (1984). *Introduction to nursing: An adaptation model* (2nd ed.). Upper Saddle River, NJ: Prentice Hall. (out of print)

Roy, C. (1988). An explication of the philosophical assumptions of the Roy Adaptation Model. *Nursing Science Quarterly, 1,* 26–24.

Roy, Sr. C. (1997a). Future of the Roy model: Challenge to redefine adaptation. *Nursing Science Quarterly, 10,* 42–48.

Roy, Sr. C. (1997b). Knowledge as universal cosmic imperative. *Proceedings of Nursing Knowledge Impact Conference 1996* (pp. 95–118). Chestnut Hill: BC Press.

Roy, C., & Andrews, H. A. (1991). *The Roy Adaptation Model: The definitive statement.* Norwalk, CT: Appleton & Lange.

Roy, Sr. C., & Andrews, H. A. (1999).*The Roy Adaptation Model* (2nd ed.). Stamford, CT: Appleton & Lange.

Roy, Sr. C., & Anway, J. (1989). Roy's Adaptation Model: Theories and propositions for administration. In Henry, B., Arndt, C., DeVincenti, M., & Marriner-Tomey, A. (Eds.), *Dimensions and issues of nursing administration.* St. Louis: Mosby.

Roy, C., & Roberts, S. (1981). *Theory construction in nursing: An adaptation model.* Upper Saddle River, NJ: Prentice Hall.

Ryan, M. C. (1996). Loneliness, social support and depression as interactive variables with cognitive status: Testing Roy's model. *Nursing Science Quarterly, 9,* 107–114.

Samarel, N., & Fawcett, J. (1992). Enhancing adaptation to breast cancer: The addition of coaching to support groups. *Oncology Nursing Forum, 19,* 591–596.

Samarel, N., Fawcett, J., Krippendorf, K., Piacentino, J. C., Eliasof, B., Hughes, P., Kowitski, C., & Ziegler, E. (1998). Women's perceptions of group support and adaptation to breast cancer. *Journal of Advanced Nursing, 28,* 1259–1268.

Samarel, N., Fawcett, J., & Tulman, L. (1997). Effect of support groups with coaching on adaptation to early stage breast cancer. *Research in Nursing and Health, 20*(1), 15–26.

Samarel, N., Fawcett, J., Tulman, L., Rothman, H., Spector, L., Spillane, P. A., Dickson, M. A., & Toole, J. H. (1999). Patient education: A resource kit for women with breast cancer: Development and evaluation. *Oncology Nursing Forum, 26,* 611–618.

Sheppard, V. A., & Cunnie, K. L. (1996). Incidence of diuresis following hysterectomy. *Journal of Post Anesthesia Nursing, 11*(1), 20–28.

Shuler, P. J. (1990). *Physical and psychosocial adaptation, social isolation, loneliness, and self-concept of individuals with cancer.* (On-line) Dissertation abstract from: CINAHL Accession No: 1991133549.

Sirapo-Ngam, Y. (1994). *Stress, caregiving demands, and coping of spousal caregivers of Parkinson's patients.* (On-line) Dissertation abstract from: CINAHL Accession No: 199803226.

Smith, C. E., Mayer, L. S., Parkhurst, C., Perkins, S. B., & Pingleton, S. K. (1991). Adaptation in families with a member requiring mechanical ventilation at home. *Heart & Lung: Journal of Critical Care, 20,* 349–356.

Spielberger, C., Gorsuch, R., Lushen, R., Vagg, P. R., & Jacobs, G.A. (1983). *Manual for State-Trait Anxiety Inventory.* Palo Alto: Consulting Psychologist Press.

Swimme, S. A., & Berry, T. (1992). *The universe story.* San Francisco: Harper.

Taylor H. J. (1997). *Self-esteem, coping, and attitude toward menopause among older rural Southern women.* (On-line) Dissertation abstract from: CINAHL Accession No: 2000029128.

Thelot, W., & Guimond-Papai, P. (2000). Physical restraints and older adults [French]. *Canadian Nurse, 96*(2), 36–40.

Tolson, D., & McIntosh, J. (1996). The Roy Adaptation Model: A consideration of its properties as a conceptual framework for an intervention study. *Journal of Advanced Nursing, 24,* 981–987.

Toye, C., Percival, P., & Blackmore, A. (1996). Satisfaction with nursing home care of a relative: Does inviting greater input make a difference? *Collegian: Journal of the Royal College of Nursing, Australia, 3*(2), 4–6, 8–11.

Vicenzi, A. E., & Thiel, R. (1992). AIDS education on the college campus: Roy's Adaptation Model directs inquiry. *Public Health Nursing, 9,* 270–276.

von Bertalanffy, L. (1968). *General system theory.* New York: Braziller.

Weiss, M. E., Hastings, W. J., Holly, D. C., & Craig, D. I. (1994). Using Roy's Adaptation Model in practice: Nurses' perspectives. *Nursing Science Quarterly, 7,* 80–86.

Willoughby, D. F. (1995). *The influence of psychosocial factors on women's adjustment to diabetes.* (On-line) Dissertation abstract from: CINAHL Accession No: 1999015006.

Woods, S. J. (1997). *Predictors of traumatic stress in battered women: A test and explication of the Roy Adaptation Model.* (On-line) Dissertation abstract from: CINAHL Accession No: 200013792.

Wright, P. S. (1993). Parents' perceptions of their quality of life. *Journal of Pediatric Oncology Nursing, 10*(4), 139–145.

Zhan, L. (2000). Cognitive adaptation and self-consistency in hearing-impaired older persons: Testing Roy's Adaptation Model. *Nursing Science Quarterly, 13,* 158–165.

Zindani, N. (1996). Managing material resources in the ED. *Nursing Management, 27*(7), 32B–D.

ANNOTATED BIBLIOGRAPHY OF SELECTED ARTICLES

Calvillo, E. R., & Flaskerud, J. H. (1993). The adequacy and scope of Roy's Adaptation Model to guide cross-cultural pain research. *Nursing Science Quarterly, 6,* 118–129.
This research investigated the operational, empirical, and pragmatic adequacy and scope of the RAM, in conjunction with the gate control theory of pain, in studying pain in 60 Mexican-American and Anglo-American women undergoing elective cholecystectomy. Operational adequacy was demonstrated through the reliability and validity of the empirical indicators used (Spielberger State-Trait Anxiety Inventory, Acculturation Scale, Pain Rating Index, Self-Esteem

Inventory, Sense of Coherence Scale, Index of Activities of Daily Living, and Support Scale). Empirical adequacy was evaluated by comparing actual findings to hypothesized results. Only partial support was found. Pragmatic adequacy was supported through the development of several innovative practice strategies. Scope was determined to be adequate.

Ducharme, F., Ricard, N., Duquette, A., Levesque, L., & Lachance, L. (1998). Empirical testing of a longitudinal model derived from the Roy Adaptation Model. *Nursing Science Quarterly, 11*, 149–159.

This article reports the results of four studies to test a theoretical longitudinal model of the psychosocial determinants of adaptation in different target groups vulnerable to mental health problems. In cross-sectional testing the model was found to be relatively stable over time. Longitudinal data indicated little consistency in relationship patterns across the studies. Important relationships were identified as those between perceived stress, passive/avoidance coping strategies, and psychological distress. Nursing interventions need to be aimed at perceived stress, conflicts in the exchange of support, and passive and avoidance coping strategies.

Ellison, K. J. (1993). *Focal and contextual stimuli influencing caregiving in spouses of older adults with diabetes.* (On-line) Dissertation abstract from: CINAHL Accession No: 1998018590.

This study investigated the interrelationships of involvement in care of a spouse, marital quality, and preparedness as they influence caregiver adaptive responses (impact on schedule, caregiver esteem, impact on health, impact on finances, family support) in a convenience sample of 51 spouse caregivers of older adult diabetics. All forms of stimuli explained 26% to 63% of the variance in responses to caregiving. The contextual stimulus of marital quality supported the RAM through its positive modification of the effects of involvement in caregiving.

Fredrickson, K., Jackson, B. S., Strauman, T., & Strauman, J. (1991). Testing hypotheses derived from the Roy Adaptation Model. *Nursing Science Quarterly, 4*, 168–174.

This study hypothesized that the translation of physiological stimuli through the cognator mechanism of perception alters biopsychosocial responses. Subjects were 45 patients who were entering an aggressive chemotherapy program. Results supported that perception of symptoms correlates positively with both psychosocial adaptation and actual physiological status. Also, perception of symptoms and psychosocial adaptation correlated with six month survival but not with actual physiological status.

Lee, A. A., & Ellenbecker, C. H. (1998). The perceived life stressors among elderly Chinese immigrants: Are they different from those of other elderly Americans? *Clincal Excellence for Nurse Practitioners, 2*(2), 96–101.

This qualitative study investigated the type and amount of stressors experienced by 30 elderly people from two Chinese churches in a northeastern metropolitan city and compared the findings with those of a similar study conducted on other elderly Americans. Findings indicated elderly Chinese immigrants in the United States report amounts and sources of stress that differ from other elderly Americans. While additional studies are needed to identify coping strategies, this study alerts the practicing nurse to the importance of carefully categorizing stimuli from the perspective of the person who is experiencing them.

Levesque, L., Ricard, N., Ducharme, F., Duquette, A., & Bonin, J. (1998). Empirial verification of a theoretical model derived from the Roy Adaptation Model: Findings from five studies. *Nursing Science Quarterly, 11*, 31–39.

This article discusses a theoretical model and the findings of five studies conducted to verify that model. Subjects in the studies included informal caregivers of demented relatives and of psychiatrically ill relatives at home, professional caregivers of elderly institutionalized patients and of aged spouses in the community. Support was found for linking the focal stimulus of perceived stress, with the contextual stimulus or conflicts in the exchange of social support and passive/avoidance coping strategies with psychological distress. Psychological distress was considered an indicator of adaptation in the self-concept mode.

Nuamah, I. F., Cooley, M. E., Fawcett, J., & McCorkle, R. (1999). Testing a theory for health-related quality of life in cancer patients: A structural equation approach. *Research in Nursing & Health, 22,* 231–242.

The study was a secondary analysis of data collected from 375 newly diagnosed cancer patients, aged 60 to 92. The analyses did not support that all four response modes are interrelated but did find a strong association between the severity of illness and adjuvant cancer treatment and biopsychosocial responses, including a reduction in health-related quality of life. Thus, the RAM proposition that environmental stimuli influence the biopsychosocial responses. Findings suggest that nursing should seek to identify the needs of those receiving adjuvant cancer treatments and to help manage the severity of the illness.

Weiss, M. E., Hastings, W. J., Holly, D. C., & Craig, D. I. (1994). Using Roy's Adaptation Model in practice: Nurses' perspectives. *Nursing Science Quarterly, 7,* 80–86.

This qualitative study investigated the use of the RAM in hospital-based nursing practice. The RAM was found to be useful in focusing, organizing, and directing nurses' thoughts and actions in relation to patient care. Nurses who used the RAM perceived an improved quality of both nursing process and patient outcomes. However, the level of integration of the RAM into practice varied among the nurses in the study. Those with prior education in the RAM who also participated in professional advancement activities had higher levels of integration while those who did not have such education and who were resistant to change were less likely to integrate the model into practice.

CHAPTER 16

THE NEUMAN SYSTEMS MODEL
BETTY NEUMAN

Julia B. George

Betty Neuman was born in 1924 on a 100-acre farm in Ohio. The middle of three children and the only daughter, she was 11 when her father died after 6 years of intermittent hospitalizations for treatment of chronic kidney disease. His praise of his nurses influenced Neuman's view of nursing and her commitment to becoming an excellent bedside nurse. Her mother's work as a rural midwife was also a significant influence.

After graduation from high school, Neuman could not afford nursing education. She worked as an aircraft instrument repair technician, as a draftsperson for an aircraft contracting company, and as a short-order cook in Dayton, Ohio, while saving for her education and helping support her mother and younger brother. The creation of the Cadet Nurse Corps Program expedited her entrance into a hospital school of nursing.

In 1947 Neuman graduated from the diploma program of Peoples Hospital (now General Hospital Medical Center), Akron, Ohio. She received a B.S. in public health nursing (1957) and an M.S. as a public health–mental health nurse consultant (1966) from the University of California, Los Angeles. In 1985 she was granted a Ph.D. in clinical psychology by Pacific Western University and has received an honorary doctorate from Grand Valley State in Michigan. She has practiced bedside nursing as a staff, head, and private duty nurse in a wide variety of hospital settings. Her work in community settings has included school and industrial nursing, office nurse in her husband Kree's private practice, and counseling and crisis intervention in community mental health settings. In 1967, six months after completion of her M.S. degree, she became the faculty chair of the program from which she graduated and began her contributions as teacher, author, lecturer, and consultant in nursing and interdisciplinary health care.

In 1973 she and her family returned to Ohio. Since then she has worked as a state mental health consultant, provided continuing education programs, and continued the development of her model. She was one of the first nurses licensed in California as a marriage and family counselor (now Marriage and Family Therapist), a Clinical Fellow of the American Association of Marriage and Family Therapists, and has maintained a limited private counseling practice. She is also a *licensed real estate agent and obtained a private pilot's license in California. In addition to her professional activities, she has exercised her interest in personal property management and other investments as well as health maintenance and promotion activities.*

The Neuman Systems Model was originally developed in 1970 in response to the request of graduate students at the University of California, Los Angeles, for an introductory course that would provide an overview of the physiological, psychological, sociocultural, and developmental aspects of human beings (Neuman, 1995). The model was developed to provide structure for the integration of this material in a wholistic manner. After a two-year evaluation, the model was first published in *Nursing Research* (Neuman & Young, 1972).

Neuman (1982, 1989, 1995) has published three editions of *The Neuman Systems Model*, which have been translated into Japanese. She also had chapters in all editions of *Conceptual models for nursing practice*, the last being the third edition edited by Riehl-Sisca (1989), and in Parker's (1990) *Nursing theories in practice*. Neuman continues work on the model but also incorporated The Neuman Systems Model Trustees Group in 1988. Neuman (1995) states that the trustees group was established for the perpetuation, preservation, and protection of the integrity of the model. Any future permanent changes in the original Neuman Systems Model diagram (see Figure 16–1), other than those made by Neuman herself, must have unanimous approval from the trustees.

DEVELOPMENT OF THE NEUMAN SYSTEMS MODEL

Neuman (1995) says that her personal philosophy of *helping each other live* was supportive in developing the wholistic systems perspective of the Neuman Systems Model. She drew upon her clinical experiences from a variety of health care and community settings and the theoretical perspectives of stress and systems. Caplan's (1964) levels of prevention were also incorporated into the model. Others whose works were drawn upon include de Chardin (1955), Cornu (1957), Edelson (1970), Emery (1969), Laszlo (1972), Lazarus (1981), Selye (1950), and von Bertalanffy (1968).

Nursing is considered a system because nursing practice contains elements in interaction with one another (Neuman, 1995). Advantages of an open-system perspective in nursing include the use of systems as a unifying force across various scientific fields, as well as the increasing complexity of nursing, which calls for an organizational system that can respond to change. A systems perspective supports recognition of the complex whole while valuing the importance of the parts. The relationships between the parts and the interactions of the parts or the whole with the environment provide a mechanism for viewing the system–environment exchanges, which support the dynamic and constantly changing nature of the system.

Neuman (1995) views wholism as both a philosophical and a biological concept. *Wholism* includes relationships that arise from wholeness, dynamic freedom, and creativity as the system responds to stressors from the internal and external environments.

THE NEUMAN SYSTEMS MODEL

The Neuman Systems Model's two major components are stress and the reaction to stress (Neuman, 1995). The client in the Neuman Systems Model is viewed as an open system in which repeated cycles of input, process, output, and feedback constitute a dynamic organizational pattern. Using the systems perspective, the client may be an individual, a group, a family, a community, or any aggregate. In their development toward growth and survival, open systems continuously become more differentiated and elaborate or complex. As they become more complex, the internal conditions of regulation become more complex. Exchanges with the environment are reciprocal; both the client and the environment may be affected either positively or negatively by the other. The system may adjust to the environment or adjust the environment to itself.

The ideal is to achieve optimal system stability. Neuman agrees with Heslin (1986) that when a system achieves stability a revitalization occurs. As an open system, the client system has a propensity to seek or maintain a balance among the various factors, both within and outside the system, that seek to disrupt it (Neuman, 1995). Neuman labels these forces as stressors and views them as capable of having either positive or negative effects. Reactions to the stressors may be possible (not yet occurring) or actual, with identifiable responses and symptoms.

The Neuman Systems Model diagram (see Figure 16–1) presents the major aspects of the model: the *basic structure and energy resources; physiological, psychological, sociocultural, developmental, and spiritual variables; lines of resistance; normal line of defense; flexible line of defense; stressors; reaction; primary, secondary, and tertiary prevention; intra-, inter-, and extrapersonal factors*; and *reconstitution*. The *environment, health*, and *nursing* are inherent parts of the model, although they are not labeled within the model. The client system is represented in the diagram by a basic structure surrounded by a series of concentric circles.

Basic Structure and Energy Resources

The basic structure, or central core, is made up of those basic survival factors common to the species (Neuman, 1995). These factors include the system variables (physiological, psychological, sociocultural, developmental, and spiritual), genetic features, and strengths and weaknesses of the system parts. If the client system is a human being, the basic structure contains such features as the ability to maintain body temperature within a normal range, genetic characteristics such as hair color and response to stimuli, and the functioning of various body systems and their interrelationships. There are also the baseline characteristics associated with each of the five variables, such as physical strength, cognitive ability, cultural perspectives, developmental stage, and value systems.

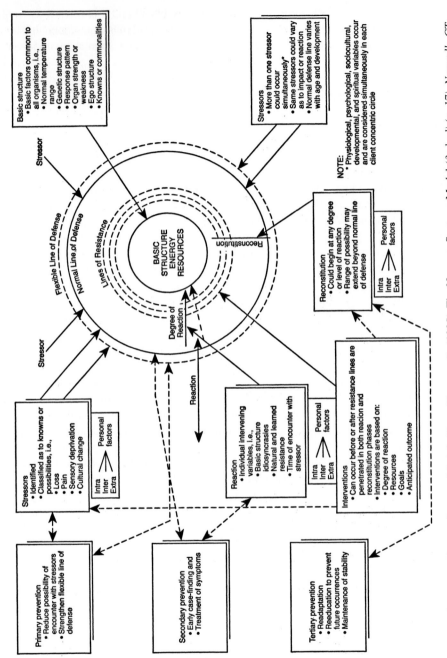

Figure 16-1. The Neuman Systems Model. *(From Neuman, B. (1995). The Neuman Systems Model (3rd ed) (p. 17). Norwalk, CT: Appleton & Lange. Used with permission.)*

Neuman (1995) identifies system stability or homeostasis as occurring when the amount of energy that is available exceeds that being used by the system. This stability preserves the character of the system. Since the system is an open system, the stability is dynamic. As output becomes feedback and input, the system seeks to regulate itself. A change in one direction is countered by a compensating movement in the opposite direction. When the system is disturbed from its normal, or stable, state, there is a rapid surge in the amount of energy needed to deal with the disorganization that results from the disturbance.

Client Variables

Neuman (1995) views the individual client wholistically and considers the variables (physiological, psychological, sociocultural, developmental, and spiritual) simultaneously and comprehensively. In the ideal situation, these variables function in harmony and stability in relation to internal and external environmental stressors. Each of the variables should be considered when assessing system reaction to stressors for each of the concentric circles in the model diagram. It is vital to avoid fragmentation if optimum stability of the client system is to be promoted through nursing care.

The *physiological* variable refers to the structure and functions of the body; the *psychological* variable to mental processes and relationships; the *sociocultural* variable to system functions that relate to social and cultural expectations and activities; the *developmental* variable to those processes related to development over the lifespan; and the *spiritual* variable to the influence of spiritual beliefs.

Neuman (1995) indicates that the first four variables are commonly understood by nursing. Because the spiritual variable was added to the model recently, she discusses it in more detail. This variable is viewed as an innate component of the basic structure that may or may not be acknowledged or developed by the client. Neuman views it as permeating all the other variables of the client system and existing on a developmental continuum from complete unawareness of the presence and potential of the variable to a highly developed spiritual understanding that supports optimal wellness. The continuum includes denial of the existence of the spiritual variable.

Lines of Resistance

The lines of resistance protect the basic structure and become activated when the normal line of defense is invaded by environmental stressors. An example of a response involving lines of resistance is the activation of the immune system mechanisms. If the lines of resistance are effective in their response, the system can reconstitute; if the lines of resistance are not effective, the resulting energy depletion may lead to death.

Normal Line of Defense

In terms of system stability, the normal line of defense represents stability over time (Neuman, 1995). It is considered to be the usual level of stability for the system or the normal wellness state and is used as the baseline for determining deviation from wellness for the client system. For the system, the normal line of defense changes over time as a result of coping with a variety of stressors. The stability represented by the normal line of defense is actually a range of responses to the environment.

Any stressor may invade the normal line of defense when the flexible line of defense offers inadequate protection. When the normal line of defense is invaded or penetrated, the client system reacts. The reaction will be apparent in symptoms of instability or illness and may reduce the system's ability to withstand additional stressors.

Flexible Line of Defense

The flexible line of defense is represented in the model diagram as the outer boundary and initial response, or protection, of the system to stressors. The flexible line of defense serves as a cushion and is described as accordionlike as it expands away from or contracts closer to the normal line of defense (Neuman, 1995). It protects the normal line of defense and acts as a buffer for the client system's usual stable state. Ideally, the flexible line of defense prevents stressors from invading the system. As the distance between the flexible and normal lines of defense increases, so does the degree of protection available to the system.

The flexible line of defense is dynamic rather than stable and can be altered over a relatively short period by factors such as inadequate nutrition or sleep. Either single or multiple stressors may invade the flexible line of defense.

Environment

Neuman (1995) defines environment as all the internal and external factors or influences that surround the client or client system. The influence of the client on the environment and the environment on the client may be positive or negative at any time. Variations in both the client system and the environment can affect the direction of the reaction. For example, individuals who experience sleep deprivation are more susceptible to viruses of the common cold from the environment than those who are well rested.

The *internal* environment exists within the client system. All forces and interactive influences that are solely within the boundaries of the client system make up this environment.

The *external* environment exists outside the client system. Those forces and interactive influences that are outside the system boundaries are identified as external.

Neuman (1989, 1990, 1995) identifies a third environment, the *created environment*. The created environment is developed unconsciously by the client and is symbolic of system wholeness. It represents the open system exchange of energy with both the internal and external environments. It is dynamic and depicts the unconscious mobilization of all system variables but particularly the psychological and sociocultural variables. The purpose of this mobilization is the integration, integrity, and stability of the system. Based on Lazarus's (1981) work, its function is seen as a protective coping shield that encompasses both the internal and external environments. Because it serves as an insulator, the created environment may change the client system's response to stressors. A major objective of the created environment is to provide a positive stimulus toward health for the client. Capers (1996) emphasizes that the created environment includes cultural factors that influence the state of wellness. The created environment is developed to be protective but may have a negative effect on the system if it uses energy needed to react to environmental stressors.

To assess the created environment, the caregiver needs to identify three aspects. First, what has been created and what is the nature of the created environment? Second, to what extent is it used, what value does the client place on it, and what are the outcomes? Third, what protection is needed or is possible, and what is the ideal that is yet to be created? The created environment is a process-based concept of perpetual adjustment that may increase or decrease the client's state of wellness (Neuman, 1995).

Stressors

Neuman (1995) defines stressors as stimuli that produce tensions and have the potential for causing system instability. The system may need to deal with one or more stressors at any given time. It is important to identify the type, nature, and intensity of the stressor; the time of the system's encounter with the stressor; and the nature of the system's reaction or potential reaction to that encounter, including the amount of energy needed. The reaction may occur in one or more subparts, or subsystems, of the system. A reaction in one subsystem may, in turn, affect the original stressor. Outcomes may be positive with the potential for beneficial system changes that may be temporary or permanent.

Stressors are present both within or outside of the system. Neuman (1995) classifies stressors as intra-, inter-, or extrapersonal in nature. *Intrapersonal* stressors are those that occur within the client system boundary and correlate with the internal environment. An example for the individual client system is the autoimmune response. *Interpersonal* stressors occur outside the client system boundary, are proximal to the system, and have an impact on the system. An example is role expectations. *Extrapersonal* stressors also occur outside the system boundaries but are at a greater distance from the system than are interpersonal stressors. An example is social policy. Interpersonal and extrapersonal stressors correlate with the external environment. The created environment includes intra-, inter-, and extrapersonal stressors.

Health

Neuman (1995) identifies health as optimal system stability, or the optimal state of wellness at a given time. Health is seen as a continuum from wellness to illness (see Figure 16–2). Health is also described as dynamic, with changing levels occurring

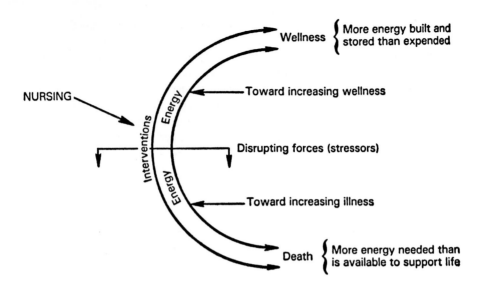

Figure 16–2. Wellness-illness based on the systems concept. *(Adapted from Neuman, B., (1982). The Neuman systems model: Applications to nursing education and practice (p. 11). Norwalk, CT: Appleton-Century-Crofts. Used with permission.)*

within a normal range for the client system over time. The levels vary because of basic structure factors and the client system's response and adjustment to environmental stressors. Wellness may be determined by identifying the actual or potential effects of invading stressors on the system's available energy levels. The client system moves toward illness and death (entropy) when more energy is needed than is available and toward wellness (negentropy) when more energy is available, or can be generated, than is needed.

Reaction

Although reaction is identified within Figure 16–1, Neuman does not discuss it separately. She points out that reactions and outcomes may be positive or negative, and she discusses system movement toward negentropy or entropy.

Prevention

Primary, secondary, and tertiary prevention as interventions are used to retain, attain, and maintain system balance. More than one prevention mode may be used simultaneously.

Primary prevention occurs before the system reacts to a stressor; it includes health promotion and maintenance of wellness. Primary prevention focuses on strengthening the flexible line of defense through preventing stress and reducing risk factors. This intervention occurs when the risk or hazard is identified but before a reaction occurs. Strategies that might be used include immunization, health education, exercise, and life style changes.

Secondary prevention occurs after the system reacts to a stressor and is provided in terms of existing symptoms. Secondary prevention focuses on strengthening the internal lines of resistance and, thus, protects the basic structure through appropriate treatment of symptoms. The intent is to regain optimal system stability and to conserve energy in doing so. If secondary prevention is unsuccessful and reconstitution does not occur, the basic structure will be unable to support the system and its interventions, and death will occur. Examples of secondary prevention include the use of analgesics or of positioning to decrease pain.

Tertiary prevention occurs after the system has been treated through secondary prevention strategies. Its purpose is to maintain wellness or protect the client system reconstitution through supporting existing strengths and continuing to conserve energy. Tertiary prevention may begin at any point after system stability has begun to be reestablished (reconstitution has begun). Tertiary prevention tends to lead back to primary prevention. An example of tertiary prevention is participation in a cardiac rehabilitation program.

Reconstitution

Reconstitution begins at any point following initiation of treatment for invasion of stressors. Neuman (1995) defines reconstitution as the increase in energy that occurs in relation to the degree of reaction to the stressor. Reconstitution may expand the normal line of defense beyond its previous level, stabilize the system at a lower level, or return it to the level that existed before the illness. It depends on successful mobilization of client resources to prevent further reaction to the stressor and represents a dynamic state of adjustment.

Nursing

Neuman (1995) also discusses nursing as part of the model. The major concern of nursing is to help the client system attain, maintain, or retain system stability. This may be accomplished through accurate assessment of both the actual and potential effects of stressor invasion and assisting the client system to make those adjustments necessary for optimal wellness. In supporting system stability, the nurse provides the linkage between the client system, the environment, health, and nursing.

Propositions of the Neuman Systems Model

In 1974, Neuman first presented the assumptions she identified as underlying the Neuman Systems Model. She has now labeled these as propositions (Neuman, 1995). These propositions follow:

1. Although each individual client or group as a client system is unique, each system is a composite of common known factors or

innate characteristics within a normal, given range of response contained within a basic structure.

2. Many known, unknown, and universal environmental stressors exist. Each differs in its potential for disturbing a client's usual stability level, or normal line of defense. The particular interrelationships of client variables—physiological, psychological, sociocultural, developmental, and spiritual—at any point in time can affect the degree to which a client is protected by the flexible line of defense against possible reaction to a single stressor or a combination of stressors.

3. Each individual client/client system has evolved a normal range of response to the environment that is referred to as a normal line of defense, or usual wellness/stability state. It represents change over time through coping with diverse stress encounters. The normal line of defense can be used as a standard from which to measure health deviation.

4. When the cushioning, accordion-like effect of the flexible line of defense is no longer capable of protecting the client/client system against an environmental stressor, the stressor breaks through the normal line of defense. The interrelationships of variables—physiological, psychological, sociocultural, developmental, and spiritual—determine the nature and degree of the system reaction or possible reaction to the stressor.

5. The client, whether in a state of wellness or illness, is a dynamic composite of the interrelationships of variables—physiological, psychological, sociocultural, developmental, and spiritual. Wellness is on a continuum of available energy to support the system in an optimal state of system stability.

6. Implicit within each client system is a set of internal resistance factors known as lines of resistance, which function to stabilize and return the client to the usual state of wellness (normal line of defense) or possibly to a higher level of stability following an environmental stressor reaction.

7. Primary prevention relates to general knowledge that is applied to client assessment and intervention in identification and reduction or mitigation of possible or actual risk factors associated with environmental stressors to prevent possible reaction. The goal of health promotion is included in primary prevention.

8. Secondary prevention relates to symptomatology following a reaction to stressors, appropriate ranking of intervention priorities, and treatment to reduce their noxious effects.

9. Tertiary prevention relates to the adjustive processes taking place as reconstitution begins and maintenance factors move the client back in a circular manner toward primary prevention.

10. The client as a system is in dynamic, constant energy exchange with the environment (pp. 20–21).

THE NEUMAN SYSTEMS MODEL AND NURSING'S METAPARADIGM

The four major concepts in nursing's metaparadigm are identified by Neuman as part of her model and have been discussed. A brief summary of each follows.

The *human being* is viewed as an open system that interacts with both internal and external environmental forces or stressors. The human is in constant change, moving toward a dynamic state of system stability or toward illness of varying degrees.

The *environment* is a vital arena that is germane to the system and its function; it includes internal, external, and created environment (Neuman, 1995). The environment may be viewed as all factors that affect and are affected by the system.

Health is defined as the condition or degree of system stability and is viewed as a continuum from wellness to illness (Neuman, 1995) (see Fig. 16–2). Stability occurs when all the system's parts and subparts are in balance or harmony so that the whole system is in balance. When system needs are met, optimal wellness exists. When needs are not satisfied, illness exists. When the energy needed to support life is not available, death occurs.

The primary concern of *nursing* is to define the appropriate action in situations that are stress-related or in relation to possible reactions of the client or client system to stressors. Nursing interventions are aimed at helping the system adapt or adjust and to retain, restore, or maintain some degree of stability between and among the client system variables and environmental stressors with a focus on conserving energy.

THE NEUMAN SYSTEMS MODEL AND THE NURSING PROCESS

Neuman (1982, 1995) presents a three-step nursing process format (see Table 16–1). The first step, entitled "Nursing Diagnosis," includes the use of a data base to identify variances from wellness and development of hypothetical interventions. The second step, "Nursing Goals," includes caregiver–client negotiation of intervention strategies to retain, attain, or maintain system stability. The third step, "Nursing Outcomes," includes nursing intervention using the prevention modes, confirming that the desired change has occurred or reformulating the nursing goals, using the outcomes of short-term goals to determine longer-term goals, and validating the nursing process through client outcomes. Neuman's first step parallels the assessment and diagnosis phases of the six-phase nursing process. Her second step equates to the outcome identification and planning phases, and her third step equates to the implementation and evaluation phases.

Using the Neuman Systems Model in the *assessment* phase of the nursing process, the nurse focuses on obtaining a comprehensive client data base to determine the existing state of wellness and the actual or potential reaction to environmental stressors.

TABLE 16–1. THE NEUMAN NURSING PROCESS FORMAT

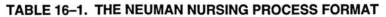

Nursing Diagnosis

Data base

Variances from wellness are determined by correlations and constraints

Hypothetical interventions are determined for prescriptive change

I. Nursing Diagnosis
   A. Data base—determined by
      1. Identification and evaluation of potential or actual stressors that pose a threat to the stability of the client/client systems.
      2. Assessment of condition and strength of basic structure factors and energy resources.
      3. Assessment of characteristics of the flexible and normal lines of defense, lines of resistance, degree of potential reaction, reaction, and/or potential for reconstitution following a reaction.
      4. Identification, classification, and evaluation of potential and/or actual intra-, inter-, and extra-personal interactions between the client and environment, considering all five variables.
      5. Evaluation of influence of past, present, and possible future life process and coping patterns on client system stability.
      6. Identification and evaluation of actual and potential internal and external resources for optimal state of wellness.
      7. Identification and resolution of perceptual differences between caregivers and client/client system.
   Note: In all the above areas of consideration the caregiver simultaneously considers five variables (dynamic interactions in the client/client system)—physiological, psychological, sociocultural, developmental, and spiritual.

(Continued)

TABLE 16–1. (CONTINUED)

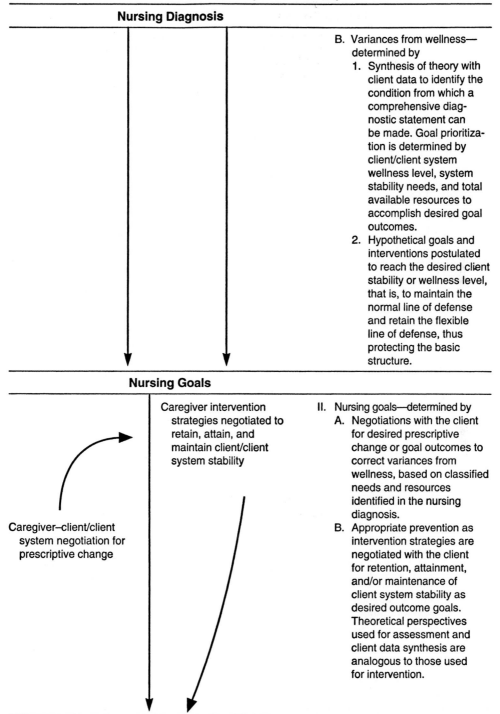

Nursing Diagnosis

B. Variances from wellness—
determined by
1. Synthesis of theory with
client data to identify the
condition from which a
comprehensive diag-
nostic statement can
be made. Goal prioritiza-
tion is determined by
client/client system
wellness level, system
stability needs, and total
available resources to
accomplish desired goal
outcomes.
2. Hypothetical goals and
interventions postulated
to reach the desired client
stability or wellness level,
that is, to maintain the
normal line of defense
and retain the flexible
line of defense, thus
protecting the basic
structure.

Nursing Goals

Caregiver intervention
strategies negotiated to
retain, attain, and
maintain client/client
system stability

Caregiver–client/client
system negotiation for
prescriptive change

II. Nursing goals—determined by
A. Negotiations with the client
for desired prescriptive
change or goal outcomes to
correct variances from
wellness, based on classified
needs and resources
identified in the nursing
diagnosis.
B. Appropriate prevention as
intervention strategies are
negotiated with the client
for retention, attainment,
and/or maintenance of
client system stability as
desired outcome goals.
Theoretical perspectives
used for assessment and
client data synthesis are
analogous to those used
for intervention.

(Continued)

TABLE 16–1. (CONTINUED)

Nursing Outcomes

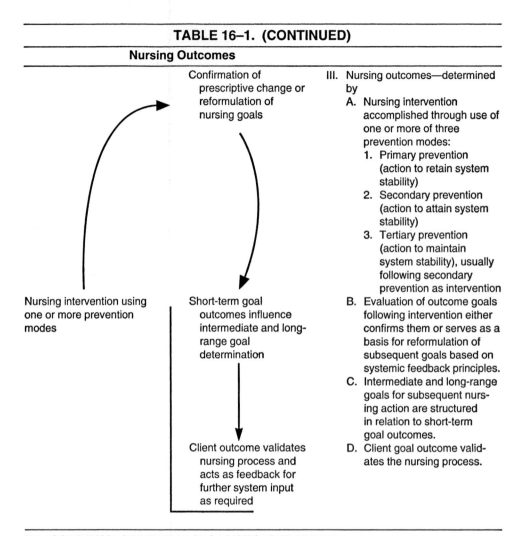

Confirmation of prescriptive change or reformulation of nursing goals

Nursing intervention using one or more prevention modes

Short-term goal outcomes influence intermediate and long-range goal determination

Client outcome validates nursing process and acts as feedback for further system input as required

III. Nursing outcomes—determined by
    A. Nursing intervention accomplished through use of one or more of three prevention modes:
       1. Primary prevention (action to retain system stability)
       2. Secondary prevention (action to attain system stability)
       3. Tertiary prevention (action to maintain system stability), usually following secondary prevention as intervention
    B. Evaluation of outcome goals following intervention either confirms them or serves as a basis for reformulation of subsequent goals based on systemic feedback principles.
    C. Intermediate and long-range goals for subsequent nursing action are structured in relation to short-term goal outcomes.
    D. Client goal outcome validates the nursing process.

A more specific guide to assessment is presented in Table 16–2, "An Assessment and Intervention Tool." The collected data are prioritized and compared to, or synthesized with, relevant theories to explain the client's condition. Variances from the usual state of wellness are identified and a summary of impressions developed. The summary includes intra-, inter-, and extrapersonal factors.

The synthesis of data with theory also provides the basis for the *nursing diagnosis*. In the Neuman model, the diagnostic statement should reflect the entire client condition.

Outcome identification and *Planning* involve negotiation between the caregiver and the client, or recipient of care. The overall goal of the caregiver is to guide the client to conserve energy and to use energy as a force to move beyond the present,

TABLE 16–2. AN ASSESSMENT AND INTERVENTION TOOL

A. Intake Summary
  1. Name_____
     Age_____
     Sex_____
     Marital status_____
  2. Referral source and related
     information_____

B. Stressors as Perceived by Client
  (If client is incapacitated, secure data from family or other resources.)
  1. What do you consider your major stress area, or areas, of health concern? (Identify these areas.)
  2. How do present circumstances differ from your usual pattern of living? (Identify life-style patterns.)
  3. Have you ever experienced a similar problem? If so, what was that problem and how did you handle it? Were you successful? (Identify past coping patterns.)
  4. What do you anticipate for yourself in the future as a consequence of your present situation? (Identify perceptual factors, that is, reality versus distortions—expectations, present and possible future coping patterns.)
  5. What are you doing and what can you do to help yourself? (Identify perceptual factors, that is, reality versus distortions—expectations, present and possible future coping patterns.)
  6. What do you expect caregivers, family, friends, or others to do for you? (Identify perceptual factors, that is, reality versus distortions—expectations, present and possible future coping patterns.)

C. Stressors as Perceived by Caregiver
  1. What do you consider to be the major stress area, or areas, of health concern? (Identify these areas.)
  2. How do present circumstances seem to differ from the client's usual pattern of living? (Identify life-style patterns versus distortions—expectations, present and possible future coping patterns).
  3. Has the client ever experienced a similar situation? If so, how would you evaluate what the client did? How successful do you think it was? (Identify past coping patterns.)
  4. What do you anticipate for the future as a consequence of the client's present situation? (Identify perceptual factors, that is, reality versus distortions—expectations, present and possible future coping patterns.)
  5. What can the client do to help him- or herself? (Identify perceptual factors, that is, reality versus distortions—expectations, present and possible future coping patterns.)
  6. What do you think the client expects from caregivers, family, friends, or other resources? (Identify perceptual factors, that is, reality versus distortions—expectations, present and possible future coping patterns.)

Summary of Impressions
Note any discrepancies or distortions between the client's perception and that of the caregiver's as relates to the situation.

D. Intrapersonal Factors
  1. Physical (Examples: degree of mobility, range of body function)
  2. Psycho-sociocultural (Examples: attitudes, values, expectations, behavior patterns, and nature of coping patterns)
  3. Developmental (Examples: age, degree of normalcy, factors related to present situation)
  4. Spiritual belief system (Examples: hope and sustaining factors)

(cont.)

TABLE 16–2. (*CONT.*)

E. Interpersonal Factors
   Examples are resources and relationships of family, friends, or caregivers that either influence or could influence Area D.

F. Extrapersonal Factors
   Examples are resources and relationship of community facilities, finances, employment, or other area which either influence or could influence Areas D and E.

G. Formulation of a Comprehensive Nursing Diagnosis
   This is accomplished by identifying and ranking the priority of needs based on total data obtained from the client's perception, the caregiver's perception, or other resources, such as laboratory reports, other caregivers, or agencies. Appropriate theory is related to the above data.

   With this format, reassessment is a continuous process and is related to the effectiveness of intervention based on the prior stated goals. Effective reassessment would include the following as they relate to the total client situation:
   a. Changes in nature of stressors and priority assignments
   b. Changes in intrapersonal factors
   c. Changes in interpersonal factors
   d. Changes in extrapersonal factors
   In reassessment it is important to note the change of priority of goals in relation to the primary, secondary, and tertiary prevention as intervention categories. An assessment tool of this nature should offer a current, progressive, and comprehensive analysis of the client's total circumstances and relationship of the five client variables (physiological, psychological, sociocultural, developmental, and spiritual) to environmental influences.

Source: Neuman, B. (1995). *The Neuman Systems Model* (pp. 59–61). Norwalk, CT: Appleton & Lange.

ideally in a way that preserves or enhances the client's wellness level. More specific outcomes will be derived from the nursing diagnoses. The perceptions of both the client and the caregiver must be considered in setting goals. Outcomes are specified under nursing goals in the Neuman Model as goal outcomes to correct variances. These are to be based on the identified needs and the available resources. Outcomes are negotiated with the client.

According to Neuman (1995), nursing actions (*implementation*) are based on the synthesis of a comprehensive data base about the client and the theory(ies) that are appropriate in light of the client's and caregiver's perceptions and possibilities for functional competence within the environment. The modes for identifying these actions are the levels of prevention as intervention. Table 16–3 presents a guide to nursing actions using prevention as intervention.

Evaluation is implied in the discussion of reassessment in Table 16–2. It is more explicitly identified in the "Nursing Outcomes" step of Neuman's three-step nursing process (see Table 16–1). According to this third step, evaluation confirms that the anticipated or prescribed change has occurred. If this is not true, then goals are reformulated. Immediate and long-range goals are then structured in relation to the short-range outcomes.

A case study example of the application of the Neuman System Model may be found in Table 16–4.

TABLE 16–3. FORMAT FOR PREVENTION AS INTERVENTION

Nursing Action		
Primary Prevention	Secondary Prevention	Tertiary Prevention
1. Classify stressors that threaten stability of the client/client system. Prevent stressor invasion.	1. Following stressor invasion, protect basic structure.	1. During reconstitution, attain and maintain maximum level of wellness or stability following treatment.
2. Provide information to retain or strengthen existing client/client system strengths.	2. Mobilize and optimize internal/external resources to attain stability and energy conservation.	2. Educate, reeducate, and/or reorient as needed.
3. Support positive coping and functioning.	3. Facilitate purposeful manipulation of stressors and reaction to stressors.	3. Support client/client system toward appropriate goals.
4. Desensitize existing or possible noxious stressors.	4. Motivate, educate, and involve client/client system in health care goals.	4. Coordinate and integrate health service resources.
5. Motivate toward wellness.	5. Facilitate appropriate treatment and intervention measures.	5. Provide primary and/or secondary preventive intervention as required.
6. Coordinate and integrate interdisciplinary theories and epidemiological input.	6. Support positive factors toward wellness.	
7. Educate or reeducate.	7. Promote advocacy by coordination and integration.	
8. Use stress as a positive intervention strategy.	8. Provide primary preventive intervention as required.	

Note: *A first priority for nursing action in each of the areas of prevention as intervention is to determine the nature of stressors and their threat to the client/client system. Some general categorical functions for nursing action are initiation, planning, organization, monitoring, coordinating, implementing, integrating, advocating, supporting, and evaluating. An example of a limited classification system for stressors is illustrated by the following four categories: (1) deprivation, (2) excess, (3) change, and (4) intolerance.*
Copyright © 1980 by Betty Neuman. Revised 1987 by Betty Neuman.

TABLE 16–4. CASE STUDY USING THE NEUMAN SYSTEMS MODEL

Intake Summary
  Name: Carolyn Miles
  Age: 35 years
  Sex: Female
  Marital Status: Married
  Referral Source: Self-referred

A. Stressors as Perceived by Client
  1. Major stress areas or areas of concern:
      a. Found out 2 weeks ago is 2 months pregnant—here for prenatal visit
      b. First child is 11 months old, wants another child, ambivalent about the timing of this pregnancy
  2. Life-style patterns
      a. Cares for home and daughter
      b. Active in church
      c. Participates in community groups related to parenting
      d. Has supportive family and friends
      e. What is different now?—experiencing nausea and fatigue
  3. Ever experienced similar problem?
      a. The nausea and fatigue are similar to the first pregnancy
      b. What helped then—crackers and lying down helped some; primarily just suffered through it
  4. Anticipations for the future
      a. Concerns about how to maintain a healthy pregnancy and care for an active toddler
         (concern greater because first pregnancy resulted in a premature delivery of a small for
         gestational age baby)
      b. Also anticipating the demands of caring for two children under the age of two
  5. What doing to help herself?
      a. Talking with friends and family about their experiences
      b. Reading articles and books on childbearing and childrearing
      c. "I need to lower my expectations of myself and try not to do so much—for me that's HARD!!"
  6. What is expected of others?
      a. Family is visiting around the time the baby is due and will help with the children and the house
      b. Husband is doing more of the cooking and helping keep the house clean
B. Stressors as Perceived by Caregiver (primary care provider who provided prenatal care with the
   first pregnancy)
  1. Major stress area
      a. History of premature delivery
      b. Type A personality who has difficulty relaxing
  2. Present circumstances differing from usual pattern of living
      a. Fatigue and nausea of pregnancy
      b. Dealing with anticipation concerns about expanding family
  3. Client's past experience with similar situation?
      a. Experienced with nausea and fatigue of pregnancy
      b. Not experienced in having 2 children under 2
  4. Future anticipations
      a. Client is capable of handling the situation—will need support and encouragement to do so
  5. What client can do to help herself?
      a. Use her support systems
      b. Concentrate on getting needed rest
      c. Remember that the goal is a healthy child and things can be done later
  6. Clients expectations of family, friends and caregivers
      a. Accurate information
      b. Support and encouragement
      c. A listening ear

Summary of Impressions: No apparent discrepancies between perceptions of client and caregiver.

TABLE 16-4. (*CONT.*)

C. Intrapersonal factors
   1. Physical
      a. Height: 5 feet, 5 inches
      b. Weight: 125 lbs (no change from prepregnancy weight)
      c. TPR 98.4 F, 76, 12
      d. B/P 118/76
      e. Urine negative for sugar and albumin
      f. Care—perform all activities of daily living for self and toddler
      g. Is current with all immunizations
      h. Sleeps 7 to 8 hours per night
      i. Does not smoke or ingest alcohol
      j. Follows a low fat, balanced diet; usually eats 3 meals per day
      k. Reports experiencing nausea and fatigue—a major stressor at this time
   2. Psycho-sociocultural
      a. 35-year-old female, married
      b. Caucasian
      c. Holds a masters degree in communications
      d. Sometimes concerned about feeling isolated—likes to have lots of friends and best friend will be moving in 6 to 12 months
      e. Knows needs to "slow down" but states that is hard for her to do, "I plan too much for any given day. I've always done this and I don't really know how to do less. The one good thing is that it doesn't bother me too much if I don't get all that I have planned done!"
      f. Lives in own home
      g. Fluent in English and Spanish
   3. Developmental
      a. "I have demonstrated my ability to be a good mother—that is reassuring that I can meet this new challenge."
      b. "How am I going to find the time to do everything?"
   4. Spiritual belief system
      a. This is an area of support, not an area of concern
      b. Active at church, regular attendance is important
      c. Has personal Bible study daily
D. Interpersonal Factors
   1. Has supportive family and friends
   2. Often speaks on the phone to family and friends, has lunch with friends regularly
   3. Shares toddler play days with friends
   4. Concerned about having 2 children under 2 in the house
   5. Is working on a project at church to improve the nursery program
   6. Cannot rest at will with toddler at home—this is different than with first pregnancy so previous coping responses are not as effective
   7. Will try to interest toddler in quiet activities on the days she is really tired
   8. Husband can work at home some days and help with the toddler
E. Extrapersonal Factors
   1. Community lacks good day care programs/facilities for toddlers so there is no real community support for when she needs a respite from child care
   2. Health care for all family members is readily available
Overall Summary:
   Physiological: Normal pregnancy with associated stressors of nausea and fatigue
   Psychosociocultural: Has supportive family and friends. Stressors related to self expectations
   Developmental: Normal for age
   Spiritual: Belief system is a positive support

(cont.)

TABLE 16–4. (*CONT.*)

F. Formulation of a Comprehensive Nursing Diagnosis:
  1. Nursing Diagnoses
     a. Nausea and fatigue related to pregnancy
     b. Lack of knowledge related to parenting two under the age of two
  2. Goals (desired outcomes)
     a. Manage nausea and fatigue so can continue normal activities of daily living
     b. Plan strategies for coping with two under the age of two
     c. Have a healthy outcome to the pregnancy—healthy mother, father, toddler, and infant
  3. Prevention as Intervention
     a. Manage nausea and fatigue
        i. primary—normal line of defense has been invaded—is having symptoms
        ii secondary—plan daily activities to include rest periods when toddler naps; explore types of foods and eating patterns that decrease nausea
        iii. tertiary—continue to encourage rest whenever possible; husband helps out as he can; plan daily intake of appropriate nutrients; keep a journal listing daily plans to demonstrate ability to plan less for each day
     b. Lack of knowledge about parenting two under two
        i. primary—discuss current parenting strategies with husband, friends, family, caregiver and explore how these strategies may be adapted; caregiver encourages discussion with friend who has two small children and works full time
        ii. secondary and tertiary—not needed as yet; flexible and normal lines of defense have functioned effectively
     c. Healthy outcome to the pregnancy
        i. The overall desired outcome—preventions as intervention listed in a and b.
  4. Evaluation

Carolyn delivered a healthy 6 pound, 8 ounce girl at 38-weeks gestation after a pregnancy she described as "much better than I thought it would be." Husband/father and older daughter are delighted with the new baby. Carolyn states, "I'm still working on not planning too much for each day." Identified outcome was achieved.

CRITIQUE OF THE NEUMAN SYSTEMS MODEL

1. What is the historical context of the theory? The assumptions that provide the basis for the Neuman Systems Model are clearly explicated in the work. These assumptions are identified as propositions and follow a logical order. Dr. Neuman identifies that she has drawn upon her own clinical experiences in nursing as well as information in the literature on stress, systems, levels of prevention, wholism within systems, coping, and gestalt theory. While study of this literature could enrich one's understanding of the relationships she has developed, such study is not vital to comprehension of the Neuman Systems Model.

The Neuman Systems Model was developed during a period when other developing nursing theories were based in general systems theory. Chronologically, it fits in the middle period of theory development in nursing during the twentieth century. Based on Parse's (1987) description of the totality paradigm, the Neuman Systems Model best fits this paradigm. The model is wholistic but emphasizes the five variables of physiological, psychological, sociocultural, developmental, and spiritual. The system's interaction with the external environment is described as responses to stressors that adapt or seek to control the stressors or the environment. Health is described as dynamic with an objective assessment of the invasion, or potential for invasion, of the lines of defense. Reconstitution and the levels of preventions may be identified as maintenance or restoration of norms. The plan of care is designed by the nurse based on skilled assessment. However, the client is viewed as unique, decision making is shared, and the care is negotiated with the client. Dr. Neuman (1995) supports the use of both quantitative and qualitative methods of research for studying relationships identified by the model.

2. What are the basic concepts and relationships presented by the theory? and **3. What major phenomena of concern to nursing are presented? These phenomena may include** *but are not limited to***: human being, environment, health, interpersonal relations, caring, goal attainment, adaptation, and energy fields.** The basic concepts of the Neuman Systems Model are the five variables (physiological, psychological, sociocultural, developmental, and spiritual), levels of prevention (primary, secondary, and tertiary), lines of defense (flexible line of defense, normal line of defense, and lines of resistance), environment (internal, external, and created), stressors (intrapersonal, interpersonal, and extrapersonal), health, reconstitution, system core and nursing. All of these are defined. The reactions to stressors are less clearly defined. These concepts are used consistently and presented in a pictorial model (see Figure 16–1). The relationships among the concepts are logical and clearly defined in the stated propositions. While the pictorial model is rather overwhelming on first view, an orderly analysis supports that it logically presents the identified relationships.

4. To whom does this theory apply? In what situations? In what ways? This model was designed for health care and applies to all recipients of nursing care—individuals, groups, organizations, and communities. Neuman's use of the term *client/client system* allows for the client to be an individual or a collection of people. The system perspective allows the user to define the system (an individual, a family, an organization . . .) and then to identify the core and lines of defense for that system. The wholistic system approach indicates the model is not situation specific but may be used in a variety of situations. It would be difficult to identify a setting where this model could not be applied.

The model explains and predicts phenomena. For example, if the lines of resistance have been activated and they are not effective and cannot be strengthened through secondary prevention as intervention strategies, then death is threatened. If the flexible lines of defense are effective, there is no immediate threat to the system but the client may be in need of primary prevention as intervention strategies to enhance responses to potential stressors.

5. By what method or methods can this theory be tested? Fawcett (1995) identifies six rules for research based on the Neuman Systems Model:

- The phenomena to be studied encompass (1) physiological, psychological, sociocultural, developmental, and spiritual variables; (2) properties of the central core of the client system; (3) properties of the flexible and normal lines of defense as well as the lines of resistance; (4) characteristics of the internal, external, and created environments; (5) characteristics of intrapersonal, interpersonal, and extrapersonal stressors; and (6) elements of primary, secondary, and tertiary prevention interventions.

- The clinical problems to be studied are those that deal with the impact of stressors on client system stability with regard to physiological, psychological, sociocultural, developmental, and spiritual variables, as well as the lines of defense and resistance. One purpose of Neuman Systems Model-based research is to predict the effect of primary, secondary, and tertiary prevention interventions on retention, attainment, and maintenance of client system stability. Another purpose is to determine the cost, benefit, and utility of prevention interventions.
- Subjects can be the client systems of individuals, families, groups, communities, organizations, or collaborative relationships between two or more individuals. Data encompass both client system and investigator perceptions and strategies for negotiated goal setting, and may be collected in inpatient, ambulatory, home, and community settings.
- This nursing model is an appropriate base for inductive and deductive research using both qualitative and quantitative research designs and associated instrumentation.
- Data analysis techniques associated with both qualitative and quantitative research designs are appropriate.
- Research will advance understanding of the influence of prevention interventions on the relationship between stressors and client system stability (p. 463).

Note particularly the fourth rule that indicates that both quantitative and qualitative research methods may be used in testing relationships identified from the Neuman Systems Model.

The Neuman Systems Model is one of the most widely used nursing models for nursing research. In 1989, Louis and Koertvelyessy reported the model was one of the three most frequently used models in nursing research. In 1999, Fawcett reported finding 200 studies published between 1982 and 1997. However, most of these studies did not include conclusions about the usability or validity of the model. Louis (1995) reports findings ranging from no significant relationships to "decisive results" (p. 478). She suggests it is important to evaluate the rigor of each study as well as the strength of the use of prevention as intervention—both in the strength of the prevention used and in the length of the time it was applied. Examples of the findings reported by Louis include:

Barrow (1992) found the stressors (job stress) to be related to lines of resistance (social support of Critical Care Registered Nurses (CCRN)) and the flexible line of defense (degree of job satisfaction) but none of these were related to the normal line of defense (CCRN behavior type of A or B). Barrow suggested further study in relation to the CCRN credential and the lines of resistance.

Fillmore (1992) used the Neuman Systems Model as a guide in creating a primary prevention of preoperative education for hysterectomy patients. The stressor was defined as the surgery and the primary prevention was intended to decrease anxiety and thus strenthen the normal line of defense. Those who received the primary prevention as intervention did demonstrate lower levels of anxiety. However, although the direction of the difference supported the model, the differences were not statistically significant.

A summary of the studies reviewed by Louis may be found in Table 16–5.

Gigliotti (1999a) points out the difficulty in making comparisons across studies as the lines of defense have not been described in a consistent manner. For example, in four cited studies, although all discussed a stressor with a specific intervention to strengthen the flexible line of defense, the associated outcome is defined differently in each. Ali and Khalil (1989) and Gigliotti (1999b) speak to the normal line of defense penetration or invasion, Louis (1989) uses the term *line of resistance not activated*, and Freiberger, Bryant, and Marino (1992) identify activated lines of resistance.

Research is active on relationships and theories derived from this model. Use of the terminology and findings are not yet consistent. Both Fawcett (1999) and Gigliotti (1999a) support the need for more consistent and explicit linkages between the concepts of the Neuman Systems Model and the variables being studied.

6. Does this theory direct critical thinking in nursing practice? Critical thinking skills are needed to understand the pictorial diagram of the relationships of the concepts within this model and to apply these concepts to nursing practice. The Neuman Systems Model provides a structure for the collection and use of assessment data. Use of the Neuman Systems Model for practice requires the use of a theoretical base of knowledge in assessing the collected data and designing/negotiating a plan of care. While there is a need for congruency in use of the terminology related to the model, the model has been tested in practice. For examples, see Table 16–5 and the annotated bibliography at the end of this chapter.

7. Does this theory direct therapeutic nursing intervention? The use of levels of prevention as intervention provide direction for therapeutic nursing intervention. A strength of the model is that there are three levels of prevention as intervention. Nursing interventions may be used to promote or maintain health status, prevent disease, and to help return people to a healthful state. A wholistic approach and viewpoint are an important part of the model, so the nurse who uses the Neuman Systems Model as a guide to the development of therapeutic nursing interventions could be using all levels of prevention as intervention over the course of the nurse and client interaction. The use of the five variables will also contribute to consideration of the whole person. Again, the use of the Neuman Systems Model for directing

TABLE 16–5. SAMPLE RESEARCH STUDIES USING THE NEUMAN SYSTEMS MODEL

Author (Date)	Focus of Study	Findings in Relation to Neuman Systems Model
Barrow (1992)	Job stress and satisfaction of Critical Care Registered Nurses (CCRN)	Stressors (job stress) related to lines of resistance (social support) and flexible line of defense (job satisfaction). None related to normal line of defense (CCRN behavior type).
Courchene, Patalski, & Martin (1991)	Health status of pediatric nurses administering cyclosporine A	The client system's (pediatric nurses) exposure to an environmental stressor (cyclosporine A) often led to indications of penetration of the flexible line of defense (complaints or symptoms) and thus were consistent with the model. Suggestions for primary prevention are provided.
Fillmore (1992)	Effects of preoperative teaching on anxiety levels of hysterectomy patients	Supported use of primary prevention as intervention (preoperative education) to strengthen the flexible line of defense (coping, lower anxiety) to decrease impact of stressor (surgery). However, the findings were not statistically significant.
Hinds (1990)	Quality of life predictor variables in persons with lung cancer	Seven quality of life variables were found to be congruent with the NSM variables of person/client, environment (including created environment), health, nursing, and intervention.
Ivey (1993)	Evaluation of social support tools with women with breast cancer	PRQ has support for reliability, concurrent and construct validity in measuring the sociocultural variables of the Neuman Systems Model. PRQ can assess intra-, inter-, and extrapersonal stressors.
Leja (1989)	Use of guided imagery before discharge of elderly postoperative patients	Use of guided imagery (primary prevention as intervention) decreased levels of depression (the line of defense). While supporting the use of primary prevention, the differences between the results of this treatment and standard discharge practices were not statistically significant.
Loescher, Clark, Attwood, Leigh, & Lamb (1990)	System stability in long-term cancer survivors	The stressor (cancer) was related to intra- and extrapersonal environments in adjusting to the situation consistent with the Neuman Systems Model. This study used both qualitative and quantitative analyses.
Mendez (1990)	College students' image of nursing as a career choice	The stressor (nursing's image) was identified as impinging on nursing's flexible line of defense and secondary preventions as intervention focusing on the public and nurses' image of nursing were presented.

TABLE 16–5. (*CONT.*)

Author (Date)	Focus of Study	Findings in Relation to Neuman Systems Model
Pardee (1992)	Family member care-givers of individuals with brain injuries	The stressor—brain injury of a family member. The client system—the caregiving family members whose flexible and normal lines of defense have been invaded by the stressor. The secondary prevention as intervention—information on cognitive dysfunction and behavioral changes. The use of the secondary prevention as intervention was supported.
Puetz (1990)	Nurse and patient perception of stressors associated with coronary artery bypass surgery (CABG)	The prevention as intervention was to align the two systems, (patient and nurse) identification of patient needs. Incongruence in these perceptions was seen as an additional stressor for the patient. Intrapersonal, interpersonal and extrapersonal stressors were identified and incongruencies between the patient and the nurse were found and related to the lack of individualized assessment by the nurse.
Robin (1991)	Use of tool for prevention as intervention in ectopic pregnancy	Primary prevention (education and health maintenance), secondary prevention (screening and case finding), and tertiary prevention (education of pregnant women about signs and symptoms of ectopic pregnancy) were included in the Ectopic Pregnancy Risk Assessment Screening Tool. The tool can be used to strengthen the lines of defense and protect the core.

Source: Adapted from Louis, M. (1995). The Neuman Model in nursing research, An update. In B. Neuman, *The Neuman Systems Model* (pp. 473–489). Stamford, CT: Appleton & Lange.

therapeutic nursing intervention has been tested (see Table 16–5 and the chapter bibliography). The third edition of *The Neuman Systems Model* has more than three dozen chapters that discuss the use of the model in curriculum, nursing practice, and nursing administration in the United States and internationally.

8. Does this theory direct communication in nursing practice? Communication is a vital component of the Neuman Systems Model. The intrapersonal stressors cannot be identified without communication. The interpersonal and extrapersonal stressors not only require communication for assessment but also may involve communication. Also, the nurse can gain an understanding of the client's created environment, a very personal attribute, only through information provided by the client. The Assessment and Intervention Tool developed by Neuman (Table 16–2) indicates that data are to be collected from the client, the family, or other resources. Communication skills are a prerequisite for the successful completion of this tool.

Not only does the model require communication, it provides guidelines to structure this activity.

9. Does this theory direct nursing actions that lead to favorable outcomes? The Neuman Systems Model directs nursing actions that lead to favorable outcomes through the use of the levels of prevention as intervention. The purpose of the levels of prevention is reconstitution, or the return to wholeness with functioning lines of defense to protect against stressors invading the system and leading to illness. The intent of the levels of prevention is to allow nursing actions to be taken as appropriate to the needs of the client system. Nursing actions are determined by asking, "What are the stressors as perceived by the client system and what has been the system's reaction been to these stressors?" By focusing on the cause and the reactions, it is possible to carry out nursing actions that are likely to lead to favorable outcomes. Because the Neuman Systems Model directs the nurse to consider the perceptions of the client and of the caregiver, when these perceptions are congruent, the frequency of favorable outcomes is enhanced. For example, Puetz (1990) found that when nurses' did not conduct an individualized assessment, the perceptions of the client and the nurse were less likely to be congruent. This lack of congruency could then be a stressor for the client and outcomes would be less favorable as the nurse has not followed the assessment guidelines of the Neuman Systems Model.

10. How contagious is this theory? The Neuman Systems Model is one of the most contagious of the nursing theories or models. It is in use worldwide in direct clinical practice and nursing administration, nursing research, and nursing education. Examples of the use of the model in these areas around the world include:

- Africa: Pediatric HIV practice (Orr, 1999); Pediatric research (Orr, 1993)
- Australia: Use in education at the University of South Australia (McCulloch, 1995).
- Canada:
  Practice in *chronic care* (Felix, Hinds, Wolfe, & Martin, 1995); *community/public health* (Beynon, 1995; Beynon & Laschinger, 1993; Bunn, 1995; Craig, 1995; Drew, Craig, & Beynon, 1989; Mytka & Beynon, 1994); *gerontology* (Gibson, 1996); *HIV* (Mill, 1997); *nursing administration* (Beynon, 1995; Craig & Morris-Coulter, 1995; Drew, Craig, & Beynon, 1989; Neuman, 1995); *orthopedics* (Shaw, 1991); and *pediatrics* (Galloway, 1993; Maligalig, 1994).
  Research related to *back pain* (McMillan, 1995); *caregiver burden* (Semple, 1995); *gender identity disorder* (Janze, Watson, & Stevenson, 1999); *hip surgery patients* (Bowman, 1997); *oncology* (Cava, 1992); *latex allergy* (Cowperthwaite, LaPlante, Mahon, & Markowski, 1997); *Nurses' Association Presidents* (Johnson, 1995); *public health nursing* (Mackenzie & Laschinger, 1995); *stress* (Montgomery & Craig, 1990); *theory based care* (Laschinger & Duff, 1991).

Education in *postdiploma and baccalaureate programs* (Beddome, 1995; Craig, 1995; Crawford, Tarko, Ting, Gunderson, & Andrews, 1999; Neuman, 1995; Peternelj-Taylor & Johnson, 1996; Tarko & Crawford, 1999).

- China: Research in *oncology* (Lin, Ku, Leu, Chen, & Lin, 1996).
- Denmark: Teaching *community health nursing* (Neuman, 1995).
- Egypt: Research in *oncology* (Ali & Khalil, 1989).
- United Kingdom:
  Practice: *breast feeding* (Evely, 1994); *community health* (Damant, 1995; Davies & Proctor, 1995); *Down syndrome* (Owens, 1995); *family nursing* (Picton, 1995); *gerontology* (Beckingham & Baumann, 1990; Haggart, 1993; Millard, 1992; Moore & Munro, 1990); *general patient care* (Goodman, 1995); *intensive care* (Black, Deeny, & McKenna, 1997; Wormald, 1995); *multiple sclerosis* (Knight, 1990); *perioperative care* (Parr, 1993); *rehabilitation* (Bowles, Oliver, & Stanley, 1995).
  Research: *Oncology* (Hinds, 1990).
  Nursing education (Ross, Bourbonnais, & Carroll, 1987; Vaughan & Gough, 1995).
- Guam: *Baccalaureate education* (Neuman, 1995).
- Hong Kong: Research in *oncology* (Molassiotis, 1997); Education (Cheung, 1997).
- Iceland: *practice* at St. Joseph's Hospital, Reykjavik (Neuman, 1995) and *baccalaureate education* at Akureye University (Neuman, 1995).
- Netherlands:
  Practice: in *mental health care* (Timmermans, 1999; Verberk, 1995).
  Research: *addiction* (Westrik, 1999).
  Education: *higher education* (de Meij & de Kuiper, 1999).
- Saudi Arabia: Research in *surgically induced menopause* (Al-Nagshabandi, 1993).
- Sweden:
  Practice: *community health* (Engberg, Bjälming, & Bertilson, 1995); *contraception* (Lindell & Olsson, 1991); *hospital care* (Neuman, 1995); *occupational health* (McGee, 1995).
  Research in *gerontology* (Lindgren & Olsson, 1999); *humor* (Carras & Olsson, 1999; Olsson & Leadersh, 1999); *slimming* (Eilert-Petersson & Olsson, 1999); *stress in student nurses* (Àgren, Fröistedt, & Olsson, 1999; Backe & Olsson, 1999).
  Education: *college* (Engberg, 1995).
- Taiwan: use in *education* (Neuman, 1995).
- Thailand: research in *cardiac care* (Pothiban, 1993).
- United States:
  Practice: *advanced practice* (Russell & Hezel, 1994); *caregivers* (Skipwith, 1994); *case management* (Bittinger, 1995; Mann, Hazel, Geer, Hurley, & Podrapovic, 1993); *cardiac care* (Lile, 1990); *cognitive*

impairment (Chiverton & Flannery, 1995); *community nursing* (Cook-fair, 1996; Frioux, Roberts, & Butler, 1995; Gellner, Landers, O'Rourke, & Schlegel, 1994; Neuman, 1995; Rodriguez, 1995); *concept analysis* (Reed, 1999); *critical care nursing* (Bueno & Sengin, 1995); *critical pathways* (Lowry, 1999); *culture* (Capers, 1996); depression (Hassell, 1996); *diabetes mellitus* (Baerg, 1991); *dialysis* (Breckenridge, 1997a; 1997b); *family assessment/nursing* (Berkey & Hanson, 1991; Flannery, 1991; Kahn, 1992; Reed, 1993; Ridgell, 1993); *gerontological nursing* (Delunas, 1990; Hiltz, 1990; Peirce & Fulmer, 1995); *health protection* (Bigbee & Jansa, 1991); *HIV care* (Miner, 1995; Pierce & Hutton, 1992; Simmons & Borgdon, 1991); *home caregivers* (Russell, Hileman, & Grant, 1995); *hospital based care* (Davidson & Myers, 1999; Neuman, 1995; Scicchitani, Cox, Heyduk, Maglicco, & Sargent, 1995); *inservice education* (Roberts, 1994); *intensive care* (Fulbrook, 1991; Kido, 1991); long term care (Schlentz, 1993); *multisystem organ failure* (Bergstrom, 1992); *neonatal intensive care* (Ware & Shannahan, 1995); *neuroscience nursing* (Foote, Piazza, & Schultz, 1990); *nurse anesthesia* (Martin, 1996); *obstetrics/battered women* (Barnes-McDowell & Freese, 1999; Bullock, 1993); *oncology* (Piazza, Foote, Wright, & Holcombe, 1992; Weinberger, 1991); *perinatal nursing* (Gigliotti, 1998; Trépanier, Dunn, & Sprague, 1995); *psychiatric nursing* (Herrick, Goodykoontz, Herrick, & Hackett, 1991; Stuart & Wright, 1995); *substance abuse* (Mynatt & O'Brien, 1993; Waters, 1993); *terminal illness* (Lile, Pase, Hoffman, & Mace, 1994); *theory-based practice* (Dale & Savala, 1990; Derstine, 1992; Neuman, 1990, 1998)

Research: *AIDS education* (Brown, 1994); *antibiotic therapy* (Herald, 1993); anxiety (Wilkey, 1990); *baccalaureate education* (Fulton, 1992; Lamb, 1998; Mirenda, 1995; Peterson, 1997; Roggensack, 1994; Speck, 1990); *back injuries/pain* (Brown, Sirles, Hilyer, & Thomas, 1992; Koku, 1992; Radwanski, 1992); *blood pressure* (Picot, Zauszniewski, Debanne, & Holston, 1999); *breast feeding* (Cagle, 1996; Marlett, 1998); *burnout* (Collins, M. A., 1996; Marsh, 1997); *cardiac* (Geiger, 1996; Harper, 1992; Kazakoff, 1990; Lijauco, 1997; Micevski, 1996; Williamson, 1992); *cerebral vascular accident* (Gifford, 1996); *chronic lung disease patients* (Narsavage, 1997); *conceptual frameworks in research* (Grant, Kinney, & Davis, 1993); *cognitive assessment* (Flannery, 1995); *critical/intensive care* (Gavigan, Kline-O'Sullivan, & Klumpp-Lybrand, 1990; Ramsey, 1999; Watson, 1991); *diabetes* (Barron, 1998); *gerontology* (Butts, 1998; Collins, C. R., 1999; Rodrigues-Fisher, Bourguignon, & Good, 1993); *head injury* (Grant & Bean, 1992; Henze, 1993; Jones, 1996; Neabel, 1998); *health promotion* (Fowler & Risner, 1994); *HIV* (Gulliver, 1997; Norman, 1990); *home care* (Peoples, 1990); *hospice* (Decker & Young, 1991); *humor* (Cullen, 1993); *immunization* (Chilton, 1996); *infant exposure to smoke* (Flanders-Stepans & Fuller, 1999); *job stress or satisfaction* (Hanson, 1997; Moody, 1996; Morris, 1991;

Peters, 1997); *long term care* (Petock, 1990); *Neonatal Intensive Care Unit* (Bass, 1991); *nursing administration* (Rowles, 1992; Walker, 1994); *nursing education* (Nortridge, Mayeux, Anderson, & Bell, 1992; Payne, 1993); *nurse-patient relations and culture* (Butrin, 1992); *nurse practitioner practice* (Larino, 1997); *nurses' values* (Cammuso, 1994); *oncology* (Allen, 1997; Jennings, 1997; Lancaster, 1991; O'Neal, 1993; Sabo & Michael, 1996; South, 1995); *orthopedics* (Nicholson, 1995; Wright, 1996); *pain control* (Vitthuhn, 1999); *parenting* (Heaman, 1991); *patient satisfaction* (Fukuzawa, 1995); *pediatrics* (Courchene, Patalski, & Martin, 1991; Freiberger, Bryant, & Marino, 1992; Gray, 1998; Rosenfeld, Goldsmith, & Madell, 1998); *perinatal care* (Higgs, 1994; Lowry, Saeger, & Barnett, 1997); *postanesthesia care* (Heffline, 1991); *psychiatric and community care* (Chiverton, Tortoretti, LaForest, & Walker, 1999; Lee, 1995); *psychiatric care* (Waddell & Demi, 1993); *quality of life* (Robinson, 1998); *sexual abuse* (Barnes, 1993; Goble, 1991); *school nursing* (Mannina, 1997); *shared governance* (George, 1997); *spinal cord injury* (Hayes, 1994); *stress and hardiness in students and educators* (Cox, 1995; Hood, 1997); *stress and nurse managers* (Holloway, 1995); *substance abuse* (Bemker, 1996; Hanson, 1995; Monahan, 1996; Poole, 1991); *Sudden Infant Death Syndrome* (Barnes-McDowell, 1997); *spiritual care* (Carrigg & Weber, 1997); *terminal illness* (Hainsworth, 1996); *trauma care* (Bueno, Redeker, & Norman, 1992); *ventilator dependent patients* (Lowry & Anderson, 1993); *women's health* (Parodi, 1997; Scalzo, 1992; Taggart & Mattson, 1996; Tarmina, 1992). Education: *associate* (Bloch & Bloch, 1995; Hilton & Grafton, 1995; Lowry & Newsome, 1995); *baccalaureate* (Bremner & Initili, 1999; Glazebrook, 1995; Klotz, 1995; Knox, Kilchenstein, & Yakulis, 1982; Kilchenstein & Yakulis, 1984; Madrid & Stefanson, 1999; McHolm & Geib, 1998; Neuman, 1995; Strickland-Seng, 1995; Walker, 1995); *baccalaureate and graduate* (Edwards & Kittler, 1991; Neuman, 1995; Stittich, Flores, & Nuttall, 1995); *interdisciplinary* (Toot, Amaya, & Memmott, 1999); and *graduate* (Neuman, 1995).
- Yugoslavia: Practice in *primary health care* (Neuman, 1995); *baccalaureate education* (Neuman, 1995).

This listing is not intended to present a comprehensive review of all use of the Neuman Systems Model, but nevertheless provides impressive documentation of the widespread contagiousness of the model.

STRENGTHS AND WEAKNESSES OF THE NEUMAN SYSTEMS MODEL

The major strength of the Neuman Systems Model is its flexibility for use in all areas of nursing—research, administration, education, and practice. The third edition of *The Neuman Systems Model* includes many chapters that discuss the use of the model in all of these areas throughout the United States and in Australia, Canada, England, Holland, Sweden, and Wales. This widespread acceptance supports the essentially universal applicability of the model.

Neuman (1995) reports that the model was designed for nursing but can be used by other health disciplines, which can be viewed as either a strength or weakness. As a strength, if multiple health disciplines use the model, a consistent approach to client care will be facilitated. If all disciplines use similar data collection techniques based on the assessment tool presented by Neuman, perhaps the client would not have to tell his or her story so many different times—at least once to each health care discipline. As a weakness, if the model is useful to a variety of disciplines, it is not specific to nursing and thus may not differentiate the practice of nursing from that of other disciplines.

The major weakness of the model is the need for further clarification of terms used. Interpersonal and extrapersonal stressors need to be more clearly differentiated. It may be that interpersonal stressors occur between two people and extrapersonal stressors occur between a group or society and the person. This differentiation is not clearly made. Other areas that require greater specification are how to identify variances of wellness and levels of wellness. Reaction also needs to be defined.

There are some inconsistencies in the presentation of the Neuman Systems Model. The pictorial diagram includes reaction; reaction is not specifically discussed in the text. Conversely, the verbal presentation incorporates health, environment, and nursing, which do not appear in the diagram. It is inferred that the diagram is considered to be the most important representation of the model because it is changes in the diagram that require unanimous agreement of the Neuman Trustees. Logically, based on this inference, the concepts in the verbal presentation should be derived from the diagram.

Other inconsistencies relate to Neuman's emphasis on a wholistic approach and a comprehensive review of the client system and her discussion of health and illness. The wholistic and comprehensive view is associated with an open system. Health and illness are presented on a continuum with movement toward health described as negentropic and toward illness as entropic. Entropy is a characteristic of a closed, rather than an open, system. She does speak of levels of wellness, rather than levels of illness, but does not make it clear if health and illness are dichotomous.

SUMMARY

The Neuman Systems Model was developed to help teach graduate students an integrated approach to client care. The model is based in general system theory and views the client as an open system that responds to stressors in the environment. The client variables are physiological, psychological, sociocultural, developmental, and spiritual. The client system consists of a basic or core structure that is protected by lines of resistance. The usual level of health is identified as the normal line of defense that is protected by a flexible line of defense. Stressors are intra-, inter-, and extrapersonal in nature and arise from the internal, external, and created environments. When stressors break through the flexible line of defense, the system is invaded, the lines of resistance are activated, and the system is described as moving into illness on a wellness–illness continuum. If adequate energy is available or can be generated, the system will be reconstituted with the normal line of defense restored at, below, or above its previous level. Nursing interventions occur through three prevention modalities: primary prevention occurs before the stressor invades the system; secondary prevention occurs after the system has reacted to an invading stressor; and tertiary prevention occurs after secondary prevention as reconstitution is being established.

This model has been widely used in all areas of nursing. Its flexibility and universality are documented in the many publications that describe its use in nursing education, research, administration, and direct patient care. Further definition of some of the concepts in the model will serve to strengthen it further.

REFERENCES

Ågren, C., Fröistedt, M., & Olsson, H. (1999). Identifying stress in trainee psychiatric care nurses using the Neuman Systems Model. Paper presented at *The 7th Biennial International Neuman Systems Model Symposia*, Vancouver, British Columbia, Canada, April 9, 1999.

Allen, K. S. (1997). The effect of cancer diagnosis information on the anxiety of patients with an initial diagnosis of first cancer. *Masters Abstracts International, 35*(04), 996. (University Microfilms No. AAG1384216)

Al-Nagshabandi, E. A. H. (1993). An exploration of the physical and psychological responses of surgically-induced menopausal Saudi women using the Neuman Systems Model. *Dissertation Abstracts International, 55*(04B), 1374. (University Microfilms No. AAG941282)

Ali, N. S., & Khalil, H. Z. (1989). Effect of psychoeducational intervention on anxiety among Egyptian bladder cancer patients. *Cancer Nursing, 12*, 236–242.

Backe, H., & Olsson, H. (1999). Stress amongst student nurses: An application of the Neuman Systems Model. Paper presented at *The 7th Biennial International Neuman Systems Model Symposia*, Vancouver, British Columbia, Canada, April 9, 1999.

Baerg, K. L. (1991). Using Neuman's model to analyze a clinical situation. *Rehabilitation Nursing, 16*(1), 38–39.

Barnes, M. E. (1993). Knowledge, experiences, attitudes, and assessment practices of nurse practitioners with regard to stressors related to childhood sexual abuse. *Masters Abstracts International, 32*(01), 223. (University Microfilms No. AAG1353486)

Barnes-McDowell, B. M. (1997). Home apnea monitoring: Family functioning, concerns, and coping (Sudden Infant Death Syndrome, parents). *Dissertation Abstracts International, 58*(03B), 1205. (University Microfilms No. AAG9726731)

Barnes-McDowell, B., & Freese, B. (1999). MEG's meeting: Dialog in diversity. Paper presented at *The 7th Biennial International Neuman Systems Model Symposia*, Vancouver, British Columbia, Canada, April 9, 1999.

Barron, L. A. (1998). Diabetes self-management and psychosocial adjustment. *Masters Abstracts International, 37*(02), 587. (University Microfilms No. AAG1392504)

Barrow, J. M. (1992). Type A behavior, job stress, social support, and job satisfaction in critical care nurses. Unpublished thesis, Northwestern State University of Lousiana, Shreveport. Louisiana.

Bass, L. S. (1991). What do parents need when their infant is a patient in the NICU? *Neonatal Network: Journal of Neonatal Nursing, 10*(4), 25–38.

Beddome, G. (1995). Community-as-client assessment: A Neuman-based guide for education and practice. In B. Neuman, *The Neuman Systems Model* (3rd ed.) (pp. 567–579). Stamford, CT: Appleton & Lange.

Bemker, M. A. (1996). Adolescent female substance abuse: Risk and resiliency factors (drug abuse, marijuana, learned helplessness, dependency). *Dissertation Abstracts International, 57*(12B), 7446. (University Microfilm No. AAG9714858)

Beynon, C. C. (1995). Neuman-based experiences of the Middlesex-London Health Unit. In B. Neuman, *The Neuman Systems Model* (3rd ed.) (pp. 537–547). Stamford, CT: Appleton & Lange.

Beynon, C., & Laschinger, H. K. (1993). Theory-based practice: Attitudes of nursing managers before and after educational sessions. *Public Health Nursing, 10*, 183–188.

Beckingham, A. C., & Baumann, A. (1990). The ageing family in crisis: Assessment and decision-making models. *Journal of Advanced Nursing, 15*, 782–787.

Bergstrom, D. (1992). Hypermetabolism in multisystem organ failure: A Neuman systems perspective. *Critical Care Nursing Quarterly, 15* (3), 63–70.

Berkey, K. M., & Hanson, S. M. (1991). *Pocket guide to family assessment and intervention.* St Louis: Mosby-Year Book.

Bigbee, J. L., & Jansa, N. (1991). Strategies for promoting health protection. *Nursing Clinics of North America, 26*, 895–913.

Bittinger, J. P. (1995). Case management and satisfaction with nursing care of patients hospitalized with congestive heart failure. *Dissertation Abstracts International, 56*(07B), 3688. (University Microfilm No. AAI9537111)

Black, P., Deeny, P., & McKenna, H. (1997). Sensoristrain: An exploration of nursing interventions in the context of the Neuman systems theory. *Intensive & Critical Care Nursing, 13,* 249–258.

Bloch, C., & Bloch, C. (1995). Teaching content and process of the Neuman Systems Model. In B. Neuman, *The Neuman Systems Model* (3rd ed.) (pp. 175–182). Stamford, CT: Appleton & Lange.

Bowles, L., Oliver, N., & Stanley, S. (1995). A fresh approach . . . Staff in two wards formed a discussion group to create a new people-centred tool of assessment for rehabilitation. *Nursing Times, 91*(1), 40–41.

Bowman, A. M. (1997). Sleep satisfaction, perceived pain and acute confusion in elderly clients undergoing orthopedic procedures. *Journal of Advanced Nursing, 26,* 550–564.

Breckenridge, D. M. (1997a). Decisions regarding dialysis treatment modality: A holistic perspective. *Holistic Nursing Practice, 12*(1), 54–61.

Breckenridge, D. M. (1997b). Patients' perceptions of why, how, and by whom dialysis treatment modality was chosen . . . including commentary by Whittaker, A. A. and Locking-Cusolito, H. with author response. *ANNA Journal, 24*, 313–321.

Bremner, M. N., & Initili, H. (1999). Development of an academic and community partnership using the Neuman Systems Model at a large urban hotel. Paper presented at *The 7th Biennial International Neuman Systems Model Symposia*, Vancouver, British Columbia, Canada, April 8, 1999.

Brown, F. A. (1994). The effects of an eight-hour affective education program on fear of AIDS and homophobia in student nurses. *Masters Abstracts International, 33*(05), 1487. (University Microfilm No. AAI1361079)

Brown, K. C., Sirles, A. T., Hilyer, J. C., & Thomas, M. J. (1992). Cost-effectiveness of a back school intervention for municipal employees. *Spine, 17*, 1224–1228.

Bueno, M. M., Redeker, N., & Norman, E. M. (1992). Analysis of motor vehicle crash data in an urban trauma center: Implications for nursing practice and research. *Heart & Lung: Journal of Critical Care, 21*, 558–567.

Bueno, M. M., & Sengin, K. K. (1995). The Neuman Systems Model for critical care nursing. In B. Neuman, *The Neuman Systems Model* (3rd ed.) (pp. 275–291). Stamford, CT: Appleton & Lange.

Bullock, L. F. C. (1993). Nursing interventions for abused women on obstetrical units. *AWHONN's Clinical Issues in Perinatal and Women's Health Nursing, 4,* 371–377.

Bunn, H. (1995). Preparing nurses for the challenge of the new focus on community mental health nursing. *Journal of Continuing Education in Nursing, 26*(2), 55–59.

Butrin, J. (1992). Cultural diversity in the nurse-client encounter. *Clinical Nursing Research, 1,* 238–251.

Butts, M. J. (1998). Outcomes of comfort touch in institutionalized elderly female residents (Nursing homes, women). *Dissertation Abstracts International, 59*(07B), 3344. (University Microfilm No. AAG9839828)

Cagle, R. (1996). The relationship between health care provider advice and the initiation of breast-feeding. *Dissertation Abstracts International, 57*(08B), 4974. (University Microfilm No. AAG9700009)

Cammuso, B. S. (1994). *Caring and accountability in nursing practice in Ireland and the United States: Helping Irish nurses bridge the gap when they choose to practice in the United States.* Unpublished doctoral dissertation. Clark University, UMI PUZ9417668

Carrigg, K. C., & Weber, R. (1997). Development of the Spiritual Care Scale. *Image: Journal of Nursing Scholarship, 29,* 293.

Capers, C. F. (1996, September/October). The Neuman Systems Model: A culturally relevant perspective. *The Association of Black Nursing Faculty Journal,* 113–117.

Caplan, G. (1964). *Principles of preventive psychiatry.* New York: Basic Books. [out of print]

Carras, C., & Olsson, H. (1999). Exploratory study of student nurse attitudes to humour using Neuman Systems Model analysis. Paper presented at *The 7th Biennial International Neuman Systems Model Symposia,* Vancouver, British Columbia, Canada, April 8, 1999.

Cava, M. A. (1992). An examination of coping strategies used by long-term cancer survivors. *Canadian Oncology Nursing Journal, 2*(3), 99–102.

Cheung, Y. L. (1997). Student forum: The application of Neuman System Model to nursing in Hong Kong. *Hong Kong Nursing Journal, 33*(4), 17–21.

Chilton, L. L. A. (1996). The influence of behavioral cues on immunization practices of elders (influenza). *Dissertation Abstracts International, 57*(09B), 5572. (University Microfilm No. AAG9704005)

Chiverton, P., & Flannery, J. C. (1995). Cognitive impairment: Use of the Neuman Systems Model. In B. Neuman, *The Neuman Systems Model* (3rd ed.) (pp. 249–261). Stamford, CT: Appleton & Lange.

Chiverton, P., Tortoretti, D., LaForest, M., & Walker, P. H. (1999). Bridging the gap between psychiatric hospitalization and community care: Cost and quality outcomes. *Journal of the American Psychiatric Nurses Association, 5*(2), 46–53.

Collins, C. R. (1999). The older widow-adult child relationship as an influence upon health promoting behaviors (Healthcare Decisions Questionnaire). *Dissertation Abstracts International, 60*(04B), 1527. (University Microfilm No. AAG9926389)

Collins, M. A. (1996). The relation of work stress, hardiness, and burnout among full-time hospital staff nurses. *Journal of Nursing Staff Development, 12*(2), 81–85.

Cookfair, J. M. (1996). *Nursing care in the community* (2nd ed.). St. Louis: Mosby-Year Book.

Cornu, A. (1957). *The origin of Marxist thought.* Springfield, IL: Thomas. [out of print]

Courchene, V. S., Patalski, E., & Martin, J. (1991). A study of the health of pediatric nurses administering cyclosporine A. *Pediatric Nursing 17,* 497–500.

Cowperthwaite, B., LaPlante, K., Mahon, B., & Markowski, T. (1997). Latex allergy in the nursing population. *Canadian Operating Room Nursing Journal, 15*(2), 23–24, 26–28, 30–32.

Cox, D. D. (1995). *The impact of stress, coping, constructive thinking and hardiness on health and academic performance of female registered nurse students pursuing a baccalaureate degree in nursing.* Unpublished doctoral dissertation, University of Pittsburgh, Pittsburgh, PA.

Craig, D. M. (1995). The Neuman Model: Examples of its use in Canadian educational programs. In B. Neuman, *The Neuman Systems Model* (3rd ed.)(pp. 521–527). Stamford, CT: Appleton & Lange.

Craig, D. M., & Morris-Coulter, C. (1995). Neuman implementation in a Canadian psychiatric facility. In B. Neuman, *The Neuman Systems Model* (3rd ed.) (pp. 397–406). Stamford, CT: Appleton & Lange.

Crawford, J., Tarko, M., Ting, B., Gunderson, J., & Andrews, H. (1999). The Neuman Systems Model: A conceptual framework for advanced psychiatric/mental health nursing education. Poster presented at *The 7th Biennial International Neuman Systems Model Symposia*, Vancouver, British Columbia, Canada, April 8, 1999.

Cullen, L. M. (1993). Nurses' perceptions of humor as a preventive intervention to promote the health of clients in a health care setting. *Masters Abstracts International, 32*(02), 592. (University Microfilm No. AAG1353482)

Dale, M. L., & Savala, S. M. (1990). A new approach to the senior practicum. *NursingConnections, 3*(1), 45–51.

Damant, M. (1995). Community nursing in the United Kingdom: A case for reconciliation using the Neuman Systems Model. In B. Neuman, *The Neuman Systems Model* (3rd ed.) (pp. 607–620). Stamford, CT: Appleton & Lange.

Davidson, J., & Myers, J. (1999). Neuman Systems Model: Application to organizational systems. Poster presented at *The 7th Biennial International Neuman Systems Model Symposia*, Vancouver, British Columbia, Canada, April 8, 1999.

Davies, P., & Proctor, H. (1995). In Wales: Using the Model in community mental health nursing. In B. Neuman, *The Neuman Systems Model* (3rd ed.) (pp. 621–627). Stamford, CT: Appleton & Lange.

de Chardin, P. T. (1955). *The phenomenon of man*. London: Collins. [out of print]

Decker, S. D., & Young, E. (1991). Self-perceived needs of primary caregivers of home-hospice clients. *Journal of Community Health, 8*, 147–154.

Delunas, L. R. (1990). Prevention of elder abuse: Betty Neuman health care systems approach. *Clinical Nurse Specialist, 4*(1), 54–58.

de Meij, J., & de Kuiper, M. (1999). The Neuman Systems Model as the basis for the curriculum of the Dutch Reformed College for Higher Education, Department of Nursing. Paper presented at *The 7th Biennial International Neuman Systems Model Symposia*, Vancouver, British Columbia, Canada, April 7, 1999.

Derstine, J. B. (1992). Theory-based advanced rehabilitation nursing: Is it a reality? *Holistic Nursing Practice, 6*(2), 1–6.

Drew, L. L., Craig, D. M., & Beynon, C. E. (1989). The Neuman Systems Model for community health administration and practice: Provinces of Manitoba and Ontario, Canada. In B. Neuman, *The Neuman Systems Model* (2nd ed.)(pp. 315–341). Norwalk, CT: Appleton & Lange.

Edelson, M. (1970). *Sociotherapy and psychotherapy*. Chicago: University of Chicago. [out of print]

Edwards, P. A., & Kittler, A. W. (1991). Integrating rehabilitation content in nursing curricula. *Rehabilitation Nursing, 16*, 70–73.

Eilert-Petersson, E., & Olsson, H. (1999). Humor and slimming related to NSM. Poster presented at *The 7th Biennial International Neuman Systems Model Symposia*, Vancouver, British Columbia, Canada, April 8, 1999.

Emery, F. (Ed.). (1969). *Systems thinking*. Baltimore: Penguin Books. [out of print]

Engberg, I. B. (1995). Brief abstracts: Use of the Neuman Systems Model in Sweden. In B. Neuman, *The Neuman Systems Model* (3rd ed.) (pp. 653–656). Stamford, CT: Appleton & Lange.

Engberg, I. B., Bjälming, E., & Bertilson, B. (1995). A structure for documenting primary health care in Sweden using the Neuman Systems Model. In B. Neuman, *The Neuman Systems Model* (3rd ed.) (pp. 637–651). Stamford, CT: Appleton & Lange.

Evely, L. (1994). A model for successful breastfeeding. *Modern Midwife, 4*(12), 25–27.

Fawcett, J. (1995). Constructing conceptual-theoretical-empirical structures for research: Future implications for use of the Neuman Systems Model. In B. Neuman, *The Neuman Systems Model* (3rd ed.) (pp. 459–471). Stamford, CT: Appleton & Lange.

Fawcett, J. (1999). An integrative review of Neuman Systems Model-based research. Paper presented at *The 7th Biennial International Neuman Systems Model Symposia*, Vancouver, British Columbia, Canada, April 9, 1999.

Felix, M., Hinds, C., Wolfe, S. C., & Martin, A. (1995). The Neuman Systems Model in a chronic care facility: A Canadian experience. In B. Neuman, *The Neuman Systems Model* (3rd ed.)(pp. 549–565). Stamford, CT: Appleton & Lange.

Fillmore, J. A. (1992). The effects of preoperative teaching on anxiety levels of hysterectomy patients. Unpublished thesis, University of Nevada, Las Vegas.

Flanders-Stepans, M. B., & Fuller, S. G. (1999). Physiological effects of infant exposure to environmental tobacco smoke: A passive observation study. *Journal of Perinatal Education, 8*(1), 10–21.

Flannery, J. (1991). FAMLI-RESCUE: A family assessment tool for use by neuroscience nurses in the acute care setting. *Journal of Neuroscience Nursing, 23,* 111–115.

Flannery, J. (1995). Cognitive assessment in the acute care setting: Reliability and validity of the Levels of Cognitive Functioning Assessment Scale (LOCFAS). *Journal of Nursing Measurement, 3*(1), 43–58.

Foote, A. W., Piazza, D., & Schultz, M. (1990). The Neuman Systems Model: Application to a patient with a cervical spinal cord injury. *Journal of Neuroscience Nursing, 22,* 302–306.

Fowler, B. A., & Risner, P. B. (1994). A health promotion program evaluation in a minority industry. *ABNF Journal, 5*(3), 72–76.

Freiberger, D., Bryant, J., & Marino, B. (1992). The effects of different central venous line dressing changes on bacterial growth in a pediatric oncology population. *Journal of Pediatric Oncology Nursing, 9,* 3–7.

Fulbrook, P. R. (1991). The application of the Neuman systems model to intensive care. *Intensive Care Nursing, 7*(1), 28–39.

Fulton, B. J. (1992). Evaluation of the effectiveness of the Neuman Systems Model as a theoretical framework for baccalaureate nursing program. *Dissertation Abstracts International, 53*(11B), 5641. (University Microfilm No. AAG9305991)

Fukuzawa, M. (1995). Nursing care behaviors which predict patient satisfaction. *Masters Abstracts International, 34*(04), 1547. (University Microfilm No. AAI1378670)

Galloway, D. A. (1993). Coping with a mentally and physically impaired infant: A self-analysis. *Rehabilitation Nursing, 18*(1), 34–36.

Gavigan, M., Kline-O'Sullivan, C., & Klumpp-Lybrand, B. (1990). The effect of regular turning on CABG patients. *Critical Care Nursing Quarterly, 12*(4), 69–76.

Geiger, P. A. (1996). Participation in a Phase II cardiac rehabilitation program and perceived quality of life. *Masters Abstracts International, 34*(04), 1548. (University Microfilm No. AAI1378753)

Gellner, P., Landers, S., O'Rourke, D., & Schlegel, M. (1994). Community health nursing in the 1990s—risky business? *Holistic Nursing Practice, 8*(2), 15–21.

George, J. (1997). Nurses' perceived autonomy in a shared governance setting. *Journal of Shared Governance, 3*(2), 17–21.

Gibson, M. (1996). Health promotion for a group of elderly clients. *Perspectives, 20*(3), 2–5.

Gifford, D. K. (1996). Monthly incidence of stroke in rural Kansas. *Kansas Nurse, 71*(5), 3–4.

Gigliotti, E. (1998). You make the diagnosis. Case study: Integration of the Neuman Systems Model with the theory of nursing diagnosis in postpartum nursing . . . including commentary by M. Lunney. *Nursing Diagnosis, The Journal of Nursing Language and Classification, 9*(1), 14, 34–38.

Gigliotti, E. (1999a) The use of Neuman's lines of defense and resistance in the published nursing research literature. Paper presented at *The 7th Biennial International Neuman Systems Model Symposia*, Vancouver, British Columbia, Canada, April 9, 1999.

Gigliotti, E. (1999b). Women's multiple role stress: Testing Neuman's flexible line of defense. *Nursing Science Quarterly, 12*, 36–44.

Glazebrook, R. S. (1995). The Neuman Systems Model in cooperative baccalaureate nursing education: The Minnesota Intercollegiate Nursing Consortium experience. In B. Neuman, *The Neuman Systems Model* (3rd ed.) (pp. 227–230). Stamford, CT: Appleton & Lange.

Goble, D. S. (1991). A curriculum framework for the prevention of child sexual abuse (sexual abuse prevention, Neuman systems, Tyler's rationale). *Dissertation Abstracts International, 52*(06A), 2004. (University Microfilm No. AAG9133480)

Goodman, H. (1995). Patients' views count as well. *Nursing Standard, 9*(40), 55.

Grant, J. S., & Bean, C. A. (1992). Self-identified needs of informal caregivers of head-injured adults. *Family & Community Health, 15*(2), 49–58.

Grant, J. S., Kinney, M. R., & Davis, L. L. (1993). Using conceptual frameworks or models to guide nursing research. *Journal of Neuroscience Nursing, 25*(1), 52–56.

Gray, R. (1998). The lived experience of children, ages 8–12 years, who witness family violence in the home. *Masters Abstracts International, 36*(05), 1327. (University Microfilm No. AAG1389149)

Gulliver, K. M. (1997). Hopelessness and spiritual well-being in persons with HIV infection (Immune Deficiency). *Masters Abstract International 35*(05), 1374. (University Microfilm No. AAG1385172)

Haggart, M. (1993). A critical analysis of Neuman's Systems Model in relation to public health nursing. *Journal of Advanced Nursing, 18*, 1917–1922.

Hainsworth, D. S. (1996). Research briefs. The effect of death education on attitudes of hospital nurses toward care of the dying. *Oncology Nursing Forum, 23*, 963–967.

Hanson, M. S. (1995). *Beliefs, attitudes, subjective norms, perceived behavioral control, and cigarette smoking in white, African-American, and Puerto Rican-American teenage women*. Unpublished doctoral dissertation, University of Pennsylvania, Philadelphia, PA.

Hanson, P. A. (1997). An application of Bowen Family Systems Theory: Triangulation, differentiation of self and nurse manager job stress responses. *Dissertation Abstracts International, 58*(11B), 5889. (University Microfilm No. AAG9815103)

Harper, B. (1992). Nurses' beliefs about social support and the effect of nursing care on cardiac clients' attitudes in reducing cardiac risk factors. *Masters Abstracts International, 31*(01), 273. (University Microfilm No. AAG1349176)

Hassell, J. S. (1996). Improved management of depression through nursing model application and critical thinking. *Journal of the American Academy of Nurse Practitioners, 8*, 161–166.

Hayes, K. V. D. (1994). Diagnostic content validation and operational definitions of risk factors for the nursing diagnosis high risk for disuse syndrome (spinal cord injury). *Dissertation Abstracts International, 55*(12B), 5284. (University Microfilm No. AAI9511772)

Heaman, D. J. (1991). Perceived stressors and coping strategies of parents with developmentally disabled children (stressors). *Dissertation Abstracts International, 52*(12B), 6316. (University Microfilms No. AAG9208071)

Heffline, M. S. (1991). Second place: A comparative study of pharmacological versus nursing interventions in the treatment of postanesthesia shivering—Mary Hanna Memorial Journalism Award winner. *Journal of Post Anesthesia Nursing, 6*, 311–320.

Henze, R. L. (1993). The relationship among selected stress variables and white blood count in severely head injured patients. *Dissertation Abstracts International, 55*(02B), 365. (University Microfilm No. AAG9419287)

Herald, P. A. (1993). Relationship between hydration status and renal function in patients receiving aminoglycoside antibiotics. *Dissertation Abstracts International, 55*(02B), 365. (University Microfilm No. AAF9419288)

Herrick, C. A., Goodykoontz, L., Herrick, R. H., & Hackett, B. (1991). Planning a continuum of care in child psychiatric nursing: A collaborative effort. *Journal of Child and Adolescent Psychiatric and Mental Health, 4*(2), 41–48.

Heslin, K. (1986). *A systems analysis of the Betty Neuman model.* Unpublished student paper. University of Western Ontario, London, Ontario, Canada.

Higgs, K. T. (1994). Preterm labor risk factors identified in an ambulatory perinatal setting with home uterine activity monitoring support. *Masters Abstracts International, 33*(05), 1490. (University Microfilm No. AAI1360323)

Hilton, S. A., & Grafton, M. D. (1995). Curriculum transition based on the Neuman Systems Model. In B. Neuman, *The Neuman Systems Model* (3rd ed.) (pp. 163–174). Stamford, CT: Appleton & Lange.

Hiltz, D. (1990). The Neuman Systems Model: An analysis of a clinical situation. *Rehabilitation Nursing, 15,* 330–332.

Hinds, C. (1990). Personal and contextual factors predicting patients' reported quality of life: Exploring congruency with Betty Neuman's assumptions. *Journal of Advanced Nursing, 15,* 456–462.

Holloway, C. (1995). Stress perceived among nurse managers in community health settings. *Masters Abstracts International, 33*(05), 1490. (University Microfilm No. AAI1361519)

Hood, L. J. (1997). The effects of nurse faculty hardiness and sense of coherence on perceived stress, scholarly productivity, and job satisfaction (stress). *Dissertation Abstracts International, 58*(09B), 4720. (University Microfilm No. AAG9809243)

Ivey, B. (1993). Evaluation of social support tools for women with diagnosed breast cancer. Unpublished thesis, University of Nevada, Las Vegas.

Jennings, K. M. (1997). Predicting intention to obtain a pap smear among African-American and Latina women (cervical cancer, cancer prevention). *Dissertation Abstracts International, 58*(07B), 3557. (University Microfilm No. AAG9800878)

Janze, T. R., Watson, D. B., & Stevenson, R. W. D. (1999). Quality of life in patients with gender identity disorder. Paper presented at *The 7th Biennial International Neuman Systems Model Symposia*, Vancouver, British Columbia, Canada, April 8, 1999.

Johnson, K. M. (1995). Stressors of local Ontario Nurses' Association presidents. *Masters Abstracts International, 34*(03), 1149. (University Microfilm No. AAI1376934)

Jones, W. R. (1996). Stressors in the primary caregivers of traumatic head injured persons. *AXON, 18*(1), 9–11.

Kahn, E. C. (1992). A comparison of family needs based on the presence or absence of DNR orders. *DCCN: Dimensions of Critical Care Nursing, 11,* 286–292.

Kazakoff, K. J. (1990). The evaluation of return to work and retention of employment of cardiac patients following cardiac rehabilitation programs. *Masters Abstracts International, 29*(03), 450. (University Microfilms No. AAG1343456)

Kido, L. M. (1991). Sleep deprivation and intensive care unit psychosis. *Emphasis: Nursing, 4*(1), 23–33.

Kilchenstein, L., & Yakulis, I. (1984). The birth of a curriculum: Utilization of the Betty Neuman Health Care Systems Model in an integrated baccalaureate program. *Journal of Nursing Education, 23,* 126–127.

Klotz, L. C. (1995). Integration of the Neuman Systems Model into the BSN curriculum at the University of Texas at Tyler. In B. Neuman, *The Neuman Systems Model* (3rd ed.) (pp. 183–195). Stamford, CT: Appleton & Lange.

Knight, J. B. (1990). The Betty Neuman Systems Model applied to practice: A client with multiple sclerosis. *Journal of Advanced Nursing, 15,* 447–455.

Knox, J. E., Kilchenstein, L., & Yakulis, I. M. (1982). Utilization of the Neuman Model in an integrated baccalaureate program: University of Pittsburgh. In B. Neuman, *The Neuman Systems Model: Application to nursing education and practice* (pp. 117–123). Norwalk, CT: Appleton-Century-Crofts.

Koku, R. V. (1992). Severity of low back pain: A comparison between participants who did and did not receive counseling. *AAOHN Journal, 40*(2), 84–89.

Lamb, K. A. (1998). Baccalaureate nursing students' perception of empathy and stress in their inter-actions with clinical instructors: Testing a theory of optimal student system stability according to the Neuman Systems Model. *Dissertation Abstracts International, 60*(03B), 1028. (University Microfilms No. AAG9923301)

Lancaster, D. R. N. (1991). Coping with appraised threat of breast cancer: Primary prevention cop-ing behaviors utilized by women at increased risk. *Dissertation Abstracts International, 53*(01B), 202. (University Microfilms No. AAG9215110)

Larino, E. A. (1997). Determining the level of care provided by the family nurse practitioner during a deployment. *Masters Abstracts International, 35*(05), 1376. (University Microfilms No. AAG1385132)

Laschinger, H. K., & Duff, V. (1991). Attitudes of practicing nurses towards theory-based nursing practice. *Canadian Journal of Nursing Administration, 4*(1), 6–10.

Laszlo, E. (1972). *The systems view of the world: The natural philosophy of the new development in the sciences.* New York: Braziller. [out of print]

Lazarus, R. (1981). The stress and coping paradigm. In C. Eisdorfer, D. Cohen, A. Kleinman, & P. Maxim (Eds.), *Models for clinical psychopathology* (pp. 177–214). New York: SP Medical and Scientific Books.

Lee, P. L. (1995). Caregiver stress as experienced by wives of institutionalized and in-home demen-tia husbands. *Dissertation Abstracts International, 56*(06B), 4241. (University Microfilms No. AAI9541861)

Leja, A. M. (1989). Using guided imagery to combat postsurgical depression. *Journal of Geronto-logical Nursing, 15*(4), 6–11.

Lijauco, C. C. (1997). Factors related to length of stay in coronary artery bypass graft patients. *Mas-ters Abstracts International, 36*(02), 512.

Lile, J. L. (1990). A nursing challenge for the 90's: Reducing risk factors for coronary heart disease in women. *Health Values: Achieving High Level Wellness, 14*(4), 17–21.

Lile, J. L., Pase, M. N., Hoffman, R. G., & Mace, M. K. (1994). The Neuman Systems Model as ap-plied to the terminally ill client with pressure ulcers. *Advances in Wound Care: The Journal for Prevention and Healing, 7*(4), 44–48.

Lin, M., Ku, N., Leu, J., Chen, J., & Lin, L. (1996). An exploration of the stress aspects, coping be-haviors, health status and related aspects in family caregivers of hepatoma patients [Chinese]. *Nursing Research [China], 4*(2), 171–185.

Lindell, M., & Olsson, H. (1991). Can combined oral contraceptives be made more effective by means of a nursing care model? *Journal of Advanced Nursing, 16*, 475–479.

Lindgren, A., & Olsson, H. (1999). Elderly and humour-An interview study with NSM as reference. Poster presented at *The 7ᵗʰ Biennial International Neuman Systems Model Symposia*, Vancouver, British Columbia, Canada, April 8, 1999.

Loescher, L. J., Clark, L., Attwood, J. R., Leigh, S., & Lamb, G. (1990). The impact of cancer expe-rience on long-term survivors. *Oncology Nursing Forum, 17*, 223–229.

Louis, M. (1989). An intervention to reduce anxiety levels for nurses working with long-term care clients using Neuman's model. In J. P. Riehl-Sisca (Ed.), *Conceptual models for nursing prac-tice* (3rd ed.) (pp. 95–103). Norwalk, CT: Appleton & Lange.

Louis, M. (1995). The Neuman model in nursing research, an update. In B. Neuman, *The Neuman Systems Model* (3rd ed.) (pp. 473–495). Stamford, CT: Appleton & Lange.

Louis, M., & Koertvelyessy, A. (1989). The Neuman Model in nursing research. In B. Neuman (Ed.), *The Neuman Systems Model* (2ⁿᵈ ed.) (pp. 93–113). San Mateo, CA: Appleton & Lange.

Lowry, L. W. (1999). Critical pathways and the Neuman Systems Model. Paper presented at *The 7ᵗʰ Biennial International Neuman Systems Model Symposia*, Vancouver, British Columbia, Canada, April 8, 1999.

Lowry, L. W., & Anderson, B. (1993). Neuman's framework and ventilator dependency: A pilot study. *Nursing Science Quarterly, 6*, 195–200.

Lowry, L. W., & Newsome, G. G. (1995). Neuman-based associate degree programs: Past, present, and future. In B. Neuman, *The Neuman Systems Model* (3rd ed.) (pp. 197–214). Stamford, CT: Appleton & Lange.

Lowry, L. W., Saeger, J., & Barnett, S. (1997). Client satisfaction with prenatal care and pregnancy outcomes. *Outcomes Management for Nursing Practice, 1*(1), 29–35.

Mackenzie, S. J., & Laschinger, H. K. (1995). Correlates of nursing diagnosis quality in public health nursing. *Journal of Advanced Nursing, 21*, 800–808.

Madrid, E., & Stafanson, D. (1999). Diversity and dialogue: Use of the Neuman Systems Model in an RN-BSN curriculum. Paper presented at *The 7th Biennial International Neuman Systems Model Symposia*, Vancouver, British Columbia, Canada, April 7, 1999.

Maligalig, R. M. (1994). Parents' perceptions of the stressors of pediatric ambulatory surgery. *Journal of Post Anesthesia Nursing, 9*, 278–282.

Marlett, L. A. (1998). The breast feeding practices of women with a history of breast cancer. *Masters Abstracts International, 37*(04), 1180. (University Microfilm No. AAG1393760)

Marsh, V. (1997). Job stress and burnout among nurses: The mediational effect of spiritual well-being and hardiness. *Dissertation Abstracts International, 58*(08B), 4142. (University Microfilms No. AAG9804907)

Martin, S. A. (1996). Applying nursing theory to the practice of nurse anesthesia. *AANA Journal, 64*, 369–372.

Mann, A. H., Hazel, C., Geer, C., Hurley, C. M. & Podrapovic, T. (1993). Development of an orthopaedic case manager role. *Orthopaedic Nursing, 12*(4), 23–27.

Mannina, J. (1997). Finding an effective hearing testing protocol to identify hearing loss and middle ear disease in school aged children. *Journal of School Nursing, 13*(5), 23–28.

McCulloch, S. J. (1995). Utilization of the Neuman Systems Model: University of South Australia. In B. Neuman, *The Neuman Systems Model* (3rd ed.) (pp. 591–597). Stamford, CT: Appleton & Lange.

McGee, M. (1995). Implications for use of the Neuman Systems Model in occupational health nursing. In B. Neuman, *The Neuman Systems Model* (3rd ed.) (pp. 657–667). Stamford, CT: Appleton & Lange.

McHolm, F. A., & Geib, K. M. (1998). Application of the Neuman Systems Model to teaching health assessment and nursing process. *Nursing Diagnosis: The Journal of Nursing Language and Classification, 9*(1), 23–33.

McMillan, D. E. (1995). Impact of therapeutic support of inherent coping strategies on chronic low back pain: A nursing intervention study. *Masters Abstracts International, 35*(02), 520. (University Microfilms No. AAGMM13363)

Mendez, D. (1990). College students' image of nursing as a career choice. Unpublished thesis, University of Nevada, Las Vegas.

Micevski, V. (1996). Gender differences in the presentation of physiological symptoms of myocardial infarction. *Masters Abstracts International, 35*(02), 520. (University Microfilms No. AAG1382268)

Mill, J. E. (1997). Clinical. The Neuman Systems Model: Application in a Canadian HIV setting. *British Journal of Nursing, 6*, 163–166.

Millard, J. (1992). Health visiting an elderly couple. *British Journal of Nursing, 1*, 772–773.

Miner, J. (1995). Incorporating the Betty Neuman Systems Model into HIV clinical practice. *AIDS Patient Care, 9*(1), 37–39.

Mirenda, R. M. (1995). A conceptual-theoretical strategy for curriculum development in baccalaureate nursing programs. *Dissertation Abstracts International, 56*(10B), 5421. (University Microfilms No. AAI9601825)

Molassiotis, A. (1997). A conceptual model of adaptation to illness and quality of life for cancer patients treated with bone marrow transplants. *Journal of Advanced Nursing, 26*, 572–579.

Monahan, G. L. (1996). A profile of pregnant drug-using female arrestees in California: The relationships among sociodemographic characteristics, reproductive and drug addiction histories, HIV/STD risk behaviors, and utilization of prenatal care services and substance abuse treatment programs (immune deficiency). *Dissertation Abstracts International, 57*(09B), 5576. (University Microfilms No. AAG9704608)

Montgomery, P., & Craig, D. (1990). Levels of stress and health practices of wives of alcoholics. *Canadian Journal of Nursing Research, 22,* 60–70.

Moody, N. B. (1996). Nurse faculty job satisfaction: A national survey. *Journal of Professional Nursing, 12,* 277–288.

Moore, S. L., & Munro, M. F. (1990). The Neuman System Model applied to mental health nursing of older adults. *Journal of Advanced Nursing, 15,* 293–299.

Morris, D. C. (1991). Occupational stress among home care first line managers. *Masters Abstracts International, 29*(03), 443. (University Microfilms No. AAG1343455)

Mynatt, S. L., & O'Brien, J. (1993). A partnership to prevent chemical dependency in nursing using Neuman's systems model. *Journal of Psychosocial Nursing and Mental Health Services, 31*(4), 27–34.

Mytka, S., & Beynon, C. (1994). A model for public health nursing in the Middlesex-London, Ontario schools. *Journal of School Health, 64*(2), 85–88.

Narsavage, G. L. (1997). Promoting function in clients with chronic lung disease by increasing their perception of control. *Holistic Nursing Practice, 12*(1), 17–26.

Neabel, B. (1998). A comparison of family needs perceived by nurses and family members of acutely brain-injured patients. *Masters Abstracts International, 37*(02), 592. (University Microfilms No. AAGMQ32546)

Neuman, B. (1974). The Betty Neuman health-care systems model: A total person approach to patient problems. In J. P. Riehl & C. Roy (Eds.), *Conceptual models for nursing practice* (pp. 99–114). New York: Appleton-Century-Crofts. [out of print]

Neuman, B. (1982). *The Neuman Systems Model.* Norwalk, CT: Appleton-Century-Crofts. [out of print]

Neuman, B. (1989). *The Neuman Systems Model* (2nd ed.). Norwalk, CT: Appleton & Lange. [out of print]

Neuman, B. (1990). Health on a continuum based on the Neuman Systems Model. *Nursing Science Quarterly, 3,* 129–135.

Neuman, B. (1995). *The Neuman Systems Model* (3rd ed.). Norwalk, CT: Appleton & Lange.

Neuman, B. (1998). Neuman Systems Model and the Omaha System. *Image: Journal of Nursing Scholarship, 30*(1), 8.

Neuman, B. M., & Young, R. J. (1972). A model for teaching total person approach to patient problems. *Nursing Research, 21,* 264–269.

Nicholson, C. H. (1995). Clients' perceptions of preparedness for discharge home following total HIP or knee replacement surgery. *Masters Abstracts International, 33*(03), 873. (University Microfilms No. AAI1359739)

Norman, S. E. (1990). The relationship between hardiness and sleep disturbances in HIV-infected men. *Dissertation Abstracts International, 51*(10B), 4780. (University Microfilms No. AAG9104437)

Nortridge, J. A., Mayeux, V., Anderson, S. J., & Bell, M. L. (1992). The use of cognitive style mapping as a predictor for academic success of first-semester diploma nursing students. *Journal of Nursing Education, 31,* 352–356.

Olsson, H., & Leadersh, E. (1999). The retirement process and humor: A Swedish explorative study using Neuman Systems Model analysis. Paper presented at *The 7ᵗʰ Biennial International Neuman Systems Model Symposia,* Vancouver, British Columbia, Canada, April 7, 1999.

O'Neal, C. A. S. (1993). Effects of BSE on depression/anxiety in women diagnosed with breast cancer. *Masters Abstracts International, 31*(04), 1747. (University Microfilms No. AAG1352556)

Orr, J. P. (1993). An adaptation of the Neuman Systems Model to the care of the hospitalized preschool child. *Curationis: South African Journal of Nursing, 16*(3), 37–44.

Orr, J. (1999). Using the Neuman Systems Model to develop a training model for caregivers of abandoned children with HIV/AIDS. Paper presented at *The 7th Biennial International Neuman Systems Model Symposia*, Vancouver, British Columbia, Canada, April 8, 1999.

Owens, M. (1995). Care of a woman with Down's syndrome using the Neuman Systems Model. *British Journal of Nursing, 4, British Journal of Disability Nursing,* 752–758.

Pardee, C. J. (1992). Evaluating family caregivers' ability to select appropriate care techniques following discharge instructions on post traumatic brain injury symptoms. Unpublished thesis, Grand Valley State University, Michigan.

Parker, M. E. (Ed.). (1990). *Nursing theories in practice* (Pub. No. 15-2350) New York: National League for Nursing.

Parodi, V. A. (1997). Neuman based analysis of women's health needs abroad a deployed Navy ship: Can nursing make a difference? *Dissertation Abstracts International, 58*(12B), 6491. (University Microfilms No. AAG9818848)

Parr, M. S. (1993). The Neuman Health Care Systems Model—an evaluation. *British Journal of Theatre Nursing, 3*(8), 20–27.

Parse, R. R. (1987). *Nursing science-Major paradigms, theories, and critiques.* Philadelphia: Saunders.

Payne, P.L. (1993). A study of the teaching of primary prevention competencies as recommended by the Report of the Pew Health Professions Commission in bachelor of science in nursing programs and associate in nursing programs. *Dissertation Abstracts International,* 54(07B), 3553.

Peirce, A. G., & Fulmer, T. T. (1995). Application of the Neuman Systems Model to gerontological nursing. In B. Neuman, *The Neuman Systems Model* (3rd ed.) (pp. 293–308). Stamford, CT: Appleton & Lange.

Peoples, L. T. (1990). The relationship between selected client, provider, and agency variables and the utilization of home care services. *Dissertation Abstracts International,* 51(08B), 3782.

Peternelj-Taylor, C. A., & Johnson, R. (1996). Custody and caring: Clinical placement of student nurses in a forensic setting. *Perspectives in Psychiatric Care: The Journal for Nurse Psychotherapists, 32*(4), 23–29.

Peters, M. R. (1997). An exploratory study of job stress and stressors in hospice administration. *Masters Abstracts International, 36*(02), 502. (University Microfilms No.AAG1387515)

Peterson, G. A. (1997). Nursing perceptions of the spiritual dimension of patient care: The Neuman Systems Model in curriculum formations. *Dissertation Abstracts International, 59*(02B), 605. (University Microfilms No. AAG9823988)

Petock, A. M. (1990). Decubitus ulcers and physiological stressors. *Masters Abstracts International, 29*(02), 267. (University Microfilms No. AAG1341348)

Piazza, D., Foote, A., Wright, P., & Holcombe, J. (1992). Neuman Systems Model used as a guide for the nursing care of an 8-year-old child with leukemia. *Journal of Pediatric Oncology Nursing, 9*(1), 17–24.

Picton, C. E. (1995). An exploration of family-centred care in Neuman's model with regard to the care of the critically ill adult in an accident and emergency setting. *Accident and Emergency Nursing, 3*(1), 33–37.

Picot, S. J., Zauszniewski, J. A., Debanne, S. M., & Holston, E. C. (1999). Mood and blood pressure in black female caregivers and noncaregivers. *Nursing Research, 48,* 150–161.

Pierce, J. D., & Hutton, E. (1992). Applying the new concepts of the Neuman Systems Model. *Nursing Forum, 27*(1), 15–18.

Poole, V. L. (1991). Pregnancy wantedness, attitude toward pregnancy, and use of alcohol, tobacco and street drugs during pregnancy. *Dissertation Abstracts International,* 52(10B), 5193.

Pothiban, L. (1993). Risk factor prevalence, risk status, and perceived risk for coronary heart disease among Thai elderly. *Dissertation Abstracts International, 54*(03B), 1337. (University Microfilms No. AAG9319896)

Puetz, R. (1990). Nurse and patient perception of stressors associated with coronary artery bypass surgery. Unpublished thesis, University of Nevada, Las Vegas.

Radwanski, M. (1992). Self-medicating practices for managing chronic pain after spinal cord injury. *Rehabilitation Nursing, 17,* 312–318.

Ramsey, B. A. (1999). Can a multidisciplinary team decrease hospital length of stay for elderly trauma patients? *Masters Abstracts International, 37*(04), 1182.

Reed, K. S. (1993). Adapting the Neuman Systems Model for family nursing. *Nursing Science Quarterly, 6,* 93–97.

Reed, K. (1999). Using Neuman's variables as a map for concept analysis. Paper presented at *The 7th Biennial International Neuman Systems Model Symposia,* Vancouver, British Columbia, Canada, April 9, 1999.

Ridgell, N. H. (1993). Home apnea monitoring: A systems approach to the family's home care needs. *Caring, 12*(12), 34–37.

Riehl-Sisca, J. (1989). *Conceptual models for nursing practice* (3rd ed.). Norwalk, CT: Appleton & Lange.

Roberts, A. G. (1994). Effective inservice education process. *Oklahoma Nurse, 39*(4), 11.

Robin, N. S. (1991). Clinical evaluation of the ectopic pregnancy risk assessment screening tool: A retrospective study. Unpublished thesis, University of Texas HealthScience Center at Houston.

Robinson, C. A. (1998). The difference in perception of quality of life in patients one year after an infrainguinal bypass for critical limb ischemia. *Masters Abstracts International, 37*(03), 914. (University Microfilms No. AAG13922664)

Rodrigues-Fisher, L., Bourguignon, C., & Good, B. V. (1993). Dietary fiber nursing intervention: Prevention of constipation in older adults. *Clinical Nursing Research, 2,* 464–477.

Roggensack, J. (1994). The influence of perioperative theory and clinical in a baccalaureate nursing program on the decision to practice perioperative nursing. *Prairie Rose, 63*(2), 6–7.

Rosenfeld, R. M., Goldsmith, A. J., & Madell, J. R. (1998). How accurate is parent rating of hearing for children with otitis media? *Archives of Otolaryngology-Head Neck Surgery, 124,* 989–992.

Ross, M. M., Bourbonnais, F. F., & Carroll, G. (1987). Curricular design and the Betty Neuman Systems Model: A new approach to learning. *International Nursing Review, 34*(3/273), 75–79.

Rowles, C. J. (1992). The relationship of selected personal and organizational variables and the tenure of directors of nursing in nursing homes. *Dissertation Abstracts International, 53*(09B), 4593. (University Microfilms No. AAG9302488)

Russell, J., & Hezel, L. (1994). Role analysis of the advanced practice nurse using the Neuman Health Care Systems Model as a framework. *Clinical Nurse Specialist, 8,* 215–220.

Russell, J., Hileman, J. W., & Grant, J. S. (1995). Assessing and meeting the needs of home caregivers using the Neuman Systems Model. In B. Neuman, *The Neuman Systems Model* (3rd ed.) (pp. 331–341). Stamford, CT: Appleton & Lange.

Sabo, C. E., & Michael, S. R. (1996). The influence of personal message with music on anxiety and side effects associated with chemotherapy. *Cancer Nursing, 19,* 283–289.

Scalzo Tarrant, T. (1992). Improving the frequency and proficiency of breast self examination. *Masters Abstracts International, 31*(03), 1211. (University Microfilms No. AAG1351247)

Scicchitani, B., Cox, J. G., Heyduk, L. J., Maglicco, P. A., & Sargent, N. A. (1995). Implementing the Neuman Model in a psychiatric hospital. In B. Neuman, *The Neuman Systems Model* (3rd ed.) (pp. 387–395). Stamford, CT: Appleton & Lange.

Schlentz, M. D. (1993). The Minimum Data Set and levels of prevention in the long-term care facility. *Geriatric Nursing: American Journal of Care for the Aging, 14,* 79–83.

Selye, H. (1950). *The physiology and pathology of exposure to stress.* Montreal, Quebec, Canada: ACTA. [out of print]

Semple, O. D. (1995). The experiences of family members of persons with Huntington's Disease. *Perspectives, 19*(4), 4–10.

Shaw, M. C. (1991). A theoretical base for orthopaedic nursing practice: The Neuman Systems Model. *CONA Journal ACIIO, 13* (2), 19–21.

Simmons, L., & Borgdon, C. (1991). The clinical nurse specialists in HIV care. *Kansas Nurse, 66*(1), 6–7.

Skipwith, D. H. (1994). Telephone counseling interventions with caregivers of elders. *Journal of Psychosocial Nursing and Mental Health Services, 32*(3), 7–12.

South, L. D. (1995). The relationship of self-concept and social support in school age children with leukemia. *Dissertation Abstracts International, 56*(04B), 1939. (University Microfilms No. AAI9527022)

Speck, B. J. (1990). The effect of guided imagery upon first semester nursing students performing their first injections. *Journal of Nursing Education, 29,* 346–350.

Stittich, E. M., Fores, F. C., & Nuttall, P. (1995). Cultural considerations in a Neuman-based curriculum. In B. Neuman, *The Neuman Systems Model* (3rd ed.) (pp. 147–162). Stamford, CT: Appleton & Lange.

Strickland-Seng, V. (1995). The Neuman Systems Model in clinical evaluation of students. In B. Neuman, *The Neuman Systems Model* (3rd ed.) (pp. 215–225). Stamford, CT: Appleton & Lange.

Stuart, G. W., & Wright, L. K. (1995). Applying the Neuman Systems Model to psychiatric nursing practice. In B. Neuman, *The Neuman Systems Model* (3rd ed.) (pp. 263–273). Stamford, CT: Appleton & Lange.

Taggart, L., & Mattson, S. (1996). Delay in prenatal care as a result of battering in pregnancy: Cross-cultural implications. *Health Care for Women International, 17*(1), 25–34.

Tarko, M., & Crawford, J. (1999). Spirituality: The core dimension of the Neuman Systems Model applied to health assessment in psychiatric nursing education. Paper presented at *The 7th Biennial International Neuman Systems Model Symposia*, Vancouver, British Columbia, Canada, April 8, 1999.

Tarmina, M. S. (1992). Self-selected diet of adult women with families. *Dissertation Abstracts International,* 53(02B), 0777.

Timmermans, O. (1999). A practical guideline for the implementation of the Neuman Systems Model in an Institute for Mental Health Care. Paper presented at *The 7th Biennial International Neuman Systems Model Symposia*, Vancouver, British Columbia, Canada, April 7, 1999.

Toot, J., Amaya, M. A., & Memmott, R. J. (1999). Interdisciplinary applications: Neuman Systems Model as a conceptual paradigm for interdisciplinary team. Paper presented at *The 7th Biennial International Neuman Systems Model Symposia*, Vancouver, British Columbia, Canada, April 10, 1999.

Trépanier, M., Dunn, S. I., & Sprague, A. E. (1995). Application of the Neuman Systems Model to perinatal nursing. In B. Neuman, *The Neuman Systems Model* (3rd ed.) (pp. 309–320). Stamford, CT: Appleton & Lange.

Vaughan, B., & Gough, P. (1995). Use of the Neuman Systems Model in England. In B. Neuman, *The Neuman Systems Model* (3rd ed.) (pp. 599–605). Stamford, CT: Appleton & Lange.

Verberk, F. (1995). In Holland: Application of the Neuman Model in psychiatric nursing. In B. Neuman, *The Neuman Systems Model* (3rd ed.) (pp. 629–636). Stamford, CT: Appleton & Lange.

Vitthuhn, K. M. (1999). Delivery of analgesics for the postoperative thoracotomy patient. *Masters Abstracts International, 37*(04), 1185. (University Microfilms No. AAG1393446)

von Bertalanffy, L. (1968). *General system theory.* New York: Braziller. [out of print]

Waddell, K. L., & Demi, A. S. (1993). Effectiveness of an intensive partial hospitalization program for treatment of anxiety disorders. *Archives of Psychiatric Nursing, 7*(1) 2–10.

Walker, P. H. (1994). Dollars and sense in health reform: Interdisciplinary practice and community nursing centers. *Nursing Administration Quarterly, 19*(1), 1–11.

Walker, P. H. (1995). Neuman-based education, practice, and research in a community nursing center. In B. Neuman, *The Neuman Systems Model* (3rd ed.) (pp. 415–430). Stamford, CT: Appleton & Lange.

Ware, L. A., & Shannahan, M. K. (1995). Using Neuman for a stable parent support group in neonatal intensive care. In B. Neuman, *The Neuman Systems Model* (3rd ed.) (pp. 321–330). Stamford, CT: Appleton & Lange.

Waters, T. (1993). Self-efficacy, change, and optimal client stability. *Addictions Nursing Network, 5*(2), 48–51.

Watson, L. A. (1991). Comparison of the effects of usual, support, and informational nursing interventions on the extent to which families of critically ill patients perceive their needs were met. *Dissertation Abstracts International, 52*(06B), 2999. (University Microfilms No. AAG9134244)

Weinberger, S. L. (1991). Analysis of a clinical situation using the Neuman Systems Model. *Rehabilitation Nursing, 16*, 278, 280–281.

Westrik, G. J. (1999). Addiction and spiritual well being in the health perspective of the Neuman Systems Model. Paper presented at *The 7th Biennial International Neuman Systems Model Symposia*, Vancouver, British Columbia, Canada, April 9, 1999.

Wilkey, S. F. (1990). The effects of an eight-hour continuing education course on the death anxiety levels of registered nurses. *Masters Abstracts International, 28*(04), 480. (University Microfilms No. AAG1340601)

Williamson, J. W. (1992). The effects of ocean sounds on sleep after coronary artery bypass graft surgery. *American Journal of Critical Care, 1*(1), 91–97.

Wormald, L. (1995). Samuel—the boy with tonsillitis. A care study. *Intensive and Critical Care Nursing, 11*, 157–160.

Wright, J. G. (1996). The impact of preoperative education on health locus of control, self-efficacy, and anxiety for patients undergoing total joint replacement surgery. *Masters Abstracts International, 35*(01), 216. (University Microfilms No. AAG1382185)

ANNOTATED BIBLIOGRAPHY*

Barker, E., Robinson, D., & Brautigan, R. (1999). The effect of psychiatric home nurse follow-up on readmission rates of patients with depression. Journal of the American Psychiatric Nurses Association, 5(4), 111–16.

This study used the Neuman Systems Model as a conceptual framework to study hospital readmission rates of patients with depression in those who had home follow-up visits by psychiatric nurses and those who did not. Findings included a substantial reduction in hospital readmissions in the group that received the in-home visits, even though both groups received similar outpatient care.

Black, P., Deeny, P., & McKenna, H. (1997). Sensoristrain: An exploration of nursing interventions in the context of the Neuman systems theory. Intensive & Critical Care Nursing, 13, 249–58.

This paper used the Neuman Systems Model to create a framework for nursing practice using prevention as intervention in comfort care, knowing the patient, and therapeutic presence of the nurse to reduce sensory strain in intensive care patients. It seeks to link nursing actions with patient outcomes.

*Selected material published in English since 1995.

Chiverton, P., Tortoretti, D., LaForest, M., & Walker, P. H. (1999). Bridging the gap between psychiatric hospitalization and community care: Cost and quality outcomes. Journal of the American Psychiatric Nurses Association, 5(2), 46–53.

This study investigated quality indicators, patient satisfaction, and costs of care related to recidivism and rehospitalization in psychiatric patients who received transitional case management services and those who received traditional care. No differences in levels of depression or in mental status were found between the groups. Those who received the transitional care management expressed high levels of satisfaction, had much lower readmission and emergency department visit rates. The costs of providing the transitional case management were significantly less than the costs for readmission and emergency department visits.

Gifford, D. K. (1996). Monthly incidence of stroke in rural Kansas. Kansas Nurse, 71(5), 3–4.

This study investigated the role of environment through studying the relationship between month of admission to a medical center and the primary medical diagnosis of cerebrovascular accident. No significant relationships were found between the total number of admissions per month and the primary diagnosis of stroke. Conclusions were that the environmental characteristics of the area possibly have no effect on the incidence of stroke.

Gigliotti, E. (1999). Women's multiple role stress: Testing Neuman's flexible line of defense. Nursing Science Quarterly, 12, 36–44.

This study used the Neuman Systems Model as conceptual framework to investigate the relations between a stressor (multiple roles: maternal and student roles), flexible line of defense (perceived social support), and normal line of defense (perceived multiple role stress). Statistically significant findings included that social support helped explain multiple role stress in women aged 37 and older. This group of women broadened its social support network, including support from children, friends at school, work associates, and clergy. Support from husband was inversely associated with multiple role stress in both the younger and older groups of women.

Hanson, M. J. (1999). Cross-cultural study of beliefs about smoking among teenaged females. Western Journal of Nursing Research, 21, 635–51.

This study used the Neuman Systems Model as a conceptual framework to study smoking behavior in African American, Puerto Rican, and non-Hispanic white females, aged 13 to 19. Statistically significant relations between beliefs and smoking behavior in each ethnic group were found. The specific beliefs differed among the groups.

Jones, W. R. (1996). Stressors in the primary caregivers of traumatic head injured patients. AXON, 18(1), 9–11.

This study used the Neuman Systems Model to identify intrapersonal, interpersonal, and extrapersonal stressors in individuals who are primary caregivers for persons who have suffered a traumatic head injury. While stressors in all three categories were identified, only intrapersonal and interpersonal stressors were positively correlated with changing levels of stress.

McHolm, F. A., & Geib, K. M. (1998). Application of the Neuman Systems Model to teaching health assessment and nursing process. Nursing Diagnosis: The Journal of Nursing Language and Classification, 9(1), 23–33.

Faculty developed a nursing theory framework for teaching health assessment to beginning level baccalaureate nursing students. The faculty concluded that students who could make connections between the Neuman Systems Model and NANDA nursing diagnoses within the nursing process would be able to make better choices about appropriate nursing diagnoses.

Marsh, V., Beard, M. T., & Adams, B. N. (1999). Job stress and burnout: The mediational effect of spiritual well-being and hardiness among nurses. Journal of Theory Construction & Testing, 3(1), 13–19.

An empirical test of a model developed from NSM and Selye's stress theory. Results supported that job stress had a direct positive effect on burnout among nurses while spiritual well-being had a direct negative effect. When operating through hardiness, spiritual well-being had an indirect negative effect on burnout. The study supported the inclusion of spiritual well-being in considering job burnout.

Molassiotis, A. (1997). A conceptual model of adaptation to illness and quality of life for cancer patients treated with bone marrow transplants. Journal of Advanced Nursing, 26, 572–79.

The Neuman Systems Model provides the basis for this model of adaptation to illness and the resultant quality of life in cancer patients who receive bone marrow transplants. The model has five stages. The first stage begins with the stressor or initial stimuli and the perception of that stressor as a threat. The second stage involves the reaction to the threat producing stressor. The third stage describes the adaptive or maladaptive coping activities related to dealing with the illness as a threat. The fourth stage includes nursing care using prevention as interventions. The fifth stage is the level of adaptation—from adaptation to illness and satisfaction with life to maladjustment and low quality of life. Included in each of these stages are the personal variables (physiological, psychological, social, development). It should be noted that the spiritual variable is not described.

Moody, N. B. (1996). Nurse faculty job satisfaction: A national survey. Journal of Professional Nursing, 12, 277–88.

In a survey of nursing faculty in universities offering a doctorate of nursing, the Neuman Systems Model was used with other theories to construct a system's framework to investigate job satisfaction of nursing faculty. Demographic variables were significantly correlated with measures of job satisfaction. The contributors to a regression model of nursing faculty job satisfaction were salary, degree level of nursing student taught, and the length of the annual contract for faculty.

Narsavage, G. L. (1997). Promoting function in clients with chronic lung disease by increasing their perception of control. Holistic Nursing Practice, 12(1), 17–26.

The Neuman Systems Model provided the format for assessing persons with chronic obstructive pulmonary disease and developing their perception of control as a secondary prevention as intervention. Control is defined as an intrapersonal component that interacts with the physiologic, sociocultural, developmental, and spiritual variables to affect stability. Methods included in the secondary prevention as intervention include use of assessment tools, diaries, relaxation, and other stress management techniques.

Picot, S. J., Zauszniewski, J. A., Debanne, S. M., & Holston, E. C. (1999). Mood and blood pressure in black female caregivers and noncaregivers. Nursing Research, 48, 150–61.

This study investigated the relationship between the mood symptoms of anger, anxiety, and sadness, and ambulatory daytime blood pressure in a group of black female caregivers of a dependent elder and in a group of noncaregivers. The findings indicated a negative relationship between anger and diastolic blood pressure, leading to a recommendation for further study of whether low anger scores represent low levels of perceived anger or suppressed anger.

Sabo, C. E., & Michael, S. R. (1996). The influence of personal message with music on anxiety and side effects associated with chemotherapy. Cancer Nursing, 19, 283–89.

This pilot study investigated the use of a recorded message with a musical background to reduce anxiety and side effects in persons receiving chemotherapy. There was no significant difference in the severity of side effects between the experimental and control groups. Those in the experimental group did demonstrate statistically significant lower levels of state anxiety.

The reader is encouraged to seek information from Dissertation Abstracts International, either in print or online, about the multitude of thesis and dissertation reports that demonstrate the use of the Neuman Systems Model in research. The numbers are too great to be included in this annotation.

CHAPTER 17

HUMANISTIC NURSING

JOSEPHINE G. PATERSON AND LORETTA T. ZDERAD*

Susan G. Praeger

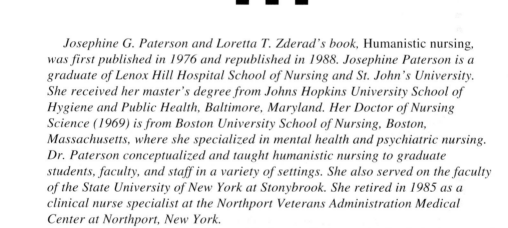

Josephine G. Paterson and Loretta T. Zderad's book, Humanistic nursing, *was first published in 1976 and republished in 1988. Josephine Paterson is a graduate of Lenox Hill Hospital School of Nursing and St. John's University. She received her master's degree from Johns Hopkins University School of Hygiene and Public Health, Baltimore, Maryland. Her Doctor of Nursing Science (1969) is from Boston University School of Nursing, Boston, Massachusetts, where she specialized in mental health and psychiatric nursing. Dr. Paterson conceptualized and taught humanistic nursing to graduate students, faculty, and staff in a variety of settings. She also served on the faculty of the State University of New York at Stonybrook. She retired in 1985 as a clinical nurse specialist at the Northport Veterans Administration Medical Center at Northport, New York.*

Loretta T. Zderad is a graduate of St. Bernard's Hospital School of Nursing and of Loyola University. She received her Master of Science degree from Catholic University, Washington, DC, and a Doctor of Philosophy (1968) from Georgetown University, Washington, DC. She has taught in several universities and has led groups on humanistic nursing. Dr. Zderad also served on the faculty of the State University of New York at Stonybrook. She retired in 1985 as the Associate Chief for Nursing Education at the Northport Veterans Administration Medical Center, Northport, New York.

---

*Paterson and Zderad use the term *man* in the generic sense to identify a human being.

385

Josephine G. Paterson and Loretta T. Zderad describe a "humanistic nursing practice" theory in several publications and presentations. Humanistic nursing practice is developed from the lived experiences of the nurse and the person receiving care. Theory becomes a response to the phenomenological experience. R. D. Laing is quoted as saying that "theory is the articulated vision of experience" (Laing, 1967, p. 23). In other words, nursing practice is the basis for our beliefs about nursing. Our experience in the world of health care is the foundation for understanding the nature of nursing and what it means to be a nurse.

Humanistic nursing is concerned with the phenomenological experiences of individuals and the exploration of human experiences. It requires entering the nursing situation fully aware of the "lenses" that we wear. We need to know what values, biases, myths, and expectations we bring to the nursing experience. And we need to fully appreciate the values, biases, myths, and expectations others bring to the nursing experience. For example, the experience between a nurse and a woman facing an unplanned pregnancy can be significantly affected by the nurse's views of childbearing choices, adoption, and pregnancy termination, as well as the client's values, experiences, expectations, and response to the nurse. The combination of these perspectives brings uniqueness to nursing.

The practice of humanistic nursing is rooted in existential thought. Existentialism is a philosophical approach to understanding life. Individuals are faced with possibilities when making choices. These choices determine the direction and meaning of one's life. Existentialism developed as a response to the dominant philosophies of positivism and determinism. A nineteenth century philosophical approach found in the writings of Kierkegaard and Nietzsche, existentialism emerged in popularity during the twentieth century with two world wars and the threat of nuclear destruction as major social concerns. Individuals needed to understand life in personally relevant terms.

The early writings of existentialists provided a basis for viewing human existence in individually meaningful terms. With the opportunity for choice, each act we choose is significant and gives meaning to our lives. One of the criticisms leveled against existentialism has been that it presents a despairing view of life (Paterson & Zderad, 1976/1988). Since individuals are faced with freedom of choice, there is always the possibility of making errors. Imagine (or remember) the experience of being an adolescent making career and personal choices while facing developmental issues related to autonomy, identity, body image, and peer acceptance. Intimacy, sexual activity, success, independence, contraception, fear of failure, and risk taking all play a part in the daily experience of a middle to late adolescent and influence the eventual outcome of this time of life. Consequently, adolescents can experience dread as well as hope in the possible consequences of their action.

According to Corey (2000), existential thought has relevance for the helping professions. Existentialism identifies individuals as (1) having the capacity for self-awareness; (2) having freedom and responsibility; (3) striving to find their own identity while being in relationships with others; (4) being involved in a search for meaning in life; (5) having to experience anxiety or dread if they are going to assume responsibility for their own lives; and finally, (6) being aware of the reality of death in order to experience the significance of living. Consequently, each individual has choices. We live in a world of possibilities, and the responsibility for making the most out of this existence rests within each of us. As a philosophy, existentialism is particularly applicable to nursing within the framework of holistic health because of the emphasis on self-determination, free choice, and self-responsibility.

Phenomenology, the study of the meaning of a phenomenon to a particular individual, is thought to have influenced the development of existentialism because existentialism requires an analysis of the human situation from the perspective of the individual's own experience (Shaffer, 1978). When combined with humanism into an existential-phenomenological-humanistic approach, we are referring to a reverence for life that values the need for human interaction in order to determine the meaning that comes from the individual's unique way of experiencing the world. Although we are ultimately alone in choosing the paths our lives will take, we can find meaning in sharing our experiences with others who are also facing the uncertain choices of daily living.

Humanistic nursing is nursing's response to existentialism, phenomenology, and the humanistic movement in psychology, which was proposed as an alternative to the two dominant psychological views of the time. Freudian psychology was seen as being limited in its orientation toward psychopathology, and behavioral psychology was seen as being too mechanistically oriented. The humanistic orientation described a broader view of the potential of human beings from the context of their experience of living in the world. Rather than trying to supplant other views, humanistic psychology sought to supplement our understanding (Bugental, 1978). Humanistic nursing care with the adolescent experiencing an unplanned pregnancy is more than presenting facts and options, more than lending a supportive ear, more than facilitating value clarification, and more than the steps of the nursing process. Nurses must acknowledge their own struggles and needs as part of the process of living. Simultaneously, they must acknowledge the importance of the struggles and needs of others. For the clients it is more than the unburdening of uncertainties and the process of choosing. It is the knowledge that their experience is unique but also shared. Only by interaction with others, by recognizing the human experience that is unique for each of us but also shared, can we truly enter into a humanistic nursing practice.

That Paterson and Zderad have been influenced by the writings of existentialists, humanistic psychologists, and phenomenologists is seen in their emphasis on the meaning of life as it is lived, the nature of dialogue, and the importance of the perceptual field. The influence of scholars such as Bergson (1946), Buber (1965), de Chardin (1961), Desan (1972), Hesse (1966), Jung (1933), Marcel (1956), and Nietzsche (1927) is readily apparent in the writings of Paterson and Zderad. Their work, *Humanistic nursing*, is a result of years of experience in clinical nursing, reflection, and exploration of their experiences as they have been lived with clients, students, nurses, and other helping professionals.

HUMANISTIC NURSING THEORY

Nursing occurs within the context of relationship. It is a nurturing response of one person to another in a time of need that aims toward the development of well-being and more-being. Nursing works toward this aim by helping to increase the possibility of making responsible choices. "The nursing situation is a particular kind of human situation in which the interhuman relating is purposely directed toward nurturing the well-being or more-being of a person with perceived needs related to the health-illness quality of living" (Paterson & Zderad, 1976/1988, p.19/18). Nursing is concerned with the individual's unique being and striving toward becoming. Nursing focuses on the whole and looks beyond the categorizations of the parts. When a person is ill and the body is manifesting certain changes, these changes influence the person's world and the experience of being in the world. The client's perspective of the world is a vital consideration in nursing. As Paterson and Zderad say:

> Nursing implies a special kind of meeting of human persons. It occurs in response to a perceived need related to the health-illness quality of the human condition. Within that domain, which is shared by other health professions, nursing is directed toward the goal of nurturing well-being and more-being (human potential). Nursing, therefore does not involve a merely fortuitous encounter but rather one in which there is purposeful call and response. In this vein, humanistic nursing may be considered as a special kind of lived dialogue (Paterson & Zderad, 1976/1988, p. 26/24).

Nursing is a unique blend of theory and methodology. The theory is articulated from the open framework that is derived from the human situation. Theory cannot exist without the practice of nursing, for it depends on the experience of nursing and the reflection of that experience. The reflection of and the practice of nursing actually revitalize each other and give meaning to each other. "Some old ideas are always new" (Paterson & Zderad, 1976/1988, p. 25/23) emphasizes the wonder of the art of humanistic nursing practice. As the young woman grapples with her choices, the nurse intimately understands how the client's decision will impact the rest of her life and is present with her in that moment of movement toward the future. As nurses, we accept and know that each action has consequences, that each person is ultimately responsible. We know this objectively as nurses. We know this subjectively as persons. But in the nursing situation, we learn it anew as an intersubjective experience between the nurse and the client.

The practice of nursing, its methodology, is a unique blend of art and science. Paterson and Zderad suggest that nurses have downplayed the art of nursing in an attempt to be accepted among other empirical disciplines. However, science and art both play critical roles in humanistic nursing. If one thinks of the rules of thermoregulation, fluid and electrolyte balance, grieving, and development as examples of our science, we can see that these rules guide us. They give direction to our nursing practice. But laws, principles, and theories remain meaningless unless they are applied to living situations. How a nurse uses theory in response to knowing a client is the art of nursing. The art of nursing is embodied in the interaction between the nurse and the client. Like all art, that interaction is often meaningful, effective, and capable of leaving a lasting impression. Nursing as an art is being able to use theories within the context of life as people struggle to become all that they are capable of becoming. The elements of the framework for humanistic nursing are:

> Incarnate men (patient and nurse) meeting (being and becoming) in a
> goal-directed (nurturing well-being and more-being), intersubjective

transaction (being with and doing with) occurring in time and space (as measured and as lived by patient and nurse) in a world of men and things (Paterson and Zderad, 1976/1988, p. 23/21).

To use this framework for a nursing practice theory the authors suggest three concepts that provide the basis (or components) of nursing: dialogue, community, and phenomenologic nursology. By coming together through dialogue, a community is formed through which nursing strives to nurture and comfort. The concepts that form this theory generate mental pictures of people touching, listening, laughing, crying, contemplating, and being in the day-to-day world. An appreciation of the importance of these people to ourselves and to those we work with provides the model of humanistic nursing.

Dialogue

Nursing is a lived dialogue. It is the nurse–nursed relating creatively. Humans need nursing. Nurses need to nurse. Nursing is an intersubjective experience in which there is real sharing. Involved in this dialogue are meeting, relating, presence, and a call and response (Paterson & Zderad, 1976/1988).

Meeting. Meeting is the coming together of human beings and is characterized by the expectation that there will be a nurse and a nursed. Factors that influence this meeting are feelings that are aroused by the anticipation of the meeting, the amount of control that the nurse or client has in coming together, the uniqueness of the nurse and the client, and the decision for disclosure and enclosure with the other.

Relating. The process of nurse–nursed "doing" with each other is relating, being with the other. Two ways of relating are described that distinguish the human situation. We are able to relate as subject to object as well as subject to subject, both of which are essential to relationships (Paterson & Zderad, 1976/1988). Subject–object relating refers to how we use objects and know others through abstractions, conceptualizations, categorizing, labeling, and so on. As a nurse I know about the developmental tasks of adolescents, their need for intimacy, their propensity for risk taking, and this tempers my relationship with a young client. But nursing also involves subject–subject relating when both the nurse and the client are open to each other as fully human, beyond the role of nurse and client, but as struggling, joyful, confused, and hopeful individuals facing the next moment. The "I–Thou" relationship described by Martin Buber (1958) provides the opportunity to develop this unique potential. Paterson and Zderad (1976/1988) describe relating as follows:

> Through the scientific objective approach, that is, subject–object relating, it is possible to gain certain knowledge about a person; through intersubjective, that is, subject–subject relating, it is possible to know a person in his unique individuality. Thus, both subject–subject and subject–object relationships are essential to the clinical nursing process. Both are integral elements of humanistic nursing (p. 30/27).

Presence. The quality of being open, receptive, ready, and available to another person in a reciprocal manner is presence. It is not merely being attentive. It is being open to the whole of the nursing experience, a sometimes difficult quality when the nurse needs to focus on specific details of the client's body or behavior. Poetically, Paterson and Zderad (1976/1988) describe the pull to be present.

> Two humans stand on the brink of the between for a precious moment filled with promise and fear. With my hand on the doorknob to open myself from within, I hesitate—should I, will I let me out, let him in? Time is suspended, then moves again as I move with resolve to recognize, to give testimony to the other presence (p. 30/28).

Presence varies depending on the nature of the interaction. When we are with family and friends our presence is different than when we are in the nursing situation and our professional presence influences our regard for the client's vulnerability. As nurses we have a responsibility to the client so that our " . . . presence flows through a filter of therapeutic tact" (p. 31/29).

Call and response. The complex nature of the lived dialogue is seen in call and response. Call and response are transactional, sequential, and simultaneous. Nurses and clients call and respond to each other both verbally and nonverbally, and there is the potential to be "all-at-once." Paterson and Zderad (1976/1988) describe "all-at-once" as nurses being able to relate simultaneously to the subjective and objective aspects of the lived situation even though we can only express this experience orally or in writing in succession.

It is through nursing acts that the dialogue of nursing is lived. The meaning of those acts to the nurse and to the client may differ and may be a potential catalyst for effecting change in the dialogue. When considering nursing as a lived dialogue, it is necessary to take into account the situation in which it occurs, the world of people and things within a framework of time and space.

Community

The phenomenon of community is the second component critical to humanistic nursing practice theory. It is two or more persons striving together, living-dying all at once. To understand community is to recognize and value uniqueness. Humanistic nursing leads to community, it occurs within a community, and is affected by community. It is through the intersubjective sharing of meaning in community that human beings are comforted and nurtured. Community is the experience of persons, and it is through community, persons relating to others, that it is possible to become. This component represents the strong humanistic influence of the theory. People find meaning in their existence by sharing and relating to others. Paterson and Zderad consider community as the "We" that occurs with clients, families, professional colleagues, and other health care providers. Traditional conceptualizations of community may be helpful for organizing one's thoughts, but the authors caution us not to limit our views. One of the greatest gifts that we can bring to the nursing experience is our " . . . ability to relate to other man, to wonder, to search, and imagine about [our] experience, to create out of what [we] come to know" (Paterson and Zderad, 1976/1988, p. 43/39).

Each community is influenced by its past, its values, its goals, and its resources. Because each of us is in a process of becoming, there is bound to be struggle within ourselves, between ourselves, and between communities. It is the responsibility of the nurse to acknowledge and value those differences in our struggles and hence in our communities. For instance, the nurse in a community with high teen pregnancy and infant morbidity rates, may value and want to institute teen pregnancy prevention measures including abstinence initiatives, local contraceptive availability, and classroom education. However, the teens may not be interested in abstinence, the church groups may have a commitment to family-based discussions of sexuality, and local pharmacies may limit over-the-counter contraception to "behind the counter" availability to limit loss from shoplifting. Humanistic nursing proposes that the nurse needs to be fully prepared to work in and with a community, exploring and valuing its reality. "Over time a merger of the values of the nurse and of the existing community would be reflected in the moreness in each. . . . Each would make an important difference in the other" (Paterson and Zderad, 1976/1988, p. 53/48).

Phenomenologic Nursology

Nursing, its practice and theory, would not be complete without a methodology that Paterson and Zderad call phenomenologic nursology. There are five phases in this approach to nursing.

   1. *Preparation of the nurse knower for coming to know*. The nurse is ever prepared and striving to be open and caring. This involves learning to take risks, being open to experiences, to one's own view of the world, and to another's perceptual framework. To achieve this, the nurse needs to be exposed to a wide range of experiences. Nurses can be prepared for this by immersing themselves in study of the humanities, where varying views about the nature of being are expressed. The wider the range of experiences the nurse has, the wider the possibility for knowing. Relating the experiences of others to the nurse's experience with clients opens the way for knowing individuals in the nursing situation. Self-knowledge, the "authenticity with self," is important to knowing and can be facilitated through clinical supervision and different forms of personal growth therapy (Paterson & Zderad, 1976/1988).

   2. *Nurse knowing the other intuitively.* This phase is the merging of the self with the rhythmic spirit of the other. Intuitive knowing requires getting "inside," into the rhythm of the other's experience, resulting in a special, difficult to express, knowledge of the other. Intuitive knowing presumes the I–Thou relationship described by Buber (1958). It also presumes a phenomenological approach of being open to the meaning of the experience for the other. In order to intuitively grasp the nursing situation, Paterson and Zderad (1976/1988) suggest going into the nursing situation without preconceived notions, avoiding expectations, labeling, and judgments. Self-awareness of one's philosophical and theoretical biases is critical. Being aware of how nursing routines dull our sensitivities can enhance our perspective.

For instance, routine testing of urine, blood pressure, and fetal heart tones during prenatal visits can reduce the pregnant woman to feeling like a weigh-and-check station. When we use closed-end questions or checklists during assessment, we limit in advance the range of responses that a client can give. Openness and a refusal to be lulled by routines help nurses better appreciate the subtle nuances involved in human interaction.

3. *Nurse knowing the other scientifically*. This phase implies a separateness from what is known. It requires taking the all-at-once phenomena that are known intuitively, then looking at them, pondering, analyzing, sorting, comparing, contrasting, relating, interpreting, naming, and categorizing them. This is taking the I–Thou and reflecting on it as an "it." Paterson and Zderad (1976/1988, p. 79–80/73) say that "The challenge of communicating a lived nursing reality demands authenticity with the self and rigorous effort in the selection of words, phrases, and precise grammar." To achieve this goal, the nurse must be adequately prepared not only in the sciences, but in the art of communication in order to seek clarification and verification from the client. Nurses need to be able to reflect critically on the experience at the same time they are immersed in the experience. For example, when working with adolescents who are struggling with home, school, and relationship problems, the unfolding of their story can be laid out in a genogram and ecomap (see Figures 17–1 and 17–2). These tools can be used to identify patterns over generations, to visualize recurrent themes, and to help the adolescent recognize areas of strengths as well as areas of risk.

4. *Nurse complementarily synthesizing known others*. This phase involves relating, comparing, and contrasting what occurs in nursing situations to enlarge one's understanding. The nurse compares and synthesizes multiple known realities and arrives at an expanded view. The nurse allows a dialogue between the realities and permits differences (Paterson & Zderad, 1976/1988). In this phase, the nurse uses not only personal experience but also the rich theoretical foundation of education and practice in order to put the clinical situation in perspective.

5. *Succession within the nurse from the many to the paradoxical one*. The fifth phase evolves from the descriptive process of a lived phenomenon. It is the articulated vision of experience that becomes expressed in a coherent whole. This phase is the process of refining the intuitive grasp, struggling with the known realities, and making an intuitive leap toward truth, thus forming a new hypothetical construct. It is a truth beyond the synthesis of the whole. The nurse starts with a general notion, an intuitive grasp; then studies it, compares, contrasts, and synthesizes it in order to arrive at a truth that is uniquely personal but has meaning for all (the paradoxical one), a descriptive theoretical construct of nursing.

These last three phases (analysis, synthesis, and description) involve many of the same techniques. In each of the phases, the nurse compares and contrasts the phenomena. Commonalities in various experiences are explored as well as the relationship between variables in the clinical situation. It is important to determine what distinguishes one phenomenon from another. For example, why do some women respond to

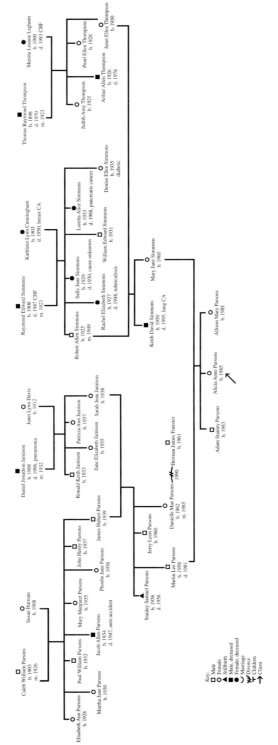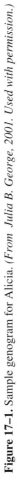

Figure 17–1. Sample genogram for Alicia. (*From Julia B. George, 2001. Used with permission.*)

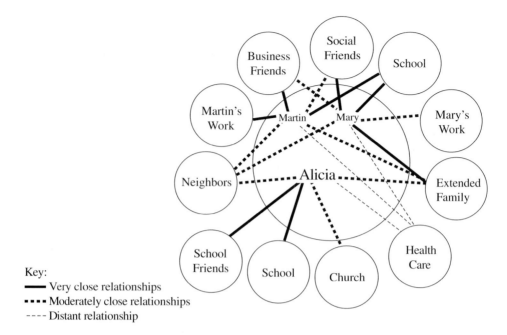

Figure 17–2. Ecomap for Alicia and her parents *(From Julia B. George, 2001. Used with permission.)*

menopause with fear and grieving, while others experience it as a time of joy and re-newed energy? Other techniques for analyzing, synthesizing, and describing a nursing phenomenon include stating what it is not, or using analogy or metaphor. These tech-niques help the nurse better understand the meaning of the experience (Paterson & Zderad, 1976/1988).

HUMANISTIC NURSING AND NURSING'S METAPARADIGM

Human Beings

In the theory of humanistic nursing practice, human beings are viewed from an existen-tial framework of becoming through choices. "Man is an individual being necessarily related to other men in time and space. As every man is beholden to other men for his birth and development, interdependence is inherent in the human situation . . . [and] human existence is coexistence" (Paterson & Zderad, 1976/1988, p. 16/15). Human beings are characterized as being capable, open to options, persons with values, and the unique manifestation of their past, present, and future. It is through relationships with others that the human being becomes, which in turn, allows for each person's unique individuality to become actualized. Implications for nursing practice are clear. People need information. They need options. They need to be viewed as competent and able to make choices. Individuals and groups need opportunities to make their own choices.

Environment

The phenomenon of society or environment comprises part of what Paterson and Zderad refer to as community. Humanistic nursing must take into account all aspects of community: the fact that we live our lives in communities of others, of time, of space, and of experiences. It is only through community that we are able to reach our full potential.

Health

Health is a matter of personal survival, a process of experiencing one's potential for well-being and more-being, a quality of living and dying. It is more than the absence of disease. Individuals have the potential for well-being but also for more-being. Well-being implies a steady state, whereas more-being refers to being in the process of becoming all that is humanly possible (Paterson & Zderad, 1978).

By understanding the existential premise of this theory, it is apparent that health is a process of finding meaning in life. Health is experienced in the process of living, of being involved in each moment. Paterson and Zderad suggest that we become more (more-being) through relationships with each other. When we relate authentically to another, we are experiencing health. This conceptualization of health implies that disease, medical diagnosis, or any form of labeling does little to determine a person's capacity for health. Health can be found in a person's willingness to be open to the experiences of life regardless of physical, social, spiritual, cognitive, or emotional status. Implications for nursing practice include being open to a wide range of definitions of health as well as possible interventions. The importance of relationships is paramount. The relationship that the nurse has with the person receiving care is critical, but even more important is the need for an appreciation of the relationships that exist for the person in daily living.

Nursing

Nursing is a nurturing response of one person to another in a time of need that aims toward the development of well-being and more-being. Nursing works toward this aim by helping to increase the possibility of making responsible choices, since this is how human beings are able to become. Nursing is concerned with the individual's unique being and striving toward becoming, focusing on the whole.

PHENOMENOLOGIC NURSOLOGY AND THE NURSING PROCESS

Case Study

Alicia is a 16-year-old high school student who participates in a variety of school activities. Her parents participate in school conferences and are supportive of her school involvement. Teachers find her to be an attentive student who succeeds in her classes. She is friends with a number of students in the school. She has come to the nursing clinic after a recent unit in health class about reproductive care that included topics related to abstinence, pregnancy prevention, and sexually transmitted diseases. She tells you that she has a friend who asked her to find out some additional information. She asks you where her friend could go if she needed to find out if she was pregnant. You know that Alicia has been steadily dating a male student. You suspect that she may be talking about herself.

Phenomenologic nursology is a methodology for understanding and describing nursing situations. It is a method of inquiry, as is the problem-solving approach of the nursing process. Phenomenologic nursology is a method of seeking to understand the nurse–nursed experience so that the nurse can be with the client in a human and therefore healing manner. The nursing process assumes the presence of a nursing problem that the nurse and client will solve together.

Phenomenologic nursology assumes a perceived health need by an individual who is involved in an interaction with a health care provider. Phenomenology is a descriptive process. It is not concerned specifically with facts (Owens, 1970), it is concerned with the nature of the facts and what they mean to the individual. Phenomenology describes phenomena but does not attempt to explain or predict their occurrence.

Preparation of the nurse knower for coming to know, the first phase of phenomenologic nursology, can be seen as a prerequisite similar to but distinct from the nursing process. The nursing process assumes that the nurse is educated in the bio-psycho-social-spiritual needs of the individual. Phenomenologic nursology makes these same assumptions but also assumes that the nurse has a sensitivity to and knowledge of the human condition and self-knowledge. Humanistic nursing requires subjectively experiencing the other. Experiencing life events through literature, drama, and the arts enriches the nurse's understanding of experiences such as love, joy, loneliness, suffering, and death. The use of guided imagery and case studies can be helpful in developing empathy, the ability to experience the other. The development of self-awareness is important if the nurse expects to encounter others in dialogue. Self-awareness can be enhanced through journaling, working in small groups, and meditation. In the case of this adolescent client, the nurse needs to understand the cognitive development as well as the physical and psychosocial changes experienced by adolescents. Knowing about the need to meet the developmental challenges of adolescence helps the nurse be aware of the kinds of behaviors that are often encountered.

Nurse knowing the other intuitively also occurs before the traditional assessment phase of the nursing process, even though intuition is indeed a kind of initial assessment. This phase is characterized by a "taking in" of the client in the human situation, the empathic encounter, the beginning of the I–Thou relationship wherein the nurse understands through an intuitive grasp the client's situation (Paterson & Zderad, 1976/1988). The use of intuition is a significant aspect of assessment that balances the often emphasized scientific and objective aspects of nursing practice. Being with the adolescent client, the nurse determines the adolescent's level of comfort in making her "call for help" to the nurse. Does she appear relaxed, inquisitive, defensive, scared, relieved, happy? Alicia appears inquisitive and a bit nervous.

The assessment phase of the nursing process can be considered analogous to the *nurse knowing the other scientifically*. This phase of nursology includes the more familiar method of looking at a phenomenon from many aspects: comparing, classifying, and looking for themes in relationships and among the parts. Dividing persons into biological, psychological, social, and spiritual parts is an example of classifying data. In the phenomenologic method of nursology the call comes first, followed by intuition and assessment, and then analysis. Assessment includes the collection of subjective and objective data about an individual obtained through observation, interaction with the client, and information from other sources such as laboratory studies. The nurse would look for signs of fatigue, ask questions about sleep and rest patterns, recent events, diet, the course of any problems, and some laboratory data. Phenomenologic nursology also includes the collection of subjective and objective data but relies on understanding the meaning of the experience to the client.

The call is Alicia's approach to the nurse with questions. Intuition is the nurse suspecting the friend is Alicia. Assessment includes that Alicia says her friend has missed one period and is going to the bathroom more often.

Analysis is similar to the phase in nursology called *nurse complementarily synthesizing known others*. During analysis the nurse compares the data with other known realities such as developmental stages, Maslow's hierarchy of needs, resiliency factors, and physiologic principles. In nursology, the nurse compares "multiple known realities" with the data and the experience of the client. In other words, the nurse examines the data and experience of the client in light of scientific and subjective knowledge and then compares, contrasts, and ultimately synthesizes to an expanded view (Paterson & Zderad, 1976/1988). Comparisons do occur in the phenomenologic method, but the purpose of the comparisons is directed toward identifying relationships and patterns with much consideration given to opposites and polarities. The phenomenologist synthesizes opposites and patterns into a larger concept, whereas the problem solver chooses a pattern and decides whether it is a problem or not (Oiler, 1982). By reflecting back to the adolescent what she has been sharing, and some possible meanings of her concerns, the nurse explores and validates the reality for the adolescent. The nurse reflects the signs and symptoms she has heard—missed one period, urinary frequency, interest in pregnancy test. Whether this situation represents a premenstrual manifestation or early pregnancy phenomenon is not the major concern. The humanistic nurse seeks to work with Alicia to determine what this means to her—what does she need to know to determine a course of action? What are her concerns about this in terms of her views of self? As dialogue continues, Alicia reveals it is herself she is concerned about and that she and her boyfriend "have only done it once." The nurse seeks further information to develop a genogram and an ecomap for Alicia (see Figures 17–1 and 17–2).

Diagnosis is the step of the nursing process in which the nurse makes a problem statement. The nurse collects data regarding the client's stated need, then analyzes the data by classifying it, comparing it to known theory and principles, and finally arriving at a conclusion that is a statement of the problem. *Succession within the nurse from the many to the paradoxical one* is comparable to identifying a diagnosis.

After synthesizing the ideas, data, and experience, the nurse reaches a conclusion that is broader than the classifications and reflects the experience of the client as well as the nurse's initial intuitive grasp of the situation. This conclusion has meaning for all and is a significant difference in emphasis from the nursing process. The problem statement needs to reflect what is of import to the client. One of the strengths of the theory is its compatibility with the use of standardized nursing language systems. Each of the diagnoses in the classification system supported by the North American Nursing Diagnosis Association (NANDA) could be used to explain the relationship of varying views of the problem expressed by the client. A possible nursing diagnosis with Alicia would be the potential for first trimester pregnancy. However, a diagnosis more compatible with phenomenologic nursology would be knowledge deficit about pregnancy tests.

The outcomes, planning, and implementation phases of the nursing process are based on one or more goals or outcomes to be reached by the client, with steps (objectives) to be accomplished toward the goal. Specific nurse and client actions are spelled out in detail. Phenomenologic nursology does not describe the formation of a goal-directed nursing care plan. Humanistic nursing is concerned with being with another who is in need. The goal of more-being or well-being is accomplished through dialogue. In the dialogue between the nurse and the nursed (client), there is the meeting and the presence of the nurse for the other, and the call and response between the nurse and the nursed, the I–Thou relationship. This is the therapeutic relationship. Allowing Alicia to express her concerns, being open to her exploration of the implications of those concerns and the consideration of a course of action is the reality of the nursing situation.

Paterson and Zderad do not elaborate on incorporating the "doing" aspects of nursing into the dialogue. The theory evolved from the authors' psychiatric nursing practice and experience where the "doing" can be construed as the interactions between the nurse and the client. Glimpses of humanistic nursing practice are available in the rich descriptions of clinical experiences throughout the text. Examples of using touch, measuring vital signs, bathing, and spending time with clients demonstrate that any nursing interaction with a client can be a vehicle for nurturing more-being.

The *evaluation* phase of the nursing process provides the support for the effectiveness of the plan by measuring outcomes in terms of client behavior. Humanistic nursing practice recognizes change in behavior but also focuses on the meaning of the experience for the client. A client who learns to make choices about health and assumes responsibility for those choices may experience personal growth and more-being. Being in a caring relationship with the adolescent who is confused and scared may allow expression of sadness, ambivalence, hopes and goals empowering her to refocus on priorities for immediate action and the future. For Alicia, this is represented by her thanking the nurse for the information she has obtained about pregnancy tests and dropping by the nursing office the next day to report that not only was a home pregnancy test negative last night, but also her period started this morning. She adds that this scare has taught her a lesson and she is going to be more careful from now on. This is in contrast to an outcome of the nursing process that is decided in advance of the nursing action, for example, that the adolescent demonstrates appropriate weight gain during the pregnancy.

CRITIQUE OF PATERSON AND ZDERAD'S HUMANISTIC NURSING THEORY

1. What is the historical context of the theory? Paterson and Zderad's book was first published in 1976 and their work is based in the traditions of existentialism and phenomenology. They define existentialism as a "philosophy based on phenomenological studies of reality; centers on the analysis of existence particularly of the individual human being, stresses the freedom and responsibility of the individual, regards human existence as not completely describable or understandable in idealistic or scientific terms" (1976/1988, 131/121). Considering the incredible losses and devastation encountered in Europe as a result of World War I and World War II, individuals sought answers to questions about the meaning of life and who was responsible. Existentialism, for some, was the logical answer; the answer that said each us is responsible for our own destiny. We have choices and they hold us accountable to ourselves. Abraham Maslow, often considered the father of humanistic psychology, wrote in 1962 that we were then ". . . in the middle of a change in the conception of man's capacities, potentialities and goals. . . . When the philosophy of man (his nature, his goals, his potentialities, his fulfillment) changes, then everything changes. Not only the philosophy of politics, of economics, of ethics and values, of interpersonal relations and of history itself change, but also the philosophy of education, the theory of how to help men become what they can and deeply need to become" (p. 34). Paterson and Zderad, in publications beginning in 1966, have taken the philosophy of existentialism and examined how it can be applied to nursing's role in helping clients achieve their maximum potential, their more-being, or as Maslow would say, their potential for self-actualization. The questions posed by a humanistic and existential frame of reference are as relevant today as they were when first framed. With increasing dependence on technology and the potential for face-to-face isolation from others, we strive to make meaningful our interactions with others.

2. What are the basic concepts and relationships presented by the theory? The basic concepts presented by Paterson and Zderad (1976/1988) are nursing, community, and phenomenologic nursology. Nursing is a lived dialogue where meeting, relating, presence, and call and response occur in the real world of people, things, time and space, nurturing more-being and well-being. What makes this a humanistic theory, beyond the existential foundation, is the underlying concept of community. Very simply put, the basis of humanistic thought is that not only is each of us struggling to find meaning in our lives, but also meaning comes from the realization that it is through each other that we more fully participate in and expand our lives. We do not exist in isolation, and as nurses our ability to open to others helps them move towards more-being while simultaneously enhancing our lives. Nursing can only exist within the community of others, recognizing and valuing our unique differences as we share the world, or a particular moment. We are able to achieve this lived dialogue through the methodology of phenomenologic nursology: preparation of the nurse knower for coming to know, knowing the other intuitively, knowing the other scientifically, complementarily synthesizing known others, and succession from the many to the paradoxical one.

3. What major phenomena of concern to nursing are presented? The existential base of this theory provides a focus on human beings as they seek well-being and more-being. Included in the nurse–nursed relationship are dialogue (meeting, relating, presence, and call and response), community, and phenomenologic nursology. A major phenomena is that of choice and the attendant responsibilities associated with making choices.

4. To whom does this theory apply? Paterson and Zderad's work can be applied to almost any nursing situation. Because it is a call and response, the nurse needs to be ready and able to hear the client's call. Regardless of whether the person is verbal and responsive or not, the nurse should always be prepared to understand basic needs, assess the situation, and determine what is needed in terms of the client. The neonate who needs nutrition, warmth, or comforting and the individual found unconscious after a drug overdose are in need of systematic assessment and affirmation as much as the adolescent father who finds himself faced with parenting responsibilities. The authors specifically address the possibility of nursing if there is no mutual response and state that even though the client may not be aware of the relationship, it exists, if it is authentic.

5. By what method can this theory be tested? Paterson and Zderad (1976/1988, p. 57/51) speak of research as " . . . an inherent component of humanistic nursing" although the nurse typically is introduced to a research methodology that demands objectivity despite the fact that so much of nursing defies controls and protocols. The nurse needs to have a sense "of wonderment, concern and responsibility" (p. 59/53). The research methodology proposed by humanistic nursing practice is " . . . phenomenology, a descriptive approach to participants in the nursing situation as a method for studying, interpreting, and attesting the nature and meaning of the lived events" (p. 60/54). Humanistic nursing must make visible to other nurses that which takes place in the nursing situation. This aspect challenges the humanistic nurse to find a way to communicate meaningfully with colleagues while protecting the privacy of clients, often through abstractions, metaphors, analogies, and parables. "Phenomenology requires vigorous investment into respectfully, appreciatively, and acceptingly making evident our lived worlds and their ramifications for the now, the past, and the anticipated future" (p. 68/61). While categorization is accepted, phenomenology requires going beyond simple labels so that the meaning of the situation to the client is of prime importance. Differences, variations, and uniqueness are valued over objective categories.

For a nurse to become a free responsible research nurse in the health arena she accepts her lived nursing world as beyond the controls valued in positivistic science. . . . To attain her potential as nurse she will discipline herself rigorously for authenticity with the self. . . . Then out of her own human social need and for the survival of nursing she will describe to propel knowledge, nursing theory, and practice forward. In this process and in its effects she will become more human as she contributes to man's humanization (p. 70/63).

6. Does this theory direct critical thinking in nursing practice? Paterson and Zderad's work has several notable strengths in relation to promoting critical thinking. The methodology is well developed and the concepts are fully described within the parameters of existential philosophy, phenomenology, and nursing. The theory broadens the possibilities for explaining and describing nursing and enhancing knowledge of nursing. An important contribution of this theory is that the methodology leads to concept formation, which is the basis of theory and the springboard of new inquiry. The theory provides a unique, unusual approach to the study of nursing. Another strength is the strong nursing focus. The theory developed from the lived experiences of clinical nurses and reflects that nursing perspective. Paterson and Zderad challenge the nurse to reflect, to synthesize, and to articulate, all of which are crucial components of critical thinking. Each nursing situation is recognized as unique, generating a unique relating between the nurse and the nursed. The steps of phenomenologic nursology challenge the nurse towards self-awareness, towards being open to another, and towards professional growth.

7. Does this theory direct therapeutic nursing interventions? Humanistic nursing theory, including phenomenologic nursology, can be used by nurses to guide and improve practice, particularly the use of therapeutic nursing interventions. What is emphasized is the importance of valuing the uniqueness of each individual and that person's situation. Routine, impersonal care would not be consistent with the message of humanistic nursing practice. The nurse must strive to be fully present during each interaction whose goal is to nurture the client.

8. Does this theory direct communication in nursing practice? Phenomenologic nursology relies on dialogue. Paterson and Zderad's theory is fundamentally rooted in communication and the importance of being open to the call of clients as well as the nature of the response. Specific attention is paid to the nature of communication and how it can be achieved. Numerous examples of lived dialogue are provided throughout the text giving direction to the role of communication in nursing practice. The authors challenge nurses to consider multiple forms of communication such as poetry, music, and writing as avenues to promote communication.

9. Does this theory direct nursing actions that lead to favorable outcomes? Humanistic nursing is designed to promote well-being and more-being, the interpretation of which is left to the individual. Clinical outcomes, per se, are not addressed since this was not a concept discussed in the literature when the theory was first published. However, the relevance of Paterson and Zderad's work is on the continued value in today's society for recognition of individual potential and search for meaning.

10. How contagious is this theory? Paterson and Zderad (1976/1988) ask, "Can an explicit philosophy of nursing allow for more meaningful quality practice, be a resource for nurses, improve service, be available for reexamination, correction, and the forwarding of knowledge?" (p. 72/67). Their answer is a committed "Yes." Their work has directed critical thinking, therapeutic nursing interventions, and communication in practice. A review of recent literature finds examples of searching for meaning based on their work in clinical practice (Coward, 1990; Lobchuck, 1996, 1999), and education (Holmes, 1990; Touhy, 1994). Specifically, one can find references that examine the nature of the dialogue and the conditions in nursing practice that facilitate client more-being (e.g., Duldt, 1995; Hinds, 1988). Much of their theory has become integrated into nursing practice without direct recognition of their work. However, their work is not without critics who find that humanistic theory is vague, inconsistent (Mulholland, 1995; Mitchell & Cody, 1992), and lacking in accountability for patient care (McKinnon, 1991).

STRENGTHS AND LIMITATIONS

This theory has several notable strengths. The methodology is well developed and the concepts are fully described within the parameters of existential philosophy, phenomenology, and nursing. This theory broadens the possibilities for explaining and describing nursing. The study of human beings and nursing using this phenomenological method is a valid approach that enhances knowledge of nursing. An important contribution of this theory is that the methodology leads to concept formation, which is the basis of theory and the springboard of new inquiry. The theory provides a unique, unusual approach to the study of nursing. Another strength is the strong nursing focus. The theory developed from the lived experiences of clinical nurses and reflects that nursing perspective.

Reading the text provides an opportunity to experience the flow and rhythm of theory development that eloquently represented the philosophical challenges facing nursing, women, and education in the 1960s and that continues to be relevant today. The text is written in a readable style that is often poetic in quality. Each chapter inspires and stimulates creative ideas for clinical practice. It is not a reference text that can be used as a quick solution to clinical practice problems, but it can be used to stimulate reflection and exploration. There are no formulas for successful nursing in their theory. This is as it should be, for the theory posits that nursing is interactive and based on the moment of the interaction.

Humanistic Nursing Theory as proposed by Josephine Paterson and Loretta Zderad resonates the sentiments of those who continue to enter the profession of nursing today: they want to make a difference in their lives and in the lives of others. They see nursing as a way to make that difference. Paterson and Zderad provide the signposts to find meaning in nursing.

SUMMARY

Paterson and Zderad were the first of the nurse theorists to base their work in existentialism. They proposed a theory of humanistic nursing that includes dialogue, community, and phenomenologic nursology. Their work is derived from nursing practice and provides a new way of viewing that practice.

REFERENCES

Bergson, H. (1946). *The creative mind*. New York: The Philosophical Library. (out of print)

Buber, M. (1958). *I and Thou* (2nd ed.). New York: Charles Scribner's Sons. (out of print)

Buber, M. (1965). Distance and relation. In M. Friedman (Ed.), & R. G. Smith (Trans.), *The knowledge of man*. New York: Harper & Row. (out of print)

Bugental, J. F. T. (1978). The third force in psychology. In D. Welch, G. Tate, & F. Richards (Eds.), *Humanistic psychology: A sourcebook*. Buffalo, NY: Prometheus Books. (out of print)

Corey, G. (2000). *Theory and practice of counseling and psychotherapy* (6th ed.). Pacific Grove, CA: Brooks/Cole.

Coward, D. D. (1990). The lived experience of self-transcendence in women with advanced breast cancer. *Nursing Science Quarterly. 3*(4), 162–169.

de Chardin, T. (1961). *The phenomenon of man*. New York: Harper & Row. (out of print)

Desan, W. (1972). *Planetary man*. New York: Macmillan. (out of print)

Duldt, B.W. (1995). Integrating nursing theory and ethics. *Perspectives in Psychiatric Care. 31*(2), 4–10.

Hesse, H. (1966). *Steppenwolf*. New York: Holt, Rinehart & Winston. (out of print)

Hinds, P. S. (1988). The relationship of nurses' caring behaviors with hopefulness and health care outcomes in adolescents. *Archives of Psychiatric Nursing, 2*(11), 21–29.

Holmes, C. A. (1990). Alternatives to natural science foundations for nursing. *International Journal of Nursing Studies. 27*, 187–198.

Jung, C. G. (1933). *Modern man in search of a soul*. New York: Harcourt, Brace & World. (out of print)

Laing, R. D. (1967). *The politics of experience*. New York: Ballantine.

Lobchuck, M. M. (1996). Humanistic nursing: Discussing nursing with myself [German]. *Pflege, 9*, 120–126.

Lobchuck, M. (1999). Humanistic reflections of a research nurse in a longitudinal study: A personal essay. *Canadian Oncology Nursing Journal, 9*, 71-73.

Marcel, G. (1956). *Being and having: An existentialist diary*. New York: Harper Torchbooks, Harper & Row. (out of print)

Maslow, A. (1962). Some basic propositions of a growth and self-actualization psychology. In *Perceiving, Behaving, Becoming: A New Focus for Education*. Washington, DC: Association for Supervision and Curriculum Development.

McKinnon, N. C. (1991). Humanistic nursing. It can't stand up to scrutiny. *Nursing & Health Care. 12*, 414–416.

Mitchell, G. J., & Cody, W. K. (1992). Nursing knowledge and human science: Ontological and epistemological considerations. *Nursing Science Quarterly, 5*(2), 54–61.

Mulholland, J. (1995). Nursing, humanism and transcultural theory: The 'bracketing-out' of reality. *Journal of Advanced Nursing, 22*, 442–449.

Nietzsche, F. (1927). Beyond good and evil. In H. Zimmern (Trans.). *The philosophy of Nietzsche*. New York: Random House. (out of print)

Oiler, C. (1982). The phenomenological approach to nursing research. *Nursing Research, 31*, 180.

Owens, T. (1970). *Phenomenology and intersubjectivity*. The Hague, Netherlands: Martinus Nijhoff. (out of print)

Paterson, J. G. (1966). Group supervision: A process and philosophy. *Community Mental Health Journal, 2,* 315–318.

Paterson, J., & Zderad, L. (1978, December). *Humanistic nursing.* Paper presented at the 2nd Annual Nurse Educator Conference, New York, NY.

Paterson, J. G., & Zderad, L. T. (1988). *Humanistic nursing* (Pub. No. 41-2218). New York: National League for Nursing. (Originally published, 1976, New York: John Wiley & Sons, Inc.)

Shaffer, J.B. (1978). *Humanistic psychology.* Upper Saddle River, NJ: Prentice Hall. (out of print)

Touhy, T. (1994). The evolution of a caring-based program. In A. Boykin (Ed.). *Living a caring-based program* (pp. 1–10) (Pub. No. 14-2536). NY: National League for Nursing Press.

Zderad, L.T. (1978). From here-and-now to theory: Reflections on "How." In *Theory development: What, why, how?* New York: National League for Nursing. (out of print)

ANNOTATED BIBLIOGRAPHY

Coward, D. D. (1990). The lived experience of self-transcendence in women with advanced breast cancer. *Nursing Science Quarterly.* 3(4), 162–169.

Phenomenological exploratory study related to the concept of self-transcendence as an indicator of more-being in women with metastatic breast cancer. The five subjects found meaning through reaching out to help others, allowing others to help them, and learning to accept the unchangeable.

Hines, D. R. (1991). *The development of the Measurement of Presence Scale* (Online). Dissertation abstract from: CINAHL Accession No.: 1993157211.

Humanistic nursing provided the conceptual framework for the development of the Measurement of Presence Scale, a self-report interval level, norm-referenced scale. This study provided initial support for internal consistency and construct validity of the scale. Nine subscales were interpreted as valuing/attending to self and others, connecting, transacting, enduring memory from past, engaging for growth, encountering, availability, person or event sustaining memory, and disclosing and enclosing.

Holmes, C. A. (1990). Alternatives to natural science foundations for nursing. *International Journal Nursing Studies.* 27(3), 187–198.

Outlines philosophical assumptions, origins, and implications of humanistic and holistic nursing theory for education and practice.

Lanza, M. L. (1996) Bibliotherapy and beyond. *Perspectives in Psychiatric Care.* 32(1), 12–14.

Anecdotal experience of the use of literature and television to promote mental health. The personal experience described supports the use of literature to promote emotional catharsis, encourage problem solving, and gain personal insight.

Lobchuck, M. M. (1996). Humanistic nursing: Discussing nursing with myself. [German] *Pflege, 9(2),* 120–126.

A presentation of two case studies with clients experiencing cancer in which the author's goal is to develop a personal authenticity. As part of her graduate study, the author conducted these interviews to explore the experience of patients with cancer, and the experience of their relatives. Her desire was to become aware of the existential experiences of both herself (during her earlier hospital nursing experience) and of the patients and their families. This awareness should help develop personal authenticity.

Touhy, T. (1994). The evolution of a caring-based program. In A. Boykin (Ed.). *Living a caring-based program* (pp. 1–10) (Pub. No. 14-2536). NY: National League for Nursing Press.

Describes the development of a curriculum based on principles of caring and influenced by Paterson and Zderad's work, among others. Of particular usefulness from the work of Paterson and Zderad were the concepts of nursing situation and call and response.

CHAPTER 18

THEORY OF TRANSPERSONAL CARING
JEAN WATSON

Jane H. Kelley and Brenda Johnson

■ ■ ■

Jean Watson (b. 1940) earned a diploma from Lewis Gale Hospital School of Nursing in Roanoke, VA; a baccalaureate in nursing degree from the University of Colorado, Boulder; a master's degree in psychiatric-mental health nursing from the University of Colorado, Denver; and a Ph.D. in educational psychology and counseling from the University of Colorado, Boulder. She has held faculty and administrative positions at the University of Colorado Health Sciences Center, including deanship of the School of Nursing from 1983 to 1990 and founding Director of the Center for Human Caring. In 1992, Dr. Watson was named Distinguished Professor at the University of Colorado, the highest honor accorded University of Colorado faculty for scholarly work. She is a widely published author and recipient of numerous awards and honors, including an international Kellogg Fellowship in Australia, a Fullbright Research Award in Sweden, and four honorary doctoral degrees as well as membership in the American Academy of Nursing and the National League for Nursing's Martha E. Rogers Award for nursing scholarship in 1993. Watson served as the president of the National League for Nursing from 1995 to 1996.

In 1998 Watson assumed the first endowed Chair in Caring Science at the University of Colorado School of Nursing. She is also Senior Scholar-Advisor for the International Center for Integrative Caring Practices (the former Center for Human Caring). The International Center has a focus on integrating caring theory and practice. It provides professional development options for visiting scholar-clinicians as well as international primary health care initiatives in caring-healing practices.

The essence of Watson's theory is authentic caring for the purpose of preserving the dignity and wholeness of humanity. She describes the theory as having emerged from her own values, beliefs, and perceptions about human life, health, and healing (Watson,

1996, p. 144). She sees nursing's "collective caring-healing role and its mission in society as attending to, and helping to sustain, humanity and wholeness" (p. 144).

Watson's theory was never meant to be prescriptive, but rather more of a worldview or ethic by which nursing could know its traditions in health and healing. Watson envisions nursing as a human science discipline as well as an academic-clinical profession with a societal mission "to caring and healing work with others during their most vulnerable moments of life's journey" (Watson, 1996, p. 145). Caring, thus, is independent of curing. According to Watson, knowledge and practice for a caring-healing discipline are primarily derived from the arts and humanities and an emerging human science that acknowledges a convergence of art and science. It calls for nursing to retain a sense of the sacred in caring for the "body physical" as a human manifestation of a soul—interconnected and in harmony with the cosmos and universal consciousness.

Since the initial publication of her theory in 1979, Watson has attempted to serve as a bridge by which nursing could transition from a biomedical/natural-science model to a postmodern/human-science perspective. Watson believes that language is essential to this endeavor. As an extension of the biomedical model, the language of nursing diagnosis is not congruent with Watson's emphasis on caring and human being as "embodied spirit." Watson sought to provide the language and structure for a transition by delineating ten carative factors as the conceptual core of nursing.

With the 1985/1988 update of her theory in *Nursing: Human science and human care*, Watson combines the humanistic with the scientific base of nursing. She is a leader in advocating for a strong liberal arts background with an emphasis on philosophy and values as the necessary educational basis for the science of caring. In the latest rendition of her theory, Watson (1999) advocates the postmodern view of science as indistinguishable from art and a vision of nursing as a discipline devoted to caring, health, and healing.

In her most recent work, Watson (1999) discusses and defines her use of the term *postmodern*. The postmodern mindset:

- Suggests there is no one Truth, but multiple truths; no one universally known reality that is defined by physical-material world;
- rather, there are multiple, constructed realities, there is attention to valuing multiple meanings;
- acknowledgment of both physical and non-physical reality and phenomena;
- . . . suggests non-linearity of thinking and acting,
- introduces relativity of time and space;
- is open to ideas that include context, critiques, challenges, multiple interpretations, stories, narratives, text and search for meaning and wholeness.

Emerging metaphors of postmodern: art, artistry, creativity, harmony, beauty, spirit-metaphysical, holographic (p. 289).

Postmodernism is a critique of cultural norms and common notions of truth and reality. It runs across disciplines and is most evident in areas such as quantum physics, ecofeminism, critical social theory, and phenomenological philosophy, where the modernist emphasis on power and domination and empirical, atomistic thought are being replaced by notions of an interconnected, balanced, and holographic universe of universal consciousness and timeless spiritual traditions. Postmodernism uses a deconstructive process to question dominant patterns of thought and governance, which have led to the modernist paternalistic system of hierarchy, followed by a reconstructive process to envision more holistic and egalitarian patterns of thought and being. Watson situates nursing within a postmodern worldview, which acknowledges the holistic and interconnected nature of the universe and the importance of subjectivity. The human science paradigm, thus, is the creation of postmodernism and contrasts with the traditional science paradigm espoused by predominant beliefs of the nineteenth and twentieth centuries and known as the modern age.

There are fundamental differences in ways of being (ontology), knowing (epistemology), and doing (praxis) within the traditional versus the human science paradigm (see Table 18–1). The purpose of traditional science is identification and prediction. Human science is predominantly concerned with the meaning of the lived experience. Thus, different approaches to knowledge development are espoused by the contrasting paradigms. Whenever nursing aligns itself within a biomedical model, key elements of a traditional science paradigm are description of symptoms, variables, and physiological or behavioral outcomes. A human science paradigm would envision the key elements to knowledge formation to be understanding of the human–environment, person–life spirit, or human–human interaction. Methodological ways by which knowledge is acquired also differ. Traditional science recognizes only the legitimacy of verifiable, objective data. This has been interpreted to mean observation of variables in controlled conditions for the purpose of identifying and determining causes of various symptoms, behaviors, and physiological manifestations. A human science approach accepts the legitimacy of multiple ways of knowing or imagining (e.g., phenomenological or aesthetic methods) in order to understand the lived experience or how human–environmental energy patterns are transformed within specific contexts.

Nursing actions (praxis) differ greatly within contrasting paradigms also. Professional nursing within a traditional science and biomedical model is focused on "doing" by controlling and manipulating physical and behavioral parameters through specific actions and environments that maintain physiological or behavioral

TABLE 18–1. A CONTRAST OF TRADITIONAL SCIENCE AND HUMAN SCIENCE

	Traditional Science Paradigm	Human Science Paradigm
Ontology	Identify Predict Human as mind/body	Meaning of the experience as lived by a person Human as embodied spirit
Epistemology	Describe outcomes in terms of physical indicators or as behaviors	Knowing about interaction of human–environment, person–life spirit, or human–human
Methodology	Structured studies relying on control of conditions and seeking to establish cause and effect	Multiple approaches seeking to understand lived experience in identified contexts
Praxis	Focus/goal is homeostasis and stability	Seeks harmony and well-being

homeostasis. Within a human science paradigm, the emphasis is on "being" and the cocreation of nurse–patient interactions on human–environmental energy patterns that restore harmony and a sense of well-being.

Watson, through the theory of caring, seeks to give nursing the epistemological and ontological structure by which to pursue a return to the sacredness and mystery of living in relationship rather than the pursuit of domination and self-determination in a health care system that mimics a society that has become fragmented and spiritually bereft.

WATSON'S THEORY OF TRANSPERSONAL CARING

Philosophical Background

In recent years, Watson's work has reflected a blend of Eastern and Western beliefs in what she refers to as the emerging/converging paradigm (Watson, 1996). In her early works, transcendental phenomenology was a strong influence on her focus on the metaphysical and spiritual nature of being human. Philosophical beliefs of several philosophers, such as Whitehead (1953), Kierkegaard (1941), and deChardin (1959), influenced her concepts of self and ontological caring. The interpersonal nature of caring was influenced by the psychological teachings of Carl Rogers (1961). Nurse theorists and philosophers who were especially influential in shaping Watson's beliefs about health, culture, environment, dignity, and caring were Nightingale (1859/1957), Henderson (1966), Leininger (1980, 1981), Martha Rogers (1970), and Gadow (1980). Eastern views on the importance of mind/body harmony as can be achieved through meditation and ritual, have influenced Watson's more recent emphasis on the power of intentionality and consciousness on health and healing. The similarities of ancient wisdoms espoused by mystics and tribal cultures and more recent beliefs of a holographic science provide the basis for "the emerging/converging paradigm," which has led to Watson's current interest in a caring/healing consciousness that transcends time and space. Watson expresses the hope that such a relational ontology can heal not only individuals, but unhealthy health care, sociopolitical, and cultural institutions as well.

Contents of the Theory

In her review of her theory, Watson (1996) presents the major conceptual elements of the original theory along with elements that have evolved over time. The major conceptual elements of the original theory are listed as: *transpersonal caring relationship; ten carative factors*; and *caring occasion/caring moment*. The latent dimensions that have evolved and emerged are:

- embodied spirit.
- Expanded views of self and person transpersonal-mindbodyspirit oneness; embodied spirit.
- Importance of caring-healing consciousness within the human-environment field.

- Positing of consciousness as energy.
- Phenomenal field/unitary consciousness: Unbroken wholeness and connectedness of all (subject-object-person-environment-nature-universe-all living things).
- Advanced caring-healing modalities/nursing arts. (Watson, 1996, p. 151)

Transpersonal Caring Relationship

Originally defined as a human-to-human connectedness occurring in a nurse–patient encounter wherein "each is touched by the human center of the other" (1989, p. 131; quoted in Watson, 1996, p. 151), the transpersonal caring relationship has taken on a multidimensional meaning not bounded by time and space.

By 1985/1988 and continuing in her 1996 work, Watson provided a list of specifications on which a transpersonal caring relationship depends:

- The moral commitment, intentionality, and consciousness needed to protect, enhance, promote, and potentiate human dignity, wholeness, and healing, wherein a person creates or cocreates his or her own meaning for existence, healing, wholeness, and caring.
- Orientation of the nurse's intent, will, and consciousness toward affirming the subjective/intersubjective significance of the person. . . .
- The nurse's ability to realize, accurately detect, and connect with the inner condition (spirit) of another. . . . .
- The nurse's ability to assess and realize another's condition of being-in-the-world and to feel a union with the other. . . . .
- The caring-healing modalities potentiate harmony, wholeness, and comfort, and promote inner healing by releasing some of the disharmony and blocked energy that interfere with the natural healing processes.
- The nurse's own life history and previous experiences. . . . To some degree, the necessary knowledge and sensitivity can be gained through work with other cultures, study of the humanities (art, drama, and literature), and exploration of one's own values, beliefs, and relationship with self . . . personal growth experiences such as psychotherapy, meditation, bioenergetics work, and spiritual awakening. . . . (Watson, 1996, pp. 153–154)

A recent elaboration on the concept of a transpersonal caring relationship describes this relationship occurring within a caring consciousness, wherein a nurse enters "into the life space or phenomenal field of another person [and] is able to detect the other person's condition of being (spirit, or soul level), feels this condition within self, and responds in such a way that the person being cared for has a release of feelings, thought, and tension" (Watson, 1996, p. 152). The concept implies a focus on the uniqueness of the persons in relationship, and the uniqueness of the "phenomena wherein the coming together can be mutual and reciprocal," and conveys a spiritual dimension influenced by the caring consciousness of the nurse (p. 152).

Ten Carative Factors

Ten carative factors were identified by Watson (1979, 1985/1988, 1996) as factors that characterize the nursing caring transaction occurring within a given caring moment or occasion. Watson notes that the carative factors are not intended to be a checklist, but to be a philosophical and conceptual guide for nursing. The ten carative factors involve

1. Forming a humanistic-altruistic system of values.
2. Enabling and sustaining faith-hope.
3. Being sensitive to self and others.
4. Developing a helping-trusting, caring relationship (seeking transpersonal connections).
5. Promoting and accepting the expression of positive and negative feelings and emotions.
6. Engaging in creative, individualized, problem-solving caring processes.
7. Promoting transpersonal teaching-learning.
8. Attending to supportive, protective, and/or corrective mental, physical, societal, and spiritual environments.
9. Assisting with gratification of basic human needs while preserving human dignity and wholeness.
10. Allowing for, and being open to, existential-phenomenological and spiritual dimensions of caring and healing that cannot be fully explained scientifically through modern Western medicine (Watson, 1996, pp. 156–157).

Watson (1996) sees the carative factors as instrumental in reintegrating a sense of harmony and dignity into interpersonal, sociopolitical, and environmental relationships.

Caring Occasion/Caring Moment

The ten carative factors have been described by Watson (1979,1985/1988, 1996) as factors that characterize the nursing–caring transaction occurring within a given caring moment or occasion. Watson defines *caring occasion* and *caring moment*, and adds descriptions of caring (healing) consciousness and the connections implicit in caring–healing consciousness and energy.

A *caring occasion/caring moment* occurs whenever nurse and other(s) come together with their unique life histories and phenomenal field in a human-to-human transaction and is "a focal point in space and time . . . has a greater field of its own that is greater than the occasion itself . . . arise[s] from aspects of itself that become part of the life history of each person, as well as part of some larger, deeper, complex pattern of life" (Watson, 1985/1988, p. 59).

Watson (1996) proposes that the caring occasion/caring moment occurs in a holographic context manifest within a field of *caring (healing) consciousness* (p. 158). Within this holographic context, the caring (healing) process is "relational and connected; transcends self, time, space, and physical dominance; and is intersubjective with transcendent possibilities that go beyond the given caring occasion" (p. 158).

The influence of quantum physics and newer models of science have led Watson (1996) to reconsider the roles of consciousness, energy, health, and well-being. She notes that the *caring–healing consciousness of a caring [occasion/caring] moment* opens up a higher, deeper energy field of consciousness "that has metaphysical and spiritual potentialities for healing and goes beyond the separate ego self and separate body (physical) self" (pp. 159–160). Watson asserts that based on these notions of *caring consciousness and energy*, nursing "collectively has the potential to enable individuals, systems, and humankind to move toward higher-frequency possibilities that offer greater harmony, wholeness, health, and spiritual evolution, while sustaining increasing diversity" (p. 160).

WATSON'S THEORY AND NURSING'S METAPARADIGM

Watson's earlier works address the metaparadigm concepts of person (human being), health, environment, and nursing as somewhat more discrete concepts than do her later works. As Watson has been inspired by quantum physics and has integrated varied ways of knowing and being and doing, her descriptions of the metaparadigm concepts have been modified. The concepts are dealt with as nondiscrete, intertwined, and discontinuous.

Person (Human Being)

Considering the individual human, Watson (1985/88) views

the human as a valued person in and of him- or herself . . . in general a philosophical view of a person as a fully functional integrated self . . . greater than, and different from, the sum of his or her parts" (p. 14). Furthermore, essential to human existence "is that the human has transcended nature—yet remains a part of it. The human can go forward, through the use of the mind, to higher levels of consciousness . . . one's soul possesses a body that is not confined by objective space and time (p. 45).

In 1996, Watson elaborated on this transcendent nature of being human. She uses a quote of de Chardin (1967):

We are not human beings having a spiritual experience.

We are spiritual beings having a human experience (quoted in Watson, p. 148).

Of the basic premises identified by Watson (1985/1988, pp. 50–51) on which her caring model is based, five relate to person:

1. A person's mind and emotions are windows to the soul . . .
2. A person's body is confined in time and space, but the mind and soul are not confined to the physical universe . . .
3. A nurse may have access to a person's mind, emotions, and inner self indirectly through any sphere—mind, body or soul—provided the physical body is not perceived or treated as separate from the mind and emotions and higher sense of self (soul) . . .
4. The spirit, inner self, or soul (geist) of a person exists in and for itself . . .
5. People need each other in a caring, loving way . . .

In more recent work (1996), Watson's focus shifts more to the connectedness of all of existence. She further develops the concept of the "unity of mindbodyspirit/nature, and of a field of connectedness between and among persons and environments at all levels, into infinity and into the universal or cosmic level of existence" (p. 147). There is an "Unbroken wholeness and connectedness of all (subject-object-person-environment-nature-universe-all living things)" (p. 151). This expanded view of what it means to be human, to be healed, and to be whole, considers person to be "embodied spirit, both immanent and transcendent" (p. 148).

Health and Illness

Watson considers *illness* to be a perceived state rather than presence of disease. Illness is defined as

> subjective turmoil or disharmony within a person's inner self or soul at some level or disharmony within the spheres of the person, for example, in the mind, body, and soul, either consciously or unconsciously. . . . Illness connotes a felt incongruence within the person such as an incongruence between the self as perceived and the self as experienced (Watson, 1985/1988, p. 48).

Watson notes that illness can result from a troubled inner soul, and illness can lead to disease, but the two concepts do not fall on a continuum and can exist apart from one another.

Watson's definition of *health*, on the other hand, does imply a health–illness continuum. As described in her 1985/1988 work:

> Health refers to unity and harmony within the mind, body, and soul. Health is also associated with the degree of congruence between the self as perceived and the self as experienced (p. 48).

Encompassing the entire nature of the individual in the physical, social, aesthetic, and moral realms, rather than limited to aspects of behavior and physiology, *health* or *illness* results from the congruence or incongruence between the self as perceived and the self as experienced. *Disease* may result from or be a causal factor in prolonged periods of incongruence. Or, disease may not be present.

Environment

In 1996, Watson reiterated the usefulness of her ten carative factors, originally presented in 1979. One of these factors speaks to *environment*. Carative factor 8 is: "Attending to supportive, protective, and/or corrective mental, physical, societal, and spiritual environments" (p. 156). However, in discussions of her more recent thought, environment is considered in the context of a human–environment field. As noted above, this field forms an "Unbroken wholeness and connectedness of all (subject-object-person-environment-nature-universe-all living things)" (Watson, 1996, p. 151). It seems, then, that environment can be perceived to be a specific context, such as social, physical, or as the greater context of interacting, nondiscrete elements within a phenomenal field.

Nursing as Profession and Praxis

In her own words, Watson (1985/1988) defined nurse to be both a noun and a verb, and nursing to consist

> of knowledge, thought, values, philosophy, commitment, and action, with some degree of passion . . . related to human care transactions and intersubjective personal human contact with the lived world of the experiencing person (p. 53).

The verb "to nurse" is carried out through human care and caring, which Watson views as the moral ideal of nursing and

> consists of transpersonal human-to-human attempts to protect, enhance, and preserve humanity by helping a person find meaning in illness, suffering, pain, and existence; to help another gain self-knowledge, control, and self-healing wherein a sense of inner harmony is restored regardless of the external circumstances (p. 54).

Human care nursing involves a reciprocal relationship between the nurse and others as coparticipants in a pattern of subjectivity–intersubjectivity evidenced in "consciousness; intentionality; perceptions and lived experiences related to caring, healing, and health-illness conditions in a given 'caring moment'; and experiences or meanings that transcend the moment and go beyond the actual experience" (Watson, 1996, p. 148).

Watson (1996) determines nursing to be both scientific and artistic, based on caring–healing knowledge and practices drawn from the arts and humanities as well as from traditional and emerging sciences (p. 142). As a profession, nursing "exists in order to sustain caring, healing, and health where, and when, they are threatened biologically, institutionally, environmentally, or politically, by local, national, or global influences" (p. 146).

The practice of nursing based on Watson's theoretical and philosophical concepts differs substantially from biomedical/natural-science based practice. The physical body is cared for, but the care is never separated from the context of the unity of mindbodyspirit/nature.

Nursing Interventions

Effective interventions are related to the goals sought through the interventions. The goals of Watson's Theory of Transpersonal Caring relate to "mental-spiritual growth for self and others, finding meaning in one's own existence and experiences, discovering inner power and control, and potentiating instances of transcendance and self-healing" (Watson, 1985/1988, p. 74). In such a theoretical context, the nurse intervenes through " 'a way of being' rather than through use of a set of behaviors for the nurse 'to do'" (Neil, 1994, p. 37). The nurse serves as a coparticipant with the patient, who is the agent of change.

Interventions, or the human care processes, within the human care context require a wide scope of knowledge:

- of human behavior and human responses to actual or potential health problems . . .
- of individual needs . . .
- of how to respond to others' needs . . .
- of our strengths and limitation . . .
- of who the other person is . . . strengths and limitations, the meaning of the situation for him or her . . .
- of how to comfort, offer compassion and empathy. (Watson, 1985/1988, p. 74)

Such interactions also require an intention, a will, a relationship, and actions. All interventions within a human care context presuppose a knowledge base and clinical competence.

Watson continues to present the combination of interventions as the list of ten carative factors. Watson (1985/1988) noted that use of these carative factors to intervene "requires the nurse to possess specific intentions, a will, values, and a commitment to an ideal of intersubjective human-to-human care transaction that is directed toward the preservation of personhood and humanity of both nurse and patient . . . whether administering an emergency intravenous treatment . . . or changing the linen of an unconscious patient)" (p. 75).

Case Study: Applying Watson's Theory of Transpersonal Caring entails first and foremost a belief in the value and dignity of each human being. The nurse must honor and respect the power of intention inherent in the caring moment. Thus, the intent with which the nurse engages in another's life-force is as important as the specific interventions and will, in fact, guide the actions taken. Using the carative factors as a guide to nursing interventions is, thus, meant not to be so much prescriptive as to be used as a guide for creativity and inspiration for restoring harmony and unity within an individual's environment and personhood.

Situation: Mr. W, 82 years old, has recently left his home of 43 years to move in with his son and daughter-in-law. Mr. W's wife died of cancer 13 months ago and his son and family have become increasingly concerned over the past few months about Mr. W's safety and well-being. His health has been gradually failing to the point that he is now very unsteady when walking, unable to hear the telephone, and eating very little. The family has also noticed that Mr. W has not been keeping up with the routine maintenance on his house (e.g., basic cleaning and yard work). Mr. W has become very suspicious of family and friends and frequently says they are trying to "take advantage" of him.

The approach to nursing care in this situation is guided by the paradigmatic perspective from which it is viewed. If it is viewed within a totality, particularistic paradigm and the nursing process is applied, the initial step of *assessment* is undertaken for the purpose of identifying problems. In Mr. W's case, the assessment identifies functional deficits in the realms of mobility, socialization, and nutrition with an identified risk to Mr. W's physical safety and emotional well-being. Nursing *diagnoses* could include: risk for social isolation r/t suspiciousness; risk for injury r/t unsteady ambulation; altered nutrition: less than body requirements r/t decreased appetite and interest in food preparation; risk for dysfunctional grieving r/t recent death of spouse and evidence of possible depression. *Goals and outcomes* would relate to physical safety and psychological well-being. *Nursing interventions* would focus on coordinating services for Mr. W for the purpose of arranging a safer environment that allows for the highest level of independent function. Nursing actions, thus, might include teaching Mr. W to use a cane or walker, and referral for an audiological exam to determine if hearing aids would improve his hearing, and thereby possibly diminish the paranoid behaviors he is exhibiting. Teaching interventions may include education to the family and client as to the possibility of a dementia. If a psychiatric referral is made, an assessment for depression may be undertaken and a possible diagnosis be followed by treatment. In this case, such a diagnosis would be labeled a "pseudodementia," since depression in the elderly frequently results in cognitive changes and behavioral changes that may appear to be a type of dementia. If antidepressant therapy is prescribed for Mr. W, another nursing intervention may be to monitor for and to teach about the possible side effects of antidepressant medication. *Evaluation* would focus on data to indicate improvements in the identified areas of functional deficit.

Nursing care that is derived from a unitary-transformative paradigm and a perspective of Watson's Theory of Transpersonal Caring, would be primarily concerned with the way in which Mr. W's situation is affecting the relationships and activities that give meaning to his everyday life. The first step would be a *mutual engagement* of the nurse and Mr. W in order to reflect on that which makes Mr. W's life meaningful. This process reflects the carative factors, humanistic-altruistic values, and sensitivity to self and others. In Mr. W's situation, the nurse learns that Mr. W had always taken special pride in his home. This had included doing all of his own home repairs and a hobby of woodworking and furniture making. In the last few years, however, Mr. W had not been doing much woodworking because he had become the primary caregiver for his ailing wife. Mr. W tells the nurse that since his wife died, he sees very little purpose to "struggling alone" and reluctantly agreed to move in with his son and family only because they "left me little choice" and because he was afraid that his house would soon be in such bad need of repairs that it would sell for "next to nothing." From this very basic and somewhat cursory understanding of Mr. W's perspective, the nurse engages the family in a discussion of some of the ways in which Mr. W's move may be expected to be a struggle and present hardships, as well as the possible enriching and fulfilling aspects to the situation. This *discussion* reflects the carative factors faith-hope; expressing positive and negative feelings, and transpersonal teaching-learning. Referrals to an audiologist and physical therapist are made for Mr. W (e.g., carative factor, human needs assistance). The nurse, however, also discusses with Mr. W and the family possible ways to enhance the nonverbal aspect to communication in order to compensate for Mr. W's hearing loss. The son and daughter-in-law also suggest that Mr. W use a part of the garage to set up a small workshop of his own—one that will be on the same level as his bedroom and to which he will have safe and ready access. The family decides that Mr. W could possibly relieve an older son and daughter-in-law of some of the yard work (reflecting the carative factors: creative problem-solving caring processes, and supportive, protective, and/or corrective mental, physical, so-

TABLE 18–2. PARADIGMATIC APPROACHES TO NURSING CARE FOR MR. W.

	Totality/Particularistic Paradigm	Holographic/Simultaneity Paradigm
Ontology (values; mission)	Identifying problems and functional deficits—mobility, socialization, and nutrition	Engagement with patient and family for purpose of identifying potential meaningful aspects of the situation—pride in his home, struggle with change
Epistemology (framework for approach)	Nursing process; nursing diagnosis—risk for social isolation r/t suspiciousness; risk for injury r/t unsteady ambulation; altered nutrition: less than body requirements r/t decreased appetite and interest in food preparation; risk for dysfunctional grieving r/t recent death of spouse and evidence of possible depression	Carative factors—faith–hope; expressing positive and negative feelings; and transpersonal teaching–learning
Praxis (knowledgeable actions and interventions)	Coordinating services Teaching Referrals	Engagement and caring occasion Teaching Referrals
Goal (purpose)	Promotion of highest level of independent function and prevention of injury	Promotion of dignity, harmony of mind/body/spirit and enhancing possibility for growth and fulfillment

cietal, and spiritual environment). Mr. W decides that he would like to have breakfast and lunch in his room, but will plan to eat dinner with the family. It is hoped that such a plan will improve his nutritional intake.

In Mr. W's case, the purpose of nursing care derived from the perspective of Watson's theory is to promote dignity and harmony of mind/body/spirit. This entails a process of mutual reflection on the possibilities for growth and fulfillment in the situation rather than mere maintenance of function. Thus, Mr. W's frailty and greater dependency are seen as an opportunity for the family to give and receive love and concern rather than merely as a greater burden and imposition (reflecting the carative factor, existential-phenomenological-spiritual forces). Please refer to Table 18–2.

CRITIQUE OF WATSON'S THEORY OF TRANSPERSONAL CARING

1. What is the historical context of the theory? A theory should be judged in light of the historical context within which it was created and the purpose for which it was intended. Jean Watson has stated that the purpose of the Theory of Transpersonal Caring is to "help others to see, to view phenomena in a new or different way, perhaps to develop or to attempt a new starting point, to use a new lens when focusing on the phenomena of human behavior in health and illness" (Watson, 1985/1988, p. 1). Watson's theory was never designed to be a theory with specific testable constructs in the natural science tradition. It began as a philosophy and with delineation of the carative factors and explication of the constructs. In Watson's 1985/1988 version, it became more of a theory at the grand or middle-range level. Watson's theory attempts to move nursing from the modernist view of the human body as machine and reality as discrete, elemental, and concrete, into a world of the metaphysical where the interdependent and nondiscrete nature of a world and the spiritual nature of humans is of paramount importance. Watson's theory is based on the Nightingale concept of a healing environment. Watson believes not only that interpersonal and environmental factors affect healing, but also that healing and a sense of well-being can occur in the presence as well as in the absence of disease. Thus, a core concept of Watson's theory is that caring is independent of curing.

2. What are the basic concepts and relationships presented by the theory? Watson's theory defines health and illness as harmony/disharmony of the mind/body/spirit. Eastern philosophies regarding the nature of the spirit and consciousness in health and healing greatly influenced Watson's original conceptualization of caring in the human health experience. The influence of Chaos Theory (Kellert, 1993) and quantum physics and quantum mechanics (Pelletier, 1985) on later twentieth century ideas about a universal consciousness and energy fields is seen in Watson's most recent thoughts on nursing as a caring ontology and the transpersonal occasion as an exchange of energy and consciousness with the capability to facilitate healing.

A common criticism of Watson's work is that by separating the person into mind, body, and spirit, Watson contradicts the core of her theory, which is that the essence of being human is wholeness and interconnectedness. This clearly is an invalid criticism in that it is not Watson's conceptualization that is flawed, but rather the language with which to express these concepts is limited. Watson has frequently stated that metaphor and poetry portray the lived experience in a much richer and more meaningful way than does the language of traditional science adopted by the medical and clinical professions. For this reason, Watson's writings are uniquely elegant as she intersperses everyday language with metaphors and images of classical literature and poetry. Often such writings are used not only to describe the ontological aspect of her theory, but also to argue for an expansion of the epistemology of nursing to include aesthetic and creative methods of discovering knowledge beyond the more traditional prescriptive methods of laboratory and social sciences.

Watson's conceptualization of the human form as an open, transforming system capable of growth and transcendence has roots in the concept of the unitary person developed by Martha Rogers (1970), as well as in existentialism. Her belief that "the body resides in a field of consciousness, rather than consciousness residing in the body" (Watson, 1999, p. 169) is based on ancient writings such as those of the twelfth century mystic Hildegard of Bingen (1985), as well as twentieth century artists such as Alex Grey (1990) and postmodern thinkers who write about the universal consciousness and the body as soul (Campbell, 1972; Wilber, 1982; Zukav, 1990). The embeddedness of body in soul is a complex concept and can be confusing in a culture that envisions the body as separate from the mind—as a mechanistic system of parts capable of replacement (consider the widespread notion of organ transplantation as a viable cure for disease and potential hope of the future for extending life). Therefore, while Watson has never excluded the "body physical" in her writings, many readers focus on the relational (e.g., transpersonal occasion) aspect of her theory instead of the connection between body and soul. In her earlier works, Watson refers to the skills and techniques of nursing as the "trim." Although she recognized the importance of the nurse to be "confident and competent in delivery of care" (Watson, 1985/1988, p. xvi), she clearly emphasized the carative factors as the core of nursing (p. xvii). Watson's recent theoretical writings emphasize to a much greater degree the human as "embodied spirit" and, thus, can no longer be misinterpreted as diminishing the importance of the body at the expense of the concepts of mind and spirit.

3. What major phenomena of concern to nursing are presented? These phenomena may include *but are not limited to*: human being, environment, health, interpersonal relations, caring, goal attainment, adaptation, and energy fields. Caring is the essence of Watson's theory. Caring, however, is not unique to nursing knowledge or practice. It is, rather, the pattern of the concepts and the way in which caring is defined in terms of specific human actions as well as the context within which it occurs that makes it unique to nursing. New worldviews reflecting ideas on energy fields, wholeness, processes, and patterns have been the basis on which theories in nursing have been built (Boykin & Schoenhofer, 1993). Regardless of whether caring is conceptualized as a human trait, a moral imperative, an affect, an interpersonal interaction, or an intervention, it is about a unique way of living caring in the world (Morse, Solberg, Neander, Bottorff, & Johnson, 1990). The focus of Watson's theory, thus, is not on an outcome such as health or wellness, but about caring for oneself, one's fellow human beings, and one's environment. Watson refers to this as "ontological caring," and believes that nurses have a moral commitment to care. Thus, while Watson uses everyday language to express the concepts of caring, the philosophical underpinnings are anything but simplistic.

Watson's theory is based on a cosmology of consciousness and possibility rather than one of matter and predictability. She posits nursing to be "metaphor for the sacred feminine archetypal energy, now critical to the healing needed in modern Western nursing and medicine" (Watson, 1999, p. 11). This cosmology is grounded in a moral ontology of caring, an epistemology open to multiple ways of being, knowing, and doing, and a postmodern quantum reality of nonlinear, complex, holographic systems. All of reality exists between the real and the possible and intentionality as consciousness and energy have the power to heal. Within this framework, the transpersonal caring occasion is not just an affect or emotion expressed between two people, but is energy with the potential for transforming and creating a new order or reality.

Thus, Watson articulates each of the metaparadigm concepts of human, health, environment, and nursing within an expanded worldview. The Nightingale emphasis on fresh air and clean water is broadened to include the healing power of the higher frequency energy transmitted by loving, caring intentions and actions. Human beings are envisioned not only as a system of cells, tissues, and organs, but as energy manifested in the ancient Hindu chakra system and the concept of the extrasensory. Energy and its balance play a role in health and healing. Within this worldview, the ontological state of the nurse is as essential to the caring/healing act as is any technological competency.

4. To whom does this theory apply? In what situations? In what ways? Watson's theory has the potential to apply to any situation in which nursing occurs. Any individual nurse in any setting can make use of the carative factors in interacting and delivering care. One demonstration of the application of this theory can be found in The Caring Center.

The Caring Center (DNPHC) was opened in 1988 as a totally nurse-directed center for clients with HIV infections/AIDS (Neil, 1990; 1994). The mission of the Center was to facilitate high quality health care for HIV-positive clients and their lovers, friends, and families. The Center believed that the healing process is fostered by the understanding, love, and concern of those who care. Each client was linked to a particular nurse who had a responsibility to be the patient's advocate. The clients had the opportunity to change nurses at their request. The Center was a model for research as praxis in that focus group meetings of staff and clients cocreated understanding and insights into the personal experience as well as the way in which the Center was operated. Programmatic decisions were based on the insights that developed out of these group meetings. Watson's theory provided the framework for the Center from the outset. In order to keep the caring theory alive and to facilitate greater consistency in applying the theory, every six months chart audits were done in which the narratives were analyzed for the way in which the carative factors had been applied in specific nurse–patient situations. In keeping with Watson's view of nursing as human science, aesthetic methods of inquiry, such as photography, were incorporated into the programmatic evaluation. The DNPHC is an excellent exemplar of how a clinical model of care uses a theory of nursing to design its purpose, organization, and program of evaluation.

5. By what method or methods can this theory be tested? Validating the concepts of Watson's theory mandates that the researcher cocreate meaning from the lived experience. Two exemplars of this type of work are Swanson's (1991) phenomenological study of caring processes identified with perinatal populations, and Neil's (1990, 1994) work with the Denver Nursing Project in Human Caring (DNPHC) for clients with HIV infections/AIDS.

Swanson's (1991) phenomenological study with three perinatal populations identified five caring processes. There was considerable cross-validation of these processes with Watson's carative factors. For example, Swanson identified one common caring process as "maintaining belief," which includes continuing to believe in another person's ability to deal with the current situation and move into a future that has meaning. Swanson correlated this process with Watson's carative factors 2 and 10 (Watson, 1985/88, p. 75) "faith-hope" and "existential-phenomenological-spiritual forces," respectively. Swanson concludes that the congruence of the five processes delineated in her study with three different perinatal populations is evidence of the validity of caring theory for nursing.

6. Does this theory direct critical thinking in nursing practice? In order to maximize the impact of Watson's theory on nursing practice, the philosophy and environment within which the nurse acts must be congruent with the cosmology that undergirds the constructs and principles of Watson's theory. In general, schools of thought that are based on linear, mechanistic models of thought, such as nursing diagnosis and critical thinking, are barriers to the enactment of Watson's theory.

7. Does this theory direct therapeutic nursing interventions? and **8. Does this theory direct communication in nursing practice?** Communication must occur for transpersonal caring to be a reality. However, in Watson's theory, communication is considered in the broadest terms possible and certainly not limited to verbal exchanges.

9. Does this theory direct nursing actions that lead to favorable outcomes? Three eras, corresponding to three paradigms that have affected nursing's progress and maturity, have been identified by nursing leaders and are discussed by Watson (1999, p. 98). Dossey (1991) described these paradigms as eras of medical science and treatment models: Era I (particulate–deterministic); Era II (integrative–interactive); and Era III (unitary-transformative). Until health care systems are congruent with the worldview identified by Era III, there is no systematic way by which the outcomes of Watson's theory may be judged.

Although the measurement of outcomes as defined within other paradigms does not fit within the Era III transformative paradigm of Watson's work, much work has been done to apply the concepts of the theory to nursing practice and research. For example, Nyman and Lutzen (1999) used Watson's ten carative factors to design a conversation guide for determining caring needs specific to the human experience of having rheumatoid arthritis and undergoing acupuncture treatment. This study is an excellent example of applying Watson's theory to evaluate caring needs that foster health in the more holistic sense of the physical, social, aesthetic, and spiritual. The caring needs identified in this study of women with rheumatoid arthritis were in the realms of seeking help, searching for meaning, uncertainty, and fear of being disappointed. It is clear from this study that when philosophically congruent methods are applied to a theory for the purpose of expanding the knowledge base of nursing as a human science with a mission of healing and health, specific and meaningful interventions by which the carative factors can be applied within a specific context may be discovered. Nyman and Lutzen's study is, thus, an exemplar for making Watson's grand theory accessible and applicable to the practice of nursing.

   10. How contagious is this theory? Clinical nurses and academic programs throughout the world use Watson's published works on the philosophy and theory of human caring and the art and science of nursing. Watson's caring philosophy is used to guide new models of caring and healing practices in diverse settings and in several different countries. In fact, educational and clinical centers in Sweden, the United Kingdom, and New Zealand have been developed and are more progressive and in line with the cosmology of Era III than has been the case, except rarely, in the United States. Watson lists numerous universities abroad using nursing education models based on ontologically congruent caring philosophies. The countries include: Sweden, Finland, Norway, Australia, New Zealand, the United Kingdom, as well as recent developments in Japan, Thailand, and South America (Watson, 1999, pp. 187–189). Both internationally and within the United States there are many models of practice being used in clinics, hospitals, home-based and community health programs that are based on a caring science and the constructs of Watson's theory (pp. 182–192).

STRENGTHS AND LIMITATIONS OF WATSON'S THEORY

Watson's work has been criticized by many who do not operate from the same Era III paradigm that serves as context for the theory. The lack of emphasis on physical as a separate entity on which to focus care disturbs those still practicing from the mechanistic medical model. Watson's "embodied spirit" does not satisfy those who perceive the world from that model.

   But Watson's work is transformative at all levels and realms of nursing. The theory directs the focus back onto the person and mandates that technology be used selectively for the betterment of humankind rather than as the sole guiding factor in health care. Watson attempts to rekindle the passion of nursing for the sacredness of being human and the sacred traditions of health and healing. The limitations of Watson's theory are not to be found in the validity of her work, but rather in the barriers to enacting these principles created by a bureaucratic health care system guided by an entirely different set of values and beliefs. The future of Watson's theory will be determined largely by the degree to which the public and the, as yet, minority of professional healers and clinicians can transform "sickness treatment systems" into the "healing/health care centers" of a caring, holographic cosmology.

SUMMARY

Jean Watson has played a major role in reorienting nursing from a biomedical, mechanistic model to one of caring as transpersonal, interactive process. While never intending to exclude the physical body from the mind/body/spirit, Watson does diminish the importance of the physical. The body is conceived to be inside consciousness. The self and person are viewed as transpersonal mindbodyspirit oneness, part of an unbroken wholeness of subject-object-person-environment-nature-universe-all living things. The role of body is best conceived as embodied spirit.

For the nurse, as coparticipant with the client as change agent, nursing care is a "way of being" rather than doing. However, all of transpersonal caring–healing is expected to take place in a context of a broad knowledge base, including physical and skill-based knowledge. It is the definitions of health and illness and the goals of caring–healing that differ and reorient nursing care. Health as unity and harmony within body, mind, and soul, and the degree of convergence between self as perceived and self as experienced determining health or illness, drive the goals of care in Watson's theory. The goals of mental–spiritual growth for self and others; finding meaning in one's existence and experiences; discovering inner power and control; and potentiating instances of transcendence and self-healing reflect a caring–healing consciousness that transcends time and space. Dr. Watson believes that the caring–healing consciousness of a caring occasion–caring moment opens up a higher energy field with potential for healing beyond body and self, with potential movement toward greater harmony, wholeness, health, and spiritual evolution.

REFERENCES

Bingen, H. (1985). *Illuminations of Hildegard of Bingen.* (Text by Hildegard of Bingen, commentary by M. Fox). Sante Fe, NM: Bear Publications.

Boykin, A., & Schoenhofer, S. (1993). *Nursing as caring: A model for transforming practice* (Pub. No. 15-2549). New York: National League for Nursing Press.

Campbell, J. (1972). *Myths to live by.* New York: Viking Press.

de Chardin, P. (1959). *The phenomenon of man.* New York: Harper & Row.

de Chardin, P. (1967). *On love.* New York: Harper & Row.

Dossey, L. (1991). *Meaning and medicine.* New York: Bantam.

Gadow, S. (1980). Existential advocacy: Philosophical foundation of nursing. In S. Spicker & S. Gadow (Eds.), *Nursing images and ideals* (pp. 86–101). New York: Springer.

Grey, A. (1990). *Sacred mirrors: The visionary art of Alex Grey.* Rochester, NY: Inner Traditions International.

Henderson, V. (1966). *The nature of nursing: A definition and its implications for practice, research, and education.* New York: Macmillan.

Kellert, S. (1993). *In the wake of chaos.* Chicago: The University of Chicago Press.

Kierkegaard, S. (1941). *Concluding: Unscientific postscript.* D. S. Swenson and W. Lowrie (trans.). Princeton, NJ: Princeton University Press.

Leininger, M. (1980). Caring: A central focus of nursing and health care. *Nursing and Health Care,* *1*(3), 135–143.

Leininger, M. (Ed.). (1981). *Caring: An essential human need.* Thorofare, NJ: Charles B. Slack.

Morse, J., Solberg, S., Neander, W., Bottorff, J., & Johnson, J. (1990). Concepts of caring and caring as a concept. *Advances in Nursing Science, 13*(1), 1–14.

Neil, R. (1990). Watson's theory of caring in nursing: The rainbow of and for people living with AIDS. In M. Parker (Ed.), *Nursing theories in practice* (pp. 289–301). New York: National League for Nursing Press.

Neil, R. (1994). Authentic caring: The sensible answer for clients and staff dealing with HIV/AIDS. *Nursing Administration Quarterly, 18*(2), 36–40.

Nightingale, F. (1957). *Notes on nursing: What it is, and what it is not* (com. ed.). Philadelphia: Lippincott. (Originally published, 1859).

Nyman, C., & Lutzen, K. (1999). Caring needs of patients with rheumatoid arthritis. *Nursing Science Quarterly, 12*(2), 164–169.

Pelletier, K. (1985). *Toward a science of consciousness.* Berkeley, CA: Celestial Arts.

Rogers, C. R. (1961). *On becoming a person: A therapist's view of psychology.* Boston: Houghton Mifflin.

Rogers, M. (1970). *An introduction to the theoretical basis of nursing.* Philadelphia: Davis.

Swanson, K. M. (1991). Empirical development of a middle range theory of caring. *Nursing Research, 40*(3), 161–166.

Watson, J. (1979). *Nursing: The philosophy and science of caring.* Boston: Little, Brown.

Watson, J. (1988). *Nursing: Human science and human care: A theory of nursing.* New York: National League for Nursing. (Originally published 1985, Appleton-Century-Crofts).

Watson, J. (1989). Keynote address: Caring theory. *Journal of Japan Academy of Nursing Science, 9*(2), 29–37.

Watson, M. J. (1996). Watson's theory of transpersonal caring. In P. H. Walker & B. Neuman (Eds.), *Blueprint for use of nursing models: Education, research, practice & administration* (pp. 141–184) (Pub. No. 14-2696). New York: National League for Nursing Press.

Watson, J. (1999). *Postmodern nursing and beyond.* New York: Harcourt, Brace.

Whitehead, A. N. (1953). *Science and the modern world.* Cambridge, England: Cambridge University Press.

Wilber, K. (Ed.). (1982). *The holographic paradigm and other paradoxes.* Boston: New Science Library.

Zukav, G. (1990). *The seat of the soul.* New York: Fireside (Simon & Schuster).

ANNOTATED BIBLIOGRAPHY

Capik, L. K. (1997). The Watson Theory of Human Care applied to ASPO/Lamaze perinatal education. *Journal of Perinatal Education, 6*(1), 43–47.
   This article links Watson's concepts of spirituality, client empowerment, caring–healing practice and ten carative factors to the philosophy of the American Society of Psychoprophylaxis in Obstetrics. Applications to perinatal education are discussed.

Chinn, P., & Watson, J. (1994). Introduction: Art and aesthetics as passage between centuries. In P. Chinn & J. Watson, *Art and aesthetics in nursing.* New York: National League for Nursing Press.
   The authors propose that the lost art of nursing is now being reclaimed and restored. They assert that art conspires with the spirit to emancipate humans and allows us to locate ourselves in another space and place, to change our perceptions and points of view. They propose to move nursing beyond the twentieth century during which spirituality has been separated from art, and art

from science. A reintegrating paradigm of caring–healing arts, with new visions, new vocabulary, and new traditions is being developed. The themes that emerge are: art as asking and knowing, art as learning, art as practice, and art as reflective experience.

Donohue, M. A. T. (1991). *The lived experience of stigma in individuals with AIDS: A phenomenological investigation.* (Online). Dissertation abstract from: CINAHL Accession Number: 1994179703.

A phenomenological analysis of the emotional and psychosocial total of being identified as having AIDS. Nine adults described their experiences with this stigma and were interviewed. A qualitative structural analysis was conducted and implications for nursing identified using Watson's theory.

McNamara, S. A. (1995). Perioperative nurses' perceptions of caring practices. *AORN Journal, 61*(2), 377, 380–382, 384–385.

Interviews were conducted with five perioperative nurses to identify how they practice caring with both conscious and unconscious patients throughout the perioperative period. The essential elements included establishing a caring relationship and providing a supportive, corrective, or protective environment for the total person.

Neil, R. (1994). Authentic caring: The sensible answer for clients and staff dealing with HIV/AIDS. *Nursing Administration Quarterly, 18*(2), 36–40.

An overview of the theory and operation of the Denver Nursing Project in Human Caring is provided. The nurse-managed outpatient community center provides integrated care and services to persons living with HIV/AIDS, their family members, and friends. Care theories of Parse and Watson are examined for areas of agreement and differences. Major tenets of existential phenomenology are described along with each theory's anchoring motifs, concepts, and principles. The theories are applied to a case study.

Schroeder, C., & Maeve, M. K. (1992). Nursing care partnerships at the Denver Nursing Project in Human Caring: An application and extension of caring theory in practice. *Advances in Nursing Science, 15*(2), 25–38.

Describes the development of nursing care partnerships as a new model of nursing practice using Watson's theory as the framework in this nurse-managed center for people living with HIV/AIDS. Includes narrative accounts from both nurses and clients to describe the relationships that are formed in this journey.

Watson, J. (1988). New dimensions of human caring theory. *Nursing Science Quarterly, 1*(4), 175–181.

Watson redefines contemporary nursing based on a caring–healing consciousness embedded in an ethic of caring as a moral ideal. She describes human caring and healing as transpersonal and intersubjective and opening up a "higher energy field-consciousness that has metaphysical, transcendent potentialities" (p. 181). A new metaparadigm for nursing is presented, consistent with holographic views of science.

Watson, J. (1990). The moral failure of the patriarchy. *Nursing Outlook, 38*(2), 62–66.

The moral failure of the patriarchal worldview in health care, in which caring is viewed as women's work and is not valued or is considered less important than men's work, is asserted. Suggestions for overcoming the patriarchy are offered.

Watson, J. (1994). Poeticizing as truth through language. In P. Chinn & J. Watson, *Art & aesthetics in nursing*. New York: National League for Nursing Press.

Because we are humans, our Truths are cocreated through a process of values and meaning-making via language. Discussed are concepts of truth and the relationship of poetry and truth, and ways of knowing. When our values become human values of caring for self, others, and all living things, and when the meaning-making of Truth involves humans and cocreation of meaning via language, then a different scenario is revealed, one of the possibilities of poeticizing as Truth. This is a way of inverting the paradigm and understanding human experiences from the inside out. This shift to a new dynamic of understanding human experience also shifts nursing's subject matter to a more authentic and poetic expression of the postmodern perspective.

Watson, J. (1995). Nursing's caring–healing paradigm as exemplar for alternative medicine? *Alternative Therapies, 1*(3), 64–69.

Provides an overview of the crisis in modern (biomedical) and postmodern (human) science and method. The evolving of nursing's caring and healing system within a unitary–transformative context is presented as an exemplar for alternative medicine.

Watson, J. (1996). United States of America: Can nursing theory and practice survive? *International Journal of Nursing Practice, 2*, 241–247.

Watson argues that the concept of caring and caring theory take on new meaning in the most contemporary discourse about theory and practice. If caring as value, ethic, concept, and theory is reconsidered, it offers a metanarrative for placing professional practice and knowledge within the distinct context of nursing. She proposes that caring theory, with its explicit philosophy and ethic of caring, context, meaning, along with its set of embedded values toward person, unity of mind/body/spirit, healing, wholeness, relation, etc., could serve as an overarching ideal for nursing, its critique of knowledge, and its application to science and practice. She calls for international models of caring–healing excellence, with communities of researchers in multiple sites, sharing assessment tools, protocols, and outcome data.

Watson, J. (1997). The theory of human caring: Retrospective and prospective. *Nursing Science Quarterly, 10*(1), 49–52.

Watson provides an overview of her original work and a description of the contemporary status of her caring theory. She offers projections for the future of the theory's use. She notes that use of the theory requires new ways of thinking, being, and acting that converge; and requires a personal, social, moral, and spiritual engagement of self. She invites users of the theory to participate as cocreators of the theory's further emergence.

Watson, J. (1999). *Postmodern nursing and beyond.* Edinburgh: Churchill Livingstone.

This work expounds and expands on Watson's philosophical concepts. She proposes that the shift from traditional, modern, Western thought to what is emerging goes beyond a paradigm shift toward an ontological shift. The elements of this ontological shift are reflected in the following paths (p. xv):

> Path of awareness, of awakening to the sacred feminine archetype/cosmology . . .;
> Path of cultivation of higher/deeper self and a higher consciousness: transpersonal self;
> Path of honoring the sacred within and without . . .;
> Path of acknowledging the metaphysical/spiritual level . . .;
> Path of acknowledging quantum concepts and phenomena such as caring-healing energy, intentionality and consciousness . . . toward . . . the evolving human consciousness;
> Path of honoring the connectedness of all . . .;
> Path of honoring the unity of mindbodyspirit . . .;
> Path of reintegrating the caring-healing arts, as an artistry of being, into healing practices . . .;
> Path of creating healing space . . .;
> Path of a relational ontology . . .;
> Path of moving beyond the modern–postmodern into the open, transpersonal space and the new thinking required for the next millennium.

Watson notes that this work is grounded in nursing, but paradoxically and simultaneously transcends nursing. The proposed ontological shift is inviting and requiring a reconstruction and revision of all medical and professional health education and practice.

CHAPTER 19

THEORY OF HUMAN BECOMING
ROSEMARIE RIZZO PARSE

Janet S. Hickman

■ ■ ■

Rosemarie Rizzo Parse earned her Bachelor of Science degree in Nursing from Duquesne University, Pittsburgh, and her Master's Degree in Nursing and Ph.D. from the University of Pittsburgh. She holds the Marcella Niehoff Chair at Loyola University in Chicago and is a Fellow of the American Academy of Nursing. Previous positions include faculty at the University of Pittsburgh; dean of the Nursing School at Duquesne University; and professor and coordinator of the Center for Nursing Research at Hunter College, City University of New York. She has been visiting professor at the University of Cincinnati; University of South Carolina; Wright State University; University of Western Sydney, Australia; and Florida Atlantic University (as the first Christine E. Lynn Eminent Scholar in Nursing).

Parse is the founding editor of Nursing Science Quarterly, *a journal that focuses on theory development and research in nursing science. She is also president of Discovery International, Inc., a firm that sponsors international theory conferences, and the founder of the Institute of Human Becoming where she teaches the ontological, epistemological, and methodological aspects of the human becoming school of thought. A recent work is* Hope: An international human perspective (1999). *Previous major works include* Man–Living–Health: A theory of nursing (1981); Nursing science: Major paradigms, theories, and critiques (1987); Nursing research: Qualitative methods (Parse, Coyne, & Smith, 1985); *and* The human becoming school of thought: A perspective for nurses and other health care providers (1998).

Parse's theory supports clinical nursing practice in a variety of settings in Canada, Finland, and Sweden as well as the United States. Her research methodology has influenced the work of nurse scholars in Australia, Canada, Denmark, Finland, Greece, Italy, Japan, South Korea, Sweden, the United Kingdom, and the United States.

In 1981, Parse presented a unique theory of nursing titled "Man–Living–Health," which synthesized principles and concepts from Rogers (1970, 1984) and concepts and tenets from existential phenomenology. Parse (1981, 1992b) said that man refers to *Homo sapiens*, a generic term for all human beings. She stated that her purpose was to posit an idea of nursing rooted in the human sciences as an alternative to ideas of nursing grounded in the natural sciences. She defined natural science-based nursing as having to do with the quantification of man and illness rather than the qualification of man's total experience with health.

In 1987, Parse refined this discussion by presenting two paradigms, or world-views, of nursing. The first discussed is the totality paradigm in which man is posited as a total summative being whose nature is a combination of bio-psycho-social-spiritual aspects. The environment is viewed as the external and internal stimuli surrounding man. Man interacts and adapts with his environment to maintain equilibrium and to achieve goals. This is a refined definition of the natural, or medical, science approach to nursing. Parse states that the works of Peplau (1952/1988), Henderson (1991), Hall (1965), Orlando (1961), Levine (1989), Johnson (1980), Roy (1984; Andrews & Roy, 1986; Roy & Andrews, 1991), Orem (1991), and King (1981, 1989) are representative of the totality paradigm.

The second worldview that Parse (1987) discusses is the simultaneity paradigm, which views man as "more than and different from the sum of the parts . . . an open being free to choose in mutual rhythmical interchange with the environment . . . gives meaning to situations and is responsible for choices in moving beyond what is . . . experiencing the what was, is, and will be, all at once . . ." (p. 136). This is a refined definition of the human science approach to nursing. Parse states that her own work and that of Rogers (1992) are representative of the simultaneity paradigm.

Parse (1998) further differentiates the paradigms by stating that the totality paradigm views nursing as an *applied* science, drawing knowledge from all other sciences, while the simultaneity paradigm views nursing as a *basic* science with its own body of distinct knowledge. Consequently, totality paradigm-based nursing practice focuses on diagnosis and treatment in curing, controlling, and preventing disease. In contrast, simultaneity paradigm-based nursing practice focuses on the optimal well-being of unitary human being (Rogers, 1970, 1992) and quality of life (Parse, 1981, 1992b, 1995, 1997a, 1998).

In the spring of 1992, Parse (1992b) changed the name of her theory of Man–Living–Health to the theory of Human Becoming. She reworded the assumptions accordingly. No other aspects of the theory were changed. The revision was made as a response to a change in the dictionary definition of the term *man*. The current dictionary definition is gender-based as opposed to the previous use of the word *man* to identify mankind.

In the preface to the 1998 revision of her work, Parse describes " . . . a global move toward more concern for the perspective of the person and family to satisfy the concerns of the public for more humane treatment, yet at the same time there is a growing trend toward diminishing services, with the blurring of disciplinary boundaries and cross-education of health care providers to lower the cost of health care" (1998, p. ix).

Parse (1998) describes her original 1981 work as a theory of nursing, which has over time evolved into a school of thought. She defines a school of thought as "a theoretical view held by a community of scholars. . . . It is a knowledge tradition, including a specific ontology (assumptions and principles), a specified epistemology (focus of inquiry), and congruent methodologies (approaches to research and practice)"(p. ix). Parse writes that the term *theory* refers to the principles of human becoming.

SUMMARY OF PARSE'S THEORY

Parse's theory makes assumptions about humans and health and deduces from them the principles, concepts, and theoretical structures of human becoming. These assumptions are based on Rogers's principles and concepts and the works of Heidegger (1962, 1972), Sartre (1963, 1964, 1966), and Merleau-Ponty (1973, 1974) on existential–phenomenological thought. Parse uses Rogers's three major principles: helicy, complementarity (now called integrality), and resonancy; and her four major concepts: energy field, openness, pattern, and organization; and four dimensionality (now called pandimensionality) as part of the theoretical basis for her own assumptions about man and health. Parse synthesizes these principles and concepts with the following tenets and concepts of existential–phenomenological thought: intentionality, human subjectivity, coconstitution, coexistence, and situated freedom. It is important to remember that the process of synthesis is, by definition, the combining of elements to create something new and different. Therefore, as will be demonstrated in the discussion of Parse's assumptions, the products of her synthesis are new and different from the original principles, tenets, and concepts on which they are based.

Parse's human becoming school of thought is a human science system of interrelated concepts describing unitary human's mutual process with the universe in cocreating becoming. The school of thought has its roots in the human sciences, which posit methodologies directed toward uncovering the meaning of phenomena as humanly experienced. The methods of inquiry lead to the creation of theories about the meaning of lived experiences. A fundamental tenet to the ontology of human becoming is the individual's participation in health (Parse, 1998).

ASSUMPTIONS

As the language of this theory has changed, it is helpful to look at the assumptions as they were originally stated. In Parse's 1981 book, *Man–Living–Health: A theory of nursing* she posited nine assumptions, each of which was based on 3 of the 12 previously identified principles, tenets, and concepts from Rogers' theory and on existential–phenomenological thought. Phillips (1987) points out that for 6 of the 9 assumptions, 2 of the 3 concepts used as the basis for each assumption come from Rogers; leaving 3 assumptions for which 2 of the 3 concepts come from existential–phenomenology. Quantitatively, Phillips implies a greater grounding of the assumptions in Rogers' theory than in existential–phenomenology. In contrast,

Winkler (1983) states that Parse's assumptions come primarily from philosophical sources and secondarily from Rogers' theory.

Parse's (1981) original nine assumptions are the following:

1. Man is coexisting while coconstituting rhythmical patterns with the environment (based on *pattern and organization, coconstitution*, and *coexistence*).
2. Man is an open being, freely choosing meaning in situation, bearing responsibility for decisions (based on *energy field, openness*, and *situated freedom*).
3. Man is a living unity continuously coconstituting patterns of relating (based on *energy field, pattern and organization*, and *coconstitution*).
4. Man is transcending multidimensionally with the possibles (based on *openness, four dimensionality*, and *situated freedom*).
5. Health is an open process of becoming, experienced by man (based on *openness, coconstitution*, and *situated freedom*).
6. Health is a rhythmically coconstituting process of the man-environment interrelationship (based on *pattern and organization, four dimensionality*, and *coconstitution*).
7. Health is man's pattern of relating value priorities (based on *openness, pattern and organization*, and *situated freedom*).
8. Health is an intersubjective process of transcending with the possibles (based on *openness, coexistence*, and *situated freedom*).
9. Health is unitary man's negentropic unfolding (based on *energy field, four dimensionality*, and *coexistence*) (pp. 25–36).

In Parse's latest revision (1998), each assumption is a synthesis of postulates with concepts in unique three-way combinations. Each of the postulates and concepts (energy field, openness, pattern, pandimensionality, coconstitution, coexistence, and situated freedom) is connected at least once with the assumptions in which they appear. The assumptions about the theory of human becoming are:

1. The human is coexisting while coconstituting rhythmical patterns with the universe.
2. The human is open, freely choosing meaning in situation, bearing responsibility for decisions.
3. The human is unitary, continuously coconstituting patterns of relating.
4. The human is transcending multidimensionally with the possibles.
5. Becoming is unitary human–living–health.
6. Becoming is a rhythmically coconstituting process of the human–universe process.
7. Becoming is the human's pattern of relating value priorities.
8. Becoming is an intersubjective process of transcending with the possibles.
9. Becoming is unitary human's emerging (pp. 19–20).

Assumption 1 (The human is coexisting while coconstituting rhythmical patterns with the universe.) This assumption means that the human lives with others mutually evolving with the universe. The human pattern and the universe pattern are unique and distinct, but are rhythmical and together coexist.

Assumption 2 (The human is open, freely choosing meaning in situation, bearing responsibility for decisions.) This assumption means " . . . that the human, in open process with the universe, chooses ways of becoming in situation and is accountable for these choices" (Parse 1998, p. 21). In choosing the meanings of situations, the human gives up other choices and is therefore both enabled and limited by the choices made. The human remains responsible for all the outcomes of choices made, even though these outcomes may be unknown at the time of the original choice.

Assumption 3 (The human is unitary, continuously coconstituting patterns of relating.) This assumption means that the human is unitary and cannot be divided into parts. It also means that "Coconstituted patterns of relating are . . . illuminated through speech, words, symbols, silence, gesture, movement, gaze, posture, and touch" (Parse, 1998, p. 22).

Assumption 4 (The human is transcending multidimensionally with the possibles.) This assumption means that the human, in conjunction with the human–universe mutual process, chooses to move beyond the actual, the contextual situation, with possibilities. This movement is unidirectional; it is not repeatable or reversible. A human moves beyond who one is via the mutual human–universe process in imaging possibilities. The human transcends the possibles by experiencing events in context. This experiencing opens or illuminates other possibilities that the human reaches toward while continually becoming through choosing.

Assumption 5 (Becoming is unitary human–living–health) This assumption means that there is continuous movement that both enables and limits becoming in the human–universe mutual process. The human's view of the options or choices one makes is based on personal history as that human knows it. An experience of a situation, though cocreated, belongs to only one person. "Choosing some options eliminates others so that possibilities are cocreated and experienced perspectively in the process of becoming—living health . . . The unique perspective of each human beings' experiencing the human–universe mutual process is health" (Parse, 1998, p. 23).

Assumption 6 (Becoming is a rhythmically coconstituting process of the human–universe process.) This assumption means that human becoming is the rhythmical process of changing through the mutual connecting–separating of human with universe. In each connecting, there is also separating, and with each separating, there is also connecting. This is paradoxical and it conconstitutes the emergence of health as a relative present.

Assumption 7 (Becoming is the human's pattern of relating value priorities.) "This assumption means that becoming is the human's style of living chosen cherished ideals, which are values—prized beliefs. Value priorities are the preferred prized beliefs. Becoming or health is a synthesis of the human's values selected from multidimensional experiences cocreated in mutual process with the universe" (Parse, 1998, p. 24).

Assumption 8 (Becoming is an intersubjective process of transcending with the possibles.) This assumption means that becoming is moving beyond with the possibles through a subject-to-subject mutual human–universe process. "Moving beyond with possibles," means experiencing the familiar while at the same time struggling with the unfamiliar of an imaged not-yet.

Assumption 9 (Becoming is unitary human's emerging.) This assumption means that becoming is the human's multidimensional changing in process with the universe. The human's coexisting multidimensional experience with the universe powers the creation of individual patterns of relating that arise as rhythms of human becoming. Therefore, human health is continuously changing in diverse ways.

The original nine assumptions are further synthesized into three assumptions on human becoming (updated from Parse 1992b, p. 38):

- Human Becoming is freely choosing personal meaning in situations in the intersubjective process of relating value priorities.
- Human Becoming is cocreating rhythmical patterns of relating in open interchange with the universe.
- Human Becoming is cotranscending multidimensionally with the unfolding possibilities (Parse, 1998, pp. 28–29).

The first assumption states that human becoming is a subject–subject or subject–universe interchange where the meaning assigned to the experience reflects one's personal values. This is a synthesis of numbers 2, 5, and 7 of her original 9, which are based on the concepts of energy field, openness, situated freedom, coconstitution, and pattern and organization.

The second assumption states that human becoming is an open interchange with the universe while *together* the human being and the environment create rhythmical patterns. This assumption appears to be a synthesis of original assumptions 1, 3, and 6, which are based on the concepts of energy fields, openness, situated freedom, pattern and organization, and coconstitution.

The third assumption states that human becoming is moving beyond the self at all levels of the universe as dreams become realities. Cotranscending is moving beyond with others and the universe multidimensionally. Multidimensionally refers to the various levels of the universe that humans experience "all at once," and choose possibles from in various situations. This is a synthesis of original assumptions 4, 8, and 9, which are based on the concepts of openness, four dimensionality, situated freedom, coexistence, and energy field. It is important to note that Parse is viewing humans as being multidimensional, not four dimensional.

Parse (1987) cites the following distinctives of her theory:

1. The belief that humans are more and different than the sum of their parts.
2. Human beings evolve mutually with the environment.
3. Human beings cocreate personal health by choosing meaning in situations.
4. Human beings convey meanings that are personal values, which reflect their dreams and hopes.

PRINCIPLES

Three main themes can be identified in Parse's (1998) assumptions: meaning, rhythmicity, and transcendence. "Meaning refers to the linguistic and imagined content of something and the interpretation that one gives to something. It arises with the human–universe process and refers to ultimate meaning or purpose in life and the meaning moments of everyday living" (p. 29).

Rhythmicity refers to the paced, paradoxical patterning of the human–universe mutual process. This can be visualized as the ebb and flow of waves coming into shore. Rhythmical patterns moving in one direction are shown and hidden all-at-once as a flowing process as cadence changes with new experiences (Parse, 1998).

Transcedence is described as reaching beyond with possibles—the hopes and dreams as seen in multidimensional experiences. The possibles are options from which to choose personal ways of becoming (Parse, 1998).

Each of Parse's themes leads to a principle of human becoming (see Fig. 19–1).

Principle I. *Structuring meaning multidimensionally is cocreating reality through the languaging of valuing and imaging.*

Parse's (1992b) first principle interrelates the concepts of *imaging, valuing,* and *languaging.* This principle indicates that human beings structure meaning to reality that is based on lived experiences. The meaning changes or is stretched to different possibilities based on lived experiences in many dimensions. Cocreating in this principle refers to the human–environment mutual participation in the creation of the pattern of each. Languaging reflects images and values through speaking and movement. Valuing is the process of living cherished beliefs while adding to one's personal worldview. Imaging refers to knowing and includes both explicit and tacit knowledge.

From this principle, Parse has identified a nursing practice dimension and a process (see Fig. 19–2). The practice dimension is illuminating meaning through discussion. This happens by explicating or making clear what is appearing now through telling about the meaning (the process). Nurses guide individuals and families to relate the meaning of a situation by making the meaning more explicit.

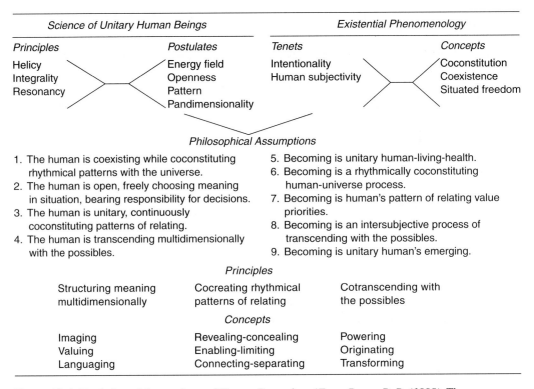

Science of Unitary Human Beings

Principles	*Postulates*
Helicy	Energy field
Integrality	Openness
Resonancy	Pattern
	Pandimensionality

Existential Phenomenology

Tenets	*Concepts*
Intentionality	Coconstitution
Human subjectivity	Coexistence
	Situated freedom

Philosophical Assumptions

1. The human is coexisting while coconstituting rhythmical patterns with the universe.
2. The human is open, freely choosing meaning in situation, bearing responsibility for decisions.
3. The human is unitary, continuously coconstituting patterns of relating.
4. The human is transcending multidimensionally with the possibles.
5. Becoming is unitary human-living-health.
6. Becoming is a rhythmically coconstituting human-universe process.
7. Becoming is human's pattern of relating value priorities.
8. Becoming is an intersubjective process of transcending with the possibles.
9. Becoming is unitary human's emerging.

Principles

Structuring meaning multidimensionally	Cocreating rhythmical patterns of relating	Cotranscending with the possibles

Concepts

Imaging	Revealing-concealing	Powering
Valuing	Enabling-limiting	Originating
Languaging	Connecting-separating	Transforming

Figure 19–1. Evolution of the ontology of Human Becoming. (*From Parse, R. R. (1998). The Human Becoming School of Thought (p. 57). Thousand Oaks, CA: Sage. Reprinted by permission of Sage Publications, Inc.*)

Principle II. *Cocreating rhythmical patterns of relating is living the paradoxical unity of revealing–concealing, and enabling–limiting, while connecting–separating.*

The second principle of the theory of Human Becoming interrelates the concepts of *revealing–concealing, enabling–limiting*, and *connecting–separating*. This principle speaks to human beings cocreating a multidimensional universe in rhythmical patterns of relating while living a paradox. The paradoxes identified are revealing–concealing, enabling–limiting, and connecting–separating. Parse (1981, 1998) states that these rhythmical patterns are not opposites; they are two aspects of the same rhythm and exist simultaneously–one in the foreground and the other in the background. In interpersonal relationships, one reveals part of the self but also conceals other parts; in revealing joy, sorrow is concealed. Making choices or decisions enables an individual in some ways but limits in others; choosing to stay at home on New Years' Eve enables one to be with family but limits one from attending the party at a friend's house. Connecting–separating is a rhythmical process of moving together and moving apart.

The practice dimension Parse (1987) describes for this principle is the synchronizing of rhythms, which happens in dwelling with the pitch, yaw, and roll of the human–universe cadence. She likens dwelling-with (the process) as moving with

DIMENSIONS

Illuminating meaning is shedding light through uncovering the what was, is, and will be, as it is appearing now; it happens in *explicating* what is.

Synchronizing rhythms happens in *dwelling with* the pitch, yaw, and roll of the interhuman cadence.

Mobilizing transcendence happens in *moving beyond* the meaning moment to what is not yet.

PROCESSES

Explicating is making clear what is appearing now through languaging.

Dwelling with is giving self over to the flow of the struggle in connecting–separating.

Moving beyond is propelng toward the possibles in transforming.

Figure 19–2. Human Becoming Practice Methodology. (*From Parse, R. R. (1987).* Nursing science: Major paradigms, theories, and critiques *(p. 167). Philadelphia: Saunders. Used with permission.*)

the flow of the individual/family leading them to recognize the harmony that exists within its own lived context. The nurse would not try to calm or balance rhythms or attempt to help the family adapt.

Principles III. *Cotranscending with the possibles is powering unique ways of originating in the process of transforming.*

The third principle of the theory of human becoming interrelates the concepts of *powering, originating,* and *transforming.* Powering is an energizing force the rhythm of which is the pushing–resisting of interhuman encounters (Parse, 1981). Originating is "inventing new ways of conforming–not conforming in the certainty–uncertainty of living" (Parse, 1998 p. 98). It is creating ways of distinguishing personal uniqueness by living out the paradoxical rhythms all-at-once. Transforming is defined as the changing of change and is recognized by increasing diversity (Parse, 1981).

The practice dimension identified by Parse (1987) for this principle is mobilizing transcendence, which happens in moving beyond the meaning of the moment with what is not yet. The process she identifies is moving beyond or "propelling toward the possibles in transforming" (p. 167). Here the nurse would guide individuals and/or families to plan for the changing of lived health patterns.

THEORETICAL STRUCTURES

The theoretical structures of the theory of human becoming are noncausal in nature and consistent with the assumptions and principles. They are designed to guide research and practice (see Fig. 19–3). To operationalize the structures for research and practice, practice propositions must be derived. Three theoretical structures are identified: (1) powering emerges with the revealing–concealing of

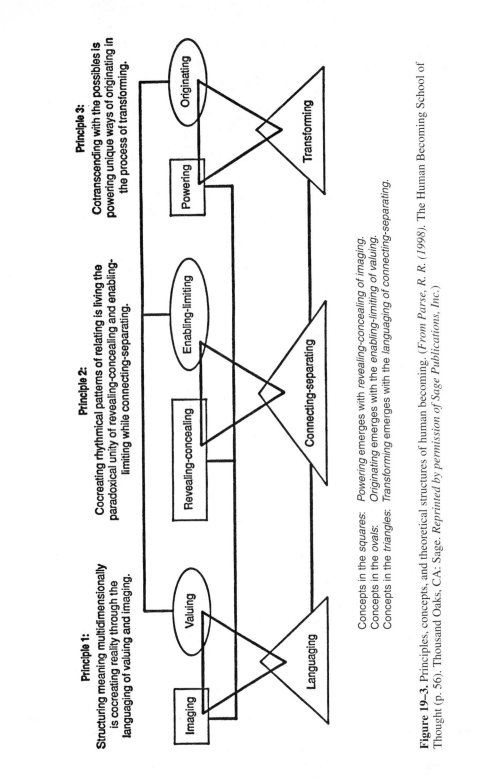

Principle 1:
Structuring meaning multidimensionally is cocreating reality through the languaging of valuing and imaging.

Principle 2:
Cocreating rhythmical patterns of relating is living the paradoxical unity of revealing-concealing and enabling-limiting while connecting-separating.

Principle 3:
Cotranscending with the possibles is powering unique ways of originating in the process of transforming.

Concepts in the *squares*:   *Powering* emerges with *revealing-concealing of imaging.*
Concepts in the *ovals*:   *Originating* emerges with the *enabling-limiting of valuing.*
Concepts in the *triangles*:   *Transforming* emerges with the *languaging of connecting-separating.*

Figure 19–3. Principles, concepts, and theoretical structures of human becoming. (*From Parse, R. R. (1998). The Human Becoming School of Thought* (p. 56). Thousand Oaks, CA: Sage. *Reprinted by permission of Sage Publications, Inc.*)

imaging, (2) originating emerges with the enabling–limiting of valuing, and (3) transforming emerges with the languaging of connecting–separating (Parse, 1998 p. 56).

In her 1987 book, Parse restates her theoretical structures at a less abstract level in order for them to be used to guide nursing practice. She explains that *powering emerges with the revealing–concealing of imaging,* "can be stated as *struggling to live goals discloses the significance of the situation*" (p. 170). The nursing practice focus "is on illuminating the process of revealing–concealing unique ways a person or family can mobilize transcendence in considering new dreams, to image new possibles" (p. 170). Parse describes a nurse–family situation in which members share their thoughts and feelings about a situation, which both reveals and conceals all they know about their struggle to meet personal goals. In disclosing the significance of the situation, the meaning of the situation changes for the family members and therefore the meaning changes for the family.

According to Parse (1987), the second theoretical structure, *originating emerges with the enabling–limiting of valuing,* can be restated as "*creating anew shows one's cherished beliefs and leads in a directional movement*" (p. 170). The nursing practice focus with a person or family would be on "illuminating ways of being alike and different from others in changing values" (p. 170). By synchronizing rhythms, the members discover opportunities and limitations created by the decisions made in choosing ways to be together. Parse states that the choices of new ways of being together mobilize transcendence.

As a restatement of the third theoretical structure, *transforming emerges with the languaging of connecting–separating.* Parse (1987) suggests "*changing views emerge in speaking and moving with others*" (p. 170). The nursing practice focus would be "on illuminating meaning of relating ways of being together as various changing perspectives shed different light on the familiar, which gives rise to new possibles" (p. 170). Parse suggests that in synchronizing rhythms in a nurse–family situation, members relate their values through speech and movement. In so doing, their views change and, through mobilizing transcendence, the ways of relating change.

HUMAN BECOMING AND THE FOUR MAJOR CONCEPTS

Human becoming will be discussed in terms of Parse's beliefs about human beings, the universe, health, and nursing. Parse (1987, 1998) identifies her theory, and that of Rogers', as being representative of the simultaneity paradigm. Hence, her assumptions about the four major concepts are congruent with those of this paradigm.

Human Beings/Universe

Parse's (1992b, 1998) first four assumptions specify the human being as an open being in mutual process with the universe, cocreating patterns of relating with others. She states that the human being "lives at multidimensional realms of the universe all at once, freely choosing ways of becoming as meaning is given to situations" (p. 37).

Human beings are central to the human becoming school of thought. Parse's views about human beings are evident in all elements of her theory—assumptions, principles, theoretical structures, practice dimensions, and research methods. She views human beings and universe as inseparable, each coparticipating in the creation of the experience of living. It is not possible or appropriate to define human beings or universe alone, for together they create a lived experience greater than and different from each seen separately.

The concept of relationships (society) is assumed under the larger view of human beings—universe. In her discussion of the concept of cotranscending, Parse (1987) speaks to "moving beyond with others and the environment multidimensionally" (p. 162). She also states that what humans choose from the multiple possibles, unfolds and surfaces in relationships with others and the universe. Although humans are described as having unique rhythmical patterns, it is difficult to interpret if Parse makes a difference in actual pattern between individuals and the human–universe interchange. If one assumes that "others" are a part of the human's universe, the interpretation becomes clearer.

Parse's view of human–universe is consistent with that of Rogers' (1984) presentation of the person–environment as inseparable, complementary, and evolving together. Parse's language revisions, however, delete general system terminology that is still evident in Rogers' work. Parse's view of human-universe is also consistent with the existentialist view of a person being in the world all-at-once and together, and the phenomenological belief that the universe is made up of everything shown to the person in the lived experience (Husserl, 1931/1962; Idie, 1967).

Winkler (1983) notes that although Parse states that all lived experiences are relevant, the omission of any references to biological manifestations of the person in his or her becoming limits Parse's theory. Phillips (1987) rejects this criticism and states that the lived experience deals with the wholeness of the person. Cody and Mitchell (1992) also reject this criticism, stating that Parse does not ignore "biological manifestations" but subsumes them within the experience of the person, which is the focus of the inquiry and practice guided by her theory.

Health

Parse (1998) describes unitary human's health as a synthesis of values, a way of living. It is not the opposite of disease or a state that a human has but rather a continuously changing process that the human cocreates in mutual process through the human–universe experience, and is incarnated as patterns of relating value priorities. Parse proposes that health is a personal commitment and that humans are the creative authors of their own unfolding (health). She emphasizes that this unfolding cannot be prescribed or described by societal norms; it can only be lived by the person. Health is viewed by Parse as a process of changing life's meanings, a personal power emerging from the individual's collective relationships with others and the universe (Parse, 1990a).

The concept of situated freedom is evident in Parse's perspective of health. Individuals choose various ways of unfolding and have personal responsibility for their choices. Phillips (1987) describes Parse's theory as a way of dealing with experience, a coming to know, rather than a product orientation. He states that the fundamental tenet of Parse's theory is that man participates in health.

Parse's theory speaks to health as man's lived experience as it unfolds negentropically. This is a very different conceptualization of health from that of the totality paradigm theorists. From the totality worldview, health is a state of balance or well-being to which man can aspire. The totality worldview infers a norm or standard of health which individuals and their health care providers aspire to attain. These two different worldviews have very different nursing practice methodologies that are presented in the next section.

Nursing

Parse (1992a, 1998) defines nursing as a basic science, the practice of which is a performing art. She places nursing in the company of drama, music, and dance, where in each, the artist creates something unique. The knowledge base of the discipline is the science of the art, and the performance is the art creatively lived. Parse states:

> So too, the nurse, an artist like the dancer, unfolds the meaning of the moment with a person or family consistent with personal knowledge and cherished beliefs. The nurse artist creatively lives knowledge about the human–universe–health connectedness (nursing's phenomenon of concern), which incarnates personal cherished beliefs. The knowledge and beliefs are *there* in the way the nurse approaches the person, the way the nurse talks and listens to the person, what the nurse is most concerned about, and how the nurse moves with the flow of the person. When the nurse artist is guided by a particular nursing theory or framework, the art form reflects that theory or framework, which represents a school of thought in nursing (Parse, 1992a, p. 147).

Parse (1981) states that nursing's responsibility to society is the guiding of individuals and families in choosing possibilities in changing the health process, which is accomplished by intersubjective participation with people. She further states that nursing practice involves innovation and creativity, which are not encumbered by prescriptive rules.

This theorist contends that the goals of nursing focus on the quality of life from the person's perspective. Nursing is practiced with all individuals and families, regardless of societal designations of health/illness status. Parse's (1987, 1992b, 1998) theory guides practice that focuses on illuminating meaning and moving beyond with the person/family relative to changing health patterns. An important aspect in regard to Parse's view of nursing is that the client, not the nurse, is the authority figure and prime decision maker in the relationship. The client, in presence with the nurse, determines the activities for changing health patterns. Nursing, according to this theory, is "loving, true presence with the other to promote health and the quality of life" (p. 169). The practice of nursing is not a prescriptive approach based on medical or nursing diagnoses, nor is it the offering of professional advice and opinions that stem from the personal value system of the nurse.

Parse (1987) has presented a practice methodology for her theory of human becoming that includes dimensions and processes (see Fig. 19–2). The dimensions are *illuminating meaning, synchronizing rhythms*, and *mobilizing transcendence*. The processes are the empirical activities of *explicating, dwelling with*, and *moving beyond*. There is a clear flow of these dimensions and processes from her assumptions and principles.

In Parse's theory the nurse is an interpersonal guide who acts in true presence, an active, energetic way of being with. Authority, responsibility, and the consequences of decisions are accorded to the client. The traditional nursing roles of care giver, advocate, counselor, and leader do not appear to be congruent with Parse's view of nursing. Teaching, however, is reflected in the dimension of illuminating meaning by explicating. The nurse as a change agent is reflected in the dimension of mobilizing transcendence by moving beyond the meaning to what is not yet.

In an editorial in *Nursing Science Quarterly*, Parse (1989) proposes a "set of fundamentals essential for fully practicing the art of nursing." These include the following:

- Know and use nursing frameworks and theories
- Be available to others
- Value the other as a human presence
- Respect differences in view
- Own what you believe and be accountable for your actions
- Move on to the new and untested
- Connect with others
- Take pride in self
- Like what you do
- Recognize the moments of joy in the struggles of living
- Appreciate mystery and be open to new discoveries
- Be competent in your chosen area
- Rest and begin anew (p. 111).

Parse (1998) defines the contextual situations of nursing practice as being nurse–person or nurse–group/community participation. She does not define specific practice settings as being more or less appropriate for practice application of the theory of human becoming. She does, however, advise the nurse to approach the client as a nurturing gardener, not as a fix-it mechanic.

PARSE'S THEORY OF HUMAN BECOMING AND NURSING PRACTICE

The Nursing Process

Parse (1987) states that the nursing process "evolves from the discipline of philosophy and does not flow from an ontological base in the discipline of nursing" (p. 166). She further states that the steps of the nursing process are the steps of the problem-solving method and are not unique to nursing. The assumptions underlying the nursing process, that the nurse is the authority on health and that the person adapts or can be "fixed," are not congruent with the theory of human becoming. Parse posits that as practice is the empirical life of a theory, the practice of one theory would be different from the practice of another.

Parse's Practice Methodology

Parse (1998) describes nursing practice as the art of living human becoming. The art of nursing is described as using nursing's body of knowledge in service to people with the goal of quality of life from the person's perspective. The practice methodology of human becoming includes dimensions and processes that were presented earlier in this chapter (see Fig. 19–2).

The human becoming nurse lives in true presence with others in the processes of illuminating meaning, synchronizing rhythms, and mobilizing transcendence. True presence is described as a special way of "being with" another person. True presence is a free-flowing attentiveness that is different from trying to attend to another—as the *trying to* distracts one from the focus. Parse states that preparation and attention are essential for true presence. "*Preparation* involves an emptying to be available . . . to the . . . other(s), . . . being flexible, . . . gracefully present, . . . and open to another. *Attention* is focus. To attend to is to focus on the moment at hand" (Parse, 1998, p. 71). Persons share with the nurse only what they choose to disclose. The nurse in true presence joins the reality of others at all realms of experience without judging or labeling.

Parse (1998) states that "the nurse is with the other(s) in true presence through face-to-face discussions, silent immersions, and lingering presence. . . . In face-to-face discussions the nurse and person or group engage in dialogue" (p. 72). The conversation may be expressed through oral discussion, poetry, music, art, movement, photographs, and other expressions. The person/group always leads the discussion, the nurse goes-with. A second way of being-with is silent immersion. This situation is "true presence without words, just 'being-with' through immediate engaging in the presence of another or through imagination with . . . the intention to bear witness to the other's becoming" (p. 73). Lingering presence, the third way of being-with another, is "living the remembered . . . recalling . . . a lingering presence that arises after the immediate engagement" (p. 73). It is a reflective recollection.

Parse (1998) states that in true presence with the nurse, people may change their health patterns when they change their value priorities. Through *creative imaging*, one pictures what a situation might be if lived a different way. This is a safe trying-on of a might-be. It enables a person to imagine the not-yet, and it is a way of changing meaning, thus changing health. Through *affirming personal becoming*, critically thinking about who one is becoming, one can uncover personal patterns of preference. Living these patterns of preference confirms the values by which the person is known. An attitude of "I can" or "I will" toward a given desire for change affirms it in a new way and changes health. Through *glimpsing the paradoxical*, one looks at the incongruence in a situation as the apparent opposites emerge. This is a way of moving beyond the moment in changing patterns of health.

Parse (1998) stresses that "for nursing practice, being in true presence with another means that all realms of the universe of the nurse and the person(s) are interconnecting"(p. 76) or cocreating becoming. It is a way of being present that values "the others' human dignity and freedom to choose within situations, and it is fundamental to living the art of human becoming, the focus of which is the quality of life from the person's or group's perspective" (p. 76).

Two examples of practice applications of the theory of human becoming will be presented.

Martin, Forchuk, Santopinto, and Butcher (1992) describe how the nurse, guided by the theory of human becoming, relates to Mrs. W, a terminally ill cancer client:

Emergent Patterns of Health for Mrs. W.

1. Mrs. W says she does not want to discuss her situation with her family, yet she makes plans to broach the subject with them.
2. Mrs. W says that this is the worst time of her life, yet she says that she has never enjoyed the natural world so much as now.

Mrs. W—Nurse Activities

1. Be truly present with Mrs. W as she imagines familiar and unfamiliar ways of engaging with and withdrawing from family during the coming days and weeks. Through presence, seek deeper levels of meaning as she describes her hopes and dreams for the days ahead. Be with her as she shares how she intends to make these hopes come to pass and what meaning these hopes hold for her. Be present with Mrs. W as she imagines new ways of being close to her family. Invite her to describe how her relationships are changing for her.
2. Be with Mrs. W while she imagines aspects of nature that have special meaning for her. Invite her to describe how she can come to enjoy these aspects in her current situation. Be with her as she creates words, images, and movements that bring her in touch with nature (p. 84).

Mitchell (1986) describes the application of the theory of human becoming to Mrs. M, an elderly woman in a long-term-care facility. In true presence with Mrs. M, Mitchell is able to tease out the multiple and complex realities the client experiences. The client transcends time and space to be all-at-once a child, a mother, and a lonely elder. All the realities lived and valued by Mrs. M continue to be lived despite the passage of time (Illuminating meaning).

In order to understand the meaning of Mrs. M's languaging, the nurse dwells with her. The nurse does not try to bring Mrs. M back to reality or to control or alter Mrs. M's experience. The nurse goes with the flow to assist the client in finding meaning. In doing so, the nurse has the opportunity to validate feelings with the client. Mrs. M states that she felt joy when her mother met her after school. The nurse then states, "You feel good when your mother is waiting for you." Mrs. M responds by saying, "Yes, she's waiting for me now too. I'm waiting to go home" (Synchronizing rhythms).

This statement helps the nurse to understand that Mrs. M perceives her present environment to be a temporary waiting area, that the client's detached behavior has occurred because she attaches little meaning to her current surroundings. Two nursing interventions are selected to guide Mrs. M's care. First, the nurse continues to facilitate the expression of Mrs. M's meaning in the present situation. Second, the nurse provides Mrs. M with information and the freedom to make choices such as participation or detachment from unit activities (Mobilizing transcendence).

Parse's approach to practice is clearly one of nurses *in presence with* people rather than doing for people. Articles detailing Parse's practice applications are presented as case studies, which, by virtue of the format, tend to be lengthy.

CRITIQUE OF PARSE'S THEORY OF HUMAN BECOMING

1. What is the historical context of the theory? Parse published the theory of Man–Living–Health in 1981. This theory is based on the work of a nurse scientist, Martha Rogers (1970), and existential phenomenology. Parse created new ways of looking at man, health, environment, and nursing. In synthesizing Rogers' principles of helicy, complementarity (now called integrality), and resonancy and her four concepts of openness, energy field, pattern and organization, and four-dimensionality with the tenets of existential–phenomemological thought, Parse created a new vision of nursing science.

Parse's theory of nursing, rooted in the human sciences and having the goal of quality of life from the perspective of the person, emerged in 1981. It was radical thinking at that time. From this view, the health–illness continuum was rendered irrelevant as were care plans based on health problems. Using this approach to care, authority, responsibility, and the consequences of decision making reside with the person, not with the nurse. This thinking was revolutionary at its inception, and now, two decades or more later, this school of thought is well supported by research findings.

In 1987, Parse differentiated the totality and simultaneity paradigms in nursing. Her work is clearly representative of the simultaneity paradigm.

Parse's human becoming theory describes a logical sequence of events. Parse (1981) presents Rogers' principles and concepts as well as tenets and concepts from existential–phenomenological thought. She then synthesizes these tenets, principles, and concepts to create her nine assumptions. The principles of the theory of human becoming are derived from the assumptions, with each principle relating three concepts to each other (see Fig. 19–3).

Parse then derived three theoretical structures, each of which uses three concepts, one from each principle (see Fig. 19–3). She defines theoretical structure as a statement that interrelates concepts in a way that can be verified (Parse, 1992b). Phillips (1987) points out that the stem of each theoretical structure is taken from the third principle. He speculates that greater importance might be attached to this principle, but qualifies this thought by saying that Parse makes it clear that other theoretical structures may be generated from her principles.

Levine (1988), Phillips (1987), and Winkler (1983) speak to the difficulty of Parse's terminology for those unfamiliar with existential–phenomenology. They concur, however, that there is consistency in meaning at each level of discourse.

2. What are the basic concepts and relationships presented by the theory? The theory of human becoming is grounded in the belief that humans coauthor their own health or becoming in mutual process with the universe, cocreating distinguishable patterns that specify the uniqueness of both humans and the universe (Parse, 1995). Parse's concepts, postulates, themes, and theoretical structures are all clearly defined and used in a consistent manner. The relationships are clear and flow with logical precision from the assumptions, to the principles, to the theoretical structures, to the practice dimensions, and to the research methodology. Concepts and relationships become more clear to the reader as one's familiarity with the terminology increases.

3. What major phenomena of concern to nursing are presented? These phenomena may include *but are not limited to*: human being, environment, health, interpersonal relations, caring, goal attainment, adaptation, and energy fields. For Parse, the central phenomenon of nursing science is the *human–universe–health process*, or the human–universe and health interrelationship. *Human* is a unitary being who coparticipates with the universe in creating becoming, and one who is open and free to choose ways of becoming (Parse, 1992b, 1998). The *universe* and human beings are viewed as being inseparable, each coparticipating in the experience of living. *Health* is viewed as the quality of life as experienced by the person (Parse, 1992b). It is a continuously changing process that the human cocreates in mutual process with the universe (Parse, 1998).

4. To whom does this theory apply? In what situations? In what ways? Parse's theory of human becoming focuses on the lived experiences of unitary human beings and therefore is applicable to all individuals, families, and communities, at all times, and in all contexts.

5. By what method or methods can this theory be tested? As Parse's theory is rooted in the human sciences rather than the natural sciences, qualitative rather than quantitative research methodologies are used to expand it. Since the early 1980s, studies about Parse's theory have been conducted using research methods borrowed from the social sciences (descriptive), psychology (van Kaam and Giorgi modifications), and anthropology (ethnography). The studies have been of two types—basic and applied. *Basic* research is conducted with the goal of uncovering the structure of lived experiences to expand knowledge of the science or may be an interpretive hermeneutic process that specifies the meaning of texts from a human becoming perspective. *Applied* research, on the other hand, has the goal of evaluating human becoming as a guide to practice (Parse, 1998).

Parse (1987) describes the theory of human becoming research methodology, which includes the identification of major entities for study, the scientific processes of investigation, and the details of the processes appropriate for inquiry. She states that the two aspects of lived experience to consider in selecting an entity for study are nature and structure. The aspect of nature refers to common lived experiences that surface in the human–universe interrelationship and are health related; examples include "being-becoming, value priorities, negentropic unfolding, and quality of life" (p. 174). Parse cites the example of "waiting" as being consistent with her definition of a common lived experience.

The second aspect of the lived experience to consider in selecting an entity for study is structure. Parse (1987) defines structure as "the paradoxical living of the remembered, the now moment and the not-yet all at once" (p. 175). Thus, the research question would be "What is the structure of the lived experience of waiting?" (p. 175). The researcher would then proceed to uncover the structure of this lived experience.

The Parse (1998) basic research methodology was constructed in congruence with the principles of human becoming. The methodology has four principles, five assumptions, and a three-step process. Parse states that her methodology "is a phenomenological–hermeneutic method in that the universal experiences [are] described by participants who lived them . . . and participants' descriptions are interpreted in light of the human becoming theory" (p. 63). The phenomena for study are lived experiences of health, such as hope, loss, happiness, laughter, sorrow, and pain. Participants are persons who can describe the meaning of the lived experience under study through words, symbols, music, metaphors, poetry, photographs, drawings, or movements.

The first process of the method is *dialogical engagement*. This is a discussion between the researcher and the participant, in true presence, that focuses on the participant's description of the lived experience under study. These dialogues are recorded, preferably on videotape. After securing the participant's signed consent, the researcher opens the dialogue by requesting that the participant describe his/her experience with the lived experience under study. The researcher does not ask specific questions, but may encourage the participant to elaborate about the lived experience.

The second process is *extraction–synthesis*, which is a sorting of the essences or patterns of the dialogue using the language of the participant. These essences are then conceptualized in the language of science to form a structure of the experience. Parse relates that this process occurs through dwelling with the transcribed dialogues in order to elicit the meaning of the experience as described by the participant. The structure, which Parse describes as "the paradoxical living of the remembered, the now moment, and the not-yet-all-at-once"(1998, p. 65), arising from this process, is the answer to the research question.

The third step of the process is *heuristic interpretation*, which "weaves the structure with the principles of human becoming and beyond to enhance the knowledge base and create ideas for further research (Parse, 1987, 1992b, 1995, 1997a). Structural transposition and conceptual integration are the processes of heuristic interpretation that move the discourse of the structure to the language of the theory" (Parse, 1998, p. 65).

The findings from studies conducted using the Parse methodology contribute new knowledge and understanding about human experiences and add to the knowledge base of nursing science. Recent studies using the Parse research methodology include: considering tomorrow (Bunkers, 1998), feeling alone while with others (Gouty, 1996), feeling uncomfortable (Baumann, 1996), grieving (Cody, 1991, 1995a; Pilkington, 1993), hope (Parse, 1990b; Thornberg, 1993; Wang, 1997), joy and sorrow (Parse, 1997b), laughing and health (Parse, 1993, 1994), persevering through the difficult time of ovarian cancer (Allchin-Petardi, 1998), quality of life for persons with Alzheimer's disease (Parse, 1996), suffering (Daly, 1995), and many more. Parse's latest book *Hope, An international human becoming perspective* presents 13 studies on hope. These studies are included in the annotated bibliographies at the end of this chapter.

A second Parse (1998) basic research methodology is called the human becoming hermeneutic method, which is a mode of inquiry focusing on interpretation and understanding. Parse describes this as a dialogical process between the researcher and the text, uncovering meaning interpreted through a particular perspective. The interpretation itself is the meaning given to the text from the frame of reference of the researcher, thus the understanding of the text incarnates that frame of reference. Cody (1995b) uses this method in interpreting selected poems by Whitman using Parse's human becoming theory. In his study he identifies three processes of hermeneutics: discoursing, interpreting, and understanding. Parse states that when a researcher is conducting a hermeneutic study from the human becoming perspective, a literary work or other text will be interpreted using the language of the principles of human becoming.

A third methodology is the applied research method. The preproject–process–postproject descriptive qualitative method is appropriate for evaluating the human becoming theory in practice. The purpose is to identify changes that occur as a result of using the theory in practice. Data are gathered prior to use of the theory, midway through the project, and at the end point of the project. Data sources include direct observation of nurse's documentation; written and taped interviews with participants regarding their beliefs about human beings, health, and nursing; and interviews with recipients of nursing care.

Frik and Polluck (1993) report the use of Parse's theory by graduate students practicing in a chronic illness setting, a community mental health setting, and an emergency department. The theory was used in promoting compliance in adults with diabetes, implementing hypertensive screening in the emergency room, promoting effective coping skills related to drug abuse, and improving the nutrition of neurologically impaired adults.

Mitchell (1991) reports successful use of Parse's theory on an acute medical–surgical unit. Cody and Mitchell (1992) report successful use of this theory by Jonas, in an outpatient setting, and by Santopinto (1989) in a long-term-care setting. Cody and Mitchell report that nurses in all of these studies identified initial difficulties in changing their approach to being with persons and giving up the urge to apply the nursing process in the traditional manner. However, increased professional satisfaction convinced them of the validity of the new approach.

More recent evaluative studies that have been conducted about the theory of human becoming include: Jonas (1995), Mitchell (1995), Santopinto and Smith (1995), and Northup and Cody (1998). Findings continue to support use of the theory of human becoming in nursing practice.

6. Does this theory direct critical thinking in nursing practice? Critical thinking in nursing practice is demonstrated by the Parse nurse in illuminating meaning, synchronizing rhythms, and mobilizing transcendence. The nurse, in true presence with the person, invites a discussion of the meaning of a situation. The process of explicating, in the presence of the nurse, sheds new light, or illuminates meaning connected with the moment. The nurse goes with the flow of the person's rhythms as she or he moves beyond the moment, reaching for hopes and dreams that have been illuminated through the process of being with the nurse. As persons, families, and communities move beyond the moment, reaching for hopes and dreams that have been illuminated through the process of being with the nurse, transcendence is mobilized.

It is important to say that the critical thinking used by the nurse in true presence with the person is thinking that guides, illuminates, synchronizes rhythms, and mobilizes transcendence *together-with* the person. It is *never* judgment or direction that the nurse gives to or requires of the person.

7. Does this theory direct therapeutic intervention? Parse's theory does not direct therapeutic intervention in the traditional sense of the term. Human becoming is a being-with, in true presence nursing relationship with another person, family, or community. The person, family, or community in true presence with the nurse determines what would be (or would not be) beneficial to their quality of life. The value system of the person directs the outcome(s), not the value system of the nurse.

8. Does this theory direct communication in nursing practice? The theory of human becoming explicitly directs communication in nursing practice. Parse (1998) describes true presence as a special way of "being with" in which the nurse is attentive to moment-to-moment changes in meaning as she or he bears witness to the person's or group's own values. "True presence is an intentional reflective love, an interpersonal art grounded in a strong knowledge base, reflecting the belief that each person knows 'the way' somewhere within self" (p. 71). *Preparation* to be in true presence involves an emptying of self to be available to bear witness to others. It also requires *attention* or focus on the moment at hand for immersion. The nurse may be in true presence with others in face-to-face discussions, silence, or in recollection.

9. Does this theory direct nursing actions that lead to satisfactory outcomes? In a review of Canadian evaluation studies of Parse's theory in practice (in a variety of health care settings from 1988 to 1994) Mitchell (1995) reports that findings indicate three main areas of change. First, with Parse's theory, nurses in all studies changed their views of human beings from seeing clients as problems, to seeing them as unique human beings in relationship with others. Secondly, nurses reported having a different respect for persons, for the meaning they gave life and for their relationships and choices. Nurses described a new appreciation for thinking about the person's perspective of what is important for their own health and quality of life. The third area of change was that nurses reported an increased morale and understanding of professional, autonomous practice. A review of the comments of persons cared for by nurses living Parse's theory indicated that they felt important, cared about, and involved in decisions.

Evaluation studies of human becoming have been conducted in various clinical settings to investigate what happens when the theory is used to guide nursing practice. The published studies include Jonas (1989, 1995), Mitchell (1995), and Santopinto and Smith (1995). The findings from all of these studies have shown that when this theory guides nursing practice, patients, families, and nurses felt greater satisfaction with care.

Northup and Cody (1998) report findings of a descriptive evaluative study of human becoming theory in practice in the acute psychiatric setting. Findings supported prior studies regarding nurses' enhanced respect for, and concern with, people as self-determining human beings who create their chosen way of being with the world. One different theme, *altered job satisfaction*, demonstrated mixed findings. Although some nurses reported enhanced job satisfaction and meaningfulness in practice, others rejected Parse's practice methodology and spoke of it as inadequate to guide practice with clients who they felt were incapable of making decisions.

10. How contagious is this theory? A short answer to this question is—very contagious!

In 1998, the South Dakota State Board of Nursing adopted a regulatory decisioning model based on Parse's theory. This model integrates the values of the Board of Nursing—vision, integrity, commitment, courage, flexibility, and collaboration with the three principles of human becoming theory and the tenets and values of public policy-making (the best interests of the practitioner, the health care institutions, and the population). This is a landmark event as it is the first regulatory adoption of nursing theory-guided professional nursing practice (Daamgard & Bunkers, 1998).

Since 1981, Parse's theory of Man–Living–Health/human becoming has generated many articles and research studies, both published and unpublished. There are currently over 300 subscribers to Parse-L on the Internet, and many more access the Parse home page for information.

More than one hundred persons from many countries belong to the International Consortium of Parse Scholars. This Consortium conducts an immersion weekend each fall, offering members an opportunity to explore issues directly with Parse and to clarify ideas regarding the theory in research and practice. Opportunities are also available to have one's own original work regarding the theory critiqued. The Consortium has produced a videotape on true presence with persons in various settings and a set of teaching modules for those interested in incorporating the theory as a guide to practice (Parse, 1997a).

In 1992, the Institute of Human Becoming was created to offer summer sessions given by Parse on the theory and its research and practice methodologies. These sessions attract international participants.

Since 1994, Parse has hosted the International Colloquium in Qualitative Research related to human becoming theory at Loyola University in Chicago. This event features doctoral students, nurse scholars, and international visiting nurse scholars who present their research.

STRENGTHS AND WEAKNESSES

A strength of Parse's theory is the logical flow from construction of her assumptions to the deductive derivation of principles, theoretical structures, practice dimensions, and research processes. Another strength of the theory of human becoming is that it focuses on all individuals, not only those defined by societal norms as being ill. The individual in the nurse–person relationship uncovers the meaning of his or her lived experience. The nurse is in true presence with the client and together they illuminate meaning, synchronize rhythms, and mobilize transcendence. This occurs as individuals/families/communities interrelate with the nurse multidimensionally.

Parse is a prolific theorist and researcher. She has developed and nurtured the theory of human becoming with great care and precision, refining it as needed since its original presentation in 1981. *Nursing Science Quarterly*, the Parse home page, and Parse-L have provided the profession with excellent and ready access to cutting edge information, discussion, and research about the theory. The International Consortium of Parse Scholars and the Institute of Human Becoming provide both education and resources for nurses to learn more about the theory.

In 1987, Phillips suggested that Parse's theory of human becoming would speed a transformation from the mechanistic approach to health care to one that has a unitary perspective of the health care of humans. Unfortunately, the current health system (or nonsystem) is focusing on cost containment and rationing of care rather than meeting human needs. Research in nursing science, however, does demonstrate the identification of common elements and themes in lived experiences that are enhancing the knowledge base of nursing science. As these common elements and themes are validated further, they will give further direction to a unitary perspective of the health care of humans.

Another strength of this theory is the assumption about humans freely choosing personal meaning in the process of relating value priorities. Coupled with this assumption is the thinking that the authority and responsibility of choices resides with the person or client, not the nurse. This is an opposing stance to the tradition of paternalistic health care, where physicians make decisions and nurses and patients accept them without question. It is a contemporary stance. Consumers *do*, in fact, question health care professionals, seek other opinions and alternative treatment modalities, and resort to the legal system for redress of their perceived damages.

A limitation of the theory of human becoming is its lack of articulation with the body of knowledge and psychomotor skills that most nurses and society generally attribute to the practice of professional nursing. It is an entirely new conceptualization of nursing practice, and is not congruent with the "assess, diagnose, and treat" language of current nurse practice acts. The South Dakota Board of Nursing recently led the nation in recognizing the simultaneity paradigm and Parse's theory of human becoming a base for professional nursing practice (Daamgard & Bunkers, 1998).

A question posed to this author by graduate students in nursing is whether you have to be a nurse to practice the theory of human becoming. Many students felt that true presence could be achieved by physicians, social workers, therapists, and members of the clergy. Parse (personal communication, 1994) responded to this idea by noting that as the knowledge base is different in each discipline, what occurs in true presence with the client will be different. She also noted that other disciplines have different goals. Different goals will affect and direct a professional's ability to be in true presence with the client.

In Parse's latest edition of her theory, *The human becoming school of thought: A perspective for nurses and other health care professionals* (1998), she states in the preface that the book " . . . is intended for professional nurses and other health care providers . . . concerned with quality of life from the perspective of the people they serve"(p. x). Phillips (1999) applauds this expansion of Parse's school of thought to other health professionals. He states that " . . . a school of thought that includes a diversity of persons transcends the current struggle in interdisciplinary and collaborative endeavors. Imagine the possible advancement in knowledge and science when people in the sciences and arts and humanities use nursing's schools of thought" (p. 87). Expansion of this school of thought to other health care professionals can only be seen as another strength of Parse's work.

Parse's theory has been criticized in the past for its exclusion of the discussion of the role of natural sciences in nursing practice. While Parse does not address this specifically in relation to her theory, she does advocate a preprofessional core curriculum that would be appropriate for the professions of law, medicine, theology, and nursing. This undergraduate preprofessional core assumes professional education to occur at the graduate level. Parse's proposed preprofessional core contains a strong natural science and liberal arts base.

Parse has clearly been successful in creating a new paradigm or worldview of nursing. Her theory of human becoming has gained considerable support both in the United States and internationally. Current definitions of nursing science (see Chapter 1) are reflective of the simultaneity paradigm, and a wealth of both basic and applied research supports the theory of human becoming.

REFERENCES

Allchin-Petardi, L. (1998). Weathering the storm: Persevering through a difficult time. *Nursing Science Quarterly, 11*, 172–177.

Andrews, H. A., & Roy, C. (1986). *Essentials of the Roy Adaptation Model.* Norwalk, CT: Appleton & Lange.

Baumann, S. L. (1996). Feeling uncomfortable: Children in families with no place of their own. *Nursing Science Quarterly, 9*, 152–159.

Bunkers, S. S. (1998). Considering tomorrow: Parse's theory-guided research. *Nursing Science Quarterly, 11*, 56–63.

Cody, W. K. (1991). Grieving a personal loss. *Nursing Science Quarterly, 4*, 61–68.

Cody, W. K. (1995a). The meaning of grieving for families living with AIDS. *Nursing Science Quarterly, 8*, 104–114.

Cody, W. K. (1995b). Of life immense in passion, pulse, and power: Dialoguing with Whitman and Parse—A hermeneutic study. In R. R. Parse (Ed.), *Illuminations: The human becoming theory in practice and research* (pp. 269–307) (Pub. No. 15-2670). New York: National League for Nursing Press.

Cody, W. K., & Mitchell, G. J. (1992). Parse's theory as a model for practice: The cutting edge. *Advances in Nursing Science, 15*, 52–65.

Daamgard, G., & Bunkers, S. S. (1998). Nursing science-guided practice and education: A state board of nursing perspective. *Nursing Science Quarterly, 11*, 142–144.

Daly, J. (1995). The lived experience of suffering. In R. R. Parse (Ed.), *Illuminations: The human becoming theory in practice and research* (pp. 243–268) (Pub. No. 15-2670). New York: National League for Nursing Press.

Frik, S. M., & Polluck, S. E. (1993). Preparation for advanced nursing practice. *Nursing and Health Care, 14*, 190–195.

Gouty, C. A. (1996). *Feeling alone while with others*. Unpublished doctoral dissertation, Loyola University, Chicago.

Hall, L. (1965). *Another view of nursing care and quality*. Address given at Catholic University Workshop, Washington, DC.

Heidegger, M. (1962). *Being and time*. New York: Harper & Row.

Heidegger, M. (1972). *On time and being*. New York: Harper & Row.

Henderson, V. A. (1991). *The nature of nursing: A definition and its implications for practice, research, and education. Reflections after 25 years*. (Pub. No. 15-2346). New York: National League for Nursing Press.

Husserl, E. (1962). *Ideas: General introduction to pure phenomenology*. New York: Collier-Macmillan. (Originally published, 1931).

Idie, J. M. (1967). Transcendental phenomenology and existentialism. In J. J. Kockelmans (Ed.), *Phenomenology*. New York: Doubleday.

Johnson, D. E. (1980). The Behavioral System Model for Nursing. In J. P. Riehl & C. Roy (Eds.), *Conceptual models for nursing practice* (2nd ed.) (pp. 207–216). New York: Appleton-Century-Crofts. (out of print)

Jonas, C. M. (1989). *Practicing Parse's theory with groups of individuals in the community*. Paper presented at The Queen Elizabeth Hospital, Toronto, Ontario, April 17, 1989.

Jonas, C. M. (1995). Evaluation of the human becoming theory in family practice. In R. R. Parse (Ed.), *Illuminations: The human becoming theory in practice and research* (pp. 347–366) (Pub. No. 15-2670). New York: National League for Nursing Press.

King, I. M. (1981). *A theory for nursing: Systems, concepts, process*. New York: Wiley. (out of print)

King, I. M. (1989). King's general systems framework and theory. In J. Riehl-Sisca (Ed.), *Conceptual models for nursing practice* (3rd ed.) (pp. 149–158). Norwalk, CT: Appleton & Lange.

Levine, M. E. (1988). [Review of the book *Nursing science*]. *Nursing Science Quarterly, 1*, 184–185.

Levine, M. E. (1989). The conservation principles of nursing: Twenty years later. In J. Riehl-Sisca (Ed.), *Conceptual models for nursing practice* (3rd ed.) (pp. 325–337). Norwalk, CT: Appleton & Lange.

Martin, M. L., Forchuk, C., Santopinto, M., & Butcher, H. K. (1992). Alternative approaches to nursing practice: Application of Peplau, Rogers, and Parse. *Nursing Science Quarterly, 5*, 80–85.

Merleau-Ponty, M. (1973). *The prose of the world*. Evanston, IL: Northwestern University Press.

Merleau-Ponty, M. (1974). *Phenomenology of perception*. C. Smith (Trans.). New York: Humanities Press.

Mitchell, G. J. (1986). Utilizing Parse's Theory of Man–Living–Health in Mrs. M's neighborhood. *Perspectives, 10*(4), 5–7.

Mitchell, G. J. (1991). Distinguishing practice with Parse's Theory. In I. E. Goertzen (Ed.), *Differentiating nursing practice: Into the 21st century*. Kansas City: American Academy of Nursing.

Mitchell, G. J. (1995). Evaluation of the human becoming theory in practice in an acute care setting. In R. R. Parse (Ed.), *Illuminations: The human becoming theory in practice and research* (pp. 367–399) (Pub. No. 15-2670). New York: National League for Nursing Press.

Northup, D. T., & Cody, W. K. (1998). Evaluation of human becoming in practice in an acute psychiatric setting. *Nursing Science Quarterly, 11*, 23–30.

Orem, D. E. (1991). *Nursing: Concepts of practice* (4th ed.). St. Louis: Mosby.

Orlando, I. J. (1961). *The dynamic nurse–patient relationship: Function, process and principles*. New York: Putnam.

Parse, R. R. (1981). *Man–living–health: A theory of nursing*. New York: Wiley.

Parse, R. R. (1987). *Nursing science—Major paradigms, theories, and critiques*. Philadelphia: Saunders.

Parse, R. R. (1989). Essentials for practicing the art of nursing. *Nursing Science Quarterly, 2*, 111.

Parse, R. R. (1990a). Health: A personal commitment. *Nursing Science Quarterly, 3*, 136–140.

Parse, R. R. (1990b). Parse's research methodology with an illustration of the lived experience of hope. *Nursing Science Quarterly, 3*, 9–17.

Parse, R. R. (1992a). Editorial: The performing art of nursing. *Nursing Science Quarterly, 5*, 147.

Parse, R. R. (1992b). Human becoming: Parse's theory of nursing. *Nursing Science Quarterly, 5*, 35–42.

Parse, R. R. (1993). The experience of laughter: A phenomenological study. *Nursing Science Quarterly, 6*, 39–43.

Parse, R. R. (1994). Laughing and health: A study using Parse's research method. *Nursing Science Quarterly, 7*, 55–64.

Parse, R. R. (1995). *Illuminations: The human becoming theory in practice and research*. (Pub. No. 15-2670). New York: National League for Nursing Press.

Parse, R. R. (1996). Quality of life for persons living with Alzheimer's disease: The human becoming perspective. *Nursing Science Quarterly, 9*, 126–133.

Parse, R. R. (1997a). Human becoming theory: The was, is, and will be. *Nursing Science Quarterly, 10*, 32–38.

Parse, R. R. (1997b). Joy–sorrow: A study using the Parse research method. *Nursing Science Quarterly, 10*, 80–87.

Parse, R. R. (1998). *The human becoming school of thought*. Thousand Oaks, CA: Sage.

Parse, R. R. (1999). *Hope: An international perspective*. Boston: Jones & Bartlett.

Parse, R. R., Coyne, A. B., & Smith, M. J. (1985). *Nursing research: Qualitative methods*. Bowie, Md.: Brady Communications.

Peplau, H. E. (1988). *Interpersonal relations in nursing*. NY: Springer. (Original work published 1952, New York: Putnam).

Phillips, J. R. (1987). A critique of Parse's Man–Living–Health Theory. In R. R. Parse (Ed.), *Nursing science: Major paradigms, theories, and critiques* (pp. 181–204). Philadelphia: Saunders.

Phillips, J. R. (1999). [Review of the book *The human becoming school of thought*]. *Nursing Science Quarterly, 12*, 87–89.

Pilkington, F. B. (1993). The lived experience of grieving the loss of an important other. *Nursing Science Quarterly, 6*, 130–139.

Rogers, M. E. (1970). *The theoretical basis of nursing*. Philadelphia: Davis. (out of print)

Rogers, M. E. (1984). *Science of Unitary Human Beings: A paradigm for nursing*. Paper presented at International Nurse Theorist Conference, Edmonton, Alberta.

Rogers, M. E. (1992). Nursing science and the space age. *Nursing Science Quarterly, 5*(1), 27–34.

Roy, C. (1984). *Introduction to nursing: An adaptation model* (2nd ed.). Upper Saddle River, NJ: Prentice Hall.

Roy, C., & Andrews, H. A. (1991). *The Roy Adaptation Model: The definitive statement*. Norwalk, CT: Appleton & Lange.

Santopinto, M. D. A. (1989). *An evaluation of Parse's practice methodology in a chronic care setting*. Paper presented at the 19th Quadrennial Congress of the International Council of Nurses, Seoul, Korea.

Santopinto, M. D. A., & Smith, M. C. (1995). Evaluation of the Human Becoming Theory in practice with adults and children. In R. R. Parse (Ed.), *Illuminations: The human becoming theory in practice and research* (pp. 309–346) (Pub. No. 15-2670). New York: National League for Nursing Press.

Sartre, J. P. (1963). *Search for a method*. New York: Alfred A. Knopf.

Sartre, J. P. (1964). *Nausea*. New York: New Dimensions.

Sartre, J. P. (1966). *Being and nothingness*. New York: Washington Square Press.

Thornberg, P. D. (1993). *The meaning of hope in parents whose infants have died from sudden death syndrome.* Unpublished doctoral dissertation, University of Cincinnati. (University Microfilms International No. 9329939).

Wang, C. E. (1997). *Mending a torn fish net: A metaphor for hope.* Unpublished doctoral dissertation, Loyola University, Chicago.

Winkler, S. J. (1983). Parse's theory of nursing. In J. J. Fitzpatrick, & A. L. Whall (Eds.), *Conceptual models of nursing—Analysis and application* (pp. 275–294). Bowie, MD: Brady.

BIBLIOGRAPHY—SINCE 1995 ONLY

Andrus, K. (1995). Parse's nursing theory and the practice of perioperative nursing. *Canadian Operating Room Nursing Journal, 13*(3), 19–22.

Arndt, M. J. (1995). Parse's theory of human becoming in practice with hospitalized adolescents. *Nursing Science Quarterly, 8,* 86–90.

Banonis, B. C. (1995). Metaphors in practice of the human becoming theory. In R. R. Parse (Ed.), *Illuminations: The human becoming theory in practice and research* (pp. 87–96) (Pub. No. 15-2670). New York: National League for Nursing Press.

Baumann, S. L. (1995). Two views of homeless children's art: Psychoanalysis and Parse's human becoming theory. *Nursing Science Quarterly, 8,* 65–70.

Baumann, S. L. (1996). Parse's research methodology and the nurse researcher–child process. *Nursing Science Quarterly, 9,* 27–32.

Baumann, S. L. (1997). Qualitative research with children as participants. *Nursing Science Quarterly, 10,* 68–69.

Baumann, S. L. (1997). Contrasting two approaches in a community-based nursing practice with older adults: The medical model and Parse's nursing theory. *Nursing Science Quarterly, 10,* 124–130.

Baumann, S. L. (2000). The lived experience of feeling loved: A study of mothers in a parolee program. *Nursing Science Quarterly, 13,* 332–338.

Blanchard, D. (1996). *Intimacy as a lived experience of health.* Unpublished doctoral dissertation. Wayne State University, Detroit.

Bunkers, S. S. (1996). Thank you, Dorothy: Now I know. *Nursing Science Quarterly, 9,* 134–135.

Bunkers, S. S. (1998). A nursing theory-guided model of health ministry: Human becoming in parish nursing. *Nursing Science Quarterly, 11,* 7–8.

Bunkers, S. S. (2000). Dialogue: A process of structuring meaning. *Nursing Science Quarterly, 13,* 210–213.

Bunting, S. M. (1995). Rosemarie Rizzo Parse: Theory of human becoming. In C. M. McQuiston. & A. A. Webb (Eds.), *Foundations of nursing theory* (pp. 302–360). Thousand Oaks, CA: Sage.

Cody, W. K. (1995). The view of family within the human becoming theory. In R. R. Parse (Ed.), *Illuminations: The human becoming theory in practice and research* (pp. 9–26) (Pub. No. 15-2670). New York: National League for Nursing Press.

Cody, W. K. (1995). True presence with families living with HIV disease. In R. R. Parse (Ed.), *Illuminations: The human becoming theory in practice and research* (pp. 115–133) (Pub. No. 15-2670). New York: National League for Nursing Press.

Cody, W. K. (1995). Intersubjectivity: Nursing's contribution to the explication of its post modern meaning. *Nursing Science Quarterly, 8,* 52–53.

Cody, W. K. (1997). The many faces of change: Discomfort with the new. *Nursing Science Quarterly, 10,* 65–67.

Cody, W. K. (2000). Parse's human becoming school of thought and families. *Nursing Science Quarterly, 13,* 281–284.

Cody, W. K., Hudepohl, J. H., & Brinkman, K. S. (1995). True presence with a child and his family. In R. R. Parse (Ed.), *Illuminations: The human becoming theory in practice and research* (pp. 133–146) (Pub. No. 15-2670). New York: National League for Nursing Press.

Daly, J. (1995). The view of suffering within the human becoming theory. In R. R. Parse (Ed.), *Illuminations: The human becoming theory in practice and research* (pp. 45–60) (Pub. No. 15-2670). New York: National League for Nursing Press.

Daly, J., Mitchell, G. J., & Jonas-Simpson, C. M. (1996). Quality of life and the human becoming theory: Exploring discipline-specific contributions. *Nursing Science Quarterly, 9*, 170–174.

Davis, D. K., & Cannava, E. (1995). The meaning of retirement for communally-living retired performing artists. *Nursing Science Quarterly, 8*, 8–16.

Huch, M. H. (1995). Nursing and the next millennium. *Nursing Science Quarterly, 8*, 38–44.

Jacono, B. J., & Jacono, J. J. (1996). The benefits of Newman and Parse in helping nurse teachers to determine methods to enhance student creativity. *Nurse Education Today, 16*, 356–362.

Jonas, C. M. (1995). True presence through music for persons living their dying. In R. R. Parse (Ed.), *Illuminations: The human becoming theory in practice and research* (pp. 97–104) (Pub. No. 15-2670). New York: National League for Nursing Press.

Jonas-Simpson, C. (1996). The patient-focused care journey: Where patients and families guide the way. *Nursing Science Quarterly, 9*, 145–146.

Jonas-Simpson, C. (1997). The Parse research method through music. *Nursing Science Quarterly, 10*, 112–114.

Jonas-Simpson, C. (1997). Living the art of the human becoming theory. *Nursing Science Quarterly, 10*, 175–179.

Kelley, L. S. (1995). Parse's theory in practice with a group in the community. *Nursing Science Quarterly, 8*, 127–132.

Kelley, L. S. (1995). The house-garden-wilderness metaphor: Caring frameworks and the human becoming theory. In R. R. Parse (Ed.), *Illuminations: The human becoming theory in practice and research* (pp. 61–76) (Pub. No. 15-2670). New York: National League for Nursing Press.

Kim, M. S., Shin, K. R., & Shin, S. R. (1998). Korean adolescents experience of smoking cessation: A prelude to research with the human becoming perspective. *Nursing Science Quarterly, 11*, 105–109.

Lee, O. J., & Pilkington, F. B. (1999). Practice with persons living their dying: A human becoming perspective. *Nursing Science Quarterly, 12*, 324–328.

Melnechenko, K. L. (1995). Parse's theory of human becoming: An alternative guide to nursing practice for pediatric oncology nurses (with commentary by R. R. Parse). *Journal of Pediatric Oncology Nursing, 12*(3), 122–128.

Mitchell, G. J. (1995). The lived experience of restriction-freedom in later life. In R. R. Parse (Ed.), *Illuminations: The human becoming theory in practice and research* (pp. 159–195) (Pub. No. 15-2670). New York: National League for Nursing Press.

Mitchell, G. J. (1995). The view of freedom within the human becoming theory. In R. R. Parse (Ed.), *Illuminations: The human becoming theory in practice and research* (pp. 27–44) (Pub. No. 15-2670). New York: National League for Nursing Press.

Mitchell, G. J. (1996). Pretending: A way to get through the day. *Nursing Science Quarterly, 9*, 92–93.

Mitchell, G. J. (1996). A reflective moment with false cheerfulness. *Nursing Science Quarterly, 9*, 53–54.

Mitchell, G. J., Closson, T., Coulis, N., Flint, F., & Gray, B. (2000). Patient-focused care and human becoming thought: Connecting the right stuff. *Nursing Science Quarterly, 13*, 216–224.

Mitchell, G. J., & Cody, W. K. (1999). Human becoming theory: A complement to medical science. *Nursing Science Quarterly, 12*, 304–310.

Parse, R. R. (1995). Again: What is nursing? *Nursing Science Quarterly, 8,* 143.

Parse, R. R. (1995). Building knowledge through qualitative research: The road less traveled. *Nursing Science Quarterly, 9,* 10–16.

Parse, R. R. (1995). Building the realm of nursing knowledge. *Nursing Science Quarterly, 8,* 51.

Parse, R. R. (1995). Nursing theories and frameworks: The essence of advanced practice nursing. *Nursing Science Quarterly, 8,* 1.

Parse, R. R. (1996). Critical thinking: What is it? *Nursing Science Quarterly, 9,* 139.

Parse, R. R. (1996). Hear ye, hear ye, novice and seasoned authors! *Nursing Science Quarterly, 9,* 1.

Parse, R. R. (1996). The human becoming theory: Challenges in practice and research. *Nursing Science Quarterly, 9,* 55–60.

Parse, R. R. (1996). Nursing theories: An original path. *Nursing Science Quarterly, 9,* 85.

Parse, R. R. (1996). Reality: A seamless symphony of becoming. *Nursing Science Quarterly, 9,* 181–184.

Parse, R. R. (1997). Concept inventing: Unitary creations. *Nursing Science Quarterly, 10,* 63–64.

Parse, R. R. (1997). The language of nursing knowledge: Saying what we mean. In I. M. King & J. Fawcett (Eds.), *The language of nursing theory and metatheory* (pp. 73–77). Indianapolis: Center for Nursing Press.

Parse, R. R. (1997). Leadership: The essentials. *Nursing Science Quarterly, 10,* 109.

Parse, R. R. (1997). New beginnings in a quiet revolution. *Nursing Science Quarterly, 10,* 1.

Parse, R. R. (1997). Transforming research and practice within the human becoming theory. *Nursing Science Quarterly, 10,* 171–174.

Parse, R. R. (1998). The art of crticism. *Nursing Science Quarterly, 11,* 43.

Parse, R. R. (1998). Moving on. *Nursing Science Quarterly, 11,* 135.

Parse, R. R. (1998). Will nursing exist tomorrow? A reprise. *Nursing Science Quarterly, 11,* 1.

Parse, R. R. (1999). Expanding the vision: Tilling the field of nursing knowledge. *Nursing Science Quarterly, 12,* 3.

Parse, R. R. (1999). Nursing: The discipline and the profession. *Nursing Science Quarterly, 12,* 275.

Parse, R. R. (2000). Into the new millennium. *Nursing Science Quarterly, 13,* 3.

Parse, R. R. (2000). Language: Words reflect and cocreate meaing. *Nursing Science Quarterly, 13,* 187.

Parse, R. R. (2000). Obfuscating: The persistent practice of misnaming. *Nursing Science Quarterly, 13,* 91.

Parse, R. R. (2000). Paradigms: A reprise. *Nursing Science Quarterly, 13,* 275.

Pilkington, F. B. (1997). Knowledge and evidence: Do they change patterns of health? *Nursing Science Quarterly, 10,* 156–157.

Rasmusson, D. L. (1995). True presence with homeless persons. In R. R. Parse (Ed.), *Illuminations: The human becoming theory in practice and research* (pp. 105–114) (Pub. No. 15-2670). New York: National League for Nursing Press.

Ray, M. A. (1990). Critical reflective analysis of Parse's and Newman's research methodologies. *Nursing Science Quarterly, 3,* 44–46.

Rendon, D. C., Sales, R., Leal, I., & Pique, J. (1995). The lived experience of aging as community-dwelling elders in Valencia, Spain: A phenomenological study. *Nursing Science Quarterly, 8,* 152–157.

Smith, C. A. (1995). The lived experience of staying healthy in rural African-American families. *Nursing Science Quarterly, 8,* 17–21.

Walker, C. A. (1996). Coalescing the theories of two nurse visionaries: Parse and Watson. *Journal of Advanced Nursing, 24,* 988–996.

Walker, K. M. (2000). Situated immersion: An experience of dialogue. *Nursing Science Quarterly, 13,* 214–215.

Wang, C. H. (1997). Quality of life and health for persons with leprosy. *Nursing Science Quarterly, 10,* 144–145.

ANNOTATED RESEARCH BIBLIOGRAPHY

Allchin-Petardi, L. (1998). Weathering the storm: Persevering through a difficult time. *Nursing Science Quarterly, 11,* 172–177.

Parse's theory and research methodology were used to uncover the structure of the lived experience of persevering through a difficult time for eight women with ovarian cancer. Three core concepts surfaced: deliberately persisting, significant engagements, and shifting life patterns. The first concept was supported in the literature on perseverance, the second concept was further clarified, and the third concept represents new knowledge to the discipline of nursing.

Allchin-Petardi, L. (1999). Hope for American women with children. In R. R. Parse (Ed.), *Hope: An international perspective* (pp. 273–286). Boston: Jones & Bartlett.

This study found that the lived experience of hope for women with children is contemplating potentials with tenacious abiding amid arduous diversity.

Banonis, B. C. (1989). The lived experience of recovering from an addiction: A phenomenological study. *Nursing Science Quarterly, 2,* 37–43.

Based on Rogers's conceptual system and Parse's theory of Man–Living–Health, this study uncovered the structure of the experience of recovering from addiction. Three recovering persons described their lived experience. Implications for nursing practice are discussed.

Baumann, S. L. (1994). No place of their own: An exploratory study. *Nursing Science Quarterly, 7,* 162–169.

The researcher used Parse's theory to explore with mothers and children the experience of having no place of their own. For the participants the experience was a sense of gratitude for protection, mingling with the discomfort of restriction and exposure, giving rise to fears and reassurances as detachment from cherished others surfaces discordance with unfamiliar patterns, while novel engagements bring pleasure as insights and struggles surface new possibles as well as disillusionment.

Baumann, S. L. (1995). Parse's research methodology and the nurse researcher-child process. *Nursing Science Quarterly, 9,* 27–32.

This study views young children as partners in the research process. In accordance with Parse's research method, children are considered the experts about their health and capable of contributing to nurses' understanding of the human–universe–health process. Children's thoughts, feelings, and imaginings are made more accessible with the aid of art, stories, and play when offered in true presence.

Baumann, S. L. (1996). Feeling uncomfortable: Children in families with no place of their own. *Nursing Science Quarterly, 9,* 152–159.

The purpose of this study was to generate a structure of the lived experience of feeling uncomfortable for children in shelters. Findings suggest that the lived experience of feeling uncomfortable is a disturbing uneasiness with the unsureness of aloneness with togetherness amidst longing for personal joyful moments.

Baumann, S. L. (1999). The lived experience of hope: Children in families struggling to make a home. In R. R. Parse (Ed.), *Hope: An international perspective* (pp. 191–210). Boston: Jones & Bartlett.

This study found that the structure of the lived experience of hope for children in families struggling to make a home in the envisioning of nurturing engagements while inventing possibilities.

Bunkers, S. S. (1998). Considering tomorrow: Parse's theory-guided research. *Nursing Science Quarterly, 11,* 56–63.

This study investigated the meaning of tomorrow for homeless females. Findings expand Parse's theory in relation to considering tomorrow, health, and quality of life. The structure of considering tomorrow is contemplating desired endeavors in longing for the cherished, while intimate alliances with isolating distance emerge, as resilient endurance surfaces amid disturbing unsureness.

Bunkers, S. S. (1999). The lived experience of hope for those working with homeless persons. In R. R. Parse (Ed.), *Hope: An international perspective* (pp. 227–250). Boston: Jones & Bartlett.

This study found that the structure of the lived experience of hope for those working with homeless persons is envisioning possibilities amid disheartenment, as close alliances with isolating turmoil surface in inventive endeavoring.

Bunkers, S. S., & Daly, J. (1999). The lived experience of hope for Australian families living with coronary disease. In R. R. Parse (Ed.), *Hope: An international perspective* (pp. 45–61). Boston: Jones & Bartlett.

The lived experience of hope for Australian families living with coronary disease is anticipating possibilities amid anguish, while enduring with vitality in intimate affiliations.

Chapman, J. S., Mitchell, G. J., & Forchuk, C. (1994). A glimpse of nursing theory-based practice in Canada. *Nursing Science Quarterly, 79*, 104–112.

A review of the literature of pre- postdescriptive qualitative research studies of the implementation of Parse's theory in hospital settings in Canada. Nurses in all the studies changed their views of human beings from seeing clients as problems to seeing them as unique persons in relation with others. Nurses described a different respect for persons, for the meanings they give life and for relationships and choices, a profound respect that according to the nurses did not exist before learning Parse's theory. Improved morale and understanding of professional, autonomous practice was also reported.

Cody, W. K. (1991). Grieving a personal loss. *Nursing Science Quarterly, 4*, 61–68.

Cody reports that the structure of the lived experience of grieving a personal loss is intense struggling in the flux of change while a shifting view fosters moving beyond the now as different possibilities surface in dwelling with and apart from the absent presence and others in light of what is cherished.

Cody, W. K. (1995). The lived experience of grieving, for families living with AIDS. In R. R. Parse (Ed.), *Illuminations: The human becoming theory in practice and research* (pp. 197–242) (Pub. No. 15-2670). New York: National League for Nursing Press.

This study found that the structure of grieving for families living with AIDS is pushing–resisting with diverse rhythms of communion–solitude evolving with certainty–uncertainty through honoring the treasured. Cody's practice proposition on grieving states that struggling with the ambiguity of change through bearing witness to absent presence sheds light on what really matters as creating new possibilities shifts priorities. This proposition is consistent with all three Parse studies on grieving.

Cody, W. K. (1995). Of life immense in passion, pulse, and power: Dialoguing with Whitman and Parse—A hermeneutic study. In R. R. Parse (Ed.), *Illuminations: The human becoming theory in practice and research* (pp. 269–308) (Pub. No. 15-2670). New York: National League for Nursing Press.

This study led to the following interpretation, which answers the research question, what does it mean to be human? To be human means to be *oneself*, embodied and sensual yet "not contained between my hat and boots." The self is one's interrelationship with the "kosmos," free and unbounded by space and time, the self includes all that is in one's universe.

Cody, W. K., & Filler, J. E. (1999). The lived experience of hope for women residing in a shelter. In R. R. Parse (Ed.), *Hope: An international perspective* (pp. 211–226). Boston: Jones & Bartlett.

This study found that the structure of the lived experience of women residing in a shelter is picturing attainment in persisting amid the arduous, while trusting in potentiality.

Daly, J. (1995). The lived experience of suffering. In R. R. Parse (Ed.), *Illuminations: The human becoming theory in practice and research* (pp. 243–268) (Pub. No. 15-2670). New York: National League for Nursing Press.

This study found that the structure of the lived experience of suffering is paralyzing anguish with glimpses of precious possibilities emerging with entanglements of engaging–disengaging while struggling in pursuit of fortification.

Davis, D. K., & Cannava, E. (1995). The meaning of retirement for communally-living retired performing artists. *Nursing Science Quarterly, 8,* 8–16.
  The meaning of retirement for retired performing artists is the emerging of an unburdening
  lightness as esthetic interconnections surface the was and will be in the now moment as the di-
  versity of everydayness enlivens through communion–solitude while anticipating the transpos-
  ing vistas of the inevitable prompts treasuring the now in confirming a perpetual artistic legacy.
  The findings are congruent with Parse's theory.
Futrell, M., Wondolowski, C., & Mitchell, G. J. (1993). Aging in the oldest old living in Scotland:
A phenomenological study. *Nursing Science Quarterly, 6,* 189–194.
  The purpose of this study was to uncover ways in which the oldest old living in a Scottish com-
  munity view the experience of aging. The research was guided by Parse's theory and followed
  the van Kaam methods to elicit the structural definition of the meaning of aging as described by
  the oldest old. It was found that the experience of aging is intensifying engagements as trans-
  figurations signify maturity tempering the unavoidable with buoyant serenity.
Jonas, C. (1992). The meaning of being an elder in Nepal. *Nursing Science Quarterly, 5,* 171–175.
  Jonas reports that the meaning of being an elder in Nepal is cherishing necessities for survival
  intermingled with the rapture of celebration with important others, as diminishing familiar patterns expand moments of respite, while regard for others affirms self, and changing customs create comfort–discomfort as what-was unfolds into new possibles. Findings are consistent with
  Parse's concepts of valuing, enabling-limiting, and transforming.
Kelley, L. S. (1991). Struggling with going along when you do not believe. *Nursing Science Quarterly, 4,* 123–129.
  Kelley reports the lived experience of going along when you do not believe to be justifi-
  able yielding, as opposing views intensify personal convictions and compel disclosure while
  suffering consequences. She reports that this phenomenon was found to be the predominant
  universal lived experience within lives of outstanding nurses in the United States. Kelley
  states that this phenomenon is comparable to Parse's notion of valuing the powering of
  revealing–concealing.
Kelley, L. S. (1999). Hope as lived by Native Americans. In R. R. Parse (Ed.), *Hope: An international perspective* (pp. 251–272). Boston: Jones & Bartlett.
  The structure of the lived experience of hope for Native Americans is a transfiguring enlightenment arising with engaging affiliations as encircling the legendary surfaces with fortification.
Mitchell, G. J. (1990). The lived experience of taking life day-by-day in later life: Research guided
by Parse's emergent method. *Nursing Science Quarterly, 3,* 29–36.
  Mitchell reports the findings of her study to be the following common concepts extracted from
  the data: affirming self through interrelationships, glimpsing a diminished now amidst expand-
  ing possibles, and the unburdened journey of moving beyond.
Mitchell, G. J. (1993). Living paradox in Parse's theory. *Nursing Science Quarterly, 6,* 44–51.
  The purpose of this study was to describe the phenomenon of living paradox as an inherent as-
  pect of human experience and health. The author demonstrates that living paradox as specified in
  Parse's theory of human becoming is a significant contribution to nursing and human science.
Mitchell, G. J. (1994). The meaning of being a senior: Phenomenological research and interpreta-
tion with Parse's theory of nursing. *Nursing Science Quarterly, 7,* 70–79.
  This study reports the findings of a phenomenological analysis on the meaning of being a senior.
  Six hundred narrative stories written by older Canadians on their personal experience in later life
  were analyzed using the van Kaam phenomenological method. The structure identified includes
  engaging the now while rolling with the vicissitudes of life as refined astuteness surfaces a buoyant unburdening, shifting rhythms propel discovery through grateful abiding in wondering
  awareness as anticipation of new possibles enlivens connectedness and altruistic commitments
  affirm self amidst the retrospective pondering of everydayness.

Mitchell, G. J. (1995). The lived experience of restriction–freedom in later life. In R. R. Parse (Ed.), *Illuminations: The human becoming theory in practice and research* (pp. 159–196) (Pub. No. 15-2670). New York: National League for Nursing Press.

This study found that the lived experience of restriction–freedom in later life is anticipating limitations amidst unencumbered self-direction as yielding to change fortifies resolve for moving beyond.

Mitchell, G. J., & Heidt, P. (1994). The lived experience of wanting to help another. *Nursing Science Quarterly, 7,* 119–127.

The purpose of this study using Parse's methodology was to generate the structure of the lived experience of nurses wanting to help another. The lived experience is directing, nurturing intentions amidst uplifting affirmations with others while dissonant constraints unfold new possibilities.

Nikitas-Costello, D. M. (1994). Choosing goals: A phenomenological study. *Nursing Science Quarterly, 7,* 87–92.

The purpose of this study was to uncover the meaning of the lived experience of choosing life goals. Seven married female nurse administrators between 27 and 37 years of age, employed in management positions in two large metropolitan hospitals, were asked to provide a written description of a situation in which they found themselves choosing life goals. Giorgi's (1975)* qualitative method of phenomenology was used to analyze the written descriptions. The major finding was choosing life goals is a struggling to fulfill competing ambitions while experiencing paradoxical feelings of calmness–turmoil, success–defeat, and security–insecurity in the process of affirming cherished beliefs. Findings support the value of the phenomenological method for nursing research and expand Parse's theory of human becoming.

*Giorgi, A. (1975). An application of phenomenological method in psychology. In A. Giorgi, C. Fischer, & E. Murray (Eds.), *Duquesne studies in phenomenological psychology* (Vol. 11, pp. 82–103). Pittsburgh, PA: Duquesne University Press.

Nokes, K. M., & Carver, K. (1991). The meaning of living with AIDS: A study using Parse's theory of Man–Living–Health. *Nursing Science Quarterly, 4,* 175–179.

This qualitative descriptive study of persons with AIDS resulted in three themes: an abrupt shift in patterns of being give rise to changing priorities, fluctuating possibilities arise in the uncertainty of being with and away from close others, and changing hopes and dreams surface from the insights of suffering.

Northrup, D. T., & Cody, W. K. (1998). Evaluation of the human becoming theory in an acute psychiatric setting. *Nursing Science Quarterly, 11,* 23–30.

This descriptive study evaluated Parse's theory of human becoming in practice in an acute psychiatric setting. A pre- mid- postimplementation design served to generate qualitative data from nurses, patients, and hospital documentation that illuminated changes in the quality of nursing care on three diverse pilot units. Findings supported prior research except about job satisfaction reactions of nurses. Some nurses felt that to be in true presence with psychotic clients was nonproductive and was an inadequate guide to psychiatric nursing practice.

Parse, R. R. (1990). Parse's research methodology with an illustration of the lived experience of hope. *Nursing Science Quarterly, 3,* 9–17.

This study used Parse's research methodology to investigate the lived experience of hope for persons on hemodialysis. The structure of the lived experience of hope is anticipating possibilities through envisioning the not-yet in harmoniously living the comfort–discomfort of everydayness while unfolding a different perspective of an expanding view.

Parse, R. R. (1993). The experience of laughter: A phenomenological study. *Nursing Science Quarterly, 6,* 39–43.

Parse reports that the structure of laughter is a buoyant immersion in the presence of unanticipated glimpsing prompting harmonious integrity which surfaces anew through contemplative visioning. She notes that the definition is congruent with her theory and expands understanding of human experience.

Parse, R. R. (1994). Laughing and health: A study using Parse's research method. *Nursing Science Quarterly, 7*, 55–64.

The purpose of this study was to uncover a structure of the lived experience of laughing—health, using Parse's research method. Twenty men and women over 65 years of age volunteered to participate in this study. The structure of the lived experience of laughing and health was found to be a potent buoyant vitality sparked through mirthful engagements prompting an unburdening delight deflecting disheartenments while emerging with blissful contentment.

Parse, R. R. (1996). Quality of life for persons living with Alzheimer's disease: The human becoming perspective. *Nursing Science Quarterly, 9*, 126–133.

The purpose of this study was to uncover the meaning of quality of life for persons with Alzheimer's disease. Findings show that quality of life for these persons is a contentment with the remembered and now affiliations that arises amidst the tedium of the commonplace, as an easy–uneasy flow of transfiguring surfaces with liberating possibilities and confining restraints, while desiring cherished intimacies yields with inevitable distance in the vicissitudes of life, as contemplating the ambiguity of the possibles emerges with yearning for successes in the moment.

Parse, R. R. (1997). Joy–sorrow: A study using the Parse research method. *Nursing Science Quarterly, 10*, 80–87.

This study found that the structure of the lived experience of joy–sorrow is the pleasure amid adversity emerging in the cherished contentment of benevolent engagements.

Parse, R. R. (1999). The lived experience of hope for family members of persons living in a Canadian chronic care facility. In R. R. Parse (Ed.), *Hope: An international perspective* (pp. 63–68). Boston: Jones & Bartlett.

The lived experience of hope for family members of persons in a Canadian chronic care home is an undaunting pursuit of the not-yet amid the wretched, as affable involvements arise with transfiguring.

Pilkington, F. B. (1993). The lived experience of grieving the loss of an important other. *Nursing Science Quarterly, 6*, 130–137.

The purpose of this study was to uncover the structure of the lived experience of grieving a loss of an important other using Parse's research methodology. Five participants described their experiences of grieving the loss of an important other through dialectical engagement with the researcher.

Pilkington, F. B., & Millar, B. (1999). The lived experience of hope with persons from Wales, U. K. In R. R. Parse (Ed.), *Hope: An international perspective* (pp. 163–190). Boston: Jones & Bartlett.

The structure of the lived experience of hope for persons in Wales, U. K., is anticipating cherished possibilities while persevering amid adversity with benevolent affiliations.

Rendon, D. C., Sales, R., Leal, I., & Pique, J. (1995). The lived experience of aging in a community-dwelling elders in Valencia, Spain: A phenomenological study. *Nursing Science Quarterly, 8*, 152–157.

Parse's theory of human becoming guided the research and van Kaam's phenomenological method of analysis was used to identify common elements and major themes. Findings revealed the meaning of aging to be confirming triumphs through the forceful enlivening of bridled potency. Findings were conceptually consistent with Parse's major themes of meaning, rhythmicity, and cotranscendence.

Santopinto, M. D. A. (1989). The relentless drive to be ever thinner: A study using the phenomenological method. *Nursing Science Quarterly, 2*, 29–36.

Santopinto reports that the structure of the lived experience to be ever thinner is a persistent struggle toward an imaged self through withdrawing–engaging.

Smith, C. A. (1995). The lived experience of staying healthy in rural African-American families. *Nursing Science Quarterly, 8,* 17–21.

Staying healthy emerged as a dynamic response to life events that involved activity and relatedness in synchrony with life's rules and emotional tranquility. Findings confirm that phenomenological research can reveal the meaning of health within the context of culture and support the conceptualization of health as a developmental process of African Americans.

Smith, M. C. (1990). Struggling through a difficult time for unemployed persons. *Nursing Science Quarterly, 3,* 18–28.

Smith reports that struggling through a difficult time is regarded by unemployed persons as sculpting new lifeways in turbulent change through affirming self while feeling expanded by assets and restricted by obstacles in the midst of grieving the loss of what was cherished.

Takahashi, T. (1999). Kibov: Hope for the person in Japan. In R. R. Parse (Ed.), *Hope: An international perspective* (pp. 115–128). Boston: Jones & Bartlett.

This study found that the structure of the lived experience of hope for persons in Japan is anticipation of expanding possibilities, while liberation amid arduous restriction arises with the contentment of desired accomplishments.

Toikkanen, T., & Muurinen, E. (1999). Toivo: Hope for persons in Finland. In R. R. Parse (Ed.), *Hope: An international perspective* (pp. 79–96). Boston: Jones & Bartlett.

This study found that the lived experience of hope for persons in Finland is persistent anticipation of contentment arising with the promise of nurturing affiliations, while inspiration emerges and easing the arduous.

Wang, C. H. (1999). Hope for persons living with leprosy in Taiwan. In R. R. Parse (Ed.), *Hope: An international perspective* (pp. 143–162). Boston: Jones & Bartlett.

This study found that the structure of hope for persons living with leprosy is anticipating an unburdening serenity amid despair, as nurturing engagements emerge in creating anew with cherished priorities.

Wondolowski, C., & Davis, D. K. (1988). The lived experience of aging in the oldest old: A phenomenological study. *American Journal of Psychoanalysis, 48,* 261–270.

This study uncovered ways in which the oldest old living in a community view the experience of aging. The study revealed that in a sample of 100 mean and women, aged 80 to 101 years, aging is creating transfiguring in the presence of unfolding euphony enhanced by moments of transcendent voyaging.

Wondolowski, C., & Davis, D. K. (1991). The lived experience of health in the oldest old: A phenomenological study. *Nursing Science Quarterly, 4,* 113–118.

This study of the lived experience of health for the oldest old found that health is regarded as an abiding vitality emanating through moments of rhapsodic reverie in generating fulfillment.

Zanotti, R., & Bournes, D. A. (1999). Speranza: A study of the lived experience of hope with persons from Italy. In R. R. Parse (Ed.), *Hope: An international perspective* (pp. 97–114). Boston: Jones & Bartlett.

This study found that the structure of hope for persons from Italy is expectancy amid the arduous, as quiescent vitality arises with expanding horizons.

CHAPTER 20

THE MODELING AND ROLE-MODELING THEORY

HELEN C. ERICKSON, EVELYN M. TOMLIN, MARY ANN P. SWAIN

Noreen Cavan Frisch
Susan Stanwyck Bowman

The Modeling and Role-Modeling Theory was developed by three individuals, Helen Cook Erickson, Evelyn M. Tomlin, and Mary Ann P. Swain. The initial publication of the theory was presented in 1983 with the text Modeling and Role-Modeling: A Theory and Paradigm for Nursing.

Helen C. Erickson completed her initial nursing education in 1957 with a diploma from Saginaw General Hospital in Saginaw, Michigan. In 1972 she returned to school to earn a bachelor of science in nursing, masters degrees in psychiatric and medical-surgical nursing, and a doctorate in educational psychology at the University of Michigan. In 1980, she received the Sigma Theta Tau Rho chapter award for excellence in nursing. Erickson was also the first president of the Society for the Advancement of Modeling and Role-Modeling from 1986 to 1990. She is a Fellow of the American Academy of Nursing and was presented an honorary certification in Holistic Nursing by the American Holistic Nurses Association for her work in guiding nursing practice toward holistic ideals. Erickson is an accomplished clinician, a scholar, and a teacher.

As a clinician, she has practiced in many different areas of nursing in both direct care and supervisory roles, in the United States and Puerto Rico. She has maintained an independent practice since 1976. The theory was developed as an outcome of her clinical practice. She continues her practice today and supervises health care providers interested in furthering their knowledge and skill in the use of Modeling and Role-Modeling as the theory base for practice.

As a scholar, Erickson initiated scientific testing of the theory, and continues to work on articulating aspects of the theory. She has been involved in relating

463

research findings and implications for practice through publications and numerous presentations. One of her current projects is to develop a Center for the Study and Practice of the Modeling and Role-Modeling theory and paradigm. Erickson is also a board member for the American Holistic Nurses Certification Corporation, which has guided the development and administration of the first national certification in holistic nursing.

Erickson is also an educator. She is an emeritus Professor of Nursing from the University of Texas at Austin. She has held both instructional and administrative positions and taught in both undergraduate and graduate curricula. She has been on the faculty of the University of Michigan, the University of South Carolina, and the University of Texas at Austin. She has received several awards for excellence in teaching, including recognition as one of two nursing faculty in the 100-year history of the University of Michigan to receive the Amoco Good Teaching Award.

Evelyn Tomlin received a baccalaureate degree in nursing from the University of Southern California and a masters in psychiatric nursing from the University of Michigan. She has extensive clinical practice experience both in the United States and Afghanistan. She has been involved in staff nursing, critical care, home health, and independent practice as well as many areas of nursing education.

In her retirement from "nursing for pay," Tomlin lives in Geneva, Illinois. She volunteers at a shelter for women and children, takes speaking engagements in Illinois and nearby states, and serves as a lay leader in several ministries (both in the United States and abroad) where she relates that remarkably expedited healings have been experienced through the power of sound teaching, truth-telling, and prayer within an interactive, interpersonal relationship with God. She published an article identifying an interface between Modeling and Role-Modeling and Judeo-Christian values in the first monograph published by the Society for the Advancement of Modeling and Role-Modeling (Tomlin, 1990).

Mary Ann Swain's educational background is in psychology with a bachelor of arts degree from DePauw University in Greencastle, Indiana, and both a masters of science and a doctoral degree from the University of Michigan. Although not a nurse, much of Swain's career has been involved with nursing. She has taught research methods and statistics as well as psychology to nurses at DePauw University and the University of Michigan. Swain has held the positions of director of the doctoral program in nursing, chairperson of nursing research, professor of nursing research, and associate vice president for academic affairs at the University of Michigan. She is presently provost and vice president for academic affairs at the State University of New York, Binghamton. She has received many awards for academic excellence and is an honorary member of Sigma Theta Tau. She is active in the Society for the Advancement of Modeling and Role-Modeling and is a past president of the Society.

The book describing the theory of Modeling and Role-Modeling presents the theory in a very informal and readable style (Erickson, Tomlin, & Swain, 1983). It includes many case studies and clinical examples of the use of this theory in nursing. The basis of the theory is always to focus on the person receiving nursing care—not on the nurse, not on the care, and not on the disease. The concept of modeling a person's world is credited to Milton H. Erickson, M.D., who was the father-in-law of the principal author of this theory, Helen Erickson. Erickson credits her father-in-law with a great deal of influence on this theory. His initial beliefs in the mind–body connection in health, healing, and disease, as well as his belief that the most important thing a nurse can do to help a client is modeling that person's world, provided the underlying themes for this theory.

Erickson returned to graduate school after many years of clinical practice to "label and articulate" practice-based knowledge that she knew was important to and consistent in nursing care. She believed this knowledge needed to be shared with other nurses. Both her master's thesis and doctoral dissertation were instrumental in developing the theory of Modeling and Role-Modeling (Erickson, 1976, 1984). Other early research that contributed to this theory was supported by two federal grants: "Influencing compliance among hypertensives" from the National Heart, Lung, and Blood Institute (HL-17045) (Erickson & Swain, 1977; Swain & Stickel, 1981) and "Health promotion among diabetics: Comparing nursing systems" from the Division of Nursing (NU-00658). More recently, Dr. Erickson was the principal investigator for a major study at the University of Texas at Austin, "Modeling and Role-Modeling with Alzheimer's patients," funded by the National Institutes of Health, the National Institute of Aging, and the National Center for Nursing Research (NIH Grant # R01NR03032–01).

The combination of talents of the three authors who collaborated at the University of Michigan in the mid-1970s was advantageous for the development of a nursing theory that was useful and related to practice, education, and research. All three of the original authors have been involved in nursing education. Two are expert nursing clinicians and remain actively involved in clinical practice, and two remain active in research and scholarly pursuits.

THE THEORY OF MODELING AND ROLE-MODELING

Modeling and role-modeling is an interpersonal and interactive theory of nursing that requires the nurse to assess *(model),* plan *(role-model),* and intervene *(five aims of intervention)* on the basis of the client's perspective of the world. The nurse always acknowledges the uniqueness and individuality of the client and appreciates that individuals, at some level, know what makes them ill and what makes them well *(self-care knowledge).* The nurse assists individuals to recognize and obtain resources that are important for their health and healing *(self-care resources),* and facilitates the use of these resources *(self-care action).* Two additional concepts important in this theory are *affiliated–individuation,* and *adaptive potential.*

Modeling

Modeling is the process used by the nurse to develop an understanding of the client's world as the client perceives it. The model of a person's world is the representation of the unique aggregation of the way an individual perceives life and all of its aspects and components; the way an individual thinks, communicates, feels, believes, and behaves; and the underlying motivation and rationale for beliefs and behaviors. This concept is based on the works of Milton Erickson, who believed that an appreciation for a client's model of the world was a prerequisite for providing holistic care (Erickson, et al., 1983). Modeling is both an art and a science. The art of modeling is the empathetic understanding of the present situation within the client's context of the world—that is, the development of a "model" of the situation from the client's perspective. The science of modeling is the analysis of the information collected about the client's world. To truly understand the client's model of the world, the nurse must have a strong theoretical base in the physical and social sciences. The client's perspective is analyzed on the basis of knowledge and theory in areas including human behavior, development, cultural diversity, interaction, pathophysiology, and human needs (Erickson, et al., 1983).

Role-Modeling

Role-modeling is the facilitation of health. It is also both an art and a science. The art of role-modeling involves the individualization of care based on the client's model of the world; the science of role-modeling is the use of theoretical bases when planning and implementing nursing care. Role-modeling is the facilitation of the individual in attaining, maintaining, or promoting health through purposeful interventions based on the individual's perceptions as well as the theoretical base for the practice of nursing (Erickson, et al., 1983).

Five Aims of Intervention

The aims of intervention are based on five principles pertaining to similarities among humans (see Table 20–1). Because each individual is unique and has his or her own model of the world, it is not possible to formulate standardized interventions. However, because all human beings have some similarities, the aims of intervention can be standardized. Individualized interventions are based on the client's model of the world and guided by the five aims of intervention defined as follows.

Build Trust. Nursing requires a trusting relationship. This relationship involves honesty, acceptance, respect, empathy, and a belief in the client's model of the world. Therapeutic communication skills are essential in building trust. Trust is basic to any interpersonal relationship and is easily threatened if clients perceive that nurses lack respect for their view of the world or feel that nurses consider the clients' concerns or beliefs to be invalid, unwarranted, erroneous, or inappropriate.

TABLE 20–1. RELATIONSHIP OF HUMAN SIMILARITY PRINCIPLES AND AIMS FOR INTERVENTION

Principle	Aim
1. The nursing process requires that a trusting and functional relationship exist between nurse and client.	Build trust
2. Affiliated–Individuation is dependent on the individual's perceiving that he or she is an acceptable, respectable, and worthwhile human being.	Promote client's positive orientation.
3. Human development is dependent on the individual's perceiving that he or she has some control over his or her life, while concurrently sensing a state of affiliation.	Promote client's control.
4. There is an innate drive toward holistic health that is facilitated by consistent and systematic nurturance.	Affirm and promote client's strengths.
5. Human growth is dependent on satisfaction of basic needs and facilitated by growth-need satisfaction.	Set mutual goals that are health-directed.

Source: From Erickson, H. C, Tomlin, E M., A Swain, M. A. P. (1983). *Modeling and role-modeling: A theory and paradigm for nursing (p. 170).* Lexington, SC: Pine Press. Used with permission.

Promote Positive Orientation. Nursing interventions need to promote each client's self-worth as well as the client's hope for the future. Reframing can be used to assist clients in changing their perception of a situation from one of threat to one of challenge, from one of hopelessness to one of hope, and from something negative to something positive. Promoting an individual's strengths promotes that individual's self-worth and perceived control. Promoting strengths also aids in building a trusting relationship between the client and the nurse.

Promote Perceived Control. Human development depends on individuals' perceiving that they have some control over their lives. Nurses may understand that clients have control over what happens to them and may understand that clients are required to give informed consent for any procedure done to them. However, many clients do not perceive that they have any control. It is not enough for the nurse to promote client control; the nurse must promote the client's *perception* of control.

Promote Strengths. Identification and promotion of strengths is a means of assisting clients to mobilize resources. In the face of stressors, individuals may become overwhelmed with their perceived weaknesses and not be able to identify or use strengths.

Set Mutual Goals That Are Health Directed. Nurses must use the individual's innate drive to be as healthy as he or she can be. The nurse's and client's goals are the same—to meet the client's basic needs. When the nurse's and client's goals appear to differ, the nurse has most likely not fully modeled the client's world. Incomplete modeling can be the result of inadequate data gathering and empathy, or a lack of knowledge for analysis and interpretation of the data collected. Incomplete modeling can also result from the nurse's focus on one subsystem (e.g., biophysical) rather than viewing the individual and health as truly holistic.

Self-Care

There are three aspects of self-care in the Modeling and Role Modeling theory: *self-care knowledge, self-care resources*, and *self-care action*.

Self-Care Knowledge. In most situations, individuals can describe what they perceive to be their health problem; they can also identify what they think will make them feel better. According to Erickson, et al. (1983), self-care knowledge is knowledge one has about "what has made him or her sick, lessened his or her effectiveness, or interfered with his or her growth. The person also knows what will make him or her well, optimize his or her effectiveness or fulfillment (given circumstances), or promote his or her growth" (p. 48). In an analysis of case studies reported by Erickson (1990a), the following four themes were found that relate to the nature of self-care knowledge:

1. An individual's perception of factors associated with his or her personal health problems are rarely obvious to the health care provider.
2. The individual's perceptions of what is needed to help him or her can best be defined by that person.
3. One nursing role is to facilitate clients to articulate what they perceive to be associated with their problem and what can be done to help them feel better.
4. Another nursing role is to assist the clients to resolve their problems in ways that meet personal needs and are health and growth directed (p. 186).

Self-Care Resources. All individuals have internal and external resources (strengths and support) that will help gain, maintain, and promote an optimum level of holistic health. It is important for the nurse to assess these resources to assist the client in self-care action.

Primary internal self-care resources for each individual result from the person having successfully negotiated developmental challenges. Characteristics that result from appropriate need satisfaction (within the context of the human needs theory by Maslow, 1970), and positive resolution of the developmental tasks (within the context of the theory of psychosocial development by Erikson, 1963), leave the individual able to mobilize resources (Erickson, 1990a). Studies have been reported that describe and expand these characteristics and their uses as self-care resources (Curl, 1992; Jensen, 1995; Keck, 1989; MacLean, 1987, 1990, 1992; Miller, 1986).

Each individual identifies external self-care resources. Characteristics of external self-care resources are being explored. These characteristics include perceptions, types of resources used when ill and well, and transitional objects, including technical devices. Kennedy (1991) discusses differences among individuals relating to perceptions of comfort and comforting care. Bowman (1998) reported that external resources used by persons when ill may be different than those used when well. Transitional objects are external resources that may be utilized to facilitate the feelings of worthiness produced by secure attachments (Erickson, 1990b). Beery and Baas (1996) describe the use of implanted technical devices such as pacemakers becoming "internal" transitional objects providing a secure attachment to facilitate health.

Self-Care Action. Self-care action is the development and use of self-care knowledge and self-care resources. The basis of nursing is assisting clients in self-care actions related to health. The concept of self-care is used differently in the Modeling and Role-Modeling theory than in Orem's (1995) Self-Care Deficit Theory. Orem's theory focuses on delineating *when* nursing is needed. In Orem's theory, self-care is a universal need met through the ability to care for one's self; nurses assist clients in meeting self-care needs when there is a deficit in the clients' ability to meet their own needs. Self-care in Modeling and Role-Modeling focuses on the individual's personal knowledge about what makes him or her well or ill. All clients have self-care knowledge, and the nurse facilitates the client's identification and use of that knowledge. Self-care, then, in Modeling and Role-Modeling is used in planning implementations rather than being used for determining the *need* for nursing implementations, as is the situation in Orem's self-care theory.

Affiliated–Individuation

All individuals are seen as having simultaneous needs to be attached to other individuals and to be separate from them. This concept is described in Modeling and Role-Modeling as "affiliated–individuation" and considered to be a motivation for human behavior. "*Affiliated–individuation* occurs when a person perceives himself or herself as simultaneously close to and separate from a significant other" (Erickson, et al., 1983, p. 68). Affiliated–individuation is different from interdependence in that it is an intrapsychic phenomenon and can occur without being reciprocated. Affiliated–individuation is a resource for healing and an important component for well-being. Acton and Miller (1996) reported no decrease in affiliated–individuation for caregivers of persons with Alzhemier's disease when the caregivers participated in a theory-based support group intervention.

Adaptive Potential

Adaptive potential refers to the individual's ability to mobilize resources to cope with stressors. The Adaptive Potential Assessment Model (APAM) has three categories: *equilibrium, arousal*, and *impoverishment*. Equilibrium has two possibilities: *adaptive equilibrium* and *maladaptive equilibrium*. Arousal and impoverishment are both stress states. They differ in that those in impoverishment must deal with stress with diminished, if not depleted, resources (Erickson, et al., 1983). Adaptive potential is dynamic, and individuals can move from any of the

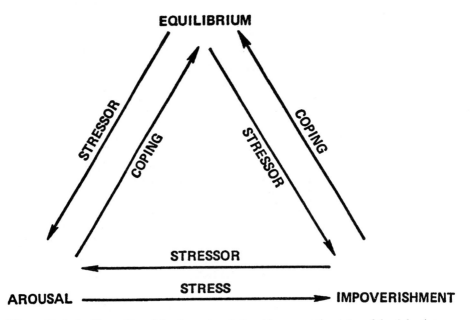

Figure 20–1. An illustration of the dynamic relationship among the states of the Adaptive Potential Assessment Model. *(From Erickson, H., Tomlin, E., & Swain, M. A. (1983). Modeling and Role-Modeling: A theory and paradigm for nursing (p. 82). Lexington, SC: Pine Press. Used with permission.)*

three states to any other of the states, as shown in Figure 20–1. Movement among the states is influenced by the individual's ability to cope. The APAM identifies states (not traits) of coping that can assist the nurse in planning interventions for the client. Assessment of adaptive potential has been well documented (Barnfather, Swain, & Erickson, 1989a, 1989b; Campbell, Finch, Allport, Erickson, & Swain, 1985; Erickson & Swain, 1982). Figure 20–2 identifies how interventions can be guided by the individual's ability to mobilize his or her own resources. A person who is impoverished is not in a situation to be an autonomous, independent person eager to learn and to perform self-care. An impoverished person requires that affiliation needs be met, internal strengths be promoted, and external resources be provided. A client in arousal is in a stress state and has difficulty mobilizing resources. This client has stronger individuation needs and responds to guidance, directions, assistance, and teaching that are all aimed at self-care. The client in equilibrium is in a nonstress state. Adaptive equilibrium is different from maladaptive equilibrium in that the adaptive client has all subsystems in harmony, whereas the maladaptive client places one or more subsystems in jeopardy to maintain equilibrium. The importance of equilibrium, whether adaptive or maladaptive, is that the client sees no reason to change because equilibrium already exists. Interventions for the client in maladaptive equilibrium need to focus on motivation strategies to develop a desire for change.

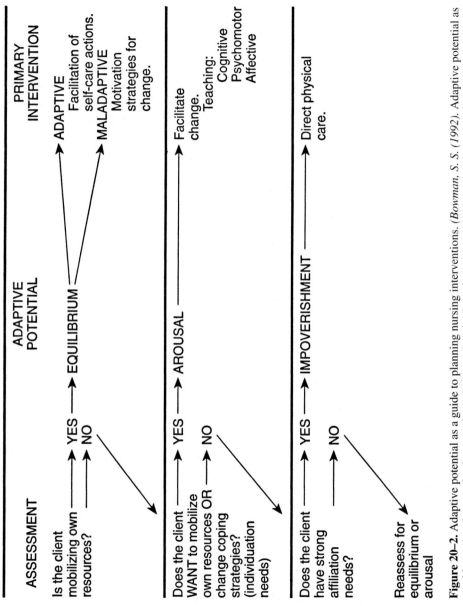

Figure 20–2. Adaptive potential as a guide to planning nursing interventions. *(Bowman, S. S. (1992). Adaptive potential as a guide to planning nursing interventions. Presented at the Fourth National Modeling and Role-Modeling Conference, Boston, MA. Used with permission.)*

MODELING AND ROLE-MODELING
AND NURSING'S METAPARADIGM

Human beings are holistic persons with interacting subsystems (biophysical, psychological, social, and cognitive) and inherent genetic bases and spiritual drive (see Fig. 20–3). "Holism" implies that the whole is greater than the sum of the parts and is differentiated from "wholism," which implies that a person is an aggregate of parts and the whole is equal to the sum of the parts (Erickson, et al., 1983). Modeling and Role-Modeling describes individuals as being born with an inherent desire to fulfill their self-potential. The developmental theories of Erik Erikson, Abraham Maslow, Jean Piaget, and George Engel are basic to describing how people are alike. People are seen as alike in that they are all holistic beings who want to de-

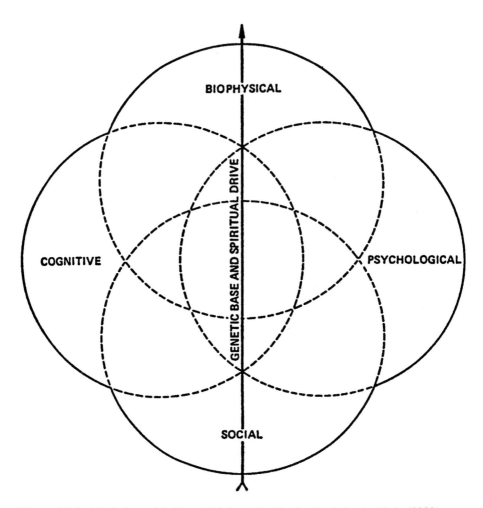

Figure 20–3. A holistic model. *(From Erickson, H., Tomlin, E., & Swain, M. A. (1983). Modeling and Role-Modeling: A theory and paradigm for nursing (p. 45). Lexington, SC: Pine Press. Used with permission.)*

velop their potential. All individuals have basic needs that motivate behavior, including a drive called *affiliated–individuation* (Erickson, et al., 1983). Although human beings share these commonalities, each individual is unique. People differ from one another as a result of their individual inherited endowment, their situational ability to mobilize their resources to respond to life's stressors, and their models of the world.

Environment is seen as internal and external and includes both stressors and resources for adapting to stressors. Stressors exist in life at all times and are necessary for overall growth and life enhancement. All individuals have both internal and external resources for dealing with stressors. Potential resources exist and individuals may need assistance in becoming aware of and constructively mobilizing them.

Within the theory, the definition of *health* is consistent with that of the World Health Organization in that Erickson, et al. (1983), write that health is a state of physical, mental, and social well-being, not merely the absence of disease or infirmity. These authors also write that health connotes a state of dynamic equilibrium among the various subsystems. This dynamic equilibrium implies an adaptive equilibrium whereby the individual learns to cope constructively with life's stressors by mobilizing internal and external coping resources and leaving no subsystem in jeopardy when adaptation occurs.

Nursing is a process between the nurse and the client and requires an interpersonal and interactive nurse–client relationship. Three characteristics of the nurse in this theory are facilitation, nurturance, and unconditional acceptance. Facilitation implies that the nurse aids the individual to identify, mobilize, and develop his or her own strengths. Rogers (1996, 1997) describes a new concept of "facilitative affiliation" that was developed within the framework of the Modeling and Role-Modeling theory to express the essence of the nurse–client relationship. The attributes of facilitative affiliation include presence, needs assessment based on the client's self-care knowledge and perception of self-care resources, interventions based on the client's model of the world, selective normative disregard, mutual trust, nurturing, and advocacy by the nurse.

Nurturance is the fusing and integrating of cognitive, psychological, and affective processes with the aim of assisting a client toward holistic health. Unconditional acceptance is the acceptance of each individual as unique, worthwhile, and important with no strings attached. The Modeling and Role-Modeling definition of nursing as given by Erickson, et al. (1983), is as follows:

> *Nursing* is the holistic helping of persons with their self-care activities in relation to their health. This is an interactive, interpersonal process that nurtures strengths to enable development, release, and channeling of resources for coping with one's circumstances and environment. The goal is to achieve a state of perceived optimum health and contentment (p. 49).

Additional statements by Erickson, et al. (1983), to define nursing are the following:

- Nursing is the nurturance of holistic self-care.
- Nursing is assisting persons holistically to use their adaptive strengths to attain and maintain optimum bio-psycho-socio-spiritual functioning.

- Nursing is helping with self-care to gain optimum health.
- Nursing is an integrated and integrative helping of persons to take better care of themselves (p. 50).

CLINICAL APPLICATION OF MODELING AND ROLE-MODELING IN NURSING PRACTICE

The authors of the Modeling and Role-Modeling theory acknowledge two distinct meanings of the nursing process. The first is the formalized, step-by-step problem-solving process that includes gathering and analyzing data, planning and implementing interventions, and evaluating outcomes. The second is a more basic use of the term and refers to an interactive process—the exchange between nurse and patient in which the nurse has a purpose of nurturing and supporting the client's self-care. Figure 20–4 illustrates these two views. The step-by-step use of the nursing process is linear and, as such, a problem-solving method frequently used in teaching to help a novice learn to think logically about nursing care. The second meaning of the nursing process is a means of reflecting on the entire nurse–client encounter. If one views nursing as an interaction, the nursing process is the means by which the nurse–client interaction takes place (Frisch, 1994). This second, more basic view of the nursing process is circular, rather than linear. The Modeling and Role-Modeling theory reminds us that experienced nurses know that one never really applies the nursing process in a step-by-step fashion. One does not assess, then diagnose, then devise outcomes, then plan, provide, and evaluate care in that order. One is diagnosing while assessing. As soon as a nurse walks into a client's room and begins interacting with a client, that nurse is intervening because the nurse's words, actions,

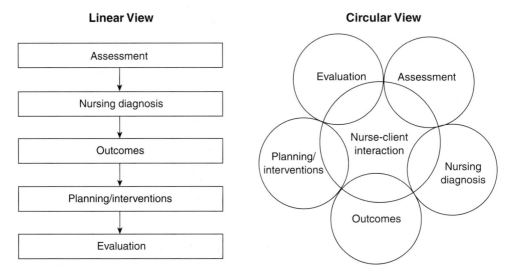

Figure 20–4. Two Views of the Nursing Process. From Frisch, N. C. & Frisch, L. E. (1998). *Psychiatric Mental Health Nursing.* Albany, NY: Delmar. Used with permission.

and presence serve as nursing interventions and are part of nursing care. The Modeling and Role-Modeling theory liberates nurses from the endless debates over use of the nursing process—the linear view of the nursing process is useful in teaching and helping nurses to think logically about care; the circular view is the *process* of carrying out nursing care grounded in person-to-person interaction.

With the primary emphasis on the interactive, interpersonal nursing process, nursing involves an ongoing exchange of information, feelings, and behaviors. Thus, the nursing process begins with the first interaction between nurse and patient. The Modeling and Role-Modeling theory accepts the view, expressed by Lucille Kinlein (1977) in the 1970s, that nursing care begins with the first patient encounter because the nurse's immediate contributions to care include the nurse himself or herself—the presence, the unconditional acceptance, and the support and comfort that are offered from one human being to another.

Because the theory directs the nurse to begin where the client is in modeling the client's world, a comprehensive assessment is rarely done to initiate nursing care. The client will always be asked to express his or her questions, concerns, and needs. Client concerns have utmost priority because a person whose immediate needs are unattended will not progress in other ways. Thus, the theory directs the nurse's priorities of care quite simply, beginning where the client requests care to begin, knowing that as one need is met, other unmet needs will emerge to direct care. At any point, assessment is dictated by client needs, and the nurse will gather whatever information is required to understand and care for the client's expressed concerns.

The interactive nursing process includes formal, logical thinking; Erickson, et al. (1983), make it clear that they value scientific thinking. However, when using Modeling and Role-Modeling, there are no preset steps in applying the nursing process. The theorists write, "When we view the nursing process predominantly as an ongoing, interactive, interpersonal relationship that *includes* use of the formal scientific mode of thought, we can regard documentation of the nursing process primarily as a valuable way to communicate with others and keep records" (p. 105). In providing care, client data are gathered to model the client's world. An evaluation of the client's stress and adaptation, as well as information on self-care knowledge, resources, and actions, are essential. Diagnoses include adaptive potential, that is, the client's potential for mobilizing resources needed to contend with stressors.

Erickson, Tomlin, and Swain do not address the use of the nursing diagnoses taxonomy developed by the North American Nursing Diagnoses Association (NANDA) with Modeling and Role-Modeling. For many nurses in practice and in education, however, Modeling and Role-Modeling has been incorporated with the NANDA taxonomy. In the early 1990s, the Brigham and Women's Hospital in Boston was the first institution in the country to adopt Modeling and Role-Modeling as the base for practice hospitalwide. Nurses there who were already using NANDA diagnoses to articulate nursing concerns readily adapted by continuing to use them to document nursing concerns while using Modeling and Role-Modeling to understand the etiology of the diagnoses. For example, the nurses may write a NANDA diagnosis of "Fatigue r/t continued state of impoverishment secondary to stressors of hospitalization and isolation." In this way, the NANDA taxonomy is used as an atheoretical labeling of a nursing concern; Modeling and Role-Modeling provides

TABLE 20–2. "HAROLD" A CASE STUDY DEMONSTRATING THE DIFFERENCE BETWEEN THE ATHEORETICAL USE OF NURSING DIAGNOSES AND THE USE OF NURSING DIAGNOSES WITH MODELING AND ROLE-MODELING AS THE THEORETICAL BASE

CASE STUDY	Nursing Care Based on Admission Data:	Revised Nursing Care Based on Modeling and Role-Modeling:
Harold is a 72-year-old unemployed truck driver who was admitted to the hospital with severe COPD, unstable angina, and severe skin lesions on his legs. He is a homeless man who lives in a nonfunctioning car on the beach. He has been admitted 7 times in the past 6 months with exacerbations of COPD, R/O sepsis, and cellulitis. He presented at this admission with a TPR of 101, 138, and 44. Laboratory results demonstrated high WBCs, abnormal blood gases, and subtherapeutic digoxin and aminophylline serum levels. Harold was dirty, odorous, and had open, draining sores on his legs. The medical regimen was aminophylline, anti-inflammatory agents, antibiotics, and his routine medications, which consisted of digoxin, brethine, etc. He was receiving oxygen but was really uncomfortable. He was also very quiet.	INITIAL DIAGNOSES Ineffective breathing pattern Altered gas exchange Self-care deficit: Bathing and hygiene Altered health maintenance Fear	REVISED DIAGNOSES Impaired mobility Fatigue Powerless
Harold was seen as "difficult" by the nurses. The nurses were frustrated by his repeated admissions. Harold was frustrated because he thought people had "judged" him and that they wanted him to "change his whole life."	INITIAL INTERVENTIONS Positioning Maintaining oxygenation	REVISED INTERVENTIONS Increasing Harold's role in his care Increasing Harold's perceived control
Additional data were gathered to model Harold's world. Harold said that he came to the hospital because he was sick and didn't want to burden his friends. He said that he believed people at the hospital didn't like him because they wanted him to change things he didn't want to change—like where he lived. Harold said that he had always had skin problems with his legs, but the new problem was that his dog had sand fleas and that he couldn't seem to manage. He ran out of medication because his car didn't work and didn't take his theophylline because he thought it altered his sexual functioning. When asked what he saw as his major problem, he said: "I can't get to the shower because I'm so tired—then my legs get worse!"	Administering the appropriate medications Skin care: bathing and hygiene Reassuring Harold	Clustering nursing activities because of fatigue Discussing Harold's specific discharge planning (dog baths; medication delivery, etc.

How did Modeling and Role Modeling-based practice change Harold's nursing care?
- Harold got holistic, individualized care.
- Harold's attitude and self-esteem improved.
- Harold participated more in self-care activities.
- There was less frustration with the nurses.
- Harold increased his adherence to treatment.
- Ten months after discharge, he had still not been readmitted.

Source: Adapted from a presentation at the Fourth National Modeling and Role-Modeling Conference. (1992) Developed by Wendy Woodward, Humboldt State University. Used with permission.

the theoretical base for understanding and intervening with that concern. A similar meshing of Modeling and Role-Modeling with NANDA has occurred at Humboldt State University, where Modeling and Role-Modeling is being used as the conceptual basis for nursing care in an undergraduate nursing curriculum. The case study "Harold" presented in Table 20–2 provides an illustration of how nursing care and diagnoses differ when using nursing diagnoses atheoretically and when using nursing diagnoses with Modeling and Role-Modeling as the theoretical base.

In carrying out nursing care, the nurse must use role-modeling, that is, help the client in attaining, maintaining, or promoting health through purposeful interventions which are consistent with the client's model of the world. Care is based on the five aims of interventions and is consistent with the client's adaptive potential (see Figure 20–2). The nurse's role is to facilitate, nurture, and provide unconditional acceptance while assisting the client to achieve health. Evaluation of nursing care is directed toward goals mutually determined between patient and client.

CRITIQUE OF THE THEORY OF MODELING AND ROLE-MODELING

1. What is the historical context of the theory? Theories long studied by nursing students—Maslow, Erikson, Piaget, Selye, and Engel—emerge in a new perspective in Modeling and Role-Modeling as these psychosocial and developmental theories become useful and immediate in understanding the client's world. Modeling and Role-Modeling provides a sense of the true meaning of client-directed care, for the client is trusted as knowing what he or she needs from the nurse to achieve health. The theory provides a unique way of understanding nursing. The client is seen in a truly holistic manner, as a person with an understandable and individual worldview. Nursing's task becomes that of knowing the client, discovering the client's needs and concerns, affirming that the client is directing all health-related actions, and facilitating the client's striving toward health. Assumptions of the theory include that human beings are each unique, but with identifiable similarities; that each person is born with a genetic base and a spiritual drive; that the individual has bio-psycho-social components, and that the whole of any person is greater than the sum of his or her parts. Further, the assumption that each person has self-care knowledge and resources such that he or she knows on some level what made him or her ill and what is needed to make him or herself better is a major divergence from traditional bio-medical views of disease. This emphasis on self-care knowledge has its roots in the work of Milton Erickson.

2. What are the basic concepts and relationships presented by the theory? Modeling and Role-Modeling provides a logical framework from which to understand nursing and from which to plan and provide care. Major concepts of the definition of the person, the meaning of health, and the client's responsibility for self-care are clear. The five aims of intervention emphasize the importance of the nurse–client relationship. Nurses who understand the interactive nature of what they are doing readily accept the view of the nursing process as an interpersonal process. Erickson

(1990b) acknowledged the functional relationships among the concepts embedded within the theory resulting in the following three major theoretical linkages:

1. Developmental task resolution and need satisfaction,
2. Basic need status, object attachment and loss, growth and development,
3. Adaptive potential and need satisfaction (p. 18).

Erickson also provided examples of theoretical propositions that can be derived from these linkages and used to direct care planning. These examples are:

1. Individuals' ability to contend with new stressors is directly related to the ability to mobilize resources needed.
2. Individuals' ability to mobilize resources is directly related to their need deficits and assets.
3. Distressors are related to unmet basic needs; stressors are related to unmet growth needs.
4. Objects that repeatedly facilitate the individual in need satisfaction take on significance for the individual. When this occurs, attachment to the object results.
5. Secure attachment produces feelings of worthiness.
6. Feelings of worthiness result in a sense of futurity.
7. Real, threatened, or perceived loss of the attachment object results in the grief process.
8. Basic need deficits coexist with the grief process.
9. An adequate alternative object must be perceived available in order for the individual to resolve the grief process.
10. Prolonged grief due to an unavailable or inadequate object results in morbid grief.
11. Unmet basic and growth needs interfere with growth processes.
12. Repeated satisfaction of basic needs is prerequisite to working through developmental tasks and resolution of related developmental crises.
13. Morbid grief is always related to need deficits (Erickson, 1990b, p. 18).

3. What major phenomena of concern to nursing are presented? These phenomena may include but are not limited to: human being, environment, health, interpersonal relations, caring, goal attainment, adaptation, and energy fields. In addition to the concepts detailed in nursing's metaparadigm (person, health, nursing, and environment) the phenomena of concern to Modeling and Role-Modeling include self-care knowledge, resources, and actions; affiliated–individuation; and adaptive-potential. These concepts direct the nurse's view of the client (i.e., one who has internal knowledge and perceptions of self that are essential to understand when working with the person to achieve health) and in understanding behavior since actions (or nonactions) are based on an individual's state of adaptive potential. Further, the concept that a person has an innate spiritual drive is a recognition of the spiritual essence of human beings. This aspect of the theory, while appealing intuitively to any holistic nurse, is less developed than the other concepts and has been identified by Erickson as one requiring further attention and development (Erickson, 1999).

4. To whom does the theory apply? In what situations? In what ways? Theories should be relatively simple but generalizable. The simplicity of Modeling and Role-Modeling is its beauty. Trusting that clients know (at some level) what they need, and planning nursing care based on each client's model of the world, as well as individual need deficits, need satisfaction, and ability to mobilize resources, is a simple, yet profound, idea. Beginning students in their first nursing course can readily understand the basic concepts, while the theory is still useful to advanced practitioners.

Modeling and Role-Modeling has been applied to clients who are individuals, families, and communities, and it has been applied to clients in all nursing specialty areas of practice. For example, the case study of *Harold* (Table 20–2) presents use of the theory to an individual client. The theory can be used in assessing a family by determining both the adaptive-potential of a family group and the adaptive-potential of the individual family members (Frisch & Kelley, 1996). Many of the families referred to as "dysfunctional" are families living in maladaptive equilibrium. According to this theory, the family would need to be pushed into a state of arousal through some kind of crisis to be motivated for change. Further, individual members of the family may be in a state of impoverishment and require direct care and nurturance in order to mobilize resources to gain a healthy state of adaptation. The theory provides the nurse with a unique way of understanding a family and, therefore, suggests unique interventions. The concepts of the theory may also be used in work with groups or communities. For example, a work-group (nurses on a hospital unit) may be understood in a manner similar to families. Likewise, a community can be assessed according to the APAM model and understood in an entirely different way.

5. By what method or methods can this theory be tested? Methodological diversity has been demonstrated through scholarly inquiry of many areas within the theory. Acton, Irvin, Jensen, Hopkins, and Miller (1997) specify advantages of combining qualitative and quantitative techniques. Investigations have been reported that test or expand the concepts of adaptive potential (Barnfather, 1990; Barnfather, et al., 1989a; 1989b; Erickson & Swain, 1982; Finch, 1990) self-care (Beery & Baas, 1996; Bowman, 1998; Erickson, 1990a; Kennedy, 1991, Rosenow, 1992), and affiliated–individuation (Acton, 1993; Acton & Miller, 1996). Studies are also reported that investigate the theoretical proposition derived from the major theoretical linkages embedded in the theory. These studies focus on developmental tasks, needs, and psychosocial developmental residual (Curl, 1992; Jensen, 1995; Keck, 1989; MacLean, 1987; 1990, 1992; Miller, 1986).

Acton, et al. (1997), describe how five researchers involved in a large research project used different data subsets and different methods to explain or affirm middle-range concepts and theories from Modeling and Role-Modeling. Acton (1993) found that affiliated–individuation was a significant predictor of well-being and further found, using Baron and Kenny's (1986) method to test for mediation, that affiliated–individuation is a resource used to mediate between the stress of care giving and the well-being of the caregiver. Irvin (1993) investigated the relationships among perceived stress of caregivers and self-care resources using path analysis with regression procedures. Irvin and Acton (1996) further employed Baron and Kenney's method to explore the mediating effect of self-care resources on stress and well-being. Jensen (1995) used case study analysis to compare the actual responses to interventions with the response patterns predicted by the theory, and found evidence of need satisfaction attainment, attachment, and resolution of loss and grief. Qualitative analysis of the case studies also showed a decrease in burden over time and an evidence of positive growth outcomes. Hopkins (1995) studied the concept of adaptive potential and utilized multivariate analysis of variance to demonstrate that caregivers in a state of equilibrium who were caring for adults with dementia showed perceived support and an increased sense of well-being. Miller's (1993) study used qualitative methods to expand knowledge of the inner spirit and Acton and Miller (1996) pursued qualitative methods and demonstrated that support group interventions had some positive effect on affiliated individuation.

6. Does this theory direct critical thinking in nursing practice? Modeling and Role-Modeling, like all nursing theories, requires reflective practice—the ability to think about and articulate nursing assessment, care, and outcomes. Modeling and Role-Modeling assists the nurse by giving direction and tools for action—beginning with the five aims of intervention. The nurse can then assess if trust has been achieved, if client strengths have been supported, and so on. Thus, the nurse has a framework to interpret and think about nursing actions. Critical thinking requires language to put into words and thoughts some of the areas of practice that can otherwise be relegated to intuition or spontaneity. Modeling and Role-Modeling directs the nurse to reflect on those intuitive moments and interpret and understand them on the basis of concepts such as adaptive potential, self-care knowledge, and modeling of another's world. Thus, practice through the use of the theory is both reflective and thoughtful.

7. Does this theory direct therapeutic nursing interventions? The concept of the five aims of intervention directs all nursing actions. While the five aims may seem simplistic, they provide a basis and a place to begin when a nurse is unsure of how to proceed. For example, in the setting of psychiatric nursing, nurses applying the theory became concerned with the notion of modeling the client's world, when the client's world was irrational and delusional. Returning to the five aims of intervention helped the nurses focus on what each knew is the basis of psychiatric nursing care—building trust and promoting positive orientation. Once the nurses adopted this focus, they began to understand that to model the client's world meant to understand the meaning of the delusions to the client. Thus, nursing interventions were based on building a positive and trusting relationship with the client and understanding the client's situations from within his own worldview.

The Adaptive Potential Assessment Model is also useful for directing therapeutic nursing interventions. A client who is impoverished cannot be expected to initiate self-care actions. Interventions for a client who is in maladaptive equilibrium need to be aimed at motivation to change rather than teaching self-care. Teaching self-care would be appropriate for someone in arousal.

The three major federally-funded research projects investigating this theory have all been intervention studies aimed at identifying the usefulness and cost effectiveness of Modeling and Role-Modeling as the basis for practice. Erickson has been the primary investigator for these projects, which have each focused on a different population of clients with chronic health problems: hypertension, diabetes, and Alzheimer's disease. There have been many examples of the use of concepts from the theory directing therapeutic interventions (Frisch & Kelley, 1996; Holl, 1992; Kinney, 1990; Walsh, Vanden Bosch, & Boehm, 1989). The examples of theoretical propositions presented by Erickson (1990b) are also useful in demonstrating how Modeling and Role-Modeling can be used to direct nursing interventions.

8. Does the theory direct communication in nursing practice? In Modeling and Role-Modeling communication between nurse and client is based on unconditional positive regard. The nurse must take the time to truly understand the client—listening is the most important communication technique a nurse can possess to begin to understand another's worldview. It is important to begin nursing practice with the client's concerns. The theory clearly states that there are many sources of information when the nurse is involved in data collection, but that the *primary and most important source is your client.* Without the client's input you will be unable to understand which nursing interventions are clearly needed" (Erickson, et al., 1983, p. 116).

9. Does the theory direct nursing actions that lead to favorable outcomes? Yes. All three of the federally-funded intervention projects led to favorable outcomes. Individuals with hypertension and those with diabetes showed improved management of these chronic conditions with the interventions of Modeling and Role-Modeling. The most recent intervention study involved a support group intervention based on the theory for individuals with Alzheimer's and their caregivers. This study demonstrated favorable outcomes for both groups.

10. How contagious is the theory? Since the initial publication of the theory in 1983, there has been increasing interest in and use of the theory. The theory has been used in multiple settings to guide nursing education, research, and practice throughout the United States. In education, the theory was adopted as the organizing framework for an undergraduate nursing curricula in California in 1990. The theory is also used as an organizing framework in RN–BSN programs in Michigan and Minnesota. While many nurses use the theory to direct their own practice, Brigham and Women's Hospital in Boston adopted the theory as a housewide framework for nursing care in the early 1990s. Research on the theory has been conducted in several medical centers and Schools of Nursing, including University of Texas at Austin, Humboldt State University in Arcata, CA, and University of Cincinnati, OH. A most recent application of the theory was presented at the 1998 Modeling and Role-Modeling conference by the Cincinnati-based independent LifeStyle Management organization, which offers behavior modification programs for smoking cessation, weight management, and management of lifestyle issues associated with specific chronic diseases. LifeStyle Management techniques have been developed based on the concepts of Modeling and Role-Modeling.

The Society for the Advancement of Modeling and Role-Modeling held its charter meeting and the first theory conference in 1986 in Ann Arbor, Michigan. The Society continues to meet biannually at different locations throughout the United States for the purpose of disseminating knowledge relating to the theory acquired through research, practice, and teaching. The seventh national conference of the Society was held in Cincinnati, Ohio, in conjunction with the University of Cincinnati College of Nursing in 1998. At that meeting 25 presentations on the research and use of the theory were made. In providing a new way of understanding nursing, the society stimulates evaluation and the study of nursing's effect on a client's health. The Society maintains a Web page at *www.globalax.com/mrm/*, and a list serv at *mrmlist@po.cwru,edu*, which is actively accessed by those using the theory in practice and conducting research on varying aspects of the theory. In the coming years, the focus of the society will be to develop a Center for the Study and Practice of Modeling and Role-Modeling theory and paradigm. The recent calls for a Center for the advancement of the theory by those actively involved with the study and use of the theory further speak to the contagiousness of the theory.

The authors of this chapter note that the theory is not as well known as other nursing theories, but that among those who have studied and used the theory, there is a growing and enthusiastic group of adherents who can no longer imagine practicing nursing without modeling their clients' worlds.

STRENGTHS AND LIMITATIONS

The theory has many strengths including a strong holistic approach and emphasis on the nurse–client interaction and client-centeredness, as has been described. Its major limitation may be that it is relatively unknown and appears simplistic. Nurses coming to learn about the theory have felt that it merely describes what they have always done intuitively, and that it is too simple merely to put the client in charge of his or her health care. A limitation in practice, particularly for inexperienced nurses, has been that the mandate to "model the client's world" leads, in some cases, to role confusion between being a caring professional and a caring friend.

Nurses at any level can quickly learn how to develop a model of the client's world and gain rewards from this practice. In practice, the development of empathetic assessment is so enticing that nurses may fail to develop the science of modeling. The science of modeling requires professional education. The scientific base for the analysis of data relating to the client's model of the world includes a broad understanding of both the physical and social sciences. To be complete in modeling the client's world, the nurse must draw on many theories in other disciplines, such as psychology, sociology, cultural anthropology, physiology, and pathophysiology.

SUMMARY

The Modeling and Role-Modeling theory suggests an interactive, interpersonal role for nursing. Modeling is the process used to develop an understanding of the client's world; role-modeling is the process of facilitating health-promoting behaviors. Nursing care is based on clients' adaptive potential and directed toward the five aims of intervention: building trust, promoting positive orientation, promoting perceived control, promoting strengths, and setting mutual, health-directed goals. From within this theory, the client is empowered to direct care, based on self-care knowledge, self-care resources, and self-care actions, as the client's perceived needs are addressed. The theory has been applied to work with clients who are individuals, families, and communities. Currently, the theory is being used in both practice and education, and research is being conducted to document and evaluate components of the theory.

REFERENCES

Acton, G. J. (1993). The relationships among stressors, stress, affiliated-individuation, burden, and well-being in caregivers of adults with dementia: A test of the theory and paradigm for nursing, Modeling and Role-Modeling. Unpublished doctoral dissertation, University of Texas at Austin.

Acton, G. J., Irvin, B. L., Jensen, B. A., Hopkins, B. A., & Miller, E. W. (1997). Explicating middle-range theory through methodological diversity. *Advances in Nursing Science, 19*(3), 78–85.

Acton, G. J., & Miller, E. W. (1996). Affiliated–individuation in caregivers of adults with dementia. *Issues in Mental Health Nursing, 17*, 245–260.

Barnfather, J. S. (1990). An overview of the ability to mobilize coping resources related to basic needs. In H. Erickson & C. Kinney (Eds.), *Modeling and Role-modeling. Theory, practice and research.* monograph, 1 (1), (pp. 156–169). Austin, TX: The Society for the Advancement of Modeling and Role-Modeling.

Barnfather, J. S., Swain, M. A. P., & Erickson, H. C. (1989a). Evaluation of two assessment techniques for adaptation to stress. *Nursing Science Quarterly, 2*, 172–182.

Barnfather, J. S., Swain, M. A. P., & Erickson, H. C. (1989b). Construct validity of an aspect of the coping process: Potential adaptation to stress. *Issues in Mental Health Nursing, 10*, 23–40.

Baron, R. M., & Kenny, D. A. (1986). The moderator–mediator variable distinction in social psychological research: Conceptual, strategic, and statistical considerations. *Journal of Personality and Social Psychology, 51*, 1173–1182.

Beery, T., & Baas, L. (1996). Medical devices and attachment: Holistic healing in the age of invasive technology. *Issues in Mental Health Nursing, 17*, 233–243.

Bowman, S. S. (1998). The human–environment relationship in self-care when healing from episodic illness. Unpublished doctoral dissertation, University of Texas at Austin.

Campbell, J., Finch, D., Allport, C., Erickson, H., & Swain, M. A. P. (1985). A theoretical approach to nursing assessment. *Journal of Advanced Nursing, 10*, 111–115.

Curl, E. D. (1992). Hope in the elderly: Exploring the relationship between psychosocial developmental residual and hope. *Dissertation Abstracts International, 53*, 1782B. (University Microfilms No. 92–25, 559).

Erickson, H. (1976). Identification of states of coping utilizing physiological and psychological data. Unpublished master's thesis, University of Michigan.

Erickson, H. (1984). Self-care knowledge: Relations among the concepts support, hope, control, satisfaction with daily life, and physical health status. *Dissertation Abstracts International, 45*, 1731 (University Microfilms No. 84–12136).

Erickson, H. C. (1990a). Self-care knowledge: An exploratory study. In H. Erickson, & E. Kinney (Eds.), *Modeling and Role-Modeling: Theory, research and practice.* monograph, 1 (1), (pp. 178–202). Austin, TX: The Society for Advancement of Modeling and Role-Modeling.

Erickson, H. C. (1990b). Theory based practice. In H. Erickson, & E. Kinney (Eds.), *Modeling and role-modeling: Theory, research and practice* monograph, 1 (1), (pp.1–27). Austin, TX: The Society for Advancement of Modeling and Role-Modeling.

Erickson, H. C. (1999). Greetings. *Modeling and Role-Modeling Newsletter, 9,* 2, 1–2.

Erickson, H., & Swain, M. A. (1977). The utilization of a nursing care model for the treatment of essential hypertension. *Circulation* (abstract).

Erickson, H., & Swain, M. A. (1982). A model for assessing potential adaptation to stress. *Research in Nursing and Health, 5,* 93–101.

Erickson, H. C., Tomlin, E. M., & Swain, M. A. P. (1983). *Modeling and Role-modeling. A theory and paradigm for nursing.* Lexington, SC: Pine Press.

Erikson, E. (1963). *Childhood and society.* New York: W.W. Norton & Co.

Finch, D. (1990). Testing a theoretically based nursing assessment. In H. Erickson & E. Kinney (Eds.), *Modeling and Role-modeling: Theory, research and practice.* monograph, 1 (1), (pp. 203–13). Austin, TX: The Society for Advancement of Modeling and Role-Modeling.

Frisch, N. (1994). The nursing process revisited. *Nursing Diagnosis, 5,* 51.

Frisch, N., & Kelley, J. (1996). *Healing life's crises: A guide for nurses.* Albany, NY: Delmar.

Holl, R. M. (1992). The effect of role-modeled visiting in comparison to restricted visiting on the well-being of clients who had open heart surgery and their significant family members in the critical care unit. *Dissertation Abstracts International, 53,* 4030B. (University Microfilms No. 92–25, 603).

Hopkins, B.A. (1995). Adaptive potential of caregivers of adults with dementia. Paper presented at the meeting of Sigma Theta Tau International, Detroit, MI.

Irvin, B. L. (1993). Social support, self-worth and hope as self-care resources for coping with caregiver status. Unpublished doctoral dissertation, University of Texas at Austin.

Irvin, B. L., & Acton, G. (1996). Stress mediation in caregivers of cognitively impaired adults: Theoretical model testing. *Nursing Research, 45*(3), 160–166.

Jensen, B. A. (1995). Caregiver responses to a theoretically based intervention program: Case study analysis. *Dissertation Abstracts International, 56*(06B), 3127. (University Microfilms No. 9534820).

Keck, V. E. (1989). Perceived social support, basic needs satisfaction, and coping strategies of the chronically ill. *Dissertation Abstracts International, 50,* 3921B. (University Microfilms No. 90–01, 655).

Kennedy, G. T. (1991). A nursing investigation of comfort and comforting care of the acutely ill patient. *Dissertation Abstracts International, 52,* 6318B. (University Microfilms No. 90–01, 655).

Kinlein, L. (1977). *Independent nursing practice with clients.* Philadelphia: Lippincott.

Kinney, C. K. (1990). Facilitating growth and development: A paradigm case for Modeling and Role-Modeling. *Issues in Mental Health Nursing, 11,* 375–395.

MacLean, T. (1987). Erikson's psychosocial development and stressors as factors in healthy lifestyle. *Dissertation Abstracts International, 48,* 1710A. (University Microfilms No. 87–20, 311).

MacLean, T. (1990). Health behaviors, developmental residual and stressors. In H. Erickson, & E. Kinney (Eds), *Modeling and Role-modeling: Theory, research and practice.* monograph, 1 (1), (pp. 147–155). Austin, TX: The Society for Advancement of Modeling and Role-Modeling.

MacLean, T. (1992). Influence of psychosocial development and life events on the health practices of adults. *Issues in Mental Health Nursing, 13,* 403–414.

Maslow, A.H. (1970). *Motivation and personality* (2nd ed.). New York: Harper & Row.

Miller, S.H. (1993). *The meaning of encouragement and its connection with the inner spirit as perceived by caregivers of the cognitively impaired.* Unpublished doctoral dissertation, University of Texas at Austin.

Miller, S. H. (1986). The relationship between psychosocial development and coping ability among disabled teenagers. *Dissertation Abstracts International, 47,* 4113B. (University Microfilms No. 87–02, 793).

Orem, D. E. (1995). *Nursing. Concepts and practice* (5th ed.). St. Louis: Mosby.

Rogers, S. (1996). Facilitative affiliation: Nurse–client interactions that enhance healing. *Issues in Mental Health Nursing, 17,* 171–184.

Rogers, S. (1997). Facilitative affiliation: A new NPR for the 21st century. *Proceedings of the First International Nursing Conference: Connecting Conversations of Nursing: Vol.1, Nursing scholarship and practice* (pp. 217–221). Reykjavik: University Press, University of Iceland.

Rosenow, D. J. (1992). Multidimensional scaling analysis of self-care actions for reintegrating holistic health after a myocardial infarction: Implications for nursing. *Dissertation Abstracts International, 53,* 1789B. (University Microfilms No. 92–25, 712).

Swain, M. A., & Stickel, S. B. (1981). Influencing adherence among hypertensives. *Research in Nursing and Health, 4,* 213–222.

Tomlin, E. M. (1990). Spiritual concerns in nursing: The interface of Modeling and Role-modeling with professional nursing's Christian roots and values. In H. Erickson, & C. Kinney (Eds.), *Modeling and Role-modeling. Theory, practice and research. monograph, 1* (1), (pp. 40–66). Austin, TX: The Society for the Advancement of Modeling and Role-Modeling.

Walsh, K. K., Vanden Bosch, T. M., & Boehm, S. (1989). Modeling and Role-Modeling: Integrating nursing theory into practice. *Journal of Advanced Nursing, 14,* 775–761.

BIBLIOGRAPHY

Acton, G. J. (1997). Affiliated–individuation as a mediator of stress and burden in caregivers of adults with dementia. *Journal of Holistic Nursing, 15,* 336–357.

Ashley, M. (1996). Differences between the attitudes and behaviors of oncology nurses: Inclusion of sexuality concerns as a component of care. *Masters Abstracts International, 35–03,* 786.

Baas, L. S. (1992). The relationships among self-care knowledge, self-care resources, activity level and life satisfaction in persons three to six months after a myocardial infarction. *Dissertation Abstracts International, 53,* 1780B. (University Microfilms No. 92–25, 512).

Barnfather, J. S. (1993). Testing a theoretical proposition for Modeling and Role-modeling: Basic need and adaptive potential status. *Issues in Mental Health Nursing, 14,* 1–18.

Barnfather, J. S., & Ronis, D. L. (2000). Test of a model of psychosocial resources, stress, and health among undereducated adults. *Research in Nursing and Health, 23,* 55–66.

Darling-Fisher, C. S. (1987). The relationship between mothers' and fathers' Eriksonian psychosocial attributes, perceptions of family support, and adaptation to parenthood. *Dissertation Abstracts International, 48,* 1640B. (University Microfilms No. 87–20, 254).

Erickson, H. (1983). Coping with new systems. *Journal of Nursing Education, 22,* 132–135.

Erickson, H. (1988). Modeling and Role-modeling: Ericksonian techniques applied to physiological problems. In J. Zeig & S. Lankton (Eds.), *Developing Ericksonian therapy: State of the art.* New York: Brunner/Mazel.

Erickson, H. (1990). Modeling and Role-modeling with psycho-physiological problems. In J. Zeig (Ed.), *Brief therapy: Myths and methods.* New York: Brunner/Mazel.

Hertz, J. E. G. (1991). The perceived enactment of autonomy scale: Measuring the potential for self-care action in the elderly. *Dissertation Abstracts International, 52,* 1953B. (University Microfilms No. 91–28, 248).

Kinney, C., & Erickson, H. (1990). Modeling the client's world: A way to holistic care. *Issues in Mental Health Nursing, 11,* 93–108.

Kline Leidy, N. (1990). A structural model of stress, psychosocial resources, and symptomatic experience in chronic physical illness. *Nursing Research, 39,* 230–236.

Landis, B. J. P. (1991). Uncertainity, spiritual well-being, and psychosocial adjustment to chronic illness. Unpublished doctoral dissertation, University of Texas at Austin.

Leidy, N. (1989). A physiologic analysis of stress and chronic illness. *Journal of Advanced Nursing, 14,* 868–876.

Leidy, N. K., & Traver, G. A. (1995). Psychological factors contributing to functional performance in people with COPD: Are there gender differences? *Research in Nursing and Health, 18,* 535–546.

Perese, E. F. (1997). Unmet needs of persons with chronic mental illnesses: Relationship to their adaptation to community living. *Issues in Mental Health Nursing, 18,* 19–34.

Robinson, K. R. (1992). Developing a scale to measure responses of clients with actual or potential myocardial infarctions. Unpublished doctoral dissertation, University of Texas at Austin.

Weber, G. J. T. (1995). Employed mothers with pre-school-aged children: An exploration of their lived experiences and the nature of their well-being. Unpublished doctoral dissertation, University of Texas at Austin.

ANNOTATED BIBLIOGRAPHY

Baas, L. S., Fontana, J. A., & Bhat, G. (1997). Relationships between self-care resources and the quality of life of persons with heart failure: A comparison of treatment groups. *Progress in Cardiovascular Nursing, 12,* 25–38.

This exploratory pilot study, based on Modeling and Role-modeling, investigated quality of life in 38 individuals with chronic heart failure in three different treatment regimens. No differences were found in resources, symptoms, total activity, or global quality of life. Physical symptoms and mental composite score predicted the health-related outcome of activity.

Baldwin, C. M., French, E. D., & Szerbiak, J. (1998). A qualitative inquiry assessing urban teachers' attitudes toward elementary school children. *Journal of Multicultural Nursing and Health, 4,* 46–51.

This naturalistic inquiry investigated the attitudes of elementary school teachers (primarily Caucasian) toward teaching minority children from impoverished environments. The teachers were found to identify with many of the concepts congruent with Modeling and Role-modeling, including unconditional acceptance, nurturance, and facilitation.

Erickson, H., & Swain, M. A. (1990). Mobilizing self-care resources: A nursing intervention for hypertension. *Issues in Mental Health Nursing, 11,* 217–235.

The purpose of this study was to investigate the potential for mobilizing self-care resources. Subjects were 10 persons with hypertension matched with 10 persons in a comparison group. Further research is needed with larger groups of subjects to validate the findings of this study that indicated treating the person rather than the symptom (hypertension) is likely to be helpful in dealing with stressors, reducing stress, and dealing with loss and grief.

Erickson, M. E. (1996). The relationships among need satisfaction, support, and maternal attachment in the adolescent mother. (Online) Dissertation abstract. Found on: CINAHL. Accession No.: 1999070568.

The underlying belief of this study is that the underlying needs of adolescent mothers must be met for these mothers to be able to attach and bond effectively with their infants. This study presents the development of the Erickson Maternal Bonding-Attachment Tool, to be used to assess maternal bonding-attachment within the context of maternal need satisfaction. The two subscales focus on the mother's orientation toward relationships. Findings supported the construct validity of the tool through indicating significant relationships among need satisfaction, support, certain demographic variables, and maternal bonding-attachment.

Frisch, N. C., & Kelley, J. (1996). *Healing life's crises: A guide for nurses.* Albany: N.Y.: Delmar.

This book of approximately 150 pages is useful as a text or reference for nurses who are new to the use of Modeling and Role-Modeling as well as those who wish to further study the application of the theory to practice. After presenting an overview of the theory in the first chapter, each subsequent chapter includes a case study with an example of using Modeling and Role-Modeling to plan care. Although the majority of chapters address individuals as clients, the final three chapters demonstrate the use of Modeling and Role-Modeling in the unique situations of the family, nursing organizations, and conflict resolution.

Sappington, J., & Kelley, J. (1996). Modeling and Role-Modeling theory: A case study for holistic care. *Journal of Holistic Nursing, 14(2)*, 130–141.

An excellent demonstration, through case study, of the use of Modeling and Role-Modeling as the theoretical base to providing care. The case presented is of a young woman recently diagnosed with diabetes mellitus who was enabled to develop her own strengths and begin the healing process.

Schultz, E. D. (1998). Academic advising from a nursing theory perspective. *Nurse Educator, 23* (2), 22–25.

A unique application of the theory of Modeling and Role-Modeling where the student is the client and the theory is the base for academic advising. Many of the major concepts of the theory are addressed and specific activities relation to the five aims of intervention are delineated.

Straub, H. G. (1993). The relationship among intellectual, psychosocial, and ego development of nursing students in associate, baccalaureate, and baccalaureate completion programs. (On-line). Dissertation abstract. Found on : CINAHL. Accession No. 1998006981.

The study investigated the readiness of nursing students to appreciate the client's perspective, a basic requirement for effective application of the theory of Modeling and Role-modeling. Subjects included 69 associate degree students, 70 baccalaureate students, and 38 RN to BSN students. No correlation was found between psychosocial development and intellectual or ego development and the type of education did not contribute to the variance in intellectual, psychosocial, or ego development.

CHAPTER 21

THEORY OF CULTURE CARE DIVERSITY AND UNIVERSALITY

MADELEINE M. LEININGER

Julia B. George

Madeleine M. Leininger was born in Nebraska and received her basic nursing education at St. Anthony's School of Nursing, Denver, CO, graduating in 1948. In 1950 she earned a bachelor of science from Mount St. Scholastica College (now known as Benedictine College), Atchison, KS; in 1954 a master of science in psychiatric-mental health nursing from The Catholic University of America, Washington, DC; and in 1965 a Ph.D. in cultural and social anthropology from the University of Washington, Seattle. She is a Fellow in the American Academy of Nursing and holds honorary doctorates from Benedictine College, the University of Indianapolis, and the University of Kuopio, Kuopio, Finland. In 1998 she was named a "Living Legend" by the American Academy of Nursing.

Dr. Leininger is the founder of transcultural nursing. She is Professor Emeritus, College of Nursing, Wayne State University, and adjunct professor at the University of Nebraska Medical Center College of Nursing, Omaha, Nebraska. She has held both faculty and administrative appointments in nursing education and has published extensively. She lectures and consults about transcultural nursing and human care theory and research worldwide. She has held visiting professorships and lectureships in Australia (Royal College of Nursing, University of Sydney), Brunei Darussalam (University of Brunei Darussalam), Finland (University of Kuopio), Germany (University of Nurnberg), The Netherlands (University of Limburg, Maastricht), Russia (Institute of Moscow), Singapore (University of Singapore), Sweden (University of Boras, Boras Health Science; University of Gothenburg), Switzerland (University of Lucern and Frieborg), Taiwan (University of Taiwan and Taipei), Thailand (University of Chulangthorn, Bangkok), and the United States (Augsberg College, Minneapolis, Minnesota; University of Memphis, Tennessee; University of Puerto Rico, San Juan; University of Tennessee, Knoxville). Her papers are housed in the Walter Ruether Archival Center, Wayne State University, Detroit, Michigan. A collection of her books is housed at Madonna University, Livonia, Michigan, the location of the home office of the Transcultural Nursing Society. Her early papers have been housed in the Boston Archives at Boston University. More information about her activities and publications can be found on the Web site for the Transcultural Nursing Society at www.tcns.org.

In the 1940s Leininger (1991) recognized the importance of caring to nursing. Statements of appreciation for nursing care made by patients alerted her to caring values and led to her longstanding focus on care as the dominant ethos of nursing. During the mid-1950s, she experienced what she describes as cultural shock while she was working in a child guidance home in the midwestern United States. While working as a clinical nurse specialist with disturbed children and their parents, she observed recurrent behavioral differences among the children, and finally concluded that these differences had a cultural base. She identified a lack of knowledge of the children's cultures as the missing link in nursing to understand the variations needed in care of clients. This experience led her to become the first professional nurse in the world to earn a doctorate in anthropology, and led to the development of the new field of transcultural nursing.

Leininger first used the terms *transcultural nursing*, *ethnonursing*, and *cross-cultural nursing* in the 1960s. In 1966, at the University of Colorado, she offered the first transcultural nursing course with field experiences and has been instrumental in the development of similar courses at a number of other institutions (Leininger, 1979). In 1995, Leininger affirmed her 1978 definition of transcultural nursing as:

> a substantive area of study and practice focused on comparative cultural care (caring) values, beliefs, and practices of individuals or groups of similar or different cultures with the goal of providing culture-specific and universal nursing care practices in promoting health or well-being or to help people to face unfavorable human conditions, illness, or death in culturally meaningful ways (p. 58).

In 1979 she defined ethnonursing as:

> the study of nursing care beliefs, values, and practices as cognitively perceived and known by a designated culture through their direct experience, beliefs, and value system (p. 15).

The term *transcultural nursing* (rather than "cross-cultural") is used today to refer to the evolving knowledge and practices related to this new field of study and practice. Leininger (1991, 1995) stresses the importance of knowledge gained from direct experience or directly from those who have experienced and labels such knowledge as *emic*, or people-centered. This is contrasted with *etic* knowledge, which describes the professional perspective. She contends that *emically* derived care knowledge is essential to establish nursing's epistemological and ontological base for practice.

Leininger built her theory of transcultural nursing on the premise that the peoples of each culture can not only know and define the ways in which they experience and perceive their nursing care world but also relate these experiences and perceptions to their general health beliefs and practices. Based on this premise, nursing care is derived and developed from the cultural context in which it is to be provided.

Leininger (1991) asserts that human care is central to nursing as a discipline and as a profession. She, and others, have studied the phenomena of care for over four decades. They recognize and are proponents of the preservation of care as the essence of nursing. With this increasing recognition of care as essential to nursing knowledge and practice, Leininger labeled her theory Culture Care. She drew upon anthropology for the culture component and upon nursing for the care component. Her belief that cultures have both health practices that are specific to one culture and prevailing patterns that are common across cultures led to the addition of the terms *diversity* and *universality* to the title of her theory. Thus, the most current title of Leininger's theory is Culture Care or Culture Care Diversity and Universality.

LEININGER'S THEORY

In 1985, Leininger (1985b) published her first presentation of her work as a theory, and in 1988b, 1991, and 1995 she presented further explication of her ideas. In the 1991 and 1995 presentations, she provided orientational definitions for the concepts of culture, culture care, culture care diversity, culture care universality, nursing, worldview, cultural and social structure dimensions, environmental context, ethnohistory, generic (folk or lay) care system, professional care system, culturally congruent nursing care, health, care/caring, culture care preservation, culture care accommodation, and culture care repatterning. Leininger points out that these definitions are provisional guides that may be altered as a culture is studied.

In addition to the definitions, she presented assumptions that support her prediction that "different cultures perceive, know, and practice care in different ways, yet there are some commonalities about care among all cultures of the world" (Leininger, 1985b, p. 210). She refers to the commonalities as universality and to the differences as diversity.

Culture is the "learned, shared, and transmitted knowledge of values, beliefs, norms and lifeways of a particular group that guides an individual or group in their thinking, decisions, and actions in patterned ways" (Leininger, 1995, p. 60). A related assumption is that the values, beliefs, and practices for culturally related care are shaped by, and often embedded in "the worldview, language, religious (or spiritual), kinship (social), political (or legal), educational, economic, technological, ethnohistorical and environmental context" of the culture (p. 104). A subculture is "closely related to culture and refers to a group that deviates in certain areas from the dominant culture in values, beliefs, norms, moral codes, and ways of living with some distinctive features of its own" (p. 60).

Culture care diversity indicates "the variabilities and/or differences in meanings, patterns, values, lifeways or symbols of care within or between collectives that are related to assistive, supportive or enabling human care expressions" (Leininger, 1995, p. 105). In contrast, *culture care universality* indicates the "common, similar, or dominant uniform care meanings, patterns, values, lifeways or symbols that are manifest among many cultures and reflect assistive, supportive, facilitative or enabling ways to help people" (p. 105). It is assumed that, while human care is universal across cultures, caring may be demonstrated through diverse expressions, actions, patterns, lifestyles, and meanings. *Culture care* is defined as "the subjectively and objectively learned and transmitted values, beliefs, and patterned lifeways that assist, support, facilitate, or enable another individual or group to maintain well-being and health, to improve the human condition and lifeway, or to deal with illness, handicaps, or death" (p. 105). A related assumption is that culture care is "the broadest holistic means to know, explain, interpret and predict nursing care phenomena to guide nursing care practices" (p. 104).

Worldview is the way in which people look at the world, or at the universe, and form a "picture or value stance" about the world and their lives (Leininger, 1995, p. 105). *Cultural and social structure dimensions* are defined as involving "the dynamic patterns and features or interrelated structural and organizational factors of a particular culture (subculture or society) which includes religious, kinship (social), political (and legal), economic, educational, technologic and cultural values, ethnohistorical factors, and how these factors may be interrelated and function to influence human behavior in different environmental contexts" (p. 105). *Environmental context* is "the totality of an event, situation or particular experiences that give meaning to human expressions, interpretations and social interactions in particular physical, ecological, sociopolitical and/or cultural settings" (p. 106). *Ethnohistory* includes "those past facts, events, instances and experiences of individuals, groups, cultures and institutions that are primarily people-centered (ethno) and which describe, explain, and interpret human lifeways within particular cultural contexts over short or long periods of time" (p. 106). "Knowledge of meanings and practices derived from world views, social structure factors, cultural values, environmental context, and language uses are essential to guide nursing decisions and actions in providing cultur[e] congruent care" (Leininger, 1988b, p. 155).

Generic (folk or lay) care systems are "culturally learned and transmitted, indigenous (or traditional), folk (home-based) knowledge and skills used to provide assistive, supportive, enabling or facilitative acts toward or for another individual, group or institution with evident or anticipated needs to ameliorate or improve a human lifeway, health condition (or well-being), or to deal with handicaps and death situations" (Leininger, 1995, p. 106). Generic or folk knowledge is emic. *Professional care system(s)* are defined as "formally taught, learned and transmitted professional care, health, illness, wellness and related knowledge and practice skills that prevail in professional institutions, usually with multidisciplinary personnel to serve consumers" (p. 106). Professional care knowledge is etic. Table 21–1 provides a comparison of the generic and professional care systems from the consumer's view. *Health* is "a state of well-being that is culturally defined, valued,

TABLE 21–1. DOMINANT (EMIC) COMPARATIVE FEATURES OF GENERIC (FOLK) AND PROFESSIONAL HEALTH CARE FROM THE CONSUMER'S VIEW*

Generic Folk, Lay Care/Caring	Professional Health Care
1. Is humanistically oriented and people-centered.	1. Is scientifically oriented and patient-illness centered.
2. Uses practical knowledge in familiar ways to care for others.	2. Uses strange or unfamiliar terms and approaches to treat patients.
3. Focuses on broad holistic lifeways, beliefs, values, and life experiences and worldviews of people.	3. Seems fragmented and focuses on symptoms, body–mind parts, specific diagnoses, and curative medical treatments with many diverse staff.
4. Has as its focus caring and curing modes with the use of home, community, or familiar resources.	4. Has as its major focus body–mind curing modes in unfamiliar medical or hospital settings.
5. Relies on lay practices and understanding cultural factors to help people regain health and for doing daily functions.	5. Relies on biophysical and emotional factors of patients with pathologies and treatment regimes.
6. Focuses on preventing illnesses and deaths by maintaining cultural rules, practices, and taboos known and tested in the culture over time.	6. Focuses on repairing body or mind conditions based on medical specialists in the profession and some care givers.
7. Focuses on how to use folk home remedies and carers or healers as they know what is best for the client. A client goes to professional staff and hospitals as a last resort.	7. Cost for services are very high and often beyond ability for many poor or minority cultures to use. Consumers tend to avoid using unless they have lots of money.
8. Reflects high cultural context modes of communication.	8. Reflects low cultural context modes of communication.
9. Limits use of high-tech tools and instruments; uses more cultural rituals.	9. Uses many high-tech tools and machines in hospital with rituals.

*These emic or local characteristics were obtained from Leininger's in-depth qualitative ethnonursing study with many different cultural informants over nearly two decades (1973–1990). The characteristics reflect the people's emic views of differences between the generic folk or lay system with those of professional care systems in 15 non-Western cultures.
Source: Leininger, M. (1995). *Transcultural nursing: Concepts, theories, research & practices* (2nd ed., p. 80). New York: McGraw-Hill. Used with permission.

and practiced, and which reflects the ability of individuals (or groups) to perform their daily role activities in culturally expressed, beneficial and patterned life-ways" (p. 106). The related assumptions are that all cultures have generic or folk health care practices, that professional practices usually vary across cultures, and that in any culture there will be cultural similarities and differences between the care-receivers (generic) and the professional care-givers.

Care as a noun is defined as those "abstract and concrete phenomena related to assisting, supporting, or enabling experiences or behaviors toward or for others with evident or anticipated needs to ameliorate or improve a human condition or lifeway" (Leininger, 1995, p. 105). Care is assumed to be a distinct, dominant, unifying, and central focus of nursing, and, while curing and healing cannot occur effectively without care, care may occur without cure. *Care* as a gerund is defined as "actions and activities directed toward assisting, supporting, or enabling another individual or group with evident or anticipated needs to ameliorate or improve a human condition or lifeway, or to face death" (p. 105). Assumptions related to care and caring include that they are essential for the survival of humans, as well as for their growth, health, well-being, healing, and ability to deal with handicaps and death. The expressions, patterns, and lifeways of care have different meanings in different cultural contexts. The phenomenon of care can be discovered or identified by examining the cultural group's view of the world, social structure, and language.

Along with the universal nature of human beings as caring beings, the cultural care values, beliefs, and practices that are specific to a given culture provide a basis for the patterns, conditions, and actions associated with human care. Knowledge of these provides the base for three modes of nursing care decisions and actions, all of which require the coparticipation of the nurse and clients. *Culture care preservation* is also known as maintenance and includes those "assistive, supporting, facilitative or enabling professional actions and decisions that help people of a particular culture to retain and/or preserve relevant care values so that they can maintain their well-being, recover from illness or face handicaps and/or death" (Leininger, 1995, p. 106). *Culture care accommodation*, also known as negotiation, includes those "assistive, supporting, facilitative, or enabling creative professional actions and decisions that help people of a designated culture adapt to or negotiate with others for a beneficial or satisfying health outcome with professional care providers" (p. 106). *Culture care repatterning*, or restructuring, includes "those assistive, supporting, facilitative or enabling professional actions and decisions that help clients reorder, change or greatly modify their lifeways for new, different and beneficial health care patterns while respecting clients' cultural values and beliefs and providing a lifeway more beneficial or healthier than before the changes were coestablished with the clients" (p. 106). Repatterning requires the creative use of an extensive knowledge of the client's culture base and must be done in a way that is sensitive to the client's lifeways while using both generic and professional knowledge.

Nursing is defined as "a learned humanistic and scientific profession and discipline focused on human care phenomena and caring activities in order to assist, support, facilitate, or enable individuals or groups to maintain or regain their health or well-being in culturally meaningful and beneficial ways, or to help individuals face handicaps or death" (Leininger, 1995, p. 59). *Professional nursing care (caring)* is defined as "formal and cognitively learned professional care knowledge and practice skills, obtained through educational institutions, that are expected to provide assistive, supportive, enabling or facilitative acts to or for another individual or group in order to improve a human health condition (or well-being), disability, lifeway, or to work with dying clients" (p. 79). *Culturally congruent (nursing) care* is defined as "those cognitive[ly] based assistive, supportive, facilitative or enabling acts or decisions that are tailor-made to fit with individual, group or institutional cultural values, beliefs and lifeways in order to provide or support meaningful, beneficial and satisfying health care or well-being services" (p. 106). Related assumptions include that nursing, as a transcultural care discipline and profession, has a central purpose to serve human beings in all areas of the world; that when culturally based nursing care is beneficial and healthy it contributes to the well-being of the client(s)—whether individuals, groups, families, communities, or institutions—as they function within the context of their environments. Also, nursing care will be culturally congruent or beneficial only when the clients are known by the nurse and the clients' patterns, expressions, and cultural values are used in appropriate and meaningful ways by the nurse with the clients. Finally, it is assumed that if clients receive nursing care that is not at least reasonably culturally congruent (i.e., compatible with and respectful of the clients' lifeways, beliefs, and values), the client will demonstrate signs of stress, noncompliance, cultural conflicts, and/or ethical or moral concerns.

Leininger named her theory Culture Care Diversity and Universality and depicts it in the Sunrise Model (see Figure 21–1). This model may be viewed as a cognitive map that moves from the most abstract to the least abstract. The top of the model is the worldview and social system level, which directs the study of perceptions of the world outside of the culture—the suprasystem in general system terms. Leininger (1985b) states this level leads to the study of the nature, meaning, and attributes of care from three perspectives. Values and social structure could be a part of each of the perspectives. The microperspective studies individuals within a culture; these studies typically would be on a small scale. The middle perspective focuses on more complex factors in one specific culture; these studies are on a larger scale than microstudies. The macrostudies investigate phenomena across several cultures and are large in scale.

The culture care worldview flows into knowledge about individuals, families, groups, communities, and institutions in diverse health care systems. This knowledge provides culturally specific meanings and expressions in relation to care and health. The next focus is on the generic or folk system, professional care system(s), and nursing care. Information about these systems includes the characteristics and the specific care features of each. This information allows for the identification of similarities and differences or culture care universality and culture care diversity.

Next are nursing care decisions and actions that involve culture care preservation/maintenance, culture care accommodation/negotiation, and culture care repatterning/restructuring. It is here that nursing care is delivered. Within the Sunrise Model, culture congruent care is developed. This care is both congruent with and valued by the members of the culture.

Leininger (1991) points out that the model is not the theory but a depiction of the components of the theory of Culture Care Diversity and Universality. The purpose of the model is to aid the study of how the components of the theory influence the health status of, and care provided to, individuals, families, groups, communities, and institutions within a culture. She points out that one may begin at any level of the model (1995). She presents cogent arguments for the use of the model to guide discovery research that uses qualitative and ethnographic methods of study. She speaks strongly against the use of operational definitions and preconceived notions, and the use of causal or linear perspectives in studying cultural care diversity and universality. She supports the importance of finding out what *is*, of exploring and discovering the essence and meanings of care.

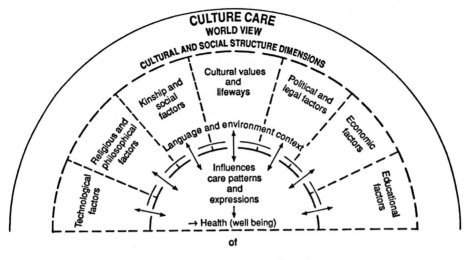

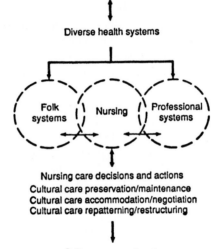

Figure 21–1. Leininger's Sunrise model depicts dimensions of Cultural Care Diversity and Universality. (*From Leininger, M. M. (Ed.). (1991). Cultural Care Diversity and Universality: A theory of nursing (p. 43). New York: National League for Nursing Press. Used with permission.*)

LEININGER'S THEORY AND THE FOUR MAJOR CONCEPTS

Leininger defines health and nursing but does not specifically define the major concepts of human being and society/environment. However, her view of these concepts can be derived from her conceptual definitions and assumptions. She also presents an argument for care as the central concept in nursing's metaparadigm (Leininger, 1991).

Human beings are best represented in her assumptions. Humans are believed to be caring and to be capable of being concerned about the needs, well-being, and survival of others. Human care is universal, that is, seen in all cultures. Humans have survived within cultures and through place and time because they have been able to care for infants, children, and the elderly in a variety of ways and in many different environments. Thus, humans are universally caring beings who survive in a diversity of cultures through their ability to provide the universality of care in a variety of ways according to differing cultures, needs, and settings. Leininger (1991) also indicates that nursing as a caring science should focus beyond traditional "nurse–patient interactions and dyads [to include] families, groups, communities, total cultures, and institutions" (p. 22) as well as worldwide health institutions and ways to develop international nursing care policies and practices. She points out that in many non-Western cultures family and institutions dominate. In these cultures, person is not an important concept. Indeed, there may be no term in the language for person. Thus, in the theory of Culture Care Diversity and Universality the focus is on human beings and not necessarily on the individual. A focus on the individual should occur only if it is appropriate to the culture in which care is being given.

Leininger defines *health*; this definition appears earlier in this chapter. She speaks of health systems, health care practices, changing health patterns, health promotion, and health maintenance. Health is an important concept in transcultural nursing. Because the emphasis is on the need for nurses to have knowledge that is specific to the culture in which nursing is being practiced, it is presumed that health is viewed as being universal across cultures but defined within each culture in a manner that reflects the beliefs, values, and practices of that particular culture. Thus, health is both universal and diverse.

Society/environment are not terms that are defined by Leininger; she speaks instead of worldview, social structure, and environmental context. However, society/environment, if viewed as being represented in culture, are a major theme of Leininger's theory. Environmental context is defined as being the totality of an event, situation, or experience. Leininger's (1991) definition of culture focuses on a particular group (society) and the patterning of actions, thoughts, and decisions that occurs as the result of "learned, shared, and transmitted values, beliefs, norms, and lifeways" (p. 47). This learning, sharing, transmitting, and patterning occur within a group of people who function in an identifiable setting or environment. Therefore, although Leininger does not use the specific terms of society or environment, the concept of culture is closely related to society/environment, and is a central theme of her theory.

Nursing is defined by Leininger; this definition appears earlier in this chapter. She also discusses that nursing, as a profession, has a societal mandate to serve people and, as a discipline, is expected to discover, develop, and use knowledge distinctive to nursing's focus on human care and caring. She expresses concern that nurses do not have adequate preparation for a transcultural perspective and that they neither value nor practice from such a perspective to the fullest extent possible. She presents three types of nursing actions that are culturally based and thus congruent with the needs and values of the clients. These are culture care preservation/maintenance, culture care accommodation/negotiation, and culture care repatterning/restructuring and have been defined earlier in this chapter. These three modes of action can lead to the delivery of nursing care that best fits with the client's culture and thus decreases cultural stress and potential for conflict between client and caregiver.

It should be noted that Leininger would add additional concepts as vital to nursing. These include human care, caring, and multiple cultural factors. These terms are defined elsewhere in this chapter and these definitions will not be repeated here.

CULTURE CARE DIVERSITY AND UNIVERSALITY AND TRANSCULTURAL NURSING

After careful review of the Sunrise Model, it becomes apparent that there are parallels between the model and the nursing process. This is true, in part, because both represent a problem-solving process. The focus of the nursing process is the client who is the recipient of nursing care. The client (whether an individual, family, group, or other aggregate of human beings) is also a focus of the Sunrise Model, but the importance of knowledge and understanding of the client's culture is a major shaping force in the Model. Major features of cultures are presented in Table 21–2.

Gaining knowledge and understanding of another's culture may be very time consuming for the nurse who is not familiar with that culture. Leininger (1978, 1991, 1995) speaks with concern about the possibility of the nurse being involved in culture shock or cultural imposition. *Culture shock* may result when an outsider attempts to comprehend or adapt effectively to a different cultural group. The outsider is likely to experience feelings of discomfort and helplessness and some degree of disorientation because of the differences in cultural values, beliefs, and practices. Culture shock may lead to anger and can be reduced by seeking knowledge of the culture before encountering that culture. *Cultural imposition* refers to efforts of the outsider, both subtle and not so subtle, to impose his or her own cultural values, beliefs, behaviors upon an individual, family, or group from another culture. Cultural imposition has been particularly prevalent in efforts to impose Western health care practices on other cultures.

In 1995, Leininger added many other concepts related to culture to those included in her earlier discussions. *Culture values* are critical to transcultural nursing as they have a strong influence on behavior. They are defined as "the powerful internal and external directive forces that give meaning and order to an individual's group's thinking, decisions, and actions" (p. 63). *Cultural relativism* is the position

TABLE 21–2. COMPLEX FEATURES OF CULTURES

- A culture reflects shared values, ideals, and meanings that are learned and guide human behavior, decisions, and actions.
  - * Group behavior is more likely to be influenced by cultural values than by individual values.
- Cultures have manifest (readily recognized) and implicit (covert and ideal) rules of behavior and expectations.
- Cultures have material items or concrete goods such as artifacts that give meaning and are special symbols of the culture.
  - * Examples in the United States include Coke and Pepsi cans and the American flag; in Papua New Guinea an example would be bows and arrows.
- Cultures also have nonmaterial expressions and symbols that characterize the culture.
  - * Native American beliefs in good and bad spirits are examples.
- Cultures have cultural traditional ceremonial practices such as religious rites and social feasts that are transmitted from one generation to another increasing the solidarity and unity of cultures.
- Cultures have their local or emic (insider's) views and knowledge about their culture that are extremely important to discover and understand.
  - * Both emic and etic knowledge are studied to guide transcultural nursing practices.
- All human cultures have intercultural variations between two or more cultures as well as intracultural variations within a particular culture.

Source: Adapted from Leininger, M. (1995). *Transcultural nursing: Concepts, theories, research & practices* (2nd ed.) (pp. 61–62). New York: McGraw-Hill. Used with permission.

that "cultures are unique and must be evaluated according to their own values and standards" (p. 66). *Ethnicity* relates to identity arising from language, religion, and national origins. *Ethnocentrism*, a universal phenomena and a core concept in transcultural nursing, is "the belief that one's own ways are the best, most superior, or preferred ways to act, believe, or behave" (p. 65). In contrast, *racism* is "derived from the concept of race, and it is usually defined as a biological feature of a discrete group, whose members share distinctive genetic traits inherited from a common ancestor" (p. 70). *Prejudice* is "preconceived ideas, beliefs, or opinions about an individual, group, or culture that limit a full and accurate understanding of the individual, culture, gender, race, event, or situation" (p. 71). *Discrimination* is "the limiting of opportunities, choices, or life experiences because of prejudices about individuals, cultures, or social groups" (p. 71). *Stereotyping* is "placing people and institutions, mentally and by attitudes, into a narrow, fixed trait, rigid pattern, or with inflexible 'boxlike' characteristics" (p. 71).

Uniculturalism (or monoculturalism) is "the belief that one's universe is largely constituted, centered upon and functions from a one-culture perspective and reflecting some cultural ethnocentric views" (p. 65). *Multiculturalism* is "a perspective and reality that there are many different cultures and subcultures in the world which need to be recognized, valued, and understood for their differences and similarities" (p. 65). *Cultural bias* is "a firm position or stance that one's own values and beliefs must govern the situation or decision" (p. 66). On the other hand, *cultural blindness* is "the inability of an individual to recognize one's own lifestyle, values and modes of behavior and those of another individual because of strong attitude to make them invisible due to ethnocentric tendencies" (p. 67). *Cultural pain* is "the suffering, discomfort, or unfavorable responses of an individual group towards an individual who has different beliefs or lifeways, usually reflecting the insensitivity of those inflicting the discomfort" (p. 67). *BiOculturalism* is "how biological, physical, and different physical environments of diverse and similar cultures relate to care, health, illness, and disabilities" (p. 68). *Culture-bound* is "specific care, health, illness, and disease conditions that are particular, highly unique, and usually specific to a designated culture or geographical area" (p. 69). Leininger (1995) uses the terms *Western* and *non-Western* for general comparative purposes in discussing transcultural nursing. Western cultures tend to be highly industrialized and dependent on technology. Non-Western (may be identified as Eastern) cultures are much less dependent on technology, have strong philosophical ideologies, and have existed for thousands of years. *Enculturation* is "in-depth learning about a culture with its specific values, beliefs, and practices in order to prepare children and adults to function or to live effective[ly] in a particular culture" (p.72). *Acculturation* is "the process by which an individual or group from culture A learns how to take on many of the behaviors, values, and lifeways of culture B" (p. 72). *Socialization* is "the social process whereby an individual or group from a particular culture learns how to become a part of and function within the larger society in order to know how to interact with others, vote, work, and live in a society" (p. 73). *Assimilation* is "the way an individual or group from one culture selectively takes on and chooses certain features of another culture without necessarily taking on the total attributes of a particular culture" (p. 73).

Terms related to culture care are:

- Configurative culture care—"pattern expectations of a culture (or subculture) and of the way these patterns fit together in meaningful clusters or characteristics"
- Culture specific care/caring—"the particularized or tailorized modes of care practices that are identified or abstracted from an individual or group of a particular culture in order to plan and implement care that fits the client's specific care needs and lifeways"
- Generalized culture care—"common professional nursing care techniques, principles, and practices that are useful to many clients as common or general human care needs"
- Culture care conflict—"areas of distress, concern or incompatibility when nursing care practices do not fit with a client's expectations, beliefs, values, or normative expectations"
- Culture care clashes—"sharp differences between the nurse and the client which occur because nursing practices are clearly incompatible, incongruent, or are perceived to be unacceptable"
- Culture time—"the dominant orientation of an individual or group to different time periods related to past, present, and future which guides one's activities and thinking"
  - Includes clock time, social time, cycle activity time
- Cultural space—"the variation of cultures in the use of body, visual, territorial, and interpersonal distance to others"
  - Includes body touching

- Cultural context—"the totality of shared meanings and life experiences in a particular social, cultural and physical environment that influence attitudes, thinking and patterns of behavior"
- Culture comforts—"diverse ways the nurse uses cultural care patterns, specific information, and previous client life experiences to ease or relieve the clients' distresses, strains, or concerns" (pp.74–78).

The upper portions of the Sunrise Model involve the development of knowledge about cultures, people, and care systems. When appropriately used, they could help prevent culture shock, cultural imposition, and culture care conflict. These levels are similar to the *assessment* and *diagnosis* phases of the nursing process. However, in the Sunrise Model, knowledge of the culture could be gained before identifying a specific client who would be the focus of the nursing process. First, one is assessing or gathering knowledge and information about the social structure and worldview of the client's culture. Other information that is needed includes the language and environmental context of the client as well as the factors of technology, religion, philosophy, kinship, social structure, cultural values and beliefs, politics, legal system, economics, and education. Much of this knowledge could be gathered before the identification of a particular client and would be useful in preventing both culture shock and cultural imposition. The principles identified by Leininger as important to conducting a cultralogical assessment are presented in Table 21–3.

Worldview and social structure knowledge needs to be applied to the situation of the client, whether that client is an individual, a family, a group, a community, or a sociocultural institution. Next, it is recognized that the client exists within a health system and the values, beliefs, and behaviors of the generic (folk), professional, and nursing care portions of that health system need to be identified. Throughout this assessment process, it is important to recognize and identify those characteristics that

TABLE 21–3. PRINCIPLES FOR USING THE SUNRISE MODEL TO GUIDE CULTURALOGICAL ASSESSMENT

- Study the Sunrise Model before doing the assessment in order to draw on the different components.
- Know own culture with its variabilities, strengths, and assets.
- Discover and remain aware of own cultural biases and prejudices.
- Show a genuine interest in the client; learn from and maintain respect for the client.
- Clarify and explain at the outset to the individual, family, or group that the focus of a culturalogical or lifeway assessment is to help clients.
- Give attention to gender differences, communication modes, special language terms, interpersonal relationships, use of space and foods, and any additional aspects the client may share.
- Be aware that the client may belong to subcultures or special groups such as the homeless, AIDS and HIV infected, drug users, lesbians, gays, the deaf, mentally retarded, and many other particular groups.
- Maintain a holistic or total view of the informant's world and environmental context by focusing on the multiple components as depicted in the Sunrise Model.

Source: Adapted from Leininger, M. (1995). *Transcultural nursing: Concepts, theories, research & practices* (2nd ed.) (pp. 122–125). New York: McGraw-Hill. Used with permission.

are universal or common across cultures and those which are diverse or specific to the culture being assessed. After identifying the culture care diversities and universalities for the culture, a nursing diagnosis can be developed based on those areas in which the client is not meeting a cultural expectation of the client's culture. A short assessment guide developed by Leininger is displayed in Table 21–4. More detailed assessment guides can be found in her 1995 text.

Once the diagnosis has been established, *planning, outcomes,* and *implementation* occur within Nursing Care Decisions and Actions. Again, the nursing care decisions and actions need to be culturally based to best meet the needs of the client and provide culture congruent care. The three modes of action are culture care preservation/maintenance, culture care accommodation/negotiation, and culture care repatterning/restructuring. In culture care preservation/maintenance, the professional actions focus on supporting, assisting, facilitating, or enabling clients to preserve or retain favorable health, to recover from illness or to face handicaps or death. An example would be facilitating an elderly person's access to grocery shopping so that the individual can continue to prepare healthful meals—or encouraging the sharing of those meals with another in a manner that is culturally acceptable.

Culture care accommodation/negotiation creates professional efforts to facilitate, enable, assist, or support actions that represent ways to negotiate with or adapt or adjust to the client's health and care patterns for a beneficial or satisfying health outcome. For example, in planning for prenatal classes for multigravidas in a Hispanic community, provision for child care needs to be included as Hispanic mothers place very high value on caring for their children and do not use babysitters as freely as do many mothers in American society. The Hispanic mother's care pattern is to provide care for her child and to have the child near her. She will choose to not attend

TABLE 21–4. LEININGER'S SHORT CULTURALOGIC ASSESSMENT GUIDE

Phase V	Develop a culturally based client–nurse care plan as a coparticipant for decisions and actions for cultural congruent care.
	⇧
Phase IV	Synthesize themes and patterns of care derived from the information obtained in phases I, II, and III.
	⇧
Phase III	Identify and document recurrent client patterns and narratives (stories) with client meanings of what has been seen, heard, or experienced.
	⇧
Phase II	Listen to and learn from the client about cultural values, beliefs, and daily (nightly) practices related to care and health in the client's environmental context. Give attention to generic (home or folk) practices and professional nursing practices.
	⇧
Phase I	Record observations of what you see, hear, or experience with clients (includes dress and appearance, body condition features, language, mannerisms and general behavior, attitudes, and cultural features).
	⇧
	Start Here

Source: From Leininger, M. (1995). *Transcultural nursing: Concepts, theories, research & practices* (2nd ed.) (p. 142). New York: McGraw-Hill. Used with permission.

the class rather than leave her child at home with a babysitter. Those who do not understand this may become involved in cultural imposition and label the mother as not caring when she does not attend meetings at which childcare is not available.

Culture care repatterning/restructuring refers to professional actions that seek to help clients change meaningful health or life patterns to patterns that will be healthier for them while respecting the client's cultural values. For example, Charles Thompson, whose dietary pattern has been to eat fried and salted foods at every meal, is found to have hypertension and elevated blood cholesterol levels. Fried chicken with a salty batter is an important element in Mr. Thompson's diet—it is a food that appears on the menu at family celebrations and one that is frequently packed in the brown bag meal he carries to work. Fortunately, the chicken itself is one of the forms of protein that is recommended in low fat and low cholesterol diets. The repatterning that can occur relates to the way in which the chicken is prepared. The food preparer in the Thompson family could be taught to skin the chicken (helps lower the fat and thus the cholesterol), use a coating of herbs (rather than salt to help with the hypertension), and bake in the microwave oven with no added fat rather than fry with a salty batter (helps with both cholesterol and hypertension). Such change would repattern the preparation of a favorite food into a way that could provide for the continued inclusion of this food in the diet on a regular basis. At the same time, important changes in the way in which Mr. Thompson eats would be supported. Similar repatterning could occur with other foods, for example, instead of cooking green beans with salt pork, the beans could be cooked with herbs and a little polyunsaturated or monosaturated oil.

The Sunrise Model does not include an area identified as *evaluation*. However, in Leininger's (1995) discussion of transcultural nursing, she places a great deal of importance on the need for nursing care to provide ways in which care will benefit the client and on the need to systematically study nursing care behaviors to determine which care behaviors are appropriate to the lifeways and behavioral patterns of the culture for healing, health, or well-being. Such study certainly is the equivalent of evaluation. Without evaluation of the outcomes of a particular plan of care that used the nursing process, or a series of such plans, the systematic study that Leininger advises cannot be completed.

Example of Transcultural Nursing Daniel Saunders, 8 years old, has been accompanied to the emergency department by his mother and grandmother. He has had acute abdominal pain for two days. The nurse notes that his mother defers questions about Daniel to him or to his grandmother and that none of the three respond immediately to questions posed or comments made by the staff or look directly at members of the staff. They sit close together but do not touch one another. The physician wants to admit Daniel for exploratory abdominal surgery. Daniel's mother will not sign the admission and surgical permission forms until his grandmother has given her approval to do so. At this point, Daniel's grandmother takes a bag of cornmeal from her pocket and begins to sprinkle it around Daniel.

The nurse who lacks transcultural knowledge, or who is unicultural, likely views this family as strange and suspicious. The lack of direct eye contact leads to questions of what they are hiding. The mother appears indecisive. The family members don't seem to care much for each other since they do not touch. And what is the deal with the cornmeal?

The transcultural nurse would recognize that this is a Navajo family and the family members are demonstrating typical characteristics as described by Phillips and Lobar (1995). The Navajo culture is a matriarchical culture whose members defer to the wisdom of elders. Thus, Daniel is accompanied by his mother and grandmother, rather than by his mother and father. Also, the grandmother is viewed as the source of wisdom so her decision and support are necessary before the permission slips are signed, even though the dominant American culture considers Daniel's mother the appropriate person to sign these permission forms. Daniel is included in responses to questions asked as a value of the culture is for the individual to speak for him or herself. The lack of direct eye contact and pauses after questions or statements are made by another are indications of respect, not of untrustworthiness. The pauses are intended to convey both respect and a degree of thought and attention being given to the content of the message. Navajo family members demonstrate their caring for one another through being physically close, but not through touching. Illness is viewed as a lack of or disturbance of one's harmony. Rituals, such as sprinkling the person with cornmeal, are important to restore harmony. The nurse needs to note that it is important to save the cornmeal to return it to the family.

After Daniel's surgery, the nurse can anticipate that he will accept pain relief. It is also likely that as many relatives as are available will want to visit—such family support is another cultural value. Finally, should Daniel be on a b.i.d. antibiotic when discharged, the timing of the administration of his medication should be tied to natural events such as sunup and sundown rather than with meals or some other activity. The Navajo sense of time tends to be casual and relative and meal times are likely to be flexible.

CRITIQUE OF CULTURE CARE DIVERSITY AND UNIVERSALITY

1. What is the historical context of the theory? Beginning with the identification of a need to understand the culture of clients, through the introduction of the terms *transcultural nursing* and *ethnonursing care*, to the presentation of the Sunrise Model, Madeleine Leininger developed the theory of Culture Care Diversity and Universality. Leininger began developing her ideas about culture and caring as nursing theory development in the United States was just beginning to occur, that is, in the 1950s and 1960s. While she has had multiple publications on these concepts annually since the mid-1960s, she first labeled her thinking a theory in 1985. Prior to the mid-1980s her publications tended to be about culture or about caring; since the mid-1980s the focus has been on transcultural nursing, culture care, and qualitative research. She provides an excellent discussion of the path she has taken in the development of the Sunrise Model and the theory of Culture Care Diversity and Universality in her 1991 book. Thus, her work has occurred during the same time frame as the major efforts in development of nursing theory. Her focus on caring is shared with many other theorists. She has provided the leadership in focusing on culture and its importance to the delivery of appropriate nursing care. She has also been in the forefront in advocating the use of qualitative research in nursing.

2. What are the basic concepts and relationships presented by the theory? Leininger developed the Sunrise Model to demonstrate the interrelationships of the concepts in her theory of Culture Care Diversity and Universality. The worldview and social structure portion of the model does not differ significantly from any other view of culture and its interaction with human beings, with the possible exception of the inclusion of care and health patterns. The Model focuses on individuals, families, groups, communities, and sociocultural institutions, which is similar to other theories of nursing. The inclusion of the term *culture* does provide a distinguishing feature since no other nursing theory has this emphasis on culture. Health systems include generic, professional, and nursing care systems. The inclusion of the generic system is unique to the culture care theory. Nursing care decisions and actions are identified as supporting, accommodating to, or repatterning current health and care practices. The focus of nursing care decisions and actions is shared with many other theories. The division of actions into supporting, accommodating, or repatterning is specific to this theory. The Sunrise Model of Culture Care Diversity and Universality in itself supports the concepts of diversity and universality. The worldview, social structure, and description of individuals, families, groups, communities, and institutions are essentially universal as they have much in common with many other theories. The identified care systems and types of nursing care actions are diverse, or more specific and unique to this particular theory. Overall, the theory of Culture Care was the first to focus specifically on human care from a transcultural perspective (Leininger, 1991). It provides a holistic rather than a fragmented view of people. This view includes "worldview; biophysical state; religious (or spiritual) orientation; kinship patterns; material (and nonmaterial) cultural phenomena; the political, economic, legal, educational, technological, and physical environment; language; and folk and professional care practices" (p. 23).

3. What major phenomena of concern to nursing are presented? These phenomena may include *but are not limited to*: human being, environment, health, interpersonal relations, caring, goal attainment, adaptation, and energy fields. The major phenomena of concern to nursing are culture, care, and culture care. The human being as an individual may or may not be important, depending on the cultural values. Environment, considered broadly, includes the multiple areas in the Sunrise Model. Health is also defined with the specifics of what is viewed as health determined again by the values of the culture. Nursing is identified as a culture.

4. To whom does this theory apply? In what situations? In what ways? Because everyone, as individuals or in groups, belongs to a culture and/or a subculture, this theory applies to anyone in any situation. For nurses, there is a special concern about being culturally appropriate in approach and in responses. Leininger particularly warns about cultural imposition and culture shock.

5. By what method or methods can this theory be tested? The theory of Culture Care Diversity and Universality is based on, and calls for, qualitative rather than quantitative research. The development of hypotheses is characteristic of positivistic, quantitative research. The development of research questions, and of relational statements, is characteristic of qualitative research. Leininger (1991) states that nursing science should be defined "as the creative study of nursing phenomena which reflects the systematization of knowledge using rigorous and explicit research methods within either the qualitative or quantitative paradigm in order to establish a new or to advance nursing's discipline knowledge" (p. 30). However, Leininger has developed a qualitative method for studying culture and care. She calls this the ethnonursing research method and indicates the qualitative methodology is the most appropriate for studying the emic views and beliefs of people. The principles that guide the ethnonursing research method are to:

- Maintain an open discovery, active listening, and a genuine learning attitude in working with informants in the total context in which the study is conducted.
- Maintain an active and curious posture about the "why" of whatever is seen, heard, or experienced, and with appreciation of whatever informants share with you.
- Record whatever is shared by informants in a careful and conscientious way for full meanings, explanations, or interpretations to preserve informant ideas.
- Seek a mentor who has experience with the ethnonursing research method to act as a guide.
- Clarify the purposes of additional qualitative research methods if they are combined with the ethnonursing method such as combining life histories, ethnography, phenomenology, or ethnoscience (Leininger, 1991, pp. 106–109).

The phases of ethnonursing research may be found in Table 21–5. Nearly 75 cultures or subcultures have been studied using this research method. The major source of information about this method, its tools, and studies conducted using it is *The Journal of Transcultural Nursing*. Other information may be found through the Transcultural Nursing Society.

6. Does this theory direct critical thinking in nursing practice? Absolutely! Critical thinking involves collecting and using data to support decisions. The focus of Leininger's leadership has been to alert, support, and inform nurses about the importance of using cultural information to understand similarities and differences as decisions are made in relationship to health and caring.

7. Does this theory direct therapeutic intervention? According to Leininger, maximum therapeutic effect will be attained only if the care given is culturally congruent. The three modes of culture care (preservation, accommodation, and

TABLE 21–5. PHASES OF LEININGER'S ETHNONURSING RESEARCH METHOD

1. Identify the general intent or purpose(s) of your study with focus on the domain(s) of inquiry phenomenon under study, area of inquiry, or research questions being addressed.
2. Identify the potential significance of the study to advance nursing knowledge and practices.
3. Review available literature on the domain or phenomena being studied.
4. Conceptualize a research plan from the beginning to the end with the following general phases or sequence factors in mind.
   a. Consider the research site, community, and people to study the phenomena.
   b. Deal with the informed consent expectations.
   c. Explore and gradually gain entry (with essential permissions) to the community, hospital, or country wherever the study is being done.
   d. Anticipate potential barriers and facilitators related to: gatekeepers expectations, language, political leaders, location, and other factors.
   e. Select and appropriately use the ethnonursing enabling tools with the research process, for example, Leininger's *Stranger-Friend Guide* and *Observation-Participation-Reflection Guide* and others (Leininger, 1985a, 1988a). Researchers may also develop enabling tools or guides for their studies.
   f. Choose key and general informants.
   g. Maintain trusting and favorable relationships with the people conferring with ethnonurse research expert(s) to prevent unfavorable developments.
   h. Collect and confirm data with observations, interviews, participant experiences, and other data. (This is a continuous process from the beginning to the end and requires the use of qualitative research criteria to confirm findings and credibility factors.)
   i. Maintain continuous data processing on computers and with field journals reflecting active analysis and reflections, and with discussions with research mentor(s). Computer processing with Leininger/Templin/Thompson's software is a helpful means to handle large amounts of qualitative data.
   j. Frequently present and reconfirm findings with the people studied to check credibility and confirmability of findings.
   k. Make plans to leave the field site, community, and informants in advance.
5. Do final analysis and writing of the research findings soon after completing the study.
6. Prepare published findings in appropriate journals.
7. Help implement the findings with nurses interested in findings.
8. Plan future studies related to this domain or other new ones.

Source: Adapted from Leininger, M. M. (Ed.). (1991). *Culture Care Diversity and Universality: A theory of nursing* (p. 105). New York: National League for Nursing Press. Used with permission.

repatterning) provide a flexible approach for providing culturally congruent care in a manner that requires the optimal amount of change and thus is more likely to be acceptable to, and continued by, the client.

8. Does this theory direct communication in nursing practice? Yes! Leininger directs the nurse to communicate with the literature as well as with the client to learn about cultural values that relate to the nursing practice situation. She encourages nurses to be aware of the importance of the culture, and the subculture, and how the client merges with and diverges from them. The emic or insider's views can only be obtained through use of appropriate means of communication. Leininger's phases of ethnonursing research (see Table 21–5) include guidelines that would be useful in relation to communication with those from a culture other than one's own.

9. Does this theory direct nursing actions that lead to satisfactory outcomes? The theory of Culture Care Diversity and Universality does not give specific direction for nursing actions such as "ambulate three times a day." However, it does provide direction on how to learn about the culture of another and how to exhibit caring in relation to another's cultural values, especially in relation to health. Leininger emphasizes that culturally congruent care is vital for lasting satisfactory outcomes.

10. How contagious is this theory? This theory is very contagious in that it is universally applicable and widely presented. Not only has Leininger spoken and consulted worldwide, many international students have come to the United States to study transcultural nursing with her. The theory has been used to guide research, education, and nursing practice about and with a wide variety of cultures and subcultures.

Research has been reported about cultures and subcultures including African American women and prenatal care (Morgan, 1996); adolescents (Rosenbaum & Carty, 1996); American gypsies (Bodnar & Leininger, 1992, 1995); American Hare Krishnas and pregnancy (Morgan, 1992); American hospital nurses (Leininger, 1995); Anglo and African American elders in long-term care (McFarland, 1997); Anglo American males in the rural Midwest (Sellers, Poduska, Propp & White, 1999); Anglo American and Philippine American nurses (Spangler, 1991); Baganda women as AIDS caregivers (MacNeil, 1994, 1996); care needs of African American male juvenile offenders (Canty-Mitchell, 1996); childbirth experiences of EuropeanAmerican women (Finn, 1994); culture and pain (Villarruel, 1995); Czech-Americans (Miller, 1997a, 1997b); diabetes education in a Hispanic community (Garcia, 1996); dying patients (Gates, 1988, 1991); elderly Anglo-Canadian caregivers (Cameron, 1990); elderly Polish Americans (McFarland, 1995); the evolution of transcultural nursing (Husting, 1991); the Gadsup of New Guinea (Leininger, 1991, 1995); the goal of culturally sensitive care (Kirkham, 1998); Greek Canadian widows (Rosenbaum, 1990, 1991); Gypsies in Portugal (Braga, 1997); health experiences of Athabascans in Galena, Alaska (Paul, 1991); health as viewed by Vietnamese immigrants in central New York state (Dean-Kelly, 1997); Iranian immigrants in New South Wales, Australia (Omeri, 1997); Japanese children with congenital heart disease (Masumori, 1997); Lebanese Muslims in the United States (Luna, 1994); Lithuanian Americans (Gelazis, 1994); male nurses in Portugal (Nobrega, Lopes Neto, Dantas, & Perez, 1996); the mentally ill (George, 1998); the Muckleshoots (Horn, 1995); Muscogee Creek Indians (Wing & Thompson, 1996); native Hawaiians (Kinney, 1985); nurse anesthesia (Horton, 1998); nursing and medicine in America (Leininger, 1995); nursing curriculum in South Africa (de Villiers & van der Wal, 1995); Old Order Amish (Wenger, 1991, 1995); perceptions of caring by Pakistanis in the United Kingdom (Cortis, 2000); Philippine Americans (Leininger, 1995); post-partum depression in Jordanian Australian women (Nahas & Amasheh, 1999); psychiatric care values in Finland (Nikkonen, 1994); quality of life (Leininger, 1994); students who study in countries other than their native country (Martsolf, 1991); The Farm and midwifery services to the Amish (Finn, 1995); trends in transcultural research (Leininger, 1997b); Tunisian hospital nurses (Lazure, Vissandjee, Pepin, & Kerouac, 1997); types of health practitioners and cultural imposition (Leininger, 1995); Ukrainian American mothers (Bohay, 1991); urban Mexican Americans (Stasiak, 1991); and viligance as a caring expression (Carr, 1998).

Discussions about the use of Culture Care Diversity and Universality in education include comparing the transcultural practices of R.N.s and baccalaureate students (Baldonado, et al., 1998); graduate curriculum in mental health nursing (Redmond, 1988); impact on nursing curricula in the United States (Andrews, 1995; Campinha-Bacote, Yahle, & Langenkamp, 1996); inclusion of African American diversity in inservice education (Dowe, 1990); incorporation in basic nursing texts in Canada (Morse & English, 1986); key references for staff development and nursing inservice (Mahon, 1997); simulation games (Talabere, 1996); undergraduate and graduate education (Haylock, 1992; Leininger, 1995); use as a context for considering education and health care in India (Basuray, 1997); use in an associate degree program (Jeffreys & O'Donnell, 1997); and use in a transcultural, transnational setting (Baker & Burkhalter, 1996).

Reports of transcultural nursing practice include the cultures and subcultures of adolescent homosexuals (Dootson, 2000); advocacy and diversity (Kavanagh, 1993); African Americans (Morgan, 1995); Anglo-Americans in the United States (Leninger, 1995); Aotearoa, New Zealand (Smith, 1997); Arab Muslims (Luna, 1995); Ayurveda medicine (Larson-Presswalla, 1994); community assessment in a Hispanic community (Ludwig-Beymer, Blankemeier, Casas-Byots, & Suarez-Baleazar, 1996); comparison and contrast with Sartre (Rajan, 1995); culturally sensitive care in the United Kingdom (McGee, 1994); the deaf (Stebnicki & Coeling, 1999); developing of a caring culture practice model in hospitals in Canada (MacDonald & Miller-Grolla, 1995); ethical, moral, and legal aspects (Leininger, 1995; Zoucha & Husted, 2000); breast cancer screening for elderly black women in the United States (Brown & Williams, 1994); care of hospitalized children in Australia (Alsop-Shields & Nixon, 1997); Chinese, Korean, and Vietnamese (Leininger, 1995); the Hausa of Northwest Africa (Chmielarczyk, 1991); health values in China (Finn & Lee, 1996); home health care in the United States (Hahn, 1997; Narayan, 1997); impact on practice (Leininger, 1996, 1997a, 1999); Japanese Americans (Leininger, 1995); Jewish Americans (Leininger, 1995); interaction with American families in relation to child-rearing (Campinha-Bacote & Ferguson, 1991); Lithuanian Americans (Gelazis, 1995); mental health nursing (Leininger, 1995); Mexican Americans (Villarruel & Leininger, 1995); Navajo child health beliefs (Phillips & Lobar, 1995); nursing administration (Leininger, 1991); nursing in Japan (Inaoka, 1997); Saudi Arabia (Luna, 1998); South Africa (Mashaba, 1995); Switzerland (Rohrbach-Viadas, 1997); and use in Germany (Brouns, 1993; Kollak & Kupper, 1998; Leininger & Gstottner, 1998).

STRENGTHS AND LIMITATIONS

A major strength of Leininger's theory is the recognition of the importance of culture and its influence on everything that involves the recipients and providers of nursing care. The development of this theory over a number of years has allowed its concepts and constructs to be tested by a number of people in a variety of settings and cultures. The Sunrise Model provides guidance for the areas in which information needs to be collected.

Some limitations, as identified by Leininger (1991), include the limited number of graduate nurses who are academically prepared to conduct the investigations needed to provide transcultural nursing care. An associated concern is that too few nursing programs include courses and planned learning experiences that provide a knowledge base for transcultural nursing practice. While there has been some increase in the number of nurses prepared in transcultural nursing, it is important to note the danger of cultural biases and cultural imposition occurring with nurses' personal cultural values. There is also a need for research funds to support continued study of caring practices—both those that are universal and those that are particular to a culture. Leininger (1997b) identifies that the three greatest continuing needs are for education of nurses to practice transcultural nursing, to use the existing findings from transcultural nursing research and to continue research to develop new knowledge and reaffirm credible findings in a continually changing world.

It is interesting to note that, in spite of Leininger's emphasis on the importance of avoiding cultural imposition and cultural shock, Domenig (1999) expresses concern that Leininger does not make interaction the main object of her theory and that nurses need to be encouraged to analyze their own cultural backgrounds. It would be difficult to identify how Leininger could have put greater emphasis on the importance of these aspects.

In some of her writings, Leininger is not consistent in her terminology. For example, in *Transcultural Nursing* (1979), she refers to ethnocultural care constructs and then to ethnonursing care constructs. In her theory presentation she refers to these same constructs as major cultural care constructs (Leininger, 1988b). Since the constructs are listed it is relatively easy to be aware that these terms all refer to the same constructs. However, the reader's mental energy could be conserved for understanding the theory and model if the terminology were more consistent.

The complexity of the Sunrise Model can be viewed as both a strength and a limitation. The complexity is a strength in that it emphasizes the importance of the inclusion of anthropological and cultural concepts in nursing education and practice. On the other hand, the complexity can lead to misinterpretation or rejection, both of which are limitations.

SUMMARY

Madeleine Leininger has been working since the 1950s on the development of her theory of Culture Care Diversity and Universality. In the 1960s, she first began to use the terms *transcultural nursing* and *ethnonursing*. While she has slightly different definitions of these terms, she often uses them interchangeably, an action that can be confusing to the reader. She defines each of her concepts and presents assumptions that she considers to be relevant. The concepts and their interrelationships provide the basis for the Sunrise Model of this theory. The Sunrise Model presents a cognitive model which, when viewed from the top down, moves from the cultural and social structure through individuals, families, groups, communities, and institutions in generic, professional, and nursing care systems to nursing care decisions and actions that are cultural care preserving, accommodating, and repatterning. The Model also indicates the need to move from knowledge generation through substantive knowledge to application of the knowledge. In discussing the Model, Leininger (1991) presents the idea that care patterns and processes may be universal or diverse. Universal care indicates care patterns, values, and behaviors that are common across cultures. Care diversities represent those patterns and processes that are unique or specific to an individual, family, or cultural group. Leininger believes, and research has supported, that care diversities are greater in number than are universal care patterns. If Nikkonen's (1994) attribution of this increasing diversity to the individualism of the 1980s is correct, this trend will continue to be demonstrated.

The theory of Culture Care Diversity and Universality is of significance in a society that is becoming more and more aware of the cultural diversity within its boundaries. While this theory does not provide specific directions for nursing care, it does provide guidelines for the gathering of knowledge and a framework for the making of decisions about what care is needed or would be of the greatest benefit to the client. Leininger has clearly identified what has been a major deficit in our provision of nursing care and provided a road map to begin to fill the gaps created by that deficit.

REFERENCES

Alsop-Shields, L., & Nixon, J. (1997). Transcultural nursing and its use in the care of children in hospital. *Australian Paediatric Nurse, 6*(2), 2–5.

Andrews, M. (1995). Transcultural nursing: Transforming the curriculum. *Journal of Transcultural Nursing, 6*(2), 4–9.

Baker, S. S., & Burkhalter, N. C. (1996). Teaching transcultural nursing in a transcultural setting. *Journal of Transcultural Nursing, 7*(2), 10–13.

Baldonado, A., Beymer, P. L., Barnes, K., Starsiak, D., Nemivant, E. B., & Anonas-Ternate, A. (1998). Transcultural nursing practice described by registered nurses and baccalaureate nursing students. *Journal of Transcultural Nursing, 9*(2), 15–25.

Basuray, J. (1997). Nurse Miss Sahib: Colonial culture-bound education in India and transcultural nursing. *Journal of Transcultural Nursing, 9*(1), 14–19.

Bodnar, A., & Leininger, M. (1992). Transcultural nursing care values, beliefs, and practices of American (USA) Gypsies. *Journal of Transcultural Nursing, 4*(1), 17–28.

Bodnar, A., & Leininger, M. (1995). Transcultural nursing care of American Gypsies. In M. Leininger, *Transcultural nursing: Concepts, theories, research & practices* (2nd ed.) (pp. 445–470). New York: McGraw-Hill.

Bohay, I. Z. (1991). Culture care meanings and experiences of pregnancy and childbirth of Ukrainians. In M. M. Leininger (Ed.), *Culture Care Diversity and Universality: A theory of nursing* (pp. 203–229) (Pub. No. 15-2402). New York: National League for Nursing Press.

Braga, C. G. (1997). Transcultural nursing and beliefs: Values and practices of the Gypsy population [Portuguese]. *Rev Esc Enferm USP, 31*, 498–516.

Brouns, G. (1993). Leininger's theory of cultural nursing diversity and universality [German]. *Pflege, 6*, 191–196.

Brown, L. W., & Williams, R. D. (1994). Culturally sensitive breast cancer screening programs for older black women. *Nurse Practitioner, 19*(3), 21, 25–26, 31.

Cameron, C. F. (1990). An ethnonursing study of the influence of extended caregiving on the health status of elderly Anglo-Canadian wives caring for physically disabled husbands. *Dissertation Abstracts International, 52(02B),* 746.

Campinha-Bacote, J., & Ferguson, S. (1991). Cultural considerations in child-rearing practices: A transcultural perspective. *Journal of National Black Nurses' Association, 5*(1), 11–17.

Campinha-Bacote, J., Yahle, T., & Langenkamp, M. (1996). The challenge of cultural diversity for nurse educators. *Journal of Continuing Education in Nursing, 2*(2), 59–64.

Canty-Mitchell, J. (1996). The caring needs of African American male juvenile offenders. *Journal of Transcultural Nursing, 8*(1), 3–12.

Carr, J. M. (1998). Vigilance as a caring expression and Leininger's theory of cultural care diversity and universality. *Nursing Science Quarterly, 11,* 74–78.

Chmielarczyk, V. (1991). Transcultural nursing: Providing culturally congruent care to the Hausa of Northwest Africa. *Journal of Transcultural Nursing, 3*(1), 15–19.

Cortis, J. D. (2000). Caring as experienced by minority ethnic patients. *International Nursing Review, 47*(1), 53–62.

Dean-Kelly, L. A. (1997). Concept and process of attaining and maintaining health for a selected Vietnamese immigrant population. *Dissertation Abstracts International, 58(07B),* 3554.

de Villiers, L., & van der Wal, D. (1995). Putting Leininger's nursing theory "Culture Care Diversity and Universality" into operation in the curriculum—Part I. *Curationis, 18*(4), 56–60.

Domenig, D. (1999). The mediation of transcultural nursing care in the clinical context: A tightrope walk [German]. *Pflege, 12,* 362–369.

Dootson, L. G. (2000). Adolescent homosexuality and culturally competent nursing. *Nursing Forum, 35*(3), 13–20.

Dowe, D. S. (1990). African-American diversity in nursing inservice programs. *Masters Abstracts International, 29-02,* 261.

Finn, J. M. (1994). Culture care of Euro-American women during childbirth: Using Leininger's theory. *Journal of Transcultural Nursing, 5*(2), 25–37.

Finn, J. (1995). Leininger's model for discoveries at The Farm and midwifery services to the Amish. *Journal of Transcultural Nursing, 7*(1), 28–35.

Finn, J., & Lee, M. (1996). Transcultural nurses reflect on discoveries in China using Leininger's Sunrise model. *Journal of Transcultural Nursing, 7*(2), 21–27.

Garcia, C. M. (1996). Diabetes education in the Hispanic community. *Masters Abstracts International, 35-02,* 517.

Gates, M. F. G. (1988). Care and cure meanings, experiences and orientations of persons who are dying in hospital and hospice settings. *Dissertation Abstracts International, 50-02B,* 493.

Gates, M. F. (1991). Culture care theory for study of dying patients in hospital and hospice contexts. In M. M. Leininger (Ed.), *Culture Care Diversity and Universality: A theory of nursing* (pp. 281–304) (Pub. No. 15-2402). New York: National League for Nursing Press.

Gelazis, R. (1994). Humor, care, and well-being of Lithuanian Americans: An ethnonursing study using Leininger's theory of Culture Care Diversity and Universality. *Dissertation Abstracts International, 55(04B),* 1377.

Gelazis, R. (1995). Lithuanian Americans and culture care. In M. Leininger, *Transcultural nursing: Concepts, theories, research & practices* (2nd ed.) (pp. 427–444). New York: McGraw-Hill.

George, T. B. (1998). Meanings, expressions, and experiences of care of chronically mentally ill in a day treatment center using Leininger's culture care theory. *Dissertation Abstracts International, 59(12B),* 6262.

Hahn, J. A. (1997). Transcultural nursing in home health care: Learning to be culturally sensitive. *Home Health Care Management & Practice, 10*(1), 66–71.

Haylock, P. J. (1992). Commentary on "Teaching cultural content: A nursing education imperative" [original article by Capers, C. F. in *Holistic Nursing Practice, 6*(3), 19–28]. *ONS Nursing Scan in Oncology, 1*(3), 20.

Horn, B. (1995). Transcultural nursing and child-rearing of the Muckleshoots. In M. Leininger, *Transcultural nursing: Concepts, theories, research & practices* (2nd ed.) (pp. 501–515). New York: McGraw-Hill.

Horton, B. J. (1998). Nurse anesthesia as a subculture of nursing in the United States. *Dissertation Abstracts International, 59(11B)*, 5786.

Husting, P. M. (1991). An oral history of transcultural nursing. *Dissertation Abstracts International, 52(07A)*, 2608.

Inaoka, F. (1997). Leininger's theory of nursing: Its meaning for nursing in Japan [Japanese]. *Kango Kenkyu, 30*(2), 3–6.

Jeffreys, M. R., & O'Donnell, M. (1997). Cultural discovery: An innovative philosophy for creative learning activities. *Journal of Transcultural Nursing, 8*(2), 17–22.

Kavanagh, K. H. (1993). Transcultural nursing: Facing the challenges of advocacy and diversity/universality. *Journal of Transcultural Nursing, 5*(1), 4–13.

Kinney, G. L. (1985). Caring values and caring practices of native Hawaiians in a Hawaiian home lands community. *Dissertation Abstracts International, 47(09B)*, 3706.

Kirkham, S. R. (1998). Nurses' descriptions of caring for culturally diverse clients. *Clinical Nursing Research, 7*, 125–146.

Kollak, I., & Kupper, H. (1998). Culturally sensitive care as an extension of Leininger's nursing theory [German]. *Pflege Aktuell, 52*, 226–228.

Larson-Presswalla, J. (1994). Insights into eastern health care: Some transcultural nursing perspectives. *Journal of Transcultural Nursing, 5*(2), 21–24.

Lazure, G., Vissandjee, B., Pepin, J., & Kerouac, S. (1997). Transcultural nursing and a care management partnership project. *Nursing Inquiry, 4*, 160–166.

Leininger, M. (1978). *Transcultural nursing: Concepts, theories, and practices.* New York: Wiley. (out of print)

Leininger, M. (1979). *Transcultural nursing.* New York: Masson. (out of print)

Leininger, M. M. (Ed.) (1985a). *Qualitative research methods in nursing.* Orlando, FL: Grune & Stratton.

Leininger, M. M. (1985b). Transcultural Care Diversity and Universality: A theory of nursing. *Nursing and Health Care, 6*, 209–212.

Leininger, M. M. (1988a). *Care: Discovery and uses in clinical and community nursing.* Detroit: Wayne State University Press.

Leininger, M. M. (1988b). Leininger's theory of nursing: Cultural Care Diversity and Universality. *Nursing Science Quarterly, 1*, 152–160.

Leininger, M. M. (Ed.) (1991). *Culture Care Diversity and Universality: A theory of nursing.* (Pub. No. 15-2402) New York: National League for Nursing Press.

Leininger, M. (1994). Quality of life from a transcultural nursing perspective. *Nursing Science Quarterly, 7*, 22–28.

Leininger, M. (1995). *Transcultural nursing: Concepts, theories, research & practices* (2nd ed.). New York: McGraw-Hill.

Leininger, M. (1996). Culture care theory, research, and practice. *Nursing Science Quarterly, 9*, 71–78.

Leininger, M. M. (1997a). Transcultural nursing as a global care humanizer, diversifier, and unifier. *Hoitotiede, 9*, 219–225.

Leininger, M. (1997b). Transcultural nursing research to transform nursing education and practice: 40 years. *Image, Journal of Nursing Scholarship, 29*, 341–347.

Leininger, M. M. (1999). Transcultural nursing: An imperative for nursing practice. *Imprint, 46*(5), 50–52.

Leininger, M., & Gstottner, E. (1998). Cultural dimensions of humane care—the Sunrise Model [German]. *Osterr Krankenpflegez, 51*(12), 26–29.

Ludwig-Beymer, P., Blankemeier, J. R., Casas-Byots, C., & Suarez-Balcazar, Y. (1996). Community assessment in a suburban Hispanic community: A description of method. *Journal of Transcultural Nursing, 8*(1), 19–27.

Luna, L. (1994). Care and cultural context of Lebanese Muslim immigrants: Using Leininger's theory. *Journal of Transcultural Nursing, 5*(2), 12–20.

Luna, L. J. (1995). Arab Muslims and culture care. In M. Leininger, *Transcultural nursing: Concepts, theories, research & practices* (2nd ed.) (pp. 317–333). New York: McGraw-Hill.

Luna, L. (1998). Culturally competent health care: A challenge for nurses in Saudi Arabia. *Journal of Transcultural Nursing, 9*(2), 1–14.

MacDonald, M. R., & Miller-Grolla, L. (1995). Developing a collective future: Creating a culture specific nurse caring practice model for hospitals. *Canadian Journal of Nursing Administration, 8*, 78–95.

MacNeil, J. M. (1994). Culture care: Meanings, patterns and expressions for Baganda women as AIDS caregivers within Leininger's theory. *Dissertation Abstracts International, 56-02B*, 743.

MacNeil, J. M. (1996). Use of Culture Care Theory with Baganda women as AIDS caregivers. *Journal of Transcultural Nursing, 7*(2), 14–20.

Mahon, P. Y. (1997). Transcultural nursing: A source guide. *Journal of Nursing Staff Development, 13*, 218–222.

Martsolf, D. S. (1991). The relationship between adjustment, health, and perception of care in two groups of cross-cultural students migrants. *Dissertation Abstracts International, 53(02B)*, 770.

Masumori, K. (1997). A study of children's experiences with congenital heart disease: Using Leininger's ethnonursing method [Japanese]. *Kango Kenkyu, 30*, 233–244.

Mashaba, G. (1995). Culturally-based health-illness patterns in South Africa and humanistic nursing care practices. In M. Leininger, *Transcultural nursing: Concepts, theories, research & practices* (2nd ed.) (pp. 591–602). New York: McGraw-Hill.

McFarland, M. (1995). Culture care theory and elderly Polish Americans. In M. Leininger, *Transcultural nursing: Concepts, theories, research & practices* (2nd ed., pp. 401–426). New York: McGraw-Hill.

McFarland, M. R. (1997). Use of culture care theory with Anglo- and African American elders in a long-term care setting. *Nursing Science Quarterly, 10*, 186–192.

McGee, P. (1994). Culturally sensitive and culturally comprehensive care . . . including commentary by Shomaker, D. *British Journal of Nursing, 3*, 789–793.

Miller, J. E. (1997a). Politics and care: A study of Czech Americans within Leininger's theory of Culture Care Diversity and Universality. *Dissertation Abstracts International, 58-03B*, 1216.

Miller, J. (1997b). Politics and care: A study of Czech Americans within Leininger's theory of Culture Care Diversity and Universality. *Journal of Transcultural Nursing, 9*(1), 3–13.

Morgan, M. G. (1992). Pregnancy and childbirth beliefs and practices of American Hare Kirshna devotees within transcultural nursing. *Journal of Transcultural Nursing, 4*(1), 5–10.

Morgan, M. (1995). African Americans and cultural care. In M. Leininger, *Transcultural nursing: Concepts, theories, research & practices* (2nd ed.) (pp. 383–400). New York: McGraw-Hill.

Morgan, M. (1996). Prenatal care of African American women in selected USA urban and rural cultural contexts. *Journal of Transcultural Nursing, 7*(2), 3–9.

Morse, J. M., & English, J. (1986). The incorporation of cultural concepts into basic nursing texts. *Nursing papers: Perspectives in nursing, 18*, 69–76.

Nahas, V., & Amasheh, N. (1999). Culture care meanings and experiences of postpartum depression among Jordanian Australian women: A transcultural study. *Journal of Transcultural Nursing, 10*(1), 37–45.

Narayan, M. C. (1997). Cultural assessment in home healthcare. *Home Healthcare Nursing, 15*, 663–670.

Nikkonen, M. (1994). Changes in psychiatric caring values in Finland. *Journal of Transcultural Nursing, 6*(1), 12–17.

Nobrega, M., Lopes Neto, D., Dantas, H. F., & Perez, V. L. (1996). Being a nurse in a transcultural context [Portuguese]. *Rev Bras Enferm, 49*, 399–408.

Omeri, A. (1997). Culture care of Iranian immigrants in New South Wales, Australia: Sharing transcultural nursing knowledge. *Journal of Transcultural Nursing, 8*(2), 5–16.

Paul, D. M. (1991). Description of the health experience of Athabascans living in Galena: A modified ethnographic approach. *Masters Abstracts International, 30-02*, 301.

Phillips, S., & Lobar, S. (1995). Navajo child health beliefs and rearing practices within a transcultural nursing framework: Literature review. In M. Leininger, *Transcultural nursing: Concepts, theories, research & practices* (2nd ed.) (pp. 485–500). New York: McGraw-Hill.

Rajan, M. J. (1995). Transcultural nursing: A perspective derived from Jean-Paul Sartre. *Journal of Advanced Nursing, 22*, 450–455.

Redmond, G. T. (1988). An examination of the influence of transcultural nursing on graduate curriculum in mental health nursing. *Dissertation Abstracts International, 49(12A)*, 3608.

Rohrbach-Viadas, C. (1997). Visit by Madeleine Leininger, June 1997. "In Switzerland transcultural nursing is indispensable" [French]. *Krankenpfl Soins Infirm, 90*(9), 65–66.

Rosenbaum, J. (1990). Cultural care of older Greek Canadian widows within Leininger's theory of culture care. *Journal of Transcultural Nursing, 2*(1), 37–47.

Rosenbaum, J. (1991). Culture care theory and Greek Canadian widows. In M. M. Leininger (Ed.), *Culture Care Diversity and Universality: A theory of nursing* (pp. 305–339) (Pub. No. 15-2402). New York: National League for Nursing Press.

Rosenbaum, J. N., & Carty, L. (1996). The subculture of adolescence: Beliefs and care, health and individuation with Leininger's theory. *Journal of Advanced Nursing, 23*, 741–746.

Sellers, S. C., Poduska, M. D., Propp, L. H., & White, S. I. (1999). The health care meanings, values, and practices of Anglo-American males in the rural Midwest. *Journal of Transcultural Nursing, 10*(4), 320–330.

Smith, M. (1997). False assumptions, ethnocentrism and cultural imposition . . . Madeleine Leininger's theory of culture care and its place in Aotearoa. *Nurs Prax NZ, 12*(1), 13–16.

Spangler, Z. D. L. (1991). Nursing care values and caregiving practices of Anglo-American and Philippine-American nurses conceptualized within Leininger's theory. *Dissertation Abstracts International, 52-04B*, 1960.

Stasiak, D. B. (1991). Culture care theory with Mexican Americans in an urban context. In M. M. Leininger (Ed.), *Culture Care Diversity and Universality: A theory of nursing* (pp. 179–201) (Pub. No. 15-2402). New York: National League for Nursing Press.

Stebnicki, J. A. M., & Coeling, H. V. (1999). The culture of the deaf. *Journal of Transcultural Nursing, 10*, 350–357.

Talabere, L. R. (1996). Meeting the challenge of culture care in nursing: Diversity, sensitivity, competence, and congruence. *Journal of Cultural Diversity, 3*(2), 53–61.

Villarruel, A. (1995). Cultural perspectives of pain. In M. Leininger, *Transcultural nursing: Concepts, theories, research & practices* (2nd ed.) (pp. 263–277). New York: McGraw-Hill.

Villarruel, A., & Leininger, M. (1995). Culture care of Mexican Americans. In M. Leininger, *Transcultural nursing: Concepts, theories, research & practices* (2nd ed.) (pp. 365–382). New York: McGraw-Hill.

Watson, J. (1988). *Nursing: Human science and human care.* (Pub. No. 15-2236) New York: National League for Nursing.

Wenger, A. F. (1991). The culture care theory and the Old Order Amish. In M. M. Leininger (Ed.), *Culture Care Diversity and Universality: A theory of nursing* (pp. 147–178) (Pub. No. 15-2402). New York: National League for Nursing Press.

Wenger, A. F. (1995). Cultural context, health and health care decision making 1994. *Journal of Transcultural Nursing, 7*(1), 3–14.

Wing, D. M., & Thompson, T. (1996). The meaning of alcohol to traditional Muscogee Creek Indians. *Nursing Science Quarterly, 9*, 175–180.

Zoucha, R., & Husted, G. L. (2000). The ethical dimensions of delivering culturally congruent nursing and health care. *Issues in Mental Health Nursing, 21*, 325–340.

SELECTED ANNOTATED BIBLIOGRAPHY

Baker, S. S., & Burkhalter, N. C. (1996). Teaching transcultural nursing in a transcultural setting. *Journal of Transcultural Nursing, 7*(2), 10–13.

> The authors present a cultural encounter between the faculty and students in a baccalaureate nursing program and the nurse–patient–community system found in the Texas–Mexico border town of Laredo. This transnational, transcultural setting provided a challenging environment for assessing the effectiveness of the theory of Culture Care Diversity and Universality and its three modes of nursing action.

Baldonado, A., Beymer, P. L., Barnes, K., Starsiak, D., Nemivant, E. B., and Anonas-Ternate, A. (1998). Transcultural nursing practice described by registered nurses and baccalaureate nursing students. *Journal of Transcultural Nursing, 9*(2), 15–25.

> This study of 767 registered nurses and senior baccalaureate nursing students found that neither group was confident about providing care to culturally diverse patients. The registered nurses did report a higher degree of use of cultural assessment data to modify care than did the students. Both groups identified an overwhelming need for transcultural nursing care and reported they seek to respond to cultural challenges through modifications of care. Care modifications were based on communication, language, perception of pain and pain relief, aspects of religious and spiritual beliefs, gender, family roles, and identified cultural values. Respondents did not identify the use of a conceptual framework to conduct these assessments and to plan the modifications of care.

Bodner, A., & Leininger, M. (1992). Transcultural nursing care values, beliefs, and practices of American (USA) gypsies. *Journal of Transcultural Nursing, 4*(1), 17–28.

> This study was based on the theory of Culture Care Diversity and Universality and used the ethnonursing research method. Findings substantiated the importance of culture to Gypsies. Care meanings identified include protective in-group caring, watching over and guarding against Gadje (outsiders), facilitating care rituals, respecting the values of the Gypsy culture, alleviating Gadje harassment, remaining suspicious of Gadje, and dealing with moral codes and rules related to purity and impurity.

Cameron, C. F. (1990). An ethnonursing study of the influence of extended caregiving on the health status of elderly Anglo-Canadian wives caring for physically disabled husbands. *Dissertation Abstracts International, 52*(02B), 746.

> This qualitative study investigated the care experiences and health status of elderly Anglo-Canadian wives as they provided care for their physically disabled spouses over an extended period of time. These women were of English, Scottish, and Irish descent. The major commonalities found included that culture care patterns of caregiving influenced the health status of the spouse; the meanings and experiences of the caregivers reflected cultural care values, social structure, and environmental context; female caregiving was culturally transmitted as caring for others throughout the life cycle; and caring activity patterns helped maintain the health of the caregivers and of others. Diversity was found in the potential for neglect, acceptance of caregiving by strangers, and culture specific planning for care in the future. Several generic care constructs were identified. These included concern for, both affectionate and spiritual love, attention, and duty. Obligation and care concepts included commitment to care, continuous caring, care enculturation, other care, and care appreciation.

Canty-Mitchell, J. (1996). The caring needs of African American male juvenile offenders. *Journal of Transcultural Nursing, 8*(1), 3–12.

This ethnonursing study investigated the social and cultural needs of male African American juvenile offenders. Five juveniles, aged 12 to 15 years old, living in a southeastern U.S. inner city participated in the interviews. A general theme was found to be survival in the face of loss. Domains of loss were family, social, and self-identity and the categories of loss in each domain were loss of caring, loss of protection, loss of discipline, and loss of support with the threat to survival dominant in each type of loss. Culturally congruent nursing actions were identified.

Cortis, J. D. (2000). Caring as experienced by minority ethnic patients. *International Nursing Review, 47*(1), 53–62.

This qualitative study reports the results of in-depth interviews with Pakistanis (20 males and 18 females) from Bradford, West Yorkshire, United Kingdom, about their perceptions of caring. In general, findings indicated a lack of congruence between the respondents' expectations of caring and their experiences of caring received from nurses.

Garcia, C. M. (1996). Diabetes education in the Hispanic community. *Masters Abstracts International, 35-02,* 517.

This master's thesis examined the effects of a community based, culturally congruent educational program on diabetes self-efficacy and hemoglobin A1C measurements in a Hispanic community. A pretest–posttest design was used with a sample of 32 subjects. The difference in diabetes self-efficacy was found to be statistically significant while a statistically significant difference in A1C was not found.

Gelazis, R. (1994). Humor, care, and well-being of Lithuanian Americans: An ethnonursing study using Leininger's theory of Culture Care Diversity and Universality. *Dissertation Abstracts International, 55(04B),* 1377.

This ethnonursing research study investigated the cultural implications of humor in Lithuanian Americans. The findings indicated that cultural humor assists in bearing life's burdens, diffusing potential confrontations, and supporting and enhancing well-being through supporting a positive outlook on life; serves a survival function; is subtle and abstract and expressed in daily life events; has a caring function to increase a sense of closeness and well being. Care themes indicate that care is a basic orientation with an attitude of concern for others, expressed as a community, and means protection with protective care modalities. Well-being themes indicated that well-being is broadly defined as a positive state of mind about self and the world, is holistic (including spiritual, emotional, physical, social, and economic aspects in balance), and the history of their culture strongly influenced identity and commitment to survival of the culture which led to a sense of well-being. The two constructs of cultural humor and culture care humor were identified.

Horton, B. J. (1998). Nurse anesthesia as a subculture of nursing in the United States. *Dissertation Abstracts International, 59(11B),* 5786.

Horton sought to demonstrate that nurse anesthesia is a subculture of nursing through this ethnonursing study of 55 registered nurse and certified registered nurse anesthetists. The five identified themes were that nurse anesthetists have a common worldview of the cultural values of nurse anesthesia; are committed to and show responsibility for the patients they serve; remain active and vigilant to defend and maintain their professional practice rights; reflect a subculture distinctly different from, while having commonalities with, the culture of nursing; have rituals and symbols that provide patient benefits and reinforce solidarity within nurse anesthesia. The findings support nurse anesthesia as a subculture of nursing.

Morgan, M. (1996). Prenatal care of African American women in selected USA urban and rural cultural contexts. *Journal of Transcultural Nursing, 7*(2), 3–9.

This ethnonursing study investigated prenatal care of African American women within their familiar cultural contexts. The impetus for the study arose from studies that connected lack of prenatal care in African American women with low birth weights and high infant mortality rates. Four major themes were identified. Cultural care meant protection, presence, and sharing. Health and well being were influenced by such social structural factors as spirituality, kinship factors, and economics. While professional prenatal care was seen as necessary, even essential, barriers, including distrust of noncaring professionals, inhibited the receipt of such care. African American women reported wide use of folk health beliefs and practices as well as indigenous health care providers.

Redmond, G. T. (1988). An examination of the influence of transcultural nursing on graduate curriculum in mental health nursing. *Dissertation Abstracts International, 49(12A)*, 3608.

The data for this study were derived from telephone interviews with Leininger and National League for Nursing Self Study reports from the "Top Twenty" schools of nursing in the United States. Findings indicated very few cultural and transcultural elements in the curricular documents studied. Data supported that faculty influence the cultural and transcultural content in graduate mental health nursing programs. Also, the philosophical foundations and curricular components of the programs studied demonstrated discontinuities, and qualitative research methods were seldom taught. In contrast, quantitative research methods were universally included in the program. Finally, those curricula that included more cultural or transcultural elements also included more content on implementation of civil rights laws.

Spangler, Z. D. L. (1991). Nursing care values and caregiving practices of Anglo-American and Philippine-American nurses conceptualized within Leininger's theory. *Dissertation Abstracts International, 52(04B)*, 1960.

This ethnonursing study sought to identify the cultural care diversities and universalities in relation to nursing care values and caregiving practices of Anglo-American and Philippine-American nurses in hospital practice. The identified diversity themes were that the care of Anglo-American nurses was characterized by promotion of autonomy (self-care), assertiveness, and situation control. The care of Philippine-American nurses was characterized by an obligation to care based on the care values of conscience, physical comfort, respect, and patience. Nurse-to-nurse conflicts were generated by cultural conflicts. Philippine-American nurses sought cultural care congruence through use of the three modes of nursing action. Two universal themes were also identified. These were the concerns associated with the nursing shortage (increased workload, frustration, inability to provide total patient care) and the influence of institutional norms, standards, and regulations on nursing practice. Implications of this study include the need to re-examine the expectation that foreign educated nurses should adopt American nursing care values, rather than American and foreign-educated nurses learning from each other.

CHAPTER 22

HEALTH AS EXPANDING CONSCIOUSNESS MARGARET NEWMAN

Julia B. George

■ ■ ■

Margaret Newman (b. 1933) received a B.S.H.E. in home economics and English from Baylor University in Texas in 1954; a B.S. in nursing from the University of Tennessee, Memphis, in 1962; an M.S. in nursing from the University of California, San Francisco, in 1964; and a Ph.D. in nursing science and rehabilitation nursing from New York University in 1971. She relates that she resisted the feeling that she should become a nurse as she completed her first bachelor's degree and during the next eight years while she served as the primary caregiver during her mother's struggle with amyotrophic lateral sclerosis. Her mother died just as Newman had prayed that she was willing to become a nurse. Within two weeks of her mother's death, Newman was a nursing major at the University of Tennessee and quickly decided that nursing was right for her.

Newman has held faculty positions at the University of Tennessee, New York University, and The Pennsylvania State University. She retired as professor in the School of Nursing at the University of Minnesota in 1996. In addition to these faculty positions, she has served as director of nursing for the University of Tennessee Clinical Research Center, acting director of nursing for the Ph.D. program in nursing science at New York University, and professor-in-charge of the graduate program in nursing at The Pennsylvania State University.

She is an active scholar and the recipient of many honors. She has served, or is serving, on the editorial boards of many scholarly nursing journals, including Advances in Nursing Science, Journal of Professional Nursing, Nursing and Health Care, Nursing Research, Nursing Science Quarterly, *and* Western Journal of Nursing Research. *She is a Fellow in the American Academy of Nursing, listed in Who's Who in American Women, and the recipient of the Outstanding Alumnus Award from the University of Tennessee College of Nursing and the Distinguished Alumnus Award and Distinguished Scholar in Nursing from the New York University Division of Nursing. She has also received the Sigma Theta Tau International Founders Award for Excellence in Nursing Research and the E. Louise Grant Award for Nursing Excellence from the University of Minnesota. She has been a Latin American Teaching*

Fellow and an American Journal of Nursing Scholar. She has conducted workshops and conferences and served as a consultant around the world, including Australia, Brazil, Canada, Czechoslovakia, France, Finland, Germany, Japan, New Zealand, Poland, and the United Kingdom, in addition to the United States.

Margaret Newman states that during her doctoral study she was interested in theory in nursing (Wallace & Coberg, 1990). More specifically, as a result of her experiences during her mother's illness, she was interested in the relationships between movement, time, and space, for she describes her mother as having been immobilized in time and space. Newman states that she did not intentionally begin to develop a theory but, rather, "slid" into theory development. Her preparations to speak at a conference in 1978 marked the beginning of her defined intention to explicate the temporal and spatial patterns of health. She says that at this time she was moving toward a theory of health. She chose health as a focus because she saw disease as a meaningful aspect of health and believed health needed better definition.

In developing her theory, Newman (1994a) was influenced by Martha Rogers (1970), Bentov (1978), Bohm (1980, 1981, 1992), Moss (1981), Prigogine (1976), and Young (1976a, 1976b). From Rogers she drew upon the concepts of pattern and the unitary nature of human beings with particular emphasis on the importance of the basic assumption of pattern. The unitary human being is open and in interaction with its environment. There are no real boundaries between human and environment; pattern is an identification of the wholeness of the person. Newman identified disease as a manifestation of pattern (Wallace & Coberg, 1990). Bentov's view of consciousness as evolving and being coextensive with the universe supported Newman's concept of health as expanding consciousness. Bohm's discussion of implicate and explicate order supported the idea of health as a pattern of the whole with a normal progression toward higher levels of organization. Moss's presentation of love as the highest level of consciousness was affirming of Newman's views of the nature of health and nursing. Prigogine's theory of dissipative structures supported the idea that seemingly negative events are part of the process of expanding consciousness (Newman, 1997a). Young's discussion of the importance of insight, pattern recognition, and choice provided the impetus for the integration of the concepts of movement, time, and space into a dynamic theory of health.

HEALTH AS EXPANDING CONSCIOUSNESS

Concepts and Assumptions

Newman (1994a, 1994b) states that she began the development of her theory with an effort to follow the demands of logical positivism. Thus, she identified concepts and assumptions for her theory. Her basic assumptions, based on Rogers and Bentov, were the following:

1. Health encompasses conditions known as disease.
2. Disease can be considered a manifestation of the underlying pattern of the person.
3. The pattern of the person that manifests itself as disease is primary and exists prior to structural or functional changes.
4. Health is the expansion of consciousness (Newman, 1997, p. 22).

The initial concepts were movement, time, space, and consciousness (Newman, 1979). Newman discussed *movement* as an essential property of matter and the change that occurs between two states of rest, but she did not define the other concepts initially. She did propose relationships among the concepts as the following:

1. Time and space have a complementary relationship.
2. Movement is a means whereby space and time become a reality.
3. Movement is a reflection of consciousness.
4. Time is a function of movement.
5. Time is a measurement of consciousness (p. 60).

More currently, Marchione (1993) states that Newman's implicit assumptions are that humans have the following characteristics:

- Open energy systems.
- In continual interconnectedness with a universe of open systems (environment).
- Continuously active in evolving their own pattern of the whole (health).
- Intuitive as well as affective and cognitive beings.
- Capable of abstract thinking as well as sensation.
- More than the sum of their parts (p. 6).

The current definition of movement remains the same as Newman's initial definition. *Time and timing* relate the rhythm of living phenomena (Newman, 1994a). Examples include the variations in the effectiveness of drug and radiation therapies throughout a 24-hour cycle. Dosages that are therapeutic at one period during the day may be fatal during another period. Individuals who refuse to adhere to the time schedule of a hospital are often identified as uncooperative even though social adherence could be detrimental to the person. For example, a newly diagnosed diabetic woman was carefully taught to follow her prescribed diet and insulin plan throughout a standard day of breakfast, lunch, and dinner. It was not until she was readmitted to regain diabetic control that it was discovered she worked nights and was having difficulty following the prescribed meal plan! Time is also seen as a symbol of status. When a person has an appointment with a physician, who is the most likely to have to wait and who is seen as having the greater status? Timing is recognized as important in the provision of nursing care, particularly in home health. A description supporting the importance of timing follows:

> When . . . [the client was] ready to express her feelings of confinement and explore options for opening her world, I made weekly home visits. When she returned to insulin use, I made weekly home visits plus three or four telephone calls per week for about one and a half months. During times when she let me know in her ways that it [was] not her time for change, I allowed the interval between visits to increase to a month and relied on her to call me if needed (Newman, Lamb & Michaels, 1992, p. 406).

Space is discussed in conjunction with time and movement and not defined separately.

Newer concepts include consciousness and expanding consciousness, pattern, pattern recognition, and transformation. *Consciousness* is "the *information* of the system; the capacity of the system to interact with the environment" (Newman, 1994a, p. 33). In humans this "informational capacity includes not only all the things we normally associate with consciousness, such as thinking and feeling, but also all the information embedded in the nervous system, the endocrine system, the immune system, the genetic code and so on" (p. 33). As human beings develop, consciousness grows, or expands. As consciousness expands, the more it coexists with the universe. Consciousness is the essence of all matter; persons do not possess consciousness, they *are* consciousness. The direction of life is ever toward higher levels of consciousness.

Pattern depicts the whole and is characterized by movement, diversity, and rhythm. Movement is constant and rhythmic, and the parts are diverse. Pattern is relatedness; the process of patterning occurs as human energy fields penetrate one another and transformation occurs. *Transformation* is change that occurs all-at-once rather than in a gradual and linear fashion. As more information is obtained, pattern evolves unidirectionally and becomes more highly organized.

Pattern recognition occurs within the observer. Although we may predict the next event in a sequence, on the basis of knowledge of the sequence to date, we cannot make such predictions *with certainty* because additional information that indicates a change in the sequence has not happened (Bateson, 1979). Thus, if given a sequence of 3, 6, 9, 12 we are likely to predict that the next number would be 15 when in reality the sequence is 3, 6, 9, 12, 16, 20, 24, 28, 33, 38, and so on. It may not be possible to see the pattern all at once. We need to remind ourselves that the piece of reality that is known to us is only a portion of the total reality. Newman (1994a) suggests that more of the pattern is revealed as the time frame is expanded. We follow this concept of increased knowledge of pattern with increased time when we need three elevated blood pressure readings taken at different times to identify an individual as hypertensive. It is also important to note that each pattern is embedded in another pattern. The pattern in the individual is embedded in the pattern of the family and of the family in the pattern of the community and so on. The more we comprehend the whole, the more knowledge of the parts becomes meaningful. Paradoxically, the whole may be seen in the parts. A change in the way an individual walks may communicate an overall mood of sadness or glee. Pattern recognition helps find meaning and understanding and in doing so speeds up the evolution of consciousness (Newman, 1997a).

Health and Disease

Newman (1994a) believes that a new view of *health* is needed. The old view that health is the absence of disease has been associated with a tendency to view those without health as inferior. She proposes that Hegel's dialectical fusion of opposites to form a synthesized new could fuse disease and nondisease to form a new concept of health. She adds Jantsch's (1980) idea that such fusion may transcend synthesis and, indeed, opposites come to include each other. Bohm (1981) states that when such synthesis is followed to its logical conclusion the opposites pass into each other, reflect each other, and are recognized as identical to each other. From these viewpoints, disease becomes "a meaningful reflection of the whole [of health]" (Newman, 1994a, p. 7). Newman states that Rogers (1970) eliminated the view of health and disease as dichotomies when she proposed persons as unitary human beings. Within such a view, health and disease are not separate entities but "*are each reflections of the larger whole*" (Newman, 1994a, p. 9). Again drawing on Bohm, Newman uses the example of the two views of the same scene provided by cameras that photograph that scene from different angles. Just as the pictures from each camera provide different pictures of the same whole, disease and nondisease provide different views of health.

Newman states that health, disease, and the pattern of the whole are consistent with Bohm's (1980) theory of implicate and explicate order. Implicate order is that "unseen, multidimensional pattern that is the ground, or basis, for all things" (Newman, 1994a, p. 10). Explicate order arises out of the implicate order and includes the tangibles—those things we can identify with our senses—of the world. Because we can see, touch, hear, feel the tangibles we tend to identify them as primary, which is contrary to Bohm's statement that implicate order is primary. In this sense, "*manifest health, encompassing disease and non-disease, can be regarded as the explication of the underlying pattern of person-environment*" (Newman, 1994a, p. 11). The explicate is a manifestation of the implicate (Newman, 1997a, p. 22).

Newman proposes that those fluctuations in patterns identified as sickness can provide the disturbance needed to reorganize the relationships of a pattern more harmoniously. Illness may achieve what people have wanted but have been unable to acknowledge; it can provide or represent the disequilibrium needed to maintain the vital active exchange with the environment. We grow or evolve through experiencing disequilibrium and learning how to attain a new sense of balance. Thus, disease may be seen as both emergent pattern and expanding consciousness. It is important to remember that although an individual may exhibit the emergent pattern labeled disease, that individual's pattern relates to and affects the patterns of others—family, friends, community. As open energy systems in constant interaction, humans influence one another's patterns and evolve together.

Newman (1994a) cites Ferguson's (1980) discussion of the paradigm shift that is occurring in the view of health. She describes it as a shift from an instrumental to a relational view. The shift includes searching for *patterns* instead of treating symptoms; perceiving pain and disease as *information* instead of seeing them as totally negative; viewing the body as a *dynamic field of energy* that is continuous with a larger field instead of as a machine in various states of repair or disrepair; and seeing disease as a *process* rather than an entity. The new paradigm of health, in its embrace of a unitary pattern of changing relationships, is essential to nursing. Within this paradigm the task is not to seek to change the pattern of another but to recognize that pattern as information that represents the whole and to seek to relate to the pattern as it unfolds. The relational paradigm of health incorporates and transforms the old instrumental paradigm. The characteristics of the instrumental paradigm—linear, causal, predictive, rational, controlling, dichotomous—need to be seen as special cases of the new relational paradigm. The characteristics of the new paradigm are pattern, emerging, unpredictable, unitary, intuitive, and innovative.

When health is seen as a pattern of the whole, disease becomes an emergent pattern that can be understood in terms of a pattern of energy (Newman, 1994a). Seeing disease as a manifestation of pattern can help people become aware of their pattern of person–environment interaction. The insight that is gained can be transforming, both for the person and the family. Newman draws on Young's (1976b) discussion of the acceleration of the evolution of consciousness to explain such transformation. Young emphasizes the process of interaction both among individuals and between people and society in reaching the goal of a higher level of development. He describes seven stages in this evolution. The first is potential freedom, which moves into the second stage, or binding. In binding, the collective is primary, the individual is not important, everything is regulated and initiative is not needed. In the third stage, centering, individual identity, self-consciousness, and self-determination develop as the person breaks with authority. The fourth stage, choice, is the turning point in which the individual learns the "law." The emphasis in choice is on science and a search for laws with a new awareness of self-limitation. When the law is learned, the fifth stage, or de-centering, begins and the emphasis shifts away from self-development to something greater than the individual. Energy is a dominant feature and one's works develop a life of their own; the experience is one of unlimited growth. The sixth stage, unbinding, involves increasing freedom from time, and the seventh stage represents complete freedom and unrestricted choice. Newman (1994a) says that most of us do not experience stages six and beyond. She does state that Young's conception of evolution and her own model of health as expanding consciousness are corollaries:

> We come into being from a state of potential consciousness, are bound in time, find our identity in space, and through movement we learn the "law" of the way things work and make choices that ultimately take us beyond space and time to a state of absolute consciousness (p. 46).

It is from Young that Newman derived her emphasis on the importance of a choice point. A choice point occurs when the old ways of doing things no longer work and new answers must be sought. The experience is one of disconnectedness—the familiar does not function in the expected way, things are falling apart. This sense of disorder is a predecessor of a transformation to a higher level of consciousness.

Such transformation is characterized by the knowledge that the old rules no longer apply and by the willingness to tolerate some degree of uncertainty and ambiguity until the emerging pattern becomes clearer.

Newman (1994a) says that disease is not necessary for evolution to higher levels of consciousness. She cites Bentov (1978) and Moss (1981) in discussing the fact that the degree of flexibility one uses to responding to stress helps to determine how disabling that stress will be. The more open and flexible one is, the more energy can flow through and the less stress has negative effects. Newman recommends that "we accept the experience as *our* experience regardless of how contrary it is to what we might have wished would happen" (p. 29).

> In the model of health as expanding consciousness it does not matter where one is in the spectrum. There is no basis for rejecting any experience as irrelevant. The important factor is to be fully present in the moment and know that whatever the experience, it is a manifestation of the process of evolving to higher consciousness (p. 68).

New Paradigm

Newman, Sime, and Corcoran-Perry (1991) have proposed a perspective for nursing that they call the unitary–transformative paradigm. The unitary–transformative paradigm views "the human being as a unitary phenomenon unfolding in an undivided universe" (Newman, 1994a, p. 82). Phenomena are identified by pattern and by interaction with the larger whole. Change is unidirectional, unpredictable, and transformative. Change occurs as systems move through periods or stages of organization and disorganization (choice points) to become more complex. Disruptive processes are seen as phases of reorganization. Health is seen as the evolving pattern of the whole, which illustrates the unfolding implicate order. The person is seen as unitary *and* continuous with the undivided wholeness of the universe. As either person or universe transforms, the other transforms and there are no identifiable boundaries. Characteristics of this paradigm may be found in Table 22–1.

The appropriate methodology for studying this paradigm is a hermenutic, dialectic approach (Newman, 1994, 1997a). Hermenutic represents the search for meaning and dialectic respresents the process and content aspects with each revealing the

TABLE 22–1. THE UNITARY–TRANSFORMATIVE PARADIGM

Moving From	To Unitary–Transformative
Attention to other as object	Attention to the "we" in relationship
Fixing things	Attending to the meaning of the whole
Hierarchical one-way interventions	Mutual process partnering
Focus on power, manipulation, and control	Reflective compassionate consciousness
Seeking cause (the past) and prediction (the future)	Process (the present) "relaxing into the uncertainty and unpredictability of this process"

Source: Adapted from Newman, M. M. (1997). *Experiencing the whole.* Advances in Nursing Science, 20(1), 34–49.

other—process as content and content as process. Newman supports research as praxis (Newman, 1990a; 1994a). She uses Wheeler and Chinn's (1984) definition of praxis as "thoughtful reflection and action that occur in synchrony, in the direction of transforming the world" (p. 2). Newman indicates that both the participants and the researchers experience growth as her interactive research methodology is carried out. She believes that research must focus on practice realities and not be limited to outcomes. It is important that the nursing research help practitioners understand and act in their unique situations. The content of the research is the process of the nursing, seeking pattern recognition. The theory of expanding consciousness is used as *a priori* theory to inform and illuminate the experiences of the participants in the research.

HEALTH AS EXPANDING CONSCIOUSNESS AND THE FOUR MAJOR CONCEPTS

Newman (1994a) deals with all the concepts in nursing's metaparadigm. *Human beings* are unitary with the *environment*. There are no boundaries. Human beings are identified by their patterns. The patterns of individuals are embedded in those of their family and, in turn, these are embedded in the patterns of the community and society. Humans are moving toward ever-increasing organization and are capable of making their own decisions. Progression to a higher level of organization often occurs after a period of disorganization, or choice point, when the older ways no longer work. Movement is a pivotal choice point in evolving consciousness and is the expression of consciousness. Restriction of movement forces one beyond space–time.

Health is expanding consciousness: "the evolving pattern of the whole, the explication of the unfolding implicate order" (Newman, 1994a, pp. 82–83). Health is a synthesis of disease and nondisease. Newman's theory is about health; further discussion of health can be found in the presentation of the theory in this chapter.

Newman (1994a) discusses *nursing* as a profession, presenting three stages in the growth of the profession. The first stage is formative. In this stage nursing was in the process of becoming, of establishing its identity, and individual practitioners were responsible for their own practice. In the second or normative stage, nursing lost some of its authority and was more competitive and persuasive in relation to the environment. During this stage, nursing moved primarily into the hospital setting and nurses became employees. The third stage is the integrative stage. Newman thinks that nursing is moving into the third stage but has not yet completed the process. In the integrative stage nursing will relate to other health care providers and to clients as partners, in a cooperative, mutual manner. Newman (1990b) suggests that three nursing roles are essential to the integrative model. The professional nursing role is the primary integrative role; Newman refers to this role as nursing clinician/case manager. The other two roles are that of nursing team leader and staff nurse. The nursing clinician/case manager embraces the whole of the nursing paradigm; the staff nurse functions primarily from the medical or disease-oriented paradigm; the nursing team leader serves as a liaison between the two to integrate and coordinate all into individualized care for every client. Notice that these three roles demonstrate the incorporation of the old (disease-oriented paradigm) within the new (nursing paradigm) with the old becoming part of the whole rather than the primary focus of activity.

Newman (1994a) defines nursing as "*caring in the human health experience*" (p. 139). She believes that caring is a moral imperative for nursing. On the basis of Moss's (1981) statement on love, she says that caring is something that transforms all of us and all that we do, rather than being something that we do. Caring reflects the whole of the person. Caring requires that we be open. Being open is being vulnerable. Being vulnerable may lead to suffering, which we tend to avoid. Avoiding suffering can impede our efforts to move to higher levels of consciousness. "The need is to let go, embrace our experience, and allow the expansion of consciousness to unfold" (Newman, 1994a, p. 142). Without caring, nursing does not occur.

HEALTH AS EXPANDING CONSCIOUSNESS AND THE NURSING PROCESS

When health is conceptualized as the expansion of consciousness in a universe of undivided wholeness, intervention aimed at producing a particular result becomes a problem. To intervene with a particular solution in mind is to say we know what form the pattern of expanding consciousness will take, and we don't. Moss (1981), who declares himself a *former* general practitioner of medicine, asks where is the world going anyway, except around in circles. Somehow this bigger picture makes it easier to relax and enjoy an authentic involvement/evolvement with another person (Newman, 1994a, p. 97).

In the relational paradigm described by Newman (1994a), the focus is not on the professional identifying what is wrong (*assessment* and *diagnosis*), or on planning and taking steps to correct the problem (*outcomes, planning, implementation, evaluation*). Rather, the professional enters into partnership with the client. The situation that brings the client to the attention of the nurse is often one of chaos and, at the minimum, involves circumstances that the client does not know how to handle. The client is at a choice point and is seeking a partner to participate in an authentic relationship. The nurse and client trust that, through the process of the unfolding of the relationship, both will emerge at a higher level of consciousness. The nurse is with the client throughout the process.

The intent of the nurse is to "enter into the process with the client to be present with it, attend to it and live it, even if it appears in the form of disharmony, catastrophe, or disease" (Newman, 1994a, p. 99). To accomplish this, the nurse must give up the compulsion to fix things, to shape the world in a previous image of what health is or should be. Newman believes that the joy of nursing is in being present with clients through disorganization and disharmony with "an unconditional acceptance of the unpredictable, paradoxical nature of life" (p. 103). Such acceptance does not mean doing nothing. Action becomes apparent as pattern becomes apparent. In the client situations Newman presents as examples, she identifies the nurse as "doing" many of the things that would be done within the old framework—providing support and information, for example. It is the intent with which these things are done that differs. In the unitary–transformative paradigm, the nurse's actions are part of the process of being with another as both nurse and client seek expanded consciousness. The actions are not oriented toward achieving a preestablished goal determined by the nurse. Newman describes successful outcomes as "a shift from concentration on self to a broader perspective that extends beyond self, a kind of universal perspective . . . manifest in congruence between inner and outer experience and a greater capacity for love and relatedness in the world. The health professional's awareness of being, rather than doing, is the primary mechanism" (p. 103).

Newman describes this nurse–client relationship as similar to the events that occur after two pebbles are thrown into a pool of water. From the entry point of each pebble ripples begin to emanate. These ripples continue to radiate, meet, interact, and develop an interference pattern. The interference pattern spreads and is part of the whole of each of the original patterns. If we substitute two people for the pebbles and the waves of each of their patterns for the ripples in the water, we have an interaction pattern similar to that shown in Figure 22–1. To be in touch with another one needs to be in touch with one's own pattern. The more we know ourselves, the clearer we can be in expressing our patterns to others and in coming to know them. There are no separate parts; the pattern is to be sensed as a whole, as a continuous flow of movement with relationships that continue to merge and move apart. "The nurse–client relationship is a rhythmic coming together and moving apart of the client and the nurse" (Newman, 1994, p. 112).

The five-step nursing process does not apply to Newman's theory. The implication of the five-step process that predictive goals can be set and that outcomes should be measured against these goals is not compatible with Newman's statements that we cannot make predictions with certainty and that we do not know what form expanding consciousness will take. For Newman, the process of nursing is one

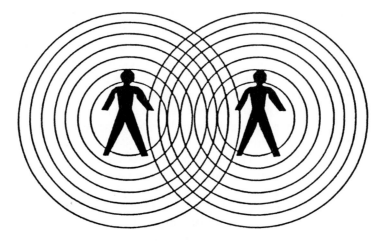

Figure 22–1. Interaction pattern of two persons: A holographic model of intervention. *(Used by permission from Newman, M. A. (1994). Health as expanding consciousness (2nd ed.). New York: National League for Nursing Press. Used with permission of National League for Nursing, New York, NY.)*

of coming together as partners during a time of chaos when the client is at a choice point. The nurse is there to be with the client and to accept the unpredictable nature of life. Accepting the circumstances decreases the stress in responding to those circumstances. Although the nurse may share knowledge, provide support, or be an organizing force in the relationship, the primary function for the nurse in this caring relationship is awareness of being. Attending to silence is at least as crucial as attending to utterances and movements. When the client is ready, the nurse and client will again move apart. It is hoped that each will have reached a higher level of consciousness through the experience.

An example of a Newman-based nurse–client experience is demonstrated in Michaels' (2000) story, "About Marie":

> I visited Marie, who was living with severe chronic obstructive pulmonary disease. Being on continuous oxygen and many medications for heart and lung disease, Marie's goal was to discontinue all the prescribed medications and shift to herbs. She was an avid shopper in health food stores and had considerable knowledge about the desired effects of herbs and other nonprescribed medications. Marie felt vulnerable and expended much of her energy taking care of herself. She was easily frightened. For example, Marie would startle when the phone rang. In dialogue with her about her life situation, Marie decided she wanted to learn to relax. She found in her closet a hand-held biofeedback device intended for a family member. She used that device continuously for more than a month and finally reached a point where she was able to relax no matter what was happening to her. Several months later she had to undergo a cholecystectomy. Her physicians wondered whether she would survive the surgery or be able to get off the ventilator. She did survive the surgery and came off the ventilator effortlessly. She attributed her success to the biofeedback device. Marie was never able to attribute success to herself alone. She relied on and gave credit to external agents for success—her medication, or herbs, or the hand-held biofeedback device. She used the hand-held biofeedback device to change her response to environmental stimuli and life events. In her efforts, Marie began to discern her pattern and meaning. She remained steadfast in believing that it was only something outside of herself that would help her. With a strong faith, Marie was not afraid of death, but she did fear dying alone. Several months later, Marie contracted pneumonia, was hospitalized, and died (Michaels, 2000, p. 29).

CRITIQUE OF NEWMAN'S THEORY OF HEALTH AS EXPANDING CONSCIOUSNESS

1. What is the historical context of the theory? Newman began the development of her theory in the late 1970s, a time during which much work was being done in the development of nursing theories. She began using the deterministic, positivist approach that was the accepted mode of knowledge development at that time. She found she was not satisfied with the results she was achieving; she was finding some evidence of support for her ideas but recognized that the knowledge development methods being used were not consistent with the paradigm underlying the theory. Therefore, the findings could not adequately guide practice.

For nearly three decades, Newman has challenged us to view the phenomenon of health in a different way. Her proposal of health as expanding consciousness, with health and disease parts of the same whole, interrelated space, time, movement, and pattern in a new way. Although concepts are present within her work, they are not primary to understanding the unitary–transformative paradigm. She indicates that she has moved beyond the interrelationship of concepts to the interrelationship of human beings.

2. What are the basic concepts and relationships presented by the theory? The basic concepts are health, expanding consciousness, the whole or unitary person, choice points, pattern, pattern recognition, movement, space, time. Newman recognizes that there are movement–time–space dimensions in the unitary evolving patterns of consciousness (Newman, 1997a, p. 25). The major relationship is that health is expanding consciousness.

3. What major phenomena of concern to nursing are presented? These phenomena may include *but are not limited to*: human being, environment, health, interpersonal relations, caring goal attainment, adaptation, and energy fields. Human beings and environment are unitary, thus inseparable. Health is a major focus of the theory. Nursing and caring are also major phenomena of concern.

4. To whom does it apply? In what situations? In what ways? Newman's theory of Health as Expanding Consciousness is not limited by person or setting. It is generalizable to anybody, anywhere. Her presentation of nursing within this theory is limited to those situations in which caring occurs. She states that without caring, nursing is not present.

5. By what method or methods can this theory be tested? Newman supports the use of the theory of health as expanding consciousness as *a priori* in research. However, she does not support the positivistic view of hypothesis development and testing. In her research methodology, the patterns that are identified through interviews with research participants are tested against the theory. Thus, the theory of health as expanding consciousness can be used in research and in testing. The hermeneutic dialectic methodology to be used does not include hypotheses, which represent a view of the world that is incongruent with the theory.

Research has been conducted by using Newman's theory. Newman has conducted studies on the needs of hospitalized patients (1966), time and movement (1972, 1976), subjective time (1982; Newman & Guadiano, 1984), and patterns in persons with coronary artery disease (Newman & Moch, 1991). These studies have both added to the general body of nursing knowledge and served to refine and develop her theory. Fryback's (1993) and Moch's (1988, 1990) studies supported Newman's thesis that disease is a part of health and that the emergence of disease allows health to unfold. Schorr, Farnham, and Ervin (1991) also report support for Newman's theory, whereas Mentzer and Schorr (1986) found that perceived duration of time was not related to age. Newman says that Engle's (1984, 1986) conclusion that the faster one moves, the healthier one is, is based on a paradigm other than Newman's even though Engle used the methodology that Newman had identified at that time. It is important to note that in the mid-1980s Newman had not yet explicated her hermeneutic dialectic methodology for the unitary–transformative paradigm.

6. Does this theory direct critical thinking in nursing practice? Newman's focus is on the process in the present, not on seeking causes from the past or defining outcomes for the future. Thus, the standard concept of critical thinking as being related to making decisions to achieve desired outcomes is not compatible with her theory. However, for the nurse to make the paradigm shift to focusing on the present and to "relax . . . into the uncertainty and unpredictability" (Newman, 1997a, p. 37) of the present requires a person who is critically aware of his or her own thought processes and behaviors. This theory requires a different focus for critical thinking rather than an abdication of its use.

7. Does this theory direct therapeutic nursing interventions? Newman's (1994a) discussion of research as praxis makes it clear that her intention and belief is that theory must be derived from practice, reflect the realities of practice, and inform practice. She has also proposed a model for practice that is derived from the theory (Newman, 1990b). Bramlett, Gueldner, and Sowell (1990) discussed consumer-centric advocacy as accomplished through the nurse–client interpersonal relationship and supported by Newman's indication of client freedom to be the decision maker. Others have spoken of the utility of Newman's work in guiding and improving practice. Areas of discussion have included parish nursing (Gustafson, 1990); caring for high-risk pregnant women (Kalb, 1990); practicing in a professional manner (Nelson, 1991); and pattern recognition as the essence of practice (Smith, M. C., 1990). The use of the theory at Carondelet St. Mary's has also been described (Ethridge, 1991; Michaels, 1992; Newman, Lamb, & Michaels, 1991). It must be remembered that the definition of therapeutic nursing interventions may differ when using this theory than in some other circumstances. Therapeutic nursing interventions in Health as Expanding Consciousness are not related to fixing something but to the relationship and the process of that relationship.

8. Does this theory direct communication in nursing practice? The theory does not provide directions for what to communicate about or how to communicate, but does place great importance on communication. Newman indicates that each nurse–client relationship will be unique and emphasizes the process. Process is dependent on communication.

9. Does this theory direct nursing actions that lead to favorable outcomes? Since the focus is on process and not on fixing what is wrong, it is difficult to define favorable outcomes in light of the theory of Health as Expanding Consciousness. The theory is not intended to be measured by outcomes.

10. How contagious is this theory? As identified in the biographical sketch at the beginning of this chapter, Newman has made worldwide presentations of her work. In her writings she has focused primarily on theory development, research, and practice. This is reflected in the areas of focus of publications about her work as there has been little mention of the use of this theory in education.

Areas of research include adolescents with diabetes mellitus (Schlotzhauer & Farnham, 1997); binge/purge behaviors (Muscari, 1992); caregiving couples (Schmitt, 1991); childhood cancer survivors (Karian, Jankowski, & Beal, 1998); chronic pain and music (Schorr, 1993); coronary heart disease (Newman & Moch, 1991); cultural diversity (Butrin, 1992); experience with breast cancer (Moch, 1988, 1990; Roux, 1993); families, in Canada and Japan, dealing with mental illness (Yamashita, 1998a, 1998b, 1999); family health (Litchfield, 1997); families with medically fragile children (Tommet, 1997); guided imagery (Gross, 1995); health in older adults (Engle, 1984; Kelley, 1990; Noveletsky-Rosenthal, 1996; Schorr, Farnham & Ervin, 1991); high-risk pregnancy (Schroeder, 1993); HIV/AIDS as expanding consciousness (Kendall, 1996; Lamendola & Newman, 1994); Japanese women with ovarian cancer and their families (Endo, 1996, 1998; Endo, et al., 2000); middle adolescent females (Shanahan, 1993); mid-life women (Picard, 1998, 2000); movement and time (Schorr & Schroeder, 1991); Native American women with breast cancer (Kiser Larson, 1999); patterns of persons with chronic obstructive pulmonary disease (Jonsdottir, 1994, 1998); peer support groups (Bruce-Barrett, 1998); perceptions of control and time duration (Mentzer & Schorr, 1986); professional identity (Brenner, 1986); rural black families (Smith, C. T., 1989); synchrony (Krejci, 1992); victimizing sexualization (Smith, S. K., 1997a, 1997b).

Publications about practice include case examples (Capasso, 1998); case management (Newman, Lamb, & Michaels, 1991); community nursing (Bunkers, Michaels, & Ethridge, 1997); an integrative model (Newman, 1990c); pattern recognition (Gustafson, 1990); pregnancy (Kalb, 1990).

Publications about research and theory development include Connor, 1998; Holmes, 1993; Newman, 1987, 1990a, 1990b, 1992, 1994b; Solari-Twadell, Bunkers, Wang, & Snyder, 1995; Wade, 1998; Wendler, 1996; Yamashita & Tall, 1998.

STRENGTHS AND LIMITATIONS

Strengths of Newman's work include that it is a work in progress, one that is evolving through the use of an identified research method. Also, Newman's presentation is logical. She presents the material from which she derived her ideas as needed and discusses with clarity those works that support her theory.

Her statement that health is expanding consciousness, seen in the evolving pattern of the whole, is relatively simple. Her ideas represent a paradigm shift in our view of health and of nursing and may be complex to those who do not comprehend the paradigm. This is true for any paradigm shift and should not be seen as a limitation of this theory.

There are some areas of potential confusion in her work. For example, she describes disease as disequilibrium or disruption and discusses the role played by disequilibrium in growth or the expansion of consciousness. At another point, she states that disease is not necessary and may not occur if human beings can be open to and accepting of the turn of events in their lives. She also describes humans and their environment as an undivided whole and speaks eloquently to the importance of viewing them in this way. Again, in another discussion, she indicates that the whole can be seen in its parts. She does discuss the fact that the smaller the piece being viewed is, the fuzzier the picture of the whole will be.

For those who seek structure and direction in providing nursing care, a limitation of this theory is its focus on the process in the present. For those to whom relationships are more important than products, this focus will be beneficial and a strength.

SUMMARY

Newman developed a theory of health as expanding consciousness in which disease and nondisease are synthesized to form a new view of health. Health is seen as the explication of the underlying pattern of person–environment. Humans are unitary beings moving in space–time and unfolding in an undivided universe toward increasing organization. Humans are ever changing in a unidirectional, unpredictable, and transformative (all-at-once) manner. Change is associated with periods of organization and disorganization. During disorganization, when old ways no longer are effective, humans face choice points. It is during such times that clients and nurses come together.

Nursing is "caring in the human health experience" (Newman, 1994a, p. 139). In the unitary–transformative paradigm, caring involves the whole of the nurse and the whole of the client. Nurse and client become partners in living through the period of disharmony and emerging at a higher level of consciousness. Newman proposes a hermeneutic dialectic approach to research and states that research is praxis. Both the participants and the researchers grow and learn in the interactive process of conducting the research. The experience of the participant and researcher is not unlike that of the client and nurse. Newman has provided a new view of the world of health in a logical manner. Her theory of health as expanding consciousness can be applied in any setting, and can be used in research and practice. Continued research is needed as this theory evolves.

REFERENCES

Bateson, G. (1979). *Mind and nature: A necessary unity.* Toronto: Bantam.
Bentov, I. (1978). *Stalking the wild pendulum.* New York: E. P. Dutton.
Bohm, D. (1980). *Wholeness and the implicate order.* London: Routledge & Kegan Paul.
Bohm, D. (1981). The physicist and the mystic—is a dialogue between them possible? A conversation with David Bohm conducted by Renee Weber. *Re-Vision, 4*(1), 22–35.
Bohm, D. (1992). On dialogue. *Noetic Sciences Review, 23,* 16–18.
Bramlett, M. H., Gueldner, S. H., & Sowell, R. L. (1990). Consumer-centric advocacy: Its connection to nursing frameworks. *Nursing Science Quarterly, 3,* 156–161.

Brenner, P. S. (1986). Temporal perspective, professional identity, and perceived well-being. *Dissertation Abstracts International, 47(12B)*, 4821.

Bruce-Barrett, C. A. (1998). Patterns of health and healing: Peer support and prostate cancer. *Masters Abstracts International, 37-01*, 233.

Bunkers, S. L., Michaels, C., & Ethridge, P. (1997). Advanced practice nursing in community: Nursing's opportunity. *Advanced Practice Nursing Quarterly, 2*, 79–84.

Butrin, J. E. (1992). Cultural diversity in the nurse–client encounter. *Clinical Nursing Research, 1*, 238–251.

Capasso, V. A. (1998). The theory is the practice: An exemplar. *Clinical Nurse Specialist, 12*, 226–229.

Connor, M. J. (1998). Expanding the dialogue on praxis in nursing research and practice. *Nursing Science Quarterly, 11*, 51–55.

Endo, E. (1996). Pattern recognition as a nursing intervention with adults with cancer. *Dissertation Abstracts International, 57(06B)*, 3653.

Endo, E. (1998). Pattern recognition as a nursing intervention with Japanese women with ovarian cancer. *Advances in Nursing Science, 20(4)*, 49–61.

Endo, E., Nitta, N., Inayoshi, M., Saito, R., Takemura, K., Minegishi, H., Kubo, S., & Kondo, M. (2000). Pattern recognition as a caring partnership in families with cancer. *Journal of Advanced Nursing, 32*, 603–610.

Engle, V. F. (1984). Newman's conceptual framework and the measurement of older adults' health. *Advances in Nursing Science, 7(1)*, 24–36.

Engle, V. F. (1986). The relationship of movement and time to older adults' functional health. *Research in Nursing and Health, 9*, 123–129.

Ethridge, P. (1991). A nursing HMO: Carondelet St. Mary's experience. *Nursing Management, 22(7)*, 22–27.

Ferguson, M. (1980). *The aquarian conspiracy: Personal and social transformation in the 1980s.* Los Angeles: J. P. Tarcher.

Fryback, P. B. (1993). Health for people with a terminal diagnosis. *Nursing Science Quarterly, 6*, 147–159.

Gross, S. W. (1995). The impact of a nursing intervention of relaxation with guided imagery on breast cancer patients' stress and health as expanded consciousness. *Dissertation Abstracts International, 56(10B)*, 5416.

Gustafson, W. (1990). Application of Newman's theory of health: Pattern recognition as nursing practice. In M. E. Parker (Ed.), *Nursing theories in practice* (pp. 141–161) (Pub. No. 15-2350). New York: National League for Nursing.

Holmes, C. A. (1993). Praxis: A case study in the depoliticization of methods in nursing research . . . including commentary by Thompson, J. L. *Scholarly Inquiry for Nursing Practice, 3(1)*, 3–15.

Jantsch, E. (1980). *The self-organizing universe.* New York: Pergamon.

Jonsdottir, H. (1994). Life patterns of people with chronic obstructive pulmonary disease: Isolation and being closed in. *Dissertation Abstracts International, 56(03B)*, 1346.

Jonsdottir, H. (1998). Life patterns of people with chronic obstructive pulmonary disease: Isolation and being closed in. *Nursing Science Quarterly, 11*, 160–166.

Kalb, K. A. (1990). The gift: Applying Newman's theory of health in nursing practice. In M. E. Parker (Ed.), *Nursing theories in practice* (pp. 163–186) (Pub. No. 15-2350). New York: National League for Nursing.

Karian, V. E., Jankowski, S. M., & Beal, J. A. (1998). Exploring the lived-experience of childhood cancer survivors. *Journal of Pediatric Oncology Nursing, 15*, 153–162.

Kelley, F. J. (1990). Spatial–temporal experiences and self-assessed health in the older adult. *Dissertation Abstracts International, 51*, 1194B.

Kendall, J. (1996). Human association as a factor influencing wellness in homosexual men with human immunodeficiency virus disease. *Applied Nursing Research, 9*, 195–203.

Kiser Larson, N. K. (1999). Life patterns of Native American women experiencing breast cancer. *Dissertation Abstracts International, 60(05B),* 2062.

Krejci, J. W. (1992). An exploration of synchrony in nursing. *Dissertation Abstracts International, 53,* 2247.

Lamendola, F. P., & Newman, M. A. (1994). The paradox of HIV/AIDS as expanding consciousness. *Advances in Nursing Science, 16*(3), 13–21.

Litchfield, M. (1997). The process of nursing partnership in family health. *Dissertation Abstracts International, 58(04B),* 1802.

Marchione, J. (1993). *Margaret Newman: Health as expanding consciousness.* Newbury Park, CA: Sage.

Mentzer, C. A., & Schorr, J. A. (1986). Perceived situational control and perceived duration of time: Expressions of life patterns. *Advances in Nursing Science, 9*(1), 12–20.

Michaels, C. (1992). Carondelet St. Mary's nursing enterprise. *Nursing Clinics of North America, 27,* 77–85.

Michaels, C. (2000). Becoming a bard: A journey to self. *Nursing Science Quarterly, 13,* 28–30.

Moch, S. D. (1988). Health in illness: Experiences with breast cancer. *Dissertation Abstracts International, 50(02B),* 497.

Moch, S. D. (1990). Health within the experience of breast cancer. *Journal of Advanced Nursing, 15,* 1426–1435.

Moss, R. (1981). *The I that is we.* Millbrae, CA: Celestial Arts.

Muscari, M. E. (1992). Binge/purge behaviors and attitudes as manifestations of relational patternings in a woman with bulimia nervosa. *Dissertation Abstracts International, 53(11B),* 5647.

Nelson, J. I. (1991). A crab or a dolphin: A new paradigm for nursing practice. *Nursing Outlook, 39,* 136–137.

Newman, M. A. (1966). Identifying and meeting patients' needs in short-span nurse–patient relationships. *Nursing Forum, 5*(1), 76–86.

Newman, M. A. (1972). Time estimation in relation to gait tempo. *Perceptual and Motor Skills, 34,* 359–366.

Newman, M. A. (1976). Movement tempo and the experience of time. *Nursing Research, 25,* 273–279.

Newman, M. A. (1979). *Theory development in nursing.* Philadelphia: Davis.

Newman, M. A. (1982). Time as an index of expanding consciousness with age. *Nursing Research, 31,* 290–293.

Newman, M. A. (1987). Aging as increasing complexity. *Journal of Gerontological Nursing, 13*(9), 16–18.

Newman, M. A. (1990a). Newman's theory of health as praxis. *Nursing Science Quarterly, 3,* 37–41.

Newman, M. A. (1990b). Shifting to higher consciousness. In M. Parker (Ed.), *Nursing theories in practice* (pp. 129–139) (Pub. No. 15-2350). New York: National League for Nursing.

Newman, M. A. (1990c). Toward an integrative model of professional practice. *Journal of Professional Nursing, 6,* 167–173.

Newman, M. A. (1992). Prevailing paradigms in nursing. *Nursing Outlook, 40,* 10–13, 32.

Newman, M. A. (1994a). *Health as expanding consciousness* (2nd ed.) (Pub. No. 14-2626). New York: National League for Nursing Press.

Newman, M. A. (1994b). Theory for nursing practice. *Nursing Science Quarterly, 7,* 153–157.

Newman, M. A. (1997a). Evolution of the theory of Health as Expanding Consciousness. *Nursing Science Quarterly, 10,* 22–25.

Newman, M. A. (1997b). Experiencing the whole. *Advances in Nursing Science, 20*(1), 34–49.

Newman, M. A., & Guadiano, J. K. (1984). Depression as an explanation for decreased subjective time in the elderly. *Nursing Research, 33,* 137–139.

Newman, M. A., Lamb, G. S., & Michaels, C. (1991). Nursing case management: The coming to-gether of theory and practice. *Nursing & Health Care, 12,* 404–408.

Newman, M. A., & Moch, S. D. (1991). Life patterns of persons with coronary artery disease. *Nursing Science Quarterly, 4,* 161–167.

Newman, M. A., Sime, A. M., & Corcoran-Perry, S. A. (1991). The focus of the discipline of nursing. *Advances in Nursing Science, 14*(1), 1–6.

Noveletsky-Rosenthal, H. T. (1996). Pattern recognition in older adults living with chronic illness. *Dissertation Abstracts International, 57(10B),* 6180.

Picard, C. A. (1998). Uncovering pattern of expanding consciousness in mid-life women: Creative movement and the narrative as modes of expression. *Dissertation Abstracts International, 59(03B),* 1049.

Picard, C. (2000). Pattern of expanding consciousness in midlife women: Creative movement and the narrative as modes of expression. *Nursing Science Quarterly, 13,* 150–157.

Prigogine, I. (1976). Order through fluctuation: Self-organization and social system. In E. Jantsch & C. H. Waddington (Eds.), *Evolution and consciousness* (pp. 93–133). Reading, MA: Addison-Wesley.

Rogers, M. (1970). *An introduction to the theoretical basis of nursing.* Philadelphia: Davis.

Roux, G. M. (1993). Phenomenologic study: Inner strength in women with breast cancer. *Dissertation Abstracts International, 55(02B),* 370.

Schlotzhauer, M., & Farnham, R. (1997). Newman's theory and insulin dependent diabetes mellitus in adolescence. *Journal of School Nursing, 13*(3), 20–23.

Schmitt, N. A. (1991). Caregiving couples: The experience of giving and receiving social support. *Dissertation Abstracts International, 52(11B),* 5761.

Schorr, J. A. (1993). Music and pattern change in chronic pain. *Advances in Nursing Science, 15*(4), 27–36.

Schorr, J. A., Farnham, R. C., & Ervin, S. M. (1991). Health patterns in aging women as expanding consciousness. *Advances in Nursing Science, 13*(4), 52–63.

Schorr, J. A., & Schroeder, C. A. (1991). Movement and time: Exertion and perceived duration. *Nursing Science Quarterly, 4,* 104–112.

Schroeder, C. A. (1993). Perceived duration of time and bed rest in high risk pregnancy: An exploration of the Newman model. *Dissertation Abstracts International, 54(04B),* 1894.

Shanahan, S. M. (1993). The lived experience of life-time passing in middle adolescent females. *Masters Abstracts International, 32-05,* 1376.

Smith, C. T. (1989). The lived experience of staying healthy in rural black families. *Dissertation Abstracts International, 50(09B),* 3925.

Smith, M. C. (1990). Pattern in nursing practice. *Nursing Science Quarterly, 3,* 57–59.

Smith, S. K. (1997a). Women's experience of victimizing sexualization, part I: Responses related to abuse and home and family environment. *Issues in Mental Health Nursing, 18,* 395–416.

Smith, S. K. (1997b). Women's experience of victimizing sexualization, part II: Community and longer term personal impacts. *Issues in Mental Health Nursing, 18,* 417–432.

Solari-Twadell, P. A., Bunkers, S. S., Wang, C. E., & Snyder, D. (1995). The Pinwheel Model of Bereavement. *Image: Journal of Nursing Scholarship, 27,* 323–326.

Tommet, P. A. (1997). Nurse–patient dialogue: Illuminating the pattern of families with children who are medically fragile. *Dissertation Abstracts International, 58(05B),* 2359.

Wade, G. H. (1998). A concept analysis of personal transformation. *Journal of Advanced Nursing, 28,* 713–719.

Wallace, D. (Producer), & Coberg, T. (Director). (1990). *Margaret Newman—The nurse theorists: Portraits of excellence* [Video tape]. Oakland, CA: Studio Three Production, Samuel Merritt College of Nursing.

Wendler, M. C. (1996). Understanding healing: A conceptual analysis. *Journal of Advanced Nursing, 24,* 836–842.

Wheeler, C. E., & Chinn, P. L. (1984). *Peace and power: A handbook of feminist process.* Buffalo: Margaret-daughters.

Yamashita, M. (1998a). Family coping with mental illness: A comparative study. *Journal of Psychiatric Mental Health Nursing, 5,* 515–523.

Yamashita, M. (1998b). Newman's theory of Health as Expanding Consciousness: Research on family caregiving in mental illness in Japan. *Nursing Science Quarterly, 11,* 110–115.

Yamashita, M. (1999). Newman's theory of health applied in family caregiving in Canada. *Nursing Science Quarterly, 12,* 73–79.

Yamashita, M., & Tall, F. D. (1998). A commentary on Newman's theory of health as expanding consciousness. *Advances in Nursing Science, 21,* 65–75.

Young, A. M. (1976a). *The geometry of meaning.* San Francisco: Robert Briggs.

Young, A. M. (1976b). *The reflective universe: Evolution of consciousness.* San Francisco: Robert Briggs.

SELECTED ANNOTATED BIBLIOGRAPHY

Bruce-Barrett, C. A. (1998). Patterns of health and healing: Peer support and prostate cancer. *Masters Abstracts International, 37-01,* 233.

This study used Newman's hermeneutic dialectic research methodology to explore the meaning and pattern of health experiences of five men diagnosed with prostate cancer. The diagnosis of cancer was identified as a choice point and the resulting expansion of consciousness included attuning to one's personal pattern; developing more authentic relationships; and transcending limitations imposed by the disease, its treatment and lack of knowledge.

Jonsdottir, H. (1994). Life patterns of people with chronic obstructive pulmonary disease: Isolation and being closed in. *Nursing Science Quarterly, 11,* 160–166.

This hermeneutic dialectic study involved 10 persons with chronic obstructive pulmonary disease. Findings included describing the life pattern as resignation, unsuccessful solution to traumatic events, and difficulties expressing oneself and relating to others. None of the participants described having experienced a choice point.

Newman, M. A. (1995). *A developing discipline: Selected works of Margaret Newman.* (Pub. No. 14-2671). New York: National League for Nursing Press.

This is a helpful volume for the student of Newman's work. Gathered in this one work are 22 previously published articles authored or coauthored by Margaret Newman. They are divided into the categories of the emerging structure of the discipline; identifying the pattern of the whole; transforming the meaning of health and practice; integrating theory, education, and practice; retrospective; and prospective.

Schmitt, N. A. (1991). Caregiving couples: The experience of giving and receiving social support. *Dissertation Abstracts International, 52(11B),* 5761.

This study investigated the experience of giving and receiving social support among spouses and spouse caregivers. Twenty older adult couples participated in the study. Results included that helping involved a readjustment of roles; the most valuable help was that keyed to what was most important to the recipient; all agreed they would rather help than be helped and saw helping as a normal part of marriage and identified the helper as a good person. Possibly the most important aspect of this study is its demonstration that the couple or family can be the unit of analysis and family patterns can be identified.

Tommet, P. A. (1997). Nurse–parent dialogue: Illuminating the pattern of families with children who are medically fragile. *Dissertation Abstracts International, 58(05B),* 2359.

This study used the hermeneutic dialectic method to investigate the pattern of families in the process of choosing an elementary school for a medically fragile child. The process of the study helped the parents identify their patterns. A major theme with these families was that of uncertainity and the families identified having moved from disruption and disorganization to reorganization in which instead of seeking to control uncertainty, they were learning to live with uncertainty. The family patterns included being isolated from other family and friends; having evolving relationships with health care providers; developing mutually supportive relationships; experiencing changes in space, time, and movement; interacting with bureaucracy; identifying personal growth and strengths; and making decisions. Developing new ways of relating within and without the family was identified as expanding consciousness.

CHAPTER 23

NURSING AS CARING
ANNE BOYKIN
AND SAVINA
SCHOENHOFER

Julia B. George

■ ■ ■

Anne Boykin (b. 1944) received her bachelors of science in nursing from Alverno College, Milwaukee, WI, her M.S. in adult nursing from Emory University and her Ph.D. in higher education administration with a nursing emphasis from Vanderbilt University. She has practiced nursing in acute care as well as community settings. She has held faculty positions at Clemson University, Valdosta State College, Marquette University, and Florida Atlantic University. She is dean of the College of Nursing, Florida Atlantic University, Boca Raton, Florida, and president of the International Association for Human Caring. She is active in numerous professional associations including the National League for Nursing, American Association of Colleges of Nursing, and the Southern Council on Collegiate Education. Her publications are in the areas of caring and nursing as a discipline.

Savina Schoenhofer (b. 1940) holds a B.A. in psychology, a B.S.N. in nursing, an M.Ed. in guidance and counseling, and an M.N. in nursing from Wichita State University, and a Ph.D. in higher education administration from Kansas State University. She has practiced nursing in community mental health and migrant health care. She has held faculty and administrative positions at Wichita State University, Florida Atlantic University, and the University of Mississippi. She is professor of graduate nursing at the Cora S. Balmat School of Nursing, Alcorn State University, Natchez, MS. She has published in the areas of nursing home management, nursing values, caring, and touch in nursing in critical care settings.

Boykin and Schoenhofer (1993) propose a grand theory of Nursing as Caring. Major influences in the development of the theory are Mayeroff's (1971) generic discussion of caring and Roach's (1984, 1987, 1992 rev.) discussions of caring person and caring in nursing. Roach's view of caring as process, rather than Mayeroff's view of caring as end, is incorporated in the theory of Nursing as Caring. Caring is a process of daily becoming, not a goal to be attained (Beckerman, Boykin, Folden, & Winland-Brown, 1994). Parker (1993) describes this theory as one that is personal rather than abstract and advises that one must know oneself as caring person to live the theory. She also points out that the theory of Nursing as Caring focuses on living caring rather than on achieving an end product and may be used alone or with other theories.

Gaut (1993) identifies the process of theory development used by Boykin and Schoenhofer as that of intension as described by Kaplan (1964). She characterizes such knowledge growth as being comparable to the gradual illumination of a room that occurs as people with lights enter a dark room. The first to enter perceive in general what is in the room. As additional people bring more light, details become clearer and clearer. Knowledge developed by intension begins with general awareness of the whole and progresses to more and more indepth identification and awareness of the specifics. Boykin and Schoenhofer (1993) write that work on their theory of Nursing as Caring began in 1983 as they worked together in curriculum development (a general view) and progressed over time to an identification of a level of detail that led them to the label of a general theory of nursing.

SUPPORTING STRUCTURES AND ASSUMPTIONS

Mayeroff's (1971) caring ingredients are drawn on in the theory of Nursing as Caring. Boykin and Schoenhofer (1993) state "when we have gone outside the discipline [of nursing] to extend possibilities for understanding, we have made an effort to go beyond application, to think through the nursing relevance of ideas that seemed, on the surface to be useful" (p. xiv). Boykin and Schoenhofer summarize Mayeroff's caring ingredients as follows (page numbers within the quotation refer to Mayeroff's work):

- Knowing—Explicitly and implicitly, knowing that and knowing how, knowing directly and knowing indirectly (p. 14).
- Alternating rhythm—Moving back and forth between a narrower and a wider framework, between action and reflection (p. 15).
- Patience—Not a passive waiting but participating with the other, giving fully of ourselves (p. 17).
- Honesty—Positive concept that implies openness, genuineness, and seeing truly (p. 18).
- Trust—Trusting the other to grow in his or her own time and own way (p. 20).
- Humility—Ready and willing to learn more about other and self and what caring involves (p. 23).
- Hope—"An expression of the plenitude of the present, alive with a sense of a possible" (p. 26).
- Courage—Taking risks, going into the unknown, trusting (p. 27). (pp. xiv-xv).

Boykin and Schoenhofer present two major perspectives for the theory of Nursing as Caring. Their perspectives are a perception of persons as caring and a conception of nursing as discipline and profession.

Perception of Persons as Caring

The basic premise of Nursing as Caring is that *all persons are caring* (Boykin & Schoenhofer, 1993, p. 3). Seven major assumptions underlie the theory, as follows:

- Persons are caring by virtue of their humanness
- Persons are caring, moment to moment
- Persons are whole or complete in the moment
- Personhood is a process of living grounded in caring
- Personhood is enhanced through participating in nurturing relationships with caring others
- Nursing is both a discipline and a profession (Boykin & Schoenhofer, 1993, p. 3)
- Persons are viewed as already complete and continuously growing in completeness, fully caring and unfolding caring possibilities moment-to-moment (p. 21)

Fundamental assumptions are person-as-person, person-as-whole in the moment, and person-as-caring (Boykin & Schoenhofer, 2000). The capacity for caring grows throughout one's life. Although the human is innately caring, not every human act is caring. Knowing oneself as caring person leads to a continuing commitment to know self and other as caring. This in turn leads to a moral obligation the quality of which is a "measure of being 'in place' in the world" (Boykin & Schoenhofer, 1993, p. 7). The ways in which one expresses caring are continually developing. The more opportunities one exercises fully to know oneself as caring, the easier it becomes to allow oneself (and others) the space and time to further develop caring. This enhances the awareness of self and consciousness that caring is lived moment to moment and directs one's "oughts." The emerging question becomes "How ought I act as caring person?" (p. 7). The degree of authentic awareness of self as caring person influences how one is with others. It requires the courage to let go of the present to discover new meaning about self and other.

Personhood, a process of living grounded in caring, recognizes the possibilities for caring in every moment and is enhanced through caring relationships with others. Caring is living in the context of relational responsibilities—responsibilities for self and other. The heart of the caring relationship is the importance of person-as-person (Boykin & Schoenhofer, 1993).

Drawing on Pribram's (1971) discussion of the uniqueness of a hologram as being that any part of a broken hologram is capable of reconstructing the total image, Boykin and Schoenhofer (1993) speak of the necessity to view the person as a whole. The person as a whole is a significant value that communicates respect for all that person is at the moment. Using the holographic perspective, it is recognized that any aspect or dimension of the person reflects the whole. Viewing the person as a whole, as caring and complete, is intentional and does not provide for dividing the other into parts or segments, such as mind, body, or spirit, at any time. The person, both self and other, is at all times whole. Unless the person is encountered as a whole, there is only a failed encounter. The person can be fully known only as a whole.

To understand the person as caring, one needs to focus on valuing, to celebrate the wholeness of humans, to view humans as both living and growing in caring, and to actively seek engagement on a personal level with others. The caring perspective of humans is basic to a view of nursing as an undertaking that focuses on humans, provides service from person to person, exists because of a social need, and is a human science (Boykin & Schoenhofer, 1993).

Conception of Nursing as a Discipline and Profession

The theory of Nursing as Caring is derived from a belief that nursing is both a discipline and a profession. The discipline of nursing originates in the unique social call to which nursing is a response and involves being, knowing, living, and valuing all at once. As a discipline, nursing is a unity of science, art, and ethic. Discipline relates to all aspects of the development of nursing knowledge.

The profession of nursing is based on understanding the social need from which the call for nursing originates and the body of knowledge that is used in creating the response known as nursing. Professions are based in everyday human experiences and responses to one another. Boykin and Schoenhofer (1993) discuss the relationship between the nurse and the nursed as a social contract that involves recognition that a basic need is present in conjunction with the availability of the knowledge and skill required to meet that need. The social call is for a group in society to make a commitment to acquire and use this knowledge and skill for the good of everyone. They also believe that nursing is in transition from social contract relationships to covenantal relationships. In contrast to the impersonal, legalistic emphasis in a social contract, the covenantal relationship emphasizes personal commitment and an always present freedom to choose commitments. The covenantal relationship leads to knowledge that each of us is related to all others as well as to the universe and that caring relationships lead to harmony. While discipline develops knowledge, as a profession nursing uses that knowledge to respond to specific human needs.

GENERAL THEORY OF NURSING AS CARING

The focus of nursing is "*nurturing persons living caring and growing in caring*" (Boykin & Schoenhofer, 1993, p. 21). Nursing is the response to the unique human need to be recognized as, and supported in being, caring person. The nurse must know the person as caring person and take those nursing actions that seek to nurture the person in living and growing in caring.

The focus of nurturing persons living caring and growing in caring is broad in statement but specific to the individual situation in practice. As the nurse seeks to know the nursed who is living and growing in caring, the individual's unique ways of living caring become known. Although it is easy to identify instances of noncaring, it is the nurse's commitment to discover the unique caring individual. For example, the nurse connects with the hope that underlies despair, hopelessness, fear, and anger and recognizes these emotions as personal expressions of the caring value. The nurse enters the world of the nursed with the intention and commitment to know the other as caring person. It is in knowing the other in this way that calls for nursing are heard (Boykin & Schoenhofer, 1993). Knowing *how* the other is living caring and expressing aspirations for growing in caring is as important as knowing the other as caring person. "The call for nursing is a call for acknowledgment and affirmation of the person living caring in specific ways in this immediate situation" (p. 24). The nursing response to this call is a caring nurturance evidenced by specific caring responses to sustain and enhance the nursed in living caring and growing in caring in the immediate situation. Boykin and Schoenhofer liken this being in relationship to a dance of caring persons (see Figure 23–1). The

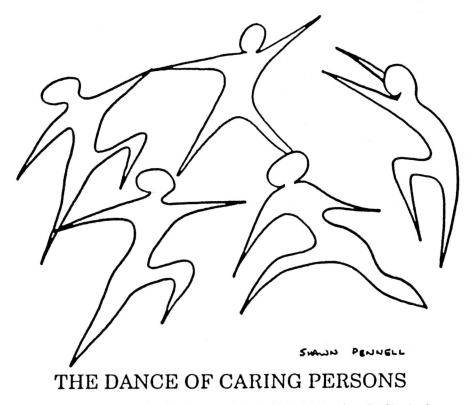

SHAWN PENNELL

THE DANCE OF CARING PERSONS

Figure 23–1. The Dance of Caring Persons. *(Used with permission from Boykin, A., & Schoenhofer, S. (1993).* Nursing as caring: A model for transforming nursing practice *(Pub. No. 15-2549).* New York: National League for Nursing Press.*)*

circle represents relating with respect for and valuing of the other in the basic dance to know self and other as caring person. Each dancer in the circle makes a contribution and moves within the dance as the nursing situation evolves. There is always room for more in the circle and dancers may move in or out as the nursed calls for services. While dancers may or may not connect by holding hands eye-to-eye contact facilitates knowing other as caring.

The *nursing situation* is defined by Boykin and Schoenhofer (1993) as "*a shared lived experience in which the caring between nurse and nursed enhances person-hood*" (p. 24). The nursing situation is the context in which nursing exists. It is through the study of the nursing situation that the content and structure of nursing knowledge is known. The nursing situation is composed whenever a nurse engages in a situation from a nursing focus. It is the intention with which the situation is approached and caring is expressed that creates the nursing situation and demonstrates nursing as caring. "As an expression of nursing, *caring is the intentional and authentic presence of the nurse with another who is recognized as person living caring and growing in caring. Here, the nurse endeavors to come to know the other as caring person and seeks to understand how that person might be supported, sustained, and strengthened in their* [sic] *unique process of living caring and growing in caring*" (p. 25).

The call for nursing comes from persons who are living caring and aspiring to grow in caring. The call is for nurturance through personal expressions of caring. The nurse responds to the call of caring person, not to a lack of caring or to noncaring. The nurse brings to this response a deliberately developed, or expert, knowledge of what it means to be human and to be caring; the nurse has made a commitment to recognize and nurture caring in all situations. The nurse risks entering the other's world, comes to know how the other is living caring in the moment, discovers unfolding possibilities for growing in caring, and thus transforms the general knowledge brought to the situation through an understanding of the uniqueness of the specific situation.

Every nursing situation is original and differs from all others because each is a lived experience that involves two individuals who do not have duplicates. The nature of this lived experience is one of reciprocity with personal investment from both the nurse and the nursed. Knowing self and other as caring, which is the crux of the nursing situation, involves a constant and mutual unfolding to discover the living of caring in the moment and the possibilities. For the nurse to enter the world of another, the other must allow such entrance. It is only through openness and willingness from both the nurse and the nursed that true presence in the situation occurs. Boykin and Schoenhofer (1993) identify the phenomenon that develops through the encountering of the nurse and the nursed as *caring between*. When caring between occurs, personhood is nurtured.

It is important that in the theory of Nursing as Caring, the call for nursing is based on neither need nor deficit. In this theory nursing does not seek to right a wrong, solve a problem, meet a need, or alleviate a deficit. Rather, Nursing as Caring is an egalitarian model of helping that celebrates the human in the fullness of being. Nursing responses are as varied as the calls for nursing (Boykin & Schoenhofer, 1993).

THE THEORY OF NURSING AS CARING
AND THE FOUR MAJOR CONCEPTS

Of the four major concepts, human beings, health, environment, and nursing, two are of primary importance in the theory of Nursing as Caring. These are human beings and nursing.

Basic beliefs about *human beings* are reflected in the major assumptions of the theory. Human beings are persons who are caring from moment to moment and are whole and complete in the moment. Humans are enhanced through their participation in nurturing relationships with caring others. All persons are caring, although not all actions are caring.

Nursing involves the nurse knowing self as caring person and coming to know the other as caring. Each expresses unique ways of living and growing in caring. The other expresses a call for caring to which the nurse attends. Nursing includes creating caring responses that nurture personhood and exists when the nurse actualizes personal and professional commitment to the belief that all persons are caring. Not all that a nurse does may express nursing. Any interpersonal experience has potential to become a nursing situation. The nursing situation occurs when the nurse presents self as offering the professional service of nursing and the other presents self as seeking, wanting, and/or accepting such professional service.

The theory of Nursing as Caring is an interpersonal process that can occur wherever nurse and other meet under circumstances that provide for the development of the nursing situation. *Environment* is not an important component of the theory itself. Aspects of the environment would be important only so far as they influence the expression of caring. Similarly, *health* is not defined as part of this theory.

THE THEORY OF NURSING AS CARING
AND THE NURSING PROCESS

The nursing process as a problem-solving approach or mechanism is incompatible with the theory of Nursing as Caring. The problem-solving focus seeks to find something to correct, which Boykin and Schoenhofer (1993) believe distracts nurses from their primary mission of caring and leads to the loss of the context of nursing. In Nursing as Caring, the challenge is to come to know the other as caring person and to nurture that person in ways that are specific to the situation rather than to discover what is missing or needed. Nursing is described as *processual* rather than a process.

Coker (1998) reports on a pilot project in a supportive residential care unit that resulted in the development of a guide to facilitate gathering and documenting information about personhood (see Table 23–1). The study supported that personhood data can be documented for use by others. A recommended extension of the study was to investigate how this information is used to individualize nursing care. A

TABLE 23–1. QUESTIONS TO ASSIST IN LEARNING ABOUT PERSONHOOD

Information about all but the last category of questions may be gathered from the person, family members, other care givers.

Respect

    What does respect of privacy mean to the individual?

    How do we know s/he is feeling disrespect?

    How does the individual wish to be addressed?

Preferences (likes/dislikes)

    Are there any cultural/religious preferences?

    What foods does s/he especially like or dislike?

    What comfort measures does s/he like?

    How does s/he like personal care (management of body functions) managed?

    What were typical sleep patterns?

    Does s/he like music? What type?

    What colors of clothing does s/he prefer?

    Does s/he like to be with others or does s/he keep to her/himself?

    Does s/he like hot beverages: tea or coffee?

    Does she like nail polish applied? Cosmetics? Earrings?

    Are there any personal hygiene preferences?

    What are her/his feelings about displays of affection (i.e., hugs, etc.)?

Interests/Activities

    What was a typical day like? Early/late riser? Early/late to bed?

    What evening activities did s/he enjoy?

    What did s/he do in spare time?

    What does s/he like doing?

    What does s/he like talking about?

Family/Social Supports

    Who is the family? Children and grandchildren?

    Who was in his or her social group? (i.e., friends, neighbors)

    What community groups was s/he involved in?

Background

    What did s/he do in life (employment, occupation, etc.)?

    What was his or her work ethic?

    Does s/he have any pictures that depict him or her in his or her life before coming here? Could someone bring them in?

    Has anyone (i.e., a grandchild) ever written a biography?

Hopes and Dreams

    What were/are some of his or her hopes?

    Are there any unfulfilled goals? Fulfilled goals?

Spirituality—Questions to be asked of the person

    Meaning of Life—What motivates you? What brings you joy? What do you want to be remembered for?

    Relationship with Higher Power—Do you communicate with a Higher Power? Do you find comfort and support from your beliefs?

    Hope—What gives you strength to go on? What are your favorite memories?

    Encouragement—From whom do you seek support? Who is a friend or advocate that is always there for you? What personal resources are available to you?

    Caring—What random acts of kindness have you done or considered doing? Who around you might benefit from a caring gesture?

    Meditation—Where is or would be a favorite place, such as in nature, to meditate? Have you tried to empty your mind of all thoughts to see what the experience would be like?

    Strive for Growth—What nurtures your spirit?

    Forgiveness—In what ways do you forgive others? What do you do to show forgiveness for yourself? How can you better accept the forgiveness of others? How do you heal your spirit?

Source: Derived from Coker, E. (1998). Does your care plan tell my story? Documenting aspects of personhood in long-term care. *Journal of Holistic Nursing, 16*, 435–452. Reprinted by permission of Sage Publications and Espeland, K. (1999). Achieving spiritual wellness: Using reflective questions. *Journal of Psychosocial Nursing, 37*(7), 36–40.

caveat in using such a tool would be that while the tool can be a helpful guide it is the caring between the nurse and the client that should be the focus, not the answering of questions and the gathering of data.

Boykin and Schoenhofer (1991, 1993) believe that the telling of stories of nursing situations make evident the service of nursing. Stories are a way to organize and communicate information about nursing in a manner that grounds the knowledge in the experience (ontology). The story represents the nursing situation, or unit of nursing knowledge. One example of such a story is:

Connections

One night as I listened to the change of shift report, I remember the strange feeling in the pit of my stomach when the evening nurse reviewed the lab tests on Tracy P. Tall, strawberry-blonde and freckle-faced, Tracy was struggling with the everyday problems of adolescence and fighting a losing battle against leukemia. Tracy rarely had visitors. As I talked with Tracy this night I felt resentment from her toward her mother, and I experienced a sense of urgency that her mother be with her. With Tracy's permission I called her mother and told her that Tracy needed her that night. I learned she was a single mother with two other small children, and that she lived several hours from the hospital. When she arrived at the hospital, distance and silence prevailed. With encouragement, the mother sat close to Tracy and I sat on the other side, stroking Tracy's arm. I left the room to make rounds and upon return found Mrs. P still sitting on the edge of the bed fighting to stay awake. I gently asked Tracy if we could lie on the bed with her. She nodded. The three of us lay there for a period of time and I then left the room. Later, when I returned, I found Tracy wrapped in her mother's arm. Her mother's eyes met mine as she whispered "she's gone." And then, "please don't take her yet." I left the room and closed the door quietly behind me. It was just after 6 o'clock when I slipped back into the room just as the early morning light was coming through the window. "Mrs. P," I reached out and touched her arm. She raised her tear-streaked face to look at me. "It's time," I said and waited. When she was ready, I helped her off the bed and held her in my arms for a few moments. We cried together. "Thank you nurse," she said as she looked into my eyes and pressed my hand between hers. Then she turned and walked away. The tears continued down my cheeks as I followed her to the door and watched her disappear down the hall.

—Gayle Maxwell (1990)

As traditionally defined, outcomes are not compatible with Nursing as Caring. However, Boykin and Schoenhofer (1997) posit that enhancing personhood is related to outcomes. The traditional definition of nursing outcomes speaks to distinct economic changes or specific end products of nursing care. However, the ethical practice of professional nursing must recognize value. Enhancing personhood does have value, can be related to change, and thus may be viewed as related to outcomes, albeit not to those that are empirically measured.

CRITIQUE OF THE THEORY OF NURSING AS CARING

1. What is the historical context of the theory? Boykin and Schoenhofer (1993) state that many theoretical works influenced the development of the theory of Nursing as Caring. They list Gaut (1983, 1984, 1985, 1986), Leininger (1978, 1981, 1991), Mayeroff (1971), Paterson and Zderad (1988), Ray (1981, 1984, 1985, 1989), Roach (1984, 1987, 1992 rev.), and Watson (1979, 1988), as major influences in their understanding of caring and caring in nursing. In a careful analysis of existing works on caring (Boykin & Schoenhofer,1990), discussed the ontological or being of caring questions, the anthropological issue of what it means to be a caring person, the ontical or function and ethic questions, the epistemological questions about how caring is known in nursing, and the pedagogical questions related to teaching and learning about caring in nursing.

King and Brownell (1976), the Nursing Development Conference Group (1979), and Phenix (1964) are identified as major influences in their understanding of nursing as a discipline. The theory of Nursing as Caring is consistent with these works. As a developing theory, Nursing as Caring leads to many as yet unanswered questions and will create new questions with each nurse–nursed caring encounter.

2. What are the basic concepts and relationships presented by the theory? The theory of Nursing as Caring identifies a focus and nursing situation rather than concepts. Boykin and Schoenhofer (1993) state that they have deliberately not presented the theory in the traditional format of concepts and propositions. Nursing as Caring presents nursing as a living caring that is personal and unique in each nursing situation. The theory does not present new and different definitions of nursing or caring but does provide a different way of looking at the phenomenon of the nursing relationship.

Their thoughts and beliefs are presented in a manner that connects them clearly and coherently. They anticipate areas in which their presentation differs from a traditional scientific format and explain their rationale for any variations.

3. What major phenomena of concern to nursing are presented? These phenomenon may include *but are not limited to*: human being, environment, health, interpersonal relations, caring, goal attainment, adaptation, and energy fields. The major phenomena are caring, persons as caring in the nursing situation, and nursing as a profession and a discipline.

4. To whom does it apply? In what situations? In what ways? There are no limitations of place or person for the application of this theory. Some might question the expression of caring with an unconscious client. Locsin (1998) helps counteract this concern in her discussion of technologic competence as caring in critical care nursing.

5. By what method or methods can this theory be tested? Qualitative, rather than a quantitative, positivistic methodology is the research methodology that is appropriate for the theory of Nursing as Caring. Boykin and Schoenhofer (1993) state that the process for coming to know nursing is dialogical rather than dialectical. The purpose of this process is enlightenment rather than control. They write about a research methodology that is totally appropriate for studying Nursing as Caring but that has not yet been developed and suggest that such a method would go beyond hermeneutics, with a phenomenological aspect in an action research orientation. Therefore, the generation of research hypotheses is not appropriate. The generation of research questions is appropriate and possible.

6. Does this theory direct critical thinking in nursing practice? Anderson (1998) describes storytelling, as recommended by Boykin and Schoenhofer, as the basis of critical thinking as stories are used by nurses to recall previous nursing situations that direct attention to what is most critical and essential in a clinical setting. It is important to remember that the purpose of critical thinking in Nursing as Caring is not to solve problems but to live caring.

7. Does this theory direct therapeutic nursing interventions? Boykin and Schoenhofer (1993) describe the theory of Nursing as Caring as a personal theory that requires knowledge of self as caring in order to interact with the other as living caring in the moment. The locus of the theory is the nursing situation. The entire reason for this theory is to guide and improve practice. Kearney and Yeager (1993) provide examples of how Nursing as Caring has guided their practices. They present nursing stories and discuss how the four major themes of Nursing as Caring (seeing the other as caring person, entering the world of the other with the intention of knowing the other, calls for caring nurturance, nursing responses that enhance personhood) have guided them.

Those who prefer to deal with the world in concrete, measurable, and impersonal terms may not view understanding living and growing in caring as directing therapeutic nursing interventions. Those who are comfortable, even excited, by a more cognitive, less measurable, and more personal approach will find the theory of Nursing as Caring with its focus on living caring in an interpersonal nursing situation to be relatively simple. The nurse brings general knowledge to the specific situation and uses that knowledge and the unique situation to inform each other. This is not generalizable to other nursing situations in the way positivistic research findings are generalizable. However, as a general theory Nursing as Caring applies whenever the nurse approaches a nursing situation from the caring perspective. This *is* generalizable to direct therapeutic nursing interventions

Locsin (1998) presents a case for technologic competence as caring in critical care nursing. She argues that it is not the knowledge of technology held by the nurse that should be important; it is the use of this knowledge in authentic presence that should take precedence. Also, competence may be described as performance or viewed as a state of being and thus a characteristic of the practitioner. This latter meaning allows for a description of competence that is distinctive to nursing as caring. In the same vein, Purnell (1998) argues that nursing is being challenged to care meaningfully for the whole person in an environment that does not support this value. She points out that the expression of a personal commitment to caring by a nurse includes a commitment to caring for self. It is the mutuality of need that provides for authentic nursing technology in which harmony is promoted.

8. Does this theory direct communication in nursing practice? Nursing as Caring depends on communication but does not provide specific directions for communication techniques. Communication, not necessarily verbal, is essential for the lived experience of the nursing situation.

9. Does this theory direct nursing actions that lead to favorable outcomes? As discussed earlier in this chapter, when value is included in outcomes, expanded personhood is a favorable outcome. Schoenhofer and Boykin (1998) reiterate this in discussing the contribution that viewing an outcome as value experienced in the nursing situation can make to the growth of the profession of nursing. However, empirically measured economic changes or specifically predicted results of nursing care are not compatible with the theory of Nursing as Caring. Also, the theory does not direct specific nursing actions but the nurse as caring participates in the relationship in the nursing situation.

10. How contagious is this theory? The development of the theory of Nursing as Caring has increased the general body of knowledge within the discipline and profession of nursing. Boykin and Schoenhofer (1993) speak to the need to develop a research methodology that is adequate to study this theory. Throughout the process of theory development, they have validated their work with practitioners of nursing. Beck (1994) reports on three phenomenological studies on the meaning of caring in a nursing program. The results of these studies have implications for nursing education.

The theory of Nursing as Caring, in itself, may be less contagious than some of the other theories and models discussed in this text. Caring is a pervasive concept and the basic foundations of Nursing as Caring are often included in discussions that do not reference Boykin and Schoenhofer but may reference those works upon which they drew. Some examples of use of the work of Boykin and Schoenhofer follow.

Anderson (1998) supports storytelling for the practice of genetics nurses as practitioners of holistic nursing. The three reasons given include that holistic practice assumes the patient is known as a whole person, that the goal in genetics of informed decision making is based on the assumption that people make the best decisions for themselves when they can integrate their values and beliefs with new knowledge, and that considering the context of being human and living a life provides a different orientation for genetics nurses in relation to the predictive value of the genetics information to be obtained.

Use of Nursing as Caring in education is discussed in Fletcher and Coffman's (1999) description of a baccalaureate nursing course on case management. The framework for this course was nursing as caring with a focus on case managers coming to know their clients and creating a climate for growth and change. Woodward (2000) speaks to the needs for the incorporation of caring in the education of nurse midwives in the United Kingdom as a result of her study of nurses in a palliative care setting and of nurse midwives. The palliative care nurses were described as responsive to the person of the other; the nurse midwives delivered care that was routine, oriented to tasks, and at times not responsive to the needs of the clients.

In Sweden, Hansebo and Kihlgren's (2000) study of nursing home caregivers telling of patient life stories supported Nursing as Caring. Included in their findings was that the life stories can act as a mediator between the patient and the caregiver in the nursing situation, and thus create a lived experience.

STRENGTHS AND LIMITATIONS

A strength of Nursing as Caring is the focus on caring, rather than problem solving, in the practice of nursing. The emphasis on the importance and strength of the client as caring provides a focus that has often been ignored or forgotten and that has been described as not being valued by the environment in which health care is delivered, in spite of the apparent value to the client.

Another strength rests in the description of Nursing as Caring as a general theory and the encouragement to use the theory in conjunction with other theories. The novice nurse particularly may find more direction and support for the knowledge that is needed in the nursing situation when combining Nursing as Caring with another nursing theory.

A limitation may be found in the qualitative nature of the theory and its approach to nursing practice. While the discussion of nursing as a discipline and a profession identifies the importance of the knowledge the nurse brings to the nursing situation, the theory itself does not provide any structure as to what that knowledge might be. Those who need structure and guidance for their nursing actions may be uncomfortable with the lack of specific structure within this theory. It does not provide an answer to the question, What am I supposed to do next?

SUMMARY

Boykin and Schoenhofer (1993) have developed the general theory of Nursing as Caring. Mayeroff's (1971) concepts of knowing, alternating rhythm, patience, honesty, trust, humility, hope, and courage provide a basis for the theory. The two major perspectives of the theory are a perception of persons as caring and a conception of nursing as discipline and profession. All persons are seen as caring. The major assumptions of the theory are that "persons are caring by virtue of their humanness; persons are caring, moment to moment; persons are whole or complete in the moment; personhood is a process of living grounded in caring; personhood is enhanced through participating in nurturing relationships with caring others; nursing is both a discipline and a profession" (Boykin & Schoenhofer, 1993, p. 3), and "persons are viewed as already complete and continuously growing in completeness, fully caring and unfolding caring possibilities moment-to-moment" (p. 21).

The discipline of nursing originates in the unique social call to which nursing is a response, and it relates to all aspects of the development of nursing knowledge. The profession of nursing is based on understanding the social need from which the social call originates and the body of knowledge used to create the response known as nursing.

The general theory of Nursing as Caring has a *focus* and a *locus*. The focus is *"nurturing persons living caring and growing in caring"* (Boykin & Schoenhofer, 1993, p. 21). The locus is the nursing situation defined as *"shared lived experience in which the caring between nursed and nursed enhances personhood"* (p. 24).

Boykin and Schoenhofer (1993) have indeed presented a different way of viewing the phenomenon of nursing in their general theory of Nursing as Caring. The relationships, which develop when this theory is lived, are dynamic and ever changing. They present this theory as one of human science that is not based on a mathematical structure but upon lived experience. Also, the theory is not congruent with the nursing process.

REFERENCES

Anderson, G. (1998). Storytelling: A holistic foundation for genetic nursing. *Holistic Nursing Practice, 12*(3), 64-76

Beck, C. T. (1994). Researching experiences of living caring. In A. Boykin (Ed.), *Living a caring-based program* (pp. 93–126) (Pub. No. 14-2536). NY: National League for Nursing Press.

Beckerman, A., Boykin, A., Folden, S., & Winland-Brown, J. (1994). The experience of being a student in a caring-based program. In A. Boykin (Ed.), *Living a caring-based program* (pp. 79–92) (Pub. No. 14-2536). NY: National League for Nursing Press.

Boykin, A., & Schoenhofer, S. (1990). Caring in nursing: Analysis of extant theory. *Nursing Science Quarterly, 3*, 149–155.

Boykin, A., & Schoenhofer, S. (1991). Story as link between nursing practice, ontology, epistemology. *Image: Journal of Nursing Scholarship, 23*, 245–248.

Boykin, A., & Schoenhofer, S. (1993). *Nursing as caring: A model for transforming practice.* (Pub. No. 15-2549). New York: National League for Nursing Press.

Boykin, A., & Schoenhofer, S. (1997). Reframing outcomes: Enhancing personhood. *Advanced Practice Nursing Quarterly, 3*(1), 60–65.

Boykin, A., & Schoenhofer, S. (2000). Invest in yourself. *Nursing Forum, 35*(4), 36–38.

Coker, E. (1998). Does your care plan tell my story? Documenting aspects of personhood in long-term care. *Journal of Holistic Nursing, 16*, 435–452.

Fletcher, I. L., & Coffman, S. (1999). Case management in the nursing curriculum. *Journal of Nursing Education, 38*, 371–377.

Gaut, D. A. (1983). Development of a theoretically adequate description of caring. *Western Journal of Nursing Research, 5*, 312–324.

Gaut, D. A. (1984). A theoretic description of caring as action. In M. Leininger (Ed.), *Care: The essence of nursing and health* (pp. 27–44). Detroit, MI: Wayne State University Press.

Gaut, D. A. (1985). Philosophical analysis as research method. In M. Leininger (Ed.), *Qualitative research methods in nursing* (pp. 73–80). Orlando, FL: Grune & Stratton.

Gaut, D. A. (1986). Evaluating caring competencies in nursing practice. *Topics in Clinical Nursing, 8*(2), 77–83.

Gaut, D. A. (1993). Introduction. In A. Boykin & S. Schoenhofer, *Nursing as caring: A model for transforming practice* (pp. xvii–xxix) (Pub. No. 15-2549). New York: National League for Nursing Press.

Hanesbro, G., & Kihlgren, M. (2000). Patient life stories and current situation as told by carers in nursing home wards. *Clinical Nursing Research, 9*, 260–279.

Kaplan, A. (1964). *The conduct of inquiry.* San Francisco: Chandler Publishing.

Kearney, C., & Yeager, V. (1993). Practical applications of Nursing as Caring theory. In M. E. Parker (Ed.), *Patterns of nursing theories in practice* (pp. 93–102) (Pub. No. 15-2548). New York: National League for Nursing Press.

King, A., & Brownell, J. (1976). *The curriculum and the disciplines of knowledge.* Huntington, NY: Publishing.

Leininger, M. (1978). *Transcultural nursing: Concepts, theories, and practices.* New York: Wiley.

Leininger, M. (1981). Some philosophical, historical and taxonomic aspects of nursing and caring in American culture. In M. Leininger (Ed.), *Caring: An essential human need* (pp. 133–143). Detroit, MI: Wayne State University Press.

Leininger, M. M. (1991). *Culture Care Diversity and Universality: A theory of nursing.* (Pub. No. 14-2402). New York: National League for Nursing Press.

Locsin, R. C. (1998). Technologic competence as caring in critical care nursing. *Holistic Nursing Practice, 12*(4), 50–56.

Maxwell, G. (1990). *Connections. Nightingale Songs, 1*(1). P.O. Box 057563, West Palm Beach, FL 33405–7563.

Mayeroff, M. (1971). *On caring.* New York: Harper & Row.

Nursing Development Conference Group. (1979). *Concept formalization in nursing: Process and product.* Boston: Little, Brown. (out of print)

Parker, M. (1993). Foreword. In A. Boykin & S. Schoenhofer, *Nursing as caring: A model for transforming practice* (pp. ix–xii) (Pub. No. 14-2549). New York: National League for Nursing Press.

Paterson, J. G., & Zderad, L. T. (1988). *Humanistic nursing.* New York: National League for Nursing.

Phenix, P. (1964). *Realms of meaning.* New York: McGraw-Hill.

Pribram, K. H. (1971). *Languages of the brain: Experimental paradoxes and principles in neuropsychology.* Upper Saddle River, NJ: Prentice Hall.

Purnell, M. J. (1998). Who really makes the bed? Uncovering technologic dissonance in nursing. *Holistic Nursing Practice, 12*(4), 12-22.

Ray, M. (1981). A philosophical analysis of caring within nursing. In M. Leininger (Ed.), *Caring: An essential human need* (pp. 25–36). Detroit, MI: Wayne State University Press.

Ray, M. (1984). The development of a classification system of institutional caring. In M. Leininger (Ed.), *Care: The essence of nursing and health* (pp. 95–112). Detroit, MI: Wayne State University Press.

Ray, M. (1985). A philosophical method to study nursing phenomena. In M. Leininger (Ed.), *Qualitative research methods in nursing* (pp. 81–92). Orlando, FL: Grune & Stratton.

Ray, M. (1989). The theory of bureaucratic caring for nursing practice in the organizational culture. *Nursing Administration Quarterly, 13*(2), 31–42.

Roach, S. (1984). *Caring: The human mode of being, implications for nursing.* Toronto: Faculty of Nursing, University of Toronto.

Roach, S. (1987). *The human act of caring.* Ottawa: Canadian Hospital Association.

Roach, S. (1992 Revised). *The human act of caring.* Ottawa: Canadian Hospital Association.

Schoenhofer, S. O., & Boykin, A. (1998). Discovering the value of nursing in high-technology environments: Outcomes revisited. *Holistic Nursing Practice, 12*(4), 31–39.

Watson, J. (1979). *Nursing: The philosophy and science of caring.* Boston: Little, Brown.

Watson, J. (1988). *Nursing: Human science and human care. A theory of nursing.* New York: National League for Nursing. (Originally published 1985, Appleton-Century-Crofts).

Woodward, V. (2000). Caring for women: The potential contribution of formal theory to midwifery practice. *Midwifery, 16*(1), 68–75.

SELECTED ANNOTATED BIBLIOGRAPHY

Boykin, A., Parker, M. E., & Schoenhofer, S. O. (1994). Aesthetic knowing grounded in an explicit conception of nursing. *Nursing Science Quarterly, 7,* 158–161.
This article highlights the value of Carper's contribution to nursing's patterns of knowing and seeks to overcome an identified limitation of that work in relation to aesthetic knowing. The expressed concern is that Carper's definition of aesthetic knowing as the art of nursing does not provide an explicit conception of nursing to serve as a guide in seeking patterns and structure of nursing knowledge. The proposed perspective is grounded in the theory of Nursing as Caring. Thus, the authors identify aesthetic knowing in nursing as creating experience in the nursing situation, expressing or communicating the experience (perhaps through the use of story), and appreciating the experience through the encounter that occurs through the expression of it.

Boykin, A., & Schoenhofer, S. (1991). Story as link between nursing practice, ontology, epistemology. *Image: Journal of Nursing Scholarship, 23,* 245–248.
Boykin and Schoenhofer define the nursing situation as a lived experience between the persons of nurse and client in which the caring between persons promotes well-being. These lived experiences provide for the generation of, conservation of, and knowing about the content of nursing knowledge. Reported segments of the lived experiences (stories) can convey the essence of the experience and thus contribute to the ability of others to participate in the lived experience and to grow and learn from it.

Boykin, A., & Winland-Brown, J. (1995). The dark side of caring: Challenges of caregiving. *Journal of Gerontological Nursing, 21*(5), 13–18.
This phenomenological research explored the caregiver burden of those providing care for loved ones diagnosed with Alzheimer's disease. The three major findings include that caregivers gradually allocated increased amounts of time and energy to care of their loved ones as the disease subtly progressed; all caregivers expressed the need to share, either formally or informally, their experience with support groups of other caregivers or with relatives or friends; the support of nurses may help the caregivers avoid viewing the loved one as an object and help prevent some of the guilt feelings that were so prevalent among the caregivers.

CHAPTER 24

USING NURSING THEORY IN CLINICAL PRACTICE

Julia B. George

■ ■ ■

A major characteristic of a profession is the identification and development of its own body of knowledge. The models and theories discussed in this book are representative of this characteristic for nursing. A body of knowledge in a practice discipline such as nursing is developed through research and through use in practice.

To assist the reader in comparing and contrasting them, this chapter provides a review of the models and theories discussed in earlier chapters. Following this review, each of these will be applied to nursing practice using the same case study. The resulting comparison should assist the reader in identifying those models and theories of greatest interest or utility for his or her own practice.

Florence Nightingale believed that the force for healing resides within the human being and, if the environment is appropriately supportive, humans will seek to heal themselves. Her thirteen canons indicate the areas of environment of concern to nursing. These are ventilation and warming, health of houses (pure air, pure water, efficient drainage, cleanliness, and light), petty management (today known as continuity of care), noise, variety, taking food, what food, bed and bedding, light, cleanliness of rooms and walls, personal cleanliness, chattering hopes and advices, and observation of the sick.

Hildegard E. Peplau focused on the interpersonal relationship between the nurse and the patient. The three phases of this relationship are orientation, working, and termination. The relationship is initiated by the patient's felt need and termination occurs when the need is met. Both the nurse and the patient grow as a result of their interaction.

Virginia Henderson first defined nursing as doing for others what they lack the strength, will, or knowledge to do for themselves and then identified 14 components of care. These components provide a guide to identifying areas in which a person may lack the strength, will, or knowledge to meet personal needs. They include breathing, eating and drinking, eliminating, moving, sleeping and resting, dressing and undressing appropriately, maintaining body temperature, keeping clean and protecting the skin, avoiding dangers and injury to others, communicating, worshiping, working, playing, and learning.

Lydia E. Hall believed that persons over the age of 16 who were past the acute stage of illness required a different focus for their care than during the acute stage. She described the circles of care, core, and cure. Activities in the care circle belong solely to nursing and involve bodily care and comfort. Activities in the core circle are shared with all members of the health care team and involve the person and therapeutic use of self. Hall believed the drive to recovery must come from within the person. Activities in the cure circle also are shared with other members of the health care team, and may include the patient's family. The cure circle focuses on the disease and the medical care.

Dorothea E. Orem identified three theories of self-care, self-care deficit, and nursing systems. The ability of the person to meet daily requirements is known as self-care, and carrying out those activities is self-care agency. Parents serve as dependent care agents for their children. The ability to provide self-care is influenced by basic conditioning factors including but not limited to age, gender, and developmental state. Self-care needs are partially determined by the self-care requisites, which are categorized as universal (air, water, food, elimination, activity and rest, solitude and social interaction, hazard prevention, function within social groups), developmental, and health deviation (needs arising from injury or illness and from efforts to treat the injury or illness). The total demands created by the self-care requisites are identified as therapeutic self-care demand. When the therapeutic self-care demand exceeds self-care agency, a self-care deficit exists and nursing is needed. Based on the needs, the nurse designs nursing systems that are wholly compensatory (the nurse provides all needed care), partly compensatory (the nurse and the patient provide care together), or supportive–educative (the nurse provides needed support and education for the patient to exercise self-care).

Dorothy E. Johnson stated that nursing's area of concern is the behavioral system that consists of seven subsystems. The subsystems are attachment or affiliative, dependency, ingestive, eliminative, sexual, aggressive, and achievement. The behaviors for each of the subsystems occur as a result of the drive, set, choices, and goal of the subsystem. The purpose of the behaviors is to reduce tensions and keep the behavioral system in balance.

Faye G. Abdellah sought to change the focus of care from the disease to the patient, and thus proposed patient-centered approaches to care. She identified 21 nursing problems, or areas vital to the growth and functioning of humans that require support from nurses when persons are for some reason limited in carrying out the activities needed to provide such growth. These areas are hygiene and comfort, activity (including exercise, rest, and sleep), safety, body mechanics, oxygen, nutrition, elimination, fluid and electrolyte balance, recognition of physiological responses to disease, regulatory mechanisms, sensory functions, emotions, interrelatedness of emotions and illness, communication, interpersonal relationships, spiritual goals, therapeutic environment, individuality, optimal goals, use of community resources, and role of society.

Ida Jean Orlando described a disciplined nursing process. Her process is initiated by the patient's behavior. This behavior engenders a reaction in the nurse, described as an automatic perception, thought, or feeling. The nurse shares the reaction with the patient, identifying it as the nurse's perception, thought, or feeling, and seeking validation of the accuracy of the reaction. Once the nurse and the patient have agreed on the immediate need that led to the patient's behavior, and to the action to be taken by the nurse to meet that need, the nurse carries out a deliberative action. Any action taken by the nurse for reasons other than meeting the patient's immediate need is an automatic action.

Ernestine Wiedenbach proposed a prescriptive theory that involves the nurse's central purpose, prescription to fulfill that purpose and the realities that influence the ability to fulfill the central purpose (the nurse, the patient, the goal, the means, and the framework or environment). Nursing involves the identification of the patient's need for help, the ministration of help, and validation that the efforts made were indeed helpful. Her principles of helping indicate the nurse should look for patient behaviors that are not consistent with what is expected, should continue helping efforts in spite of encountering difficulties, and should recognize personal limitations and seek help from others as needed. Nursing actions may be reflex or spontaneous and based on sensations, conditioned or automatic and based on perceptions, impulsive and based on assumptions, or deliberate or responsible and based on realization, insight, design and decision that involves discussion and joint planning with the patient.

Myra Estrin Levine described adaptation as the process by which conservation is achieved with the purpose of conservation being integrity, or preservation of the whole of the person. Adaptation is based on past experiences of effective responses (historicity), the use of responses specific to the demands being made (specificity), and more than one level of response (redundancy). Adaptation seeks the best fit between the person and his environment. The principles of conservation deal with conservation of energy, structural integrity, personal integrity, and social integrity of the individual.

Imogene M. King presented both a systems-based conceptual framework of personal, interpersonal, and social systems and a theory of goal attainment. The concepts of the theory of goal attainment are interaction, perception, communication, transaction, self, role, stress, growth and development, time, and personal space. The nurse and the client usually meet as strangers. Each brings to this meeting perceptions and judgments about the situation and the other; each acts and then reacts to the other's action. The reactions lead to interaction, which, when effective, leads to transaction or movement toward mutually agreed on goals. She emphasizes that both the nurse and the patient bring important knowledge and information to this goal attainment process.

Martha E. Rogers identified the basic science of nursing as the Science of Unitary Human Beings. The human being is a whole, not a collection of parts. She presented the human being and the environment as energy fields that are integral with each other. The human being does not have an energy field but is an energy field. These fields can be identified by their pattern, described as a distinguishing characteristic that is perceived as a single wave. These patterns occur in a pandimensional world. Rogers' principles are resonancy or continuous change to higher frequency, helicy or unpredictable movement toward increasing diversity, and integrality or the continuous mutual process of the human field and the environmental field.

Sister Callista Roy proposed the Roy Adaptation Model. The person or group responds to stimuli from the internal or external environment through control processes or coping mechanisms identified as the regulator and cognator (stabilizer and innovator for the group) subsystems. The regulator processes are essentially automatic while the cognator processes involve perception, learning, judgment, and emotion. The results of the processing by these coping mechanisms are behaviors in one of four modes. These modes are the physiological–physical mode (oxygenation; nutrition; elimination; activity and rest; protection; senses; fluid, electrolyte, and acid-base balance; and endocrine function for individuals; resource adequacy for groups), self-concept–group identity mode, role function mode, and interdependence mode. These behaviors may be either adaptive (promoting the integrity of the human system) or ineffective (not promoting such integrity). The nurse assesses the behaviors in each of the modes and identifies those adaptive behaviors that need support and those ineffective behaviors that require intervention. For each of these behaviors the nurse then seeks to identify the associated stimuli. The stimulus most directly associated with the behavior is the focal stimulus; all other stimuli that are verified as influencing the behavior are contextual stimuli. Any stimuli that may be influencing the behavior, but that have not been verified as doing so, are residual stimuli. Once the stimuli are identified, the nurse, in cooperation with the patient, plans and carries out interventions to alter stimuli and support adaptive behaviors. The effectiveness of the actions taken is evaluated.

Betty Neuman developed the Neuman Systems Model. Systems have three environments—the internal, the external, and the created environment. Each system, whether an individual or a group, has several structures. The basic structure or core is where the energy resources reside. This core is protected by lines of resistance that in turn are surrounded by the normal line of defense, and finally the flexible line of defense. Each of the structures consists of the five variables of physiological, psychological, sociocultural, developmental, and spiritual characteristics. Each variable is influenced by intrapersonal, interpersonal, and extrapersonal factors. The system seeks a state of equilibrium that may be disrupted by stressors. Stressors, either existing or potential, first encounter the flexible line of defense. If the flexible line of defense cannot counteract the stressor, then the normal line of defense is activated. If the normal line of defense is breached, the stressor enters the system and leads to a reaction, associated with the lines of resistance. This reaction is what is usually termed *symptoms*. If the lines of resistance allow the stressor to reach the core, depletion of energy resources and death are threatened. In the Neuman Systems Model, there are three levels of prevention. Primary prevention occurs before a stressor enters the system and causes a reaction. Secondary prevention occurs in response to the symptoms, and tertiary prevention seeks to support maintenance of stability and to prevent future occurrences.

Josephine E. Paterson and *Loretta T. Zderad* presented humanistic nursing. Humans are seen as becoming through choices and health is a personal value of more-being and well-being. Humanistic nursing involves dialogue, community, and phenomenologic nursology. Dialogue occurs through meeting the other, relating with the other, being in presence together, and sharing through call and response. Community is the sense of "we." Phenomenolgic nursology involves the nurse preparing to know another, having intuitive responses to another, learning about the other scientifically, synthesizing information about the other with information already known, and developing a truth that is both uniquely personal and generally applicable.

Jean Watson described nursing as human science and human care. Her ten carative factors include a humanistic–altruistic system of values; faith–hope; sensitivity to self and others; transpersonal connections; expression of feelings and emotions; creative problem solving caring processes; transpersonal teaching–learning; environments that support, protect, or correct; human needs gratification in a manner that preserves dignity and wholeness; and existential–phenomenological–spiritual dimensions of caring and healing. These carative factors occur within a transpersonal caring relationship and a caring occasion and caring moment as the nurse and other come together and share with each other. The transpersonal caring relationship seeks to provide mental and spiritual growth for both participants while seeking to restore or improve the harmony and unity within the personhood of the other.

Rosemarie Rizzo Parse developed the theory of Human Becoming within the simultaneity paradigm that views human beings as developing meaning through freedom to choose and more than and different from a sum of parts. Her practice methodology has three dimensions, each with a related process. The first is illuminating meaning is explicating, or making clear through talking about it, what was, is, and will be. The second is synchronizing rhythms is dwelling with, or being immersed with the process of connecting and separating, within the rhythms of the exchange between the human and the universe. The third is mobilizing transcendence is moving beyond, or moving toward what is envisioned, the moment to what has not yet occurred. In the theory of Human Becoming, the nurse is an interpersonal guide with the responsibility for decision making (or making of choices) residing in the client. The nurse provides support but not counseling. However, the traditional role of teaching does fall within illuminating meaning and serving as a change agent is congruent with mobilizing transcendence.

Helen C. Erickson, Evelyn M. Tomlin, and *Mary Ann P. Swain* presented the theory of Modeling and Role-Modeling. Both modeling and role-modeling involve an art and a science. Modeling requires the nurse to seek an understanding of the client's view of the world. The art of modeling involves the use of empathy in developing this understanding. The science of modeling involves the use of the nurse's knowledge in analyzing the information collected to create the model. Role-modeling seeks to facilitate health. The art of role-modeling lies in individualizing the facilitations while the science lies in the use of the nurse's theoretical knowledge base to plan and implement care. The aims of intervention are to build trust, promote the client's positive orientation of self, promote the client's perception of being in control, promote the client's strengths, and set mutual health directed goals. The client has self-care knowledge about what his or her needs are, self-care resources to help meet these needs, and takes self-care action to use the resources to meet the needs. In addition, a major motivation for human behavior is the drive for affliliated–individuation or having a personal identity while being connected to others. The individual's ability to mobilize resources is identified as adaptive potential. Adaptive potential may be identified as adaptive equilibrium (a nonstress state in which resources are utilized appropriately), maladaptive equilibrium (a nonstress state in which resource utilization is placing one or more subsystem in jeopardy), arousal (a stress state in which the client is having difficulty mobilizing resources), or impoverishment (a stress state in which resources are diminished or depleted). Interventions differ according to the adaptive potential. Those in adaptive equilibrium can be encouraged to continue and may require only facilitation of their self-care actions. Those is maladaptive equilibrium present the challenge of seeing no reason to change, since they are in equilibrium. Here motivation strategies to seek to change are needed. Those in arousal are best supported by actions that facilitate change and support individuation; these are likely to include teaching, guidance, direction, and other assistance. Those in impoverishment have strong affiliation needs, need their internal strengths promoted, and need to have resources provided.

Madeleine M. Leininger provided a guide to the inclusion of culture as a vital aspect of nursing practice. Her Sunrise Model posits that important dimensions of culture and social structure are technology, religion, philosophy, kinship and other related social factors, cultural values and lifeways, politics, law, economics, and education within the context of language and environment. All of these influence care patterns and expressions that impact the health or well being of individuals, families, groups, and institutions. The diverse health systems include the folk care systems and the professional care systems that are linked by nursing. To provide culture congruent care, nursing decisions and actions should seek to provide culture care preservation or maintenance, culture care accommodation or negotiation, or culture care repatterning or restructuring.

Margaret Newman described health as expanding consciousness. Important concepts are movement (an essential property of matter), time (the rhythm of living), space (related to time and movement), consciousness (the information capacity of the system), pattern (movement, diversity and rhythm of the whole), pattern recognition (identification within the observer of the whole of another), and transformation (change). Health and disease are seen as reflections of the larger whole rather than as different entities. She proposed (with Sime and Corcoran-Perry) the unitary–transformative paradigm in which human beings are viewed as unitary phenomenon. These phenomenon are identified by pattern and change is unpredictable, towards diversity, and transformative. Stages of disorganization, or choice points, lead to change and health is the evolving pattern of the whole as the system moves to higher levels of consciousness. The nurse enters into process with a client and does not serve as a problem solver.

Anne Boykin and *Savina Schoenhofer* present nursing as caring in a grand theory that may be used in combination with other theories. Persons are caring by virtue of being human; are caring, moment to moment; whole and complete in the moment; and already complete while growing in completeness. Personhood is the process of living grounded in caring and is enhanced through nurturing relationships. Nursing as a discipline is a being, knowing, living, and valuing response to a social call. As a profession, nursing is based on a social call and uses a body of knowledge to respond to that call. The focus of nursing is nurturing persons living in caring and growing in caring. This nurturing occurs in the nursing situation, or the lived experience shared between the nurse and the nursed in which personhood is enhanced. The call for nursing is not based on a need or a deficit and thus focuses on helping the other celebrate the fullness of being rather than seeking to fix something. Boykin and Schoenhofer encourage the use of story telling to make evident the service of nursing.

Each of these models or theories will be applied to clinical practice with the following case study:

> May Allenski, an 84-year-old white female, had emergency femoral-popliteal bypass surgery 2 days ago. She has severe peripheral vascular disease and a clot blocked 90% of the circulation to her right leg one week ago. The grafts were taken from her left leg so there are long incisions in each leg. She lives in a small town about 75 miles from the medical center. The initial clotting occurred late on Friday night; she did not see a doctor until Monday. The first physician referred her to a vascular specialist who then referred her to the medical center. Her 90-year-old husband drove her to the medical center on Tuesday. You anticipate she will be discharged to home on the 4th postoperative day, as is standard procedure. She is learning to transfer to and from bed and toilet to wheelchair.

The following examples of application in clinical practice are not complete but are intended to provide only a partial example for each. Study of these examples can provide ideas or suggestions for use in clinical practice. Each reader is encouraged to develop further detail as appropriate to his or her practice.

TABLE 24–1. APPLICATION OF THEORIES IN CLINICAL PRACTICE

Assessment	Diagnosis	Outcomes	Planning	Implementation	Evaluation
			Florence Nightingale's Environmental Focus		
Ventilation and warming: Room is temperature controlled; uses an extra blanket because she is "always cold"	Sleep pattern disturbance related to noisy environment.	Adequate amount of sleep to support healing.	Encourage night staff to hold all conversations quietly. Close door to room. Be certain lights are dimmed in room and that call light is within reach. Offer earplugs.	Planned activities were carried out— ear plugs refused.	On 4th postoperative day, reported "slept better last night"
Health of houses (pure air, pure water, efficient drainage, cleanliness, and light), bed and bedding, cleanliness of rooms and walls: Hospital environment meets these satisfactorily					
Petty management: There is a written plan of care for the nursing staff					
Noise: 2-bed room is located near nurses' station; MA states she has trouble sleeping at night due to the noise					
Variety: Able to move about the unit in wheelchair					
Taking food: Can feed herself; states she is not very hungry					
What food: On a low-sodium diet					
Light: Large window in the room provides natural lighting; well lit at night					
Personal cleanliness: Able to bathe with assistance					
Chattering hopes and advices: Only visitor is her husband.					
Observation of the sick: Vital signs are near her baseline data; wounds are healing normally.					

Hildegard E. Peplau's Interpersonal Relationships

Orientation:	Orientation:	Working:	Working:	Working:	Termination:
MA's expressed felt need is to go home.	Relocation stress syndrome related to hospitalization	To have access to needed care at home	Home health nurse in hometown to provide support	Referral made to appropriate home health agency	MA discharged from medical center on 4th post op day (a Sunday). Monday is a holiday; home health agency personnel not available before Tuesday—outcome only partially met

Virginia Henderson's Definition and 14 Components

				Working:	Termination:
	Risk of constipation related to low fiber and fluid intake and to decrease in exercise	Restoration of normal bowel function	Have fluid and fiber intake adequate to restore normal bowel functioning within one week.	Identify favorite foods and fluids. Identify who will be fixing meals at home. Ascertain her knowledge about fluid and fiber intake (her college education was in home economics). Mutually develop a plan of tempting sources of fiber and fluids to increase her intake.	By discharge had increased fluid intake to 250 cc daily; fiber intake remained limited. Stated not hungry or interested in food. *Reassessment:* Need to investigate if this disinterest is evidence of depression.

Breathing: R 18; skin pink

Eating and drinking: States not very hungry; fluid intake 100 cc

Eliminating: Voiding without discomfort; no bowel movement since surgery, normally has at least one daily

Moving: Able to move self about in bed; learning to transfer to wheelchair

Sleeping and resting: States not sleeping well due to noisy environment

Dressing and undressing appropriately: Dressed in hospital gown and own robe and slippers

Maintaining body temperature: T 98.9° F.

Keeping clean and protecting the skin: Needs assistance with washing back and feet.

Avoiding dangers and injury to others: Learning safe transfer techniques; needs information on dressing changes

TABLE 24–1. (*CONT.*)

Assessment	Diagnosis	Outcomes	Planning	Implementation	Evaluation
		Virginia Henderson's Definition and 14 Components (*cont.*)			
Communicating: Hears best when wearing glasses; expresses self clearly					
Worshiping: No information available					
Working: Has always cared for own home					
Playing: Enjoys reading and watching tennis on television					
Learning: Reads for information; avid TV news watcher					
		Lydia E. Hall's Care, Core, and Cure			
Care: Able to provide most of own hygiene, needs help bathing back and feet. Having little pain from surgical sites but needs pain relief for arthritis pain in hands and hips. *Core:* Does not like being in hospital, wants to be at home. Will not discuss how she will be cared for at home. *Cure:* Incisions are healing normally, pedal pulses present in both feet although diminished on the right.	Relocation stress syndrome related to hospitalization	Have MA involved in solving the challenges associated with her care needs at home	Develop a plan of care to be used at home	Identify with MA what she can do for herself. Identify with MA what she will need help doing (for example, dressing changes, preparing meals, housekeeping chores). Include MA in problem solving how these needs can be met—e.g., home health referral.	MA agreed to home health referral and indicated her husband will find someone to help with the housekeeping. Also, he can cook.

Dorothea E. Orem's Theories of Self-Care

Universal self-care requisites: Air—Breathing normally, lung sounds clear Water—Fluid intake of 100cc qd Food—States has no appetite, eating about ¼ of what is served on each meal tray Elimination—Voiding adequately; no bowel movement since surgery Activity and rest—Can position self in bed, learning to transfer to and from wheelchair *Solitude and social interaction*—Only visitor is her husband. No family living in area. Interacts with roommate *Hazard prevention*—bed rails are kept up, call bell within reach *Function within social groups*—at home interacts with friends through their visits to her home; used to play bridge but she and husband are the only members of the group still living *Development self-care requisites:* See function within social groups *Health deviation self-care requisites:* Cannot walk due to surgical involvement of both legs; has fresh incision bilaterally, history of hypertension	Self-care deficit in ability to continue to care for self and home independently	Safe and adequate care at home for self and husband	Identify changed areas of self-care needs. Identify sources of meeting each of these needs. Assist the family in making contact with these sources.	Discuss with MA and her husband how they can handle meal preparation, housekeeping, and health deviation care needs.	After they return home, Mr. A. will find a house-keeper who can help will meals, housecleaning, laundry, and MA's dressing and hygiene needs.

TABLE 24–1. *(CONT.)*

Assessment	Diagnosis	Outcomes	Planning	Implementation	Evaluation
			Dorothy E. Johnson's Behavioral System		
Attachment or affiliative: Husband drove her to the medical center and has stayed in a nearby motel. He visits daily. *Dependency:* MA hesitates to ask for needed help—states she is used to being able to care for herself and it is hard to have others do for her. *Ingestive:* Likes her coffee hot and ice cream cold. *Eliminative:* Usually has a bowel movement every morning after breakfast. *Sexual:* Kisses her husband each time he leaves. *Aggressive:* No data *Achievement:* No data	Discrepancy in dependency subsystem: has difficulty asking for needed help	Able to seek help appropriately	MA will identify areas in which she needs help. MA will plan how to seek the needed help.	Discuss with MA what she can do for herself, and what she needs help to do. Discuss what would make her more comfortable in accepting help Plan with her how she can seek and accept help in a way that is acceptable to her.	By discharge, MA is calling the nurse for supervision in transferring from bed to chair and is clearly verbalizing exactly what she needs.
			Faye G. Abdellah's Patient-Centered Approach to Care		
Hygiene and comfort: Can position self in bed; needs medication for arthritis pain; needs assistance washing back and feet. *Activity (including exercise, rest, and sleep):* Cannot walk on own at present; states not sleeping well due to noise from nurses' station *Safety:* Bed rails are up when in bed; call bell in reach *Body mechanics:* Learning appropriate transfer techniques. *Oxygen:* R 18, lung sounds clear, skin pink	Risk for activity intolerance	Able to carry out activities of daily living independently	Will be able to transfer to and from wheelchair safely by discharge Will gradually resume walking, first using a walker and then independently	Physical therapy twice daily to teach about and prepare muscles for transfer activities Home health referral for physical therapy at home to assist in walking	Able to safely transfer by time of discharge. Home health referral made for physical therapy at home

Nutrition: Eating about ¼ of food served at each meal; fluid intake 100 cc in 24 hours

Elimination: Voiding adequately, urine clear and yellow; no bowel movement since surgery

Fluid and electrolyte balance: Lab values WNL

Recognition of physiological responses to disease: Reduced pedal pulse on right

Regulatory mechanisms: Lab values WNL

Sensory functions: Wears glasses, slightly hard of hearing, states often cannot tell if she has a good grip on an object or not

Emotions: Teary about this sudden change in her ability to be independent

Interrelatedness of emotions and illness: Recognizes her emotional responses to this illness

Communication: Communicates clearly

Interpersonal relationships: Husband visits daily

Spiritual goals: Not expressed

Therapeutic environment: Says would feel better at home

Individuality: Able to select desired foods—little other opportunity to express her individuality

Optimal goals: To function independently and care for her own home again

Use of community resources: Will need home health referral

Role of society: No apparent social contribution to current problems

TABLE 24–1. (CONT.)

Assessment	Diagnosis	Outcomes	Planning	Implementation	Evaluation
Ida Jean Orlando's Disciplined Nursing Process					
MA's behavior: Rubbing one hand with the other *Nurse's reaction:* Perception—she is anxious or worried. Perception is shared—MA says, no, her joints hurt from arthritis and she has not had her medication for it.	*Immediate need:* Relief from arthritis pain	Comfort	Within one hour after receiving pain medication, the joint pain will be alleviated.	*Deliberative action:* MA and the nurse agree that the ordered NSAID would be appropriate; the nurse obtains the medication for MA.	In one hour, MA reports her hands feel much better.
Ernestine Wiedenbach's Prescriptive Theory of Nursing					
The nurse's central purpose is to educate her patients so they can care for themselves effectively. The nurse (the agent) assesses that MA (the recipient) will need to know how to assess healing of her incisions (the goal).	Altered protection related to compromised circulation secondary to severe peripheral vascular disease	Cleanly healed surgical incisions .	MA will describe the signs and symptoms of healing and of delayed healing.	The means: teach MA about the signs and symptoms to be observed and actions to be taken to support healing or in response to delayed healing.	By discharge, the nurse had not been able to have this discussion with MA due to the time MA spent in physical therapy and the nurse's days off.
Myra E. Levine's Adaptation and Principles of Conservation					
Conservation of energy: Vital signs and lab values WNL. MA naps in room after returning from physical therapy. *Conservation of structural integrity:* Surgical wounds are seeping and are slightly reddened *Conservation of personal integrity:* MA does not want to talk about herself *Conservation of social integrity:* MA's husband brought her to the medical center and visits daily.	Need to conserve structural integrity: ensure wound healing	Clean healing of surgical wounds.	Avoid infection of surgical wounds	Keep wounds clean, expose to air at least 4 hours a day. Position with legs elevated to encourage circulation	At discharge, wounds are seeping serous fluid, no indication of infection.

Imogene M. King's Theory of Goal Attainment

Growth and development: "Senior citizen," accustomed to caring for self and home *View of self:* Independently functioning, self-sufficient person *Perception of current health status:* Ability to care for self and home now limited due to mobility difficulties *Communication patterns:* Does not talk much about self and her emotions *Role:* Wife, homemaker, mother, and grandmother *Sensory system:* At times cannot tell if she has a grip on an object, wears glasses, slightly hard of hearing, very sensitive skin on shoulder where had shingles *Education:* College graduate, taught in a one-room school before marriage. Reads and watches TV to keep current *Drug history:* Has taken medication for high blood pressure for 40 years, also takes NSAIDs for arthritis. *Diet history:* Has followed low-fat, low-sodium diet for 35 to 40 years.	Altered role performance related to surgery	Will be able to work with support services at home	Help MA identify what would increase her comfort level with having help at home—how to let them know what she would like done and how she would like for it to be done without feeling she is being too demanding.	At time of discharge MA not able to make such identifications— included as a need in home health referral

Martha E. Rogers' Science of Unitary Human Beings

Pattern manifestation knowing indicates that the energy field patterns of the human and environmental fields point to a disruption due to environmental noise disturbing sleep. Voluntary mutual patterning indicates MA's preference is to go home but in the meantime she suggests closing the door to the room during the night hours and asks for pain medication at hs. After the first night, she indicates she slept a little bit better.

TABLE 24–1. (*CONT.*)

Assessment	Diagnosis	Outcomes	Planning	Implementation	Evaluation
		Sister Callista Roy's Adaptation Model			
Physiological-physical mode:	Sleep pattern disruption	Adequate rest to support healing	Will sleep 7 to 8 hours at night by time of discharge.	Since she is stable postoperatively, move her to a room farther from the nurses' station.	On day of discharge, indicates she slept better last night— at least 6 hours, more like at home.
Oxygenation— R 18, skin pink, lung sounds clear				Offer pain medication at hs.	
Nutrition—eating about ¼ of food served, fluid intake 100 cc				Close door to room at hs.	
Elimination—voiding adequately, no bowel movement since surgery					
Activity and rest—reports not sleeping well at night; learning to transfer to and from wheelchair					
Protection—protective dressings on leg wounds					
Senses—wears glasses, slightly hard of hearing					
Fluid, electrolyte, and acid-base balance— Lab values WNL					
Endocrine function—Lab values WNL					
Self-concept-group identity mode: A senior citizen					
Role function mode: Married, has cared for own home					
Interdependence mode: Social contact with others occurs through visits to her home and via telephone. Primary relationship is with husband.					
Focal stimulus: Noise at night					
Contextual stimuli: Different bed, postoperative discomfort					
Residual stimuli: Arthritis					

Betty Neuman's Systems Model

Major stressor: Blood clot that led to secondary prevention of emergency surgery	To regain system stability, need to heal surgical incisions, regain strength to walk again and regain independence	Regain independence	By two weeks after surgery, incisions will be healing without sign of infection.	Teach AM how to care for incisions and observations to make.	At time of discharge, signs of healing were appropriate. Data not yet available for longer time frames.
Life-style patterns: Maintained own home with husband			By one month after surgery will be ambulatory.	Make referral for home health physical therapy.	
Coping patterns: "Grin and bear it," do what is necessary			By two months after surgery, will be independent except for housecleaning.		
Perception of future: Hope to return to independence					
Ability to help self: Will do what doctors say					
Care from others: Husband will help and maybe daughter, who is a nurse, will be able to come help out for a few days					
Physical factors: History of hypertension, severe peripheral vascular disease. Bilateral incisions on legs					
Psycho-sociocultural factors: Lives with husband in own home					
Development: Normal for age					
Spiritual beliefs: No information					
Resources: Adequate finances; on Medicare					

TABLE 24-1. (CONT.)

Assessment	Diagnosis	Outcomes	Planning	Implementation	Evaluation
Josephine E. Paterson and Loretta T. Zderad's Humanistic Nursing					
Nurse preparing to know: The nurse has a B.S.N. and five-years experience on the vascular surgery unit. *Nurse knowing other intuitively:* Nurse perceives MA as unhappy to be in the hospital and dealing with the stress as best she can. *Nursing knowing other scientifically:* Notes history of hypertension, lab values within normal limits.	*Synthesizing information about the other with information already known, and developing a truth that is both uniquely personal and generally applicable:* Normal reaction to emergency surgery	Be with MA and encourage and support her efforts to regain well-being and develop more-being. Consider educational needs of MA and her family members.			
Jean Watson's Theory of Transpersonal Caring					
Caring interaction identifies functional deficits in relation to food and fluid intake, bowel elimination, mobility.	*Altered nutrition:* Less than body requirements related to decreased appetite	Nutritional intake adequate to support healing and regaining function	By time of discharge, fluid intake will be at least 500 cc daily and nutrient intake will be at least 1200 calories.	Explore with MA what foods and fluids are among her favorites. Provide them in frequent, small amounts.	By discharge, fluid intake 250 cc, nutrient intake 900 calories. Movement toward desired outcome but goal not reached.
Rosemarie Rizzo Parse's Theory of Human Becoming					

The nurse seeks to be in true presence with MA—the nurse prepares to be open to MA and to focus on the moment at hand. In illuminating meaning, MA indicates this surgery is "the pits" because it limits her ability to continue in her accustomed life style; in synchronizing rhythms, MA is not willing (or not yet able) to discuss the changes she will be making in her lifestyle, and in mobilizing transcendence, MA is able to talk about what it might be like to prepare to go home.

Helen C. Erickson, Evelyn M. Tomlin, and Mary Ann P. Swain's Modeling and Role-modeling

MA is in a stress state due to the emergency surgery. She has not yet mobilized resources but is interested in doing so.	MA is in a state of arousal.	MA's self-care actions will provide for appropriate use of resources and coping mechanisms.	MA will be facilitated in changing how she reaches her goals. MA will be informed about techniques she can use to meet her self-care needs.	As MA identifies her self-care needs, teaching and support will be provided to help her meet those needs.	Discharge 4 days postoperatively occurred before MA felt confident in her ability to meet her self-care needs. She could identify the needs but did not yet feel comfortable about the resources to meet them.

Madeleine M. Leininger's Theory of Culture Care Diversity and Universality

In addition to the information she already has about MA, the nurse learns that MA's culture places emphasis on the importance of independence and taking care of one's self and one's family. She believes in seeking professional care when symptoms lie outside the range of her folk care system knowledge. She also believes that it is important to follow the directions of the professional care provider.	Altered role performance related to surgery	Regain ability to perform role	Through culture congruent care, heal from surgery and walk again.	*Culture care preservation:* Provide foods she likes prepared in the manner she prefers. *Culture care accommodation:* Provide small frequent meals to tempt failing appetite *Culture care repatterning:* If she is not able to walk, provide ramp for the front porch so she can enter and exit the house.	At time of discharge, appetite remained poor. Activities need to be ongoing.

TABLE 24-1. (*CONT.*)

Assessment	Diagnosis	Outcomes	Planning	Implementation	Evaluation

Margaret Newman's Health as Expanding Consciousness

MA is at a choice point as she must function differently, at least temporarily. The nurse seeks to be present with her, providing support and information as called for by MA's pattern.

Anne Boykin and Savina Schoenhofer's Theory of Nursing as Caring

MA says she cannot sleep. The nurse offers a brief back rub to help her relax. After the back rub, the nurse straightens the linens and helps MA achieve a position of comfort in bed—on her side with a pillow at her back and another supporting her upper leg. The next morning MA reports having slept as well as she does at home and credits the caring response of the nurse, including the experience of human touch that occurred through the back rub, as making a major contribution to her ability to rest.

CHAPTER 25

NURSING THEORY AND PRACTICE WITH OTHER DISCIPLINES

■ ■ ■

Whether called collaborative, interdisciplinary, interprofessional, or transdisciplinary, practice and education involving members of more than one of the helping professions has become increasingly popular and even necessary. A CINAHL search investigated the occurrence of these terms in all listings, between 1982 and 1989, 1990 and 1999, and in 2000–2001. Table 25–1 presents the findings, along with the results from PubMed. It is of interest to note that for the approximately 15-month period of 2000–2001, in all instances there are more references than for the 8 years of 1982–1989. Also, the term *transdisciplinary* is consistently used with less frequency than any of the other terms.

The literature also is not consistent in defining these terms. Ducanis and Golin (1979) indicated they chose to use interdisciplinary, rather than multidisciplinary or transdisciplinary, as they believed interdisciplinary best described teamwork among individuals from a variety of disciplines who work together to coordinate their activities in providing service and that interdisciplinary was the term most frequently used in the literature current at that time. Casto, et al. (1994), use interprofessional to describe the interaction of persons from different professions working together with intention, mutual respect, and commitment to find a more adequate response to a human problem. They identify transdisciplinary as identifying work that involves a number of professions but does not necessarily indicate the members of those professions working together and multidisciplinary as simply indicating that more than one profession is interested in the problem and members of these professions may consult but their actions are sequential and not interactive. Massey (2001) agrees that multidisciplinary indicates the involvement of members of many disciplines who make contributions independent of each other. However, Massey describes interdisciplinary as involving mutual effort in planning and priority setting but independent in assessment and intervention and transdisciplinary as involving members of many professions who work together to address the needs of the whole person and let the problem choose the lead profession in each situation. Kuehn (1998) describes multidisciplinary as involving interaction among professionals across many disciplines, interdisciplinary as involving professionals from many disciplines working together in relation to a shared vision, and transdisciplinary as representing interaction that exists without professional boundaries.

TABLE 25–1. OCCURRENCES OF USE OF MULTIPLE PRACTICE TERMINOLOGY

Term	CINAHL				PubMed
	General	**1982–1989**	**1990–1999**	**2000–2001**	**General**
Collaboration	7165	20	706	82	12378
Interdisciplinary	2977	51	1210	154	7166
Transdisciplinary	164	2	133	12	79
Interprofessional	2452	83	420	53	22183

In spite of these differences in definitions, the value of members of various professions working together for a common goal appears as desirable. Many use the term *collaboration*, but often do not define it. This chapter will discuss collaborative practice. For the purposes of this chapter, Sullivan's (1998) definition will be used:

> Collaboration is defined as a dynamic, transforming process of creating a power sharing partnership for pervasive application in . . . practice, education, research, and organizational settings for the purposeful attention to needs and problems in order to achieve likely successful outcomes (p. 6).

Many of those whose work is found in CINAHL references discuss collaborative practice only within health care. Decanis and Golin (1979) included respiratory therapy, hospital administrators, dentists, dental assistants, dental hygienists, dieticians, physicians, medical record librarians, medical technologists, nurses, occupational therapists, optometrists, personnel and guidance counselors, physical therapists, podiatrists, psychologists, medical technologists, speech and hearing therapists, social workers and rehabilitation counselors. Sullivan (1998), in her title, limits her discussion to health care providers but includes consumers in her discussions. Corser (1998) focused on nurse–physician collaboration. Massey (2001) describes a transdisciplinary model for educating those in the health professions of nursing, respiratory therapy, physical therapy, and occupational therapy. However, others expand their discussion of collaborative practice to include helping professionals outside of health care. Casto, et al. (1994), describe the work of the Commission on Interprofessional Education and Practice in Ohio, which includes lawyers, nurses and nurse anesthetists, pastors and theologians, physicians, physical therapists, psychologists, public health practitioners, social workers, and teacher educators and teachers. Gropper and Shepard-Tew (2000) describe an educational project that involved educators, nurses, school counselors, social workers, and school psychologists. If nurses are truly interested in collaborative practice that seeks to serve the whole person, the members of the collaborative team must include helping professionals beyond health care providers.

NURSING THEORIES AND COLLABORATIVE EDUCATION AND PRACTICE

As is apparent in the chapters on the individual theories in this text, many of the nursing theories were developed with a focus on the relationship of the nurse and the patient. How do these fit with the concept of collaborative practice that involves not only other health care providers but also members of other helping professions? In some instances, the theories were developed with an eye toward including helpers other than nursing. In other instances, the theories are amenable to expansion to including others. Please note that this expansion does not necessarily make them less nursing theories, as the knowledge brought to the use of the theory will differ between disciplines or professions. Is it not interesting to consider others "borrowing" nursing theory? A review of the theories from this perspective follows.

Florence Nightingale wrote *Notes on nursing* for all women who had care of others. Since nursing was a woman's activity at that time, it is logical that she limited the application to women. However, her focus on environment and her belief that the energy for healing or improvement comes from within the person is certainly applicable by any of the helping professions.

Hildegard Peplau described interpersonal relationships and applied them to nursing. Certainly all helping professionals are involved in interpersonal relationships and Peplau's ideas could be useful to them.

Virginia Henderson sought to differentiate nursing as a separate profession and thus other professions do not as readily use some of her work. However, the concept of doing for another what he or she lacks the strength, will, or knowledge to do, and to seek to return that person to independence as soon as possible is useful to all the helping professions. The differences would come in the areas in which the professional could provide help. For example, the social worker could help with applying for food stamps for someone who lacks the knowledge of how to do this and the teacher could help a family identify a tutor to assist a child who is struggling with a subject in school.

Lydia Hall stated that the core and cure circle were shared with other members of the health professions. While care is strictly nursing's domain, and cure relates best to health care practitioners, the activities in the core circle could be relevant to other helping professionals. The professional in juvenile justice could use core to help the juvenile offender explore the motivations that led to the offense, for example.

Dorothea Orem's theories of self-care and self-deficit, while written in language that describes nursing, can be used by any helping professional. The theory of nursing systems may be less useful to others. The purpose of many collaborative efforts is to help the individual or family to regain the ability to provide self-care.

Dorothy Johnson indicated that the behavioral system, and its subsystems, were the domain of nursing and differentiated nursing from other professions. While behaviors play a role in the work of all helping professionals, the definitions provided by Johnson are less useful in a collaborative effort, unless the focus of the collaboration is on an individual.

Faye Abdellah sought to increase the focus on the patient, rather than on the disease. This basic idea, and the identification of problems as overt or covert, is useful to all helping professions. The listing of the 21 nursing problems may be of less utility.

Ida Jean Orlando and Ernestine Wiedenbach both focused on responding to a validated need of a patient. Again, the concept of validating what the client wants or needs, as well as identifying what capabilities the client has, is an important concept in collaborative practice.

Myra Levine's ideas about adaptation and conservation, while typically focused on the individual in her writings, could be expanded to families and communities. Such expansion would make the ideas quite useful for collaborative practice.

Imogene King's theory of goal attainment has resulted in the development of a goal-oriented record that has been used by health care practitioners hospital wide. Thus, it has been demonstrated to be useful to practitioners other than nurses. The concept of goals, and of outcomes, is currently one of importance to many inside and outside of health care.

Martha Rogers stated the Science of Unitary Human Beings was a basic science of nursing. While she spoke to this as differentiating nursing as a profession, the concept of energy fields is not unique to nursing and can provide a communication link with other professions.

Callista Roy's ideas of adaptive and ineffective behaviors and the need to identify the associated stimuli can be applied to individuals and groups. These are ideas that can be understood and utilized by a variety of practitioners.

Betty Neuman's Neuman Systems Model was developed with the intent that the health care team could use it. Anyone with an understanding of system theory and of the differentiation of primary, secondary, and tertiary prevention can find utility in this model.

Josephine Paterson and Loretta Zderad sought to differentiate humanistic nursing from other practices. However, their emphasis on caring is applicable to the helping professions in general.

Jean Watson also emphasizes caring, including her carative factors. Many can provide caring, although it seems that caring is often forgotten. Perhaps the use of one of the caring theories would the greatest contribution nursing could make to a collaborative model.

Rosemarie Parse also developed a basic theory of nursing. Her theory is not compatible with problem solving and thus is not as useful to a collaborative practice model.

Erickson, Tomlin, and Swain's ideas of modeling and role-modeling originated with a physician and have been developed for application in nursing practice. This supports the utility of these concepts for practitioners in the helping professions.

Madeleine Leininger's emphasis on the importance of cultural knowledge and of shaping care practices to be culturally congruent are applicable beyond nursing practice. Her three areas of preservation, accommodation, and repatterning can be used in a wide variety of situation.

Margaret Newman focuses on health and thus is more appropriate for health care professions. However, similar to Parse, her argument against serving as problem solvers limits its usefulness with collaborative practice.

Boykin and Schoenhofer's concept of caring also can be as useful as the earlier theories about caring. While they speak against problem solving, they do suggest their theory can be used with other theories that might make it more useful in a collaborative setting. Certainly their assumptions about living caring could be very helpful in establishing and growing relationships in a collaborative practice.

MODELS OF COLLABORATIVE EDUCATION OR PRACTICE

Many models for collaboration exist in both education and practice. Three will be presented here. The first, the Collaborative Care Model, was developed to support theory-based collaborative professional practice in an acute care setting. The second, the Collaborative Seminars, was developed to provide a collaborative educational experience for practitioners and practitioners-to-be in five disciplines. The third, the Negotiated Process Approach, was developed as a practice model to facilitate interactions between a health professions group and a community group. It has utility both in practice and in education.

COLLABORATIVE CARE MODEL

Lake, Keeling, Weber, & Olade (1999), describe the development of a professional practice model of health care delivery that supports the practice of many disciplines in an acute care facility. This model is known as the Collaborative Care Model (CCM) (see Figure 25–1). The model represents a system that is based in theory and standards with an emphasis on attaining optimal patient care delivery outcomes. The vision of the institution is "creating healthy lives for people and communities" (p. 53). The theoretical bases of the model were derived from the nursing theories of Neuman, Watson, and Orem.

The major focus of the model is patient-centered care. The professional practice needed to achieve this care is supported through: "standards and systems, innovation and improvement, process and pathways, clinical standards, protocols, practice standards, and care management" (Lake, et al., 1999, p. 53). Key terms in the model are outcomes and research/patient outcome information management, systems, care delivery and operations, care management, lines of defense, caring, and governance and practice. *Outcomes* and research/patient outcome information management include the identification of measurable outcomes in relation to both patient and staff satisfaction. These measurements had to be compatible with the existing information system. There are overall outcomes for the institution and individual units have developed specific outcomes, based on theories and standards of care for that unit's population. *Systems* reflect the interaction of all components of the institution in relation to the delivery of patient care. Along with standards of care and outcome measurements, systems create the umbrella from which the rest of the model components flow. *Care delivery and operations* are monitored from the unit level upward using care management, standards of practice, and protocols. *Care management* (note, not

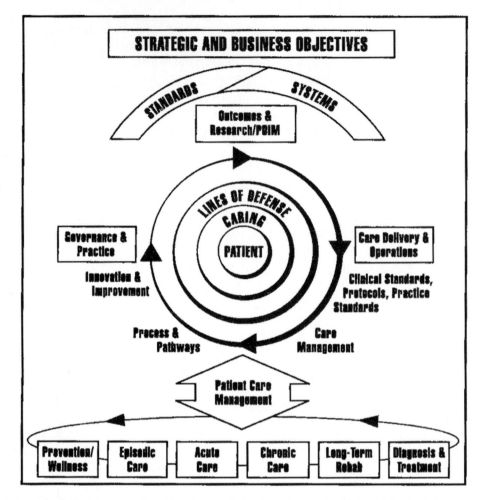

Figure 25–1. Collaborative Care Model. From Lake, M., Keeling, P., Weber G. J., & Olade, R. (1999). Collaborative care: A professional practice model. *Journal of Nursing Administration, 29*(9), 51-56.

case management) is the broad philosophical approach that supports the involvement of multiple disciplines into patient management decisions and the delivery of care. Patient care management focuses on self-care (Orem) and the restoration of health. *Defenses* are derived from the Neuman Systems Model and emphasize that patient-centered care recognizes the uniqueness of the holistic person and provides care specific to the context of that person. *Caring* is derived from Watson' theory of human caring and from Orem's theory of self-care. Caring is reflected in collaborating with the patient in meeting the patient's needs with the goals of achieving self-harmony, self-knowledge, and self-healing. *Governance and practice* is an evolving component of the model as it is based in continuous quality improvement.

The planning, implementation, and evaluation of the CCM are done by all levels of staff and has included 100% of the staff. Decision making responsibility for patient care resides in the professional nurse, based on a therapeutic relationship appropriate to the patient's individual needs. Communication occurs through collaborative care teams that include all disciplines. These teams deal with issues related to the semantics of all forms of communication, staff management and use of resources, expectations of managers, how to monitor cost-effectiveness and quality of care, and how to support professional development.

The CCM is both a model created for a specific institution and a model of how collaborative practice can be conducted. The development of this model began as a collaborative effort and continues to reflect the achievements that may be obtained through working together.

Collaborative Seminars

In contrast to the CCM, the Collaborative Seminars are an educational effort to prepare practitioners for collaborative practice. In a semester based institution, faculty from five disciplines (child and adolescent studies, criminal justice, human services, nursing [RN to BSN], and teacher education [post-baccalaureate]) each schedule one course to meet at the same time. The faculty then plan their courses so the students can meet in the collaborative seminars three times during the semester. These meetings are spaced several weeks apart so the students can process the information from them with their course materials. For example, the nursing course is Community Health Nursing and the importance of collaboration is woven throughout the course. Examples from clinical experience are frequently used to reinforce the idea from the collaborative seminars that, in many cases, care can be delivered in a manner that is cost-effective and, in particular, is less stressful for the recipient of care, if coordination of that care occurs through collaboration by the providers.

The first seminar provides an overview of the purpose of the Collaborative Seminars—to serve as a model of collaboration and to facilitate conversations among developing professionals. The students are placed in integrated groups, preassigned by major to assure each group has representation from each of the disciplines. Group size is limited to 8 to 10 students so the number of students enrolled in the five courses determines the number of groups. Each group is assigned a vignette and time is provided for small group discussion. A sample vignette is presented in Figure 25–2. All the collaborative groups return to the full seminar in time for each vignette to be presented and discussed. The purpose of this seminar is for each student to begin to learn about what other disciplines have to offer, and to learn about what members of other disciplines need to know about the student's discipline.

The second seminar has the students working in the same collaborative groups. This time the assignment is to design an agency that will provide collaborative (or integrated) services to children and families. They are to assume there are no barriers or constraints from rules, regulations, or resources. The material to be presented to the full seminar at the end of the session is to include the services to be provided, where these services will be physically located, how families will access them, and how the services will be provided by following a hypothetical family from entry into the services through returning to self-care. The purpose of this seminar is to think about what could be in a manner that can help overcome existing barriers rather than focusing on the barriers to the exclusion of creating solutions.

COLLABORATIVE ACTIVITY VIGNETTE

Min is a 5-year-old girl whose family recently immigrated from Vietnam. At school, Min appeared uncomfortable. When her friend tried to hug her, Min screamed out sharply in pain. Her teacher sent Min to the school nurse. Upon examination the nurse found Min's entire back was red and abraded, with several lacerations 2 cm long and bleeding. When asked what had happened to her, Min replied that her grandmother had "coined" her to keep her from becoming sick. Coining is an ancient ritualized practice of scraping the skin with a coin. The intent of coining is to exorcise evil spirits that could bring disease or illness to those they inhabit.

Discussion Questions:

1. From the perspective of your assumed professional position (e.g., nurse, teacher, child development professional, probation worker, therapist, and so forth), what role and responsibilities might you have for Min, or the family as a unit?
2. How would collaboration among some or all of the professionals represented in your small group change the delivery of services to these children, individually or as part of a family unit?
3. From what you know of current service delivery policies and procedures (for the professional services you represent), what encourages collaboration between and among professionals? What makes it difficult for professionals to collaborate?

Figure 25–2. Collaborative Seminars Vignette. From Julia B. George, California State University Fullerton, 1996. Used with permission.

The third seminar provides presentations from area practitioners who are involved in collaborative practice situations. The purpose of this seminar is to demonstrate the reality of collaborative practice with comparison between the real and the desired as designed in the previous seminar.

Each of the first two seminars has an out-of-class activity that helps shape the content. For example, the questions for the first seminar are "What did you learn about each discipline?" and "What questions would you like to have addressed in the next seminars?" The third seminar includes an in-class evaluation of the seminars. Contents of this evaluation are used to fine-tune the next offering of the collaborative seminars.

These seminars have provided a model of collaboration and integration as the faculty from five disciplines have worked together to plan and present them. The students have had a collaborative experience as part of their education. Feedback from employers has indicated that this knowledge of and experience with collaboration has given the graduates of these seminars an edge over others who have not had such experience.

While these seminars do not identify specific nursing theories, the nursing students do bring their theoretical approach to practice to their discussions in the small groups. The Neuman Systems Model is often mentioned, probably because of its high degree of compatibility with community health nursing. Leininger's cultural diversity and universality is also very useful, as can be seen from reading the vignette in Figure 25–2. The caring theories are also very useful in these discussions.

Negotiated Process Approach

Reeves (1987, 1990) describes her Negotiated Process Approach as a practice model of interactions between a group of health professionals and a community group. She presents basic components, assumptions, guiding principles, and a conceptual framework (see Figure 25–3).

The components are overall goal, collaboration, education/process consultation, structured joint-group interactions, negotiated agreements, joint decisions, joint par-

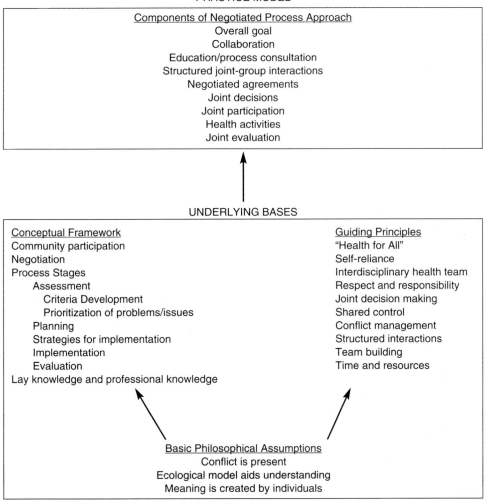

PRACTICE MODEL

Components of Negotiated Process Approach
Overall goal
Collaboration
Education/process consultation
Structured joint-group interactions
Negotiated agreements
Joint decisions
Joint participation
Health activities
Joint evaluation

UNDERLYING BASES

Conceptual Framework
Community participation
Negotiation
Process Stages
   Assessment
     Criteria Development
     Prioritization of problems/issues
   Planning
   Strategies for implementation
   Implementation
   Evaluation
Lay knowledge and professional knowledge

Guiding Principles
"Health for All"
Self-reliance
Interdisciplinary health team
Respect and responsibility
Joint decision making
Shared control
Conflict management
Structured interactions
Team building
Time and resources

Basic Philosophical Assumptions
Conflict is present
Ecological model aids understanding
Meaning is created by individuals

Figure 25–3. The Negotiated Process Approach. From Joan S. Reeves, 1987. Used with permission.

ticipation, health activities, and joint evaluation. The *overall goal* is to have interactions between a group of health professionals and members of a community group that will promote health activities to achieve higher levels of sustainable community health. *Collaboration* in this model means that the members of each group agree to work together and to try to use the negotiated process approach in doing so. The *education/process consultation* involves each group meeting separately for activities that provide information about primary health care, the Negotiated Process Approach, negotiation principles, group dynamics, and simulated negotiations and team building before they begin interaction. This consultation process is a vital initial step. The process consultant remains available to both groups and yet independent from them. *Structured joint-group interactions* are scheduled meetings for the purpose of negotiating joint decisions. *Negotiated agreements* are made through a process in which differences are recognized and explored. Conflict is viewed as a natural occurrence and the goal is to manage conflict so that differences are accepted and enhanced. The process consultant and negotiation activities are crucial in dealing with differences so that mutual agreement is reached. The method of negotiation used is that of principled negotiation as described by Fisher and Ury (1981). *Joint decisions* occur when both groups share influence. Joint decisions may or may not be negotiated decisions. *Joint participation* indicates that the groups work together by participating in the process and working on activities. *Health activities* are the community health activities that evolve from the joint group planning process. *Joint evaluation* is planned and conducted by the two groups together.

The conceptual framework for the Negotiated Process Approach consists of four concepts. *Community participation* involves participation in which each group has influence or the opportunity to influence decisions. *Negotiation* occurs through a series of actions to manage conflict. The aim in not conflict resolution but rather recognition of differences. This recognition is then used to enhance the group interactions and to manage the conflict. As the groups move toward mutual decisions, the differences narrow. The principled negotiation process to be used includes a focus on the problem and on the interests of each party and asks the involved parties to create options for mutual gain as well to use objective criteria. The planning process has five *process stages* of assessment, including criteria development and prioritization of issues; planning; implementation strategies; implementation; and evaluation. *Lay knowledge and professional knowledge* is similar to Madeleine Leininger's description of emic and etic views.

The assumptions of the Negotiated Process Approach are:

- Conflict will be present
- An ecological model provides the best approach for understanding the relationships
- Meaning is created by individuals as they interact

The guiding principles of the NPA are:

- The groups should use a social philosophy that endorses "Health for All"
- Community health activities should increase the self-reliance of community participants

- An interdisciplinary health team with flexible membership should be used in working with a community group
- A social ethic should be supported that respects the abilities of the community members and recognizes their responsibility for improving their health status.
- Joint decision making should be supported through all the process stages
- Perceptions of shared control should be promoted throughout the process
- Conflict management should be used
- The process should be based on structured interactions between the groups
- Team building should be promoted within each group
- The time and resources available to each group should be taken into consideration.

Reeves (1990) provides a detailed example of the use of the NPA by a group of graduate student health professionals and a team of women from a Hispanic community. This NPA occurred within the time constraints of the students' quarter-long field experience and resulted in an educational forum about the issue of battered women in this community.

SUMMARY

Examples of collaborative education and practice are becoming increasingly common. This chapter has sought to link such education and practice to nursing theory and demonstrate that the use of theory-based nursing practice is compatible with nursing's participation in collaborative practice. Three examples of collaborative models have been presented for further consideration by the reader.

REFERENCES

Casto, R. M., Julia, M. C., Platt, L. J., Harbaugh, G. L., Waugaman, W. R., Thompson, A., Jost, T. S., Bope, E. T., Williams, T., & Lee, D. H. (1994). *Interprofessional care and collaborative practice*. Pacific Grove, CA: Brooks/Cole.

Corser, W. D. (1998). A conceptual model of collaborative nurse–physician interactions: The management of traditional influences and personal tendencies. *Scholarly Inquiry for Nursing Practice, 12*, 325–341.

Ducanis, A. J., & Golin, A. K. (1979). *The interdisciplinary health care team: A handbook*. Germantown, MD: Aspen Systems Corporation.

Fisher, R., & Ury, W. (1981). *Getting to yes*. Boston: Houghton Mifflin.

Gropper, R. G., & Shepard-Tews, D. (2000). Project EFFECT: A case study of collaboration and cooperation. *Nursing Outlook, 48,* 276-280.

Kuehn, A. F. (1998). Collaborative health professional education: An interdisciplinary mandate for the third millennium. In T. J. Sullivan (Ed.), *Collaboration: A health care imperative.* (pp. 419-465). New York: McGraw-Hill.

Lake, M., Keeling, P., Weber, G. J., & Olade, R. (1999). Collaborative care: A professional practice model. *Journal of Nursing Administration, 29*(9), 51–56.

Massey, C. M. (2001). A transdisciplinary model for curricular revision. *Nursing and Health Care Perspectives, 22*, 85–88.

Reeves, J. S. (1987). The negotiated process approach in lay group–professional group interactions. *Dissertation Abstracts International, 49*(02B), 379.

Reeves, J. S. (1990). The use of a negotiated approach in health care: University–community group interaction. In B. B. Cassara (Ed.), *Adult education in a multicultural society* (pp. 186–195). London: Routledge.

Sullivan, T. J. (1998). *Collaboration: A health care imperative.* New York: McGraw-Hill.

GLOSSARY

Abstract concept.   An image of something neither observable nor measurable.

Achievement subsystem.   (Johnson) The behavioral subsystem relating to behaviors that attempt to control the environment and lead to personal accomplishment.

Adaptation.   (Levine) Process of adjusting or modifying behavior or functioning to fit the situation and to achieve conservation; life process by which people maintain wholeness.

Adaptation.   (Roy) Process and outcome of the use, by thinking and feeling people as individuals and groups, of conscious awareness and choice to create human and environmental integration.

Adaptation level.   (Roy) Internal pooling of stimuli with three levels:

Integrated processes working as a whole to meet human system needs.

Compensatory processes occur when response systems have been activated.

Compromised processes occur when the integrated and compensatory processes are not providing for adaptation.

Adaptive potential.   (Erickson, Tomlin, and Swain) The person's ability to mobilize resources to cope with stressors.

Adaptive responses.   (Roy) Behaviors that positively affect health through promotion of the integrity of the person in terms of survival, growth, reproduction, mastery, and transformation of the system and environment.

Affiliated-individuation.   (Erickson, Tomlin, and Swain) The individual's simultaneous needs to be attached to others and separate from them.

Agent.   (Wiedenbach) The practicing nurse, or the nurse's delegate, who serves as the propelling force in goal-directed behavior.

Aggressive subsystem.   (Johnson) The behavioral subsystem that relates to behaviors concerned with protection and self-preservation.

Arousal.   (Erickson, Tomlin, and Swain) A stress state in which the person needs assistance to moblize resources.

Assumption.   Statement or view that is widely accepted as true.

Assumption.   (Wiedenbach) The meaning a nurse attaches to an interpretation of a sensory impression.

Attachment or affiliative subsystem.   (Johnson) The behavioral subsystem that is the first formed and provides for a strong social bond.

Authority.   (King) An active, reciprocal relationship that involves values, experience, and perceptions in defining, validating, and accepting the right of an individual to act within an organization.

Automatic activities.   (Orlando) Nursing actions decided on for reasons other than the patient's immediate need.

---

*When a term relates specifically to a theorist, the name of the theorist appears in parentheses after the term.

588 NURSING THEORIES: THE BASE FOR PROFESSIONAL NURSING PRACTICE

Basic conditioning factors. (Orem) Aspects that influence the individual's self-care ability; include age, gender, stage of development, state of health, sociocultural orientation, health care system and family system factors, patterns of living, environment, availability and adequacy of resources.

Body image. (King) Individuals' perceptions of their own bodies, influenced by the reactions of others.

Call and response. (Paterson and Zderad) Simultaneous, sequential transactions, possibly all-at-once.

Care. (Hall) The exclusive aspect of nursing that provides the patient bodily comfort through "laying on of hands" and provides an opportunity for closeness.

Care. (Leininger) (noun) Phenomena related to assistive, supportive, or enabling behavior toward or for another individual (or group) with evident or anticipated needs to ameliorate or improve a human condition or lifeway.

Care. (Leininger) (gerund) Action directed toward assisting, supporting, or enabling behavior of another individual (or group) with evident or anticipated needs to ameliorate or improve a human condition or lifeway.

Caring. (Boykin and Schoenhofer) Intentional and authentic presence recognizing the other as living and growing in caring.

Caring (healing) consciousness. (Watson) The field within which caring occasions occur.

Caring occasion/moment. (Watson) The coming together of a nurse and another in human-to-human transaction.

Central purpose. (Wiedenbach) The commitment of the individual nurse, based on a personal philosophy, that defines the desired quality of health and specifies the nurse's special responsibility in providing care to assist others in achieving or sustaining that quality.

Clustering of data. The grouping of data pieces that fit together and show relationships.

Cocreating. (Parse) Participation of human and environment in creating the pattern of each.

Cognator mechanism. (Roy) Coping mechanism or control subsystem that relates to the higher brain functions of perception, information processing, learning, judgment, and emotion.

Communication. (King) A direct or indirect process in which one person gives information to another.

Community. (Paterson and Zderad) Two or more persons striving together, living–dying all-at-once.

Concept. An abstract notion; a vehicle of thought that involves images; words that describe objects, properties, or events.

Connecting–separating. (Parse) The rhythmical process of moving together and apart.

Consciousness. (Newman) The information of the system; the system's capacity to interact with the environment.

Conservation. (Levine) Defense of the wholeness of a living system through the most economical use of resources; ensures ability to confront change appropriately and retain unique identity.

Conservation of energy. (Levine) Balancing energy output with energy input to avoid excessive fatigue.

Conservation of personal integrity. (Levine) Maintaining or restoring the patient's sense of identity and self-worth.

Conservation of social integrity. (Levine) Acknowledging the patient as a social being.

Conservation of structural integrity. (Levine) Maintaining or restoring the structure of the body.

Contextual stimuli. (Roy) Stimuli of the human system's internal or external world, other than those immediately confronting the system, that influence the situation and are observable, measurable, or subjectively reported by the system as having a positive or negative effect.

Core. (Hall) The aspect of client interaction shared with any health professional who therapeutically uses a freely offered closeness to help the patient discover who he or she is.

Core. (Neuman) The basic structure and energy resources of the system.

Covert problem. Hidden or concealed condition of concern.

Cultural imposition. (Leininger) Efforts of an outsider, subtle and not so subtle, to impose his or her own cultural values, beliefs, or behaviors upon an individual, family, or group from another culture.

Cultural values. (Leininger) Values that are derived from the culture, identify desirable ways of acting or knowing, guide decision making, and are often held over long periods.

Culture. (Leininger) Learned, shared, and transmitted values, beliefs, norms, and lifeway practices of a particular group that guide thinking, decisions, and actions in patterned ways.

Culture Care. (Leininger) The subjectively and objectively learned and transmitted values, beliefs, and patterned expressions that assist, support, facilitate, or enable another individual or group to maintain well-being, improve a human condition or lifeway, or face death and disabilities.

Culture care accommodation/negotiation. (Leininger) Assistive, supportive, or enabling professional actions and decisions that help clients of a particular culture to adapt to, or negotiate for a beneficial or satisfying health status, or to face death.

Culture care diversity. (Leininger) The variability of meanings, patterns, values, lifeways, or symbols of care that are culturally derived by humans for their well-being, through assisting, supporting, facilitating, or enabling.

Culture care preservation/maintenance. (Leininger) Assistive, supportive, or enabling professional actions and decisions that help clients of a particular culture to preserve or maintain a state of health, or to recover from illness, and to face death.

Culture care repatterning/restructuring. (Leininger) Assistive, supportive, or enabling professional actions or decisions that help clients change their lifeways for new or different patterns that are culturally meaningful and satisfying, or that support beneficial and healthy life patterns.

Culture care universality. (Leininger) Common, similar, dominant, or uniform meanings, patterns, values, or symbols of care that are culturally derived by humans for their well-being or to improve a human condition and lifeway or to face death.

Culture shock. (Leininger) Experiencing feelings of discomfort, helplessness, disorientation while attempting to comprehend or adapt effectively to a different cultural group.

Cure. (Hall) An aspect of nursing shared with medical personnel in which the nurse helps the patient and family through medical, surgical, and rehabilitative care.

Decision making in organizations. (King) An active process in which choice, directed by goals, is made and acted upon.

Deliberative actions. (Orlando) Nursing actions that ascertain or meet the patient's immediate need.

Dependency subsystem. (Johnson) The behavioral subsystem in which behaviors evoke nurturing behaviors in others.

Dialogue. (Paterson and Zderad) An intersubjective experience in which individuals relate creatively and have a real sharing.

Discrepancy. (Johnson) Action that does not achieve the intended goal.

Dominance. (Johnson) Primary use of one behavioral subsystem to the detriment of the other subsystems and regardless of the situation.

Drive. (Johnson) Stimulus to behavior.

Eliminative subsystem. (Johnson) The behavioral subsystem that relates to socially acceptable behaviors surrounding the excretion of waste products from the body.

Emic. (Leininger) Personal knowledge or explanation of behavior; indigenous, not universal.

Empirical. Measured or observed through the senses.

Enabling–limiting. (Parse) Making choices results in enabling an individual in some ways while limiting in others.

Energy field. (Rogers) The dynamic, infinite, fundamental unit of both the living and nonliving.

Environment. (Neuman) Those forces that surround humans at any given point in time; may be internal, external, or created.

Environment. (Nightingale) External conditions and influences that affect life and development.

Environment. (Rogers) Pan-dimensional, negentropic energy field identified by pattern and integral with the human energy field.

Environment. (Roy) All conditions, circumstances, and influences surrounding and affecting the development and behavior of human systems. Special attention is to be paid to person and earth resources.

Environmental context. (Leininger) The totality of an event, situation, or particular experience that gives meaning to human expressions, including physical, ecological, social interactions, emotional, and cultural dimensions.

Epistemology. The study of the history of knowledge, including the origin, nature, methods, and limitations of knowledge development.

Equifinality. An open system that may attain a state independent of time or initial conditions and determined only by the system parameters.

Equilibrium. (Erickson, Tomlin, and Swain) A nonstress state. In adaptive equilibrium all subsystems are in harmony. In maladaptive equilibrium, one or more subsystems are placed in jeopardy to maintain the nonstress state.

Ethnonursing. (Leininger) The study of nursing care beliefs, values, and practices as cognitively perceived and known by a designated culture through their direct experience, beliefs, and value system.

Existential psychology. The study of human existence using phenomenological analysis.

Extrapersonal stressors. (Neuman) Forces occurring outside the system that generate a reaction or response from the system.

First-level assessment. (Roy) Behavioral assessment; the gathering of output behaviors of the person in relation to the four adaptive modes.

Flexible line of defense. (Neuman) Variable and constantly changing biological-psychological-sociocultural-developmental and spiritual ability to respond to stressors.

Focal stimulus. (Roy) Stimulus of the human system's internal or external world that immediately confronts the system.

Framework. (Wiedenbach) The human, environmental, professional, and organizational facilities that make up the context in which nursing is practiced and that constitute its currently existing limits.

General system theory. A general science of wholeness.

Generic care system. (Leininger) Traditional or local indigenous health care or cure practices that have special meanings and uses to heal or assist people and are generally offered in familiar home or community environmental contexts with their local practitioners.

Goal. (Wiedenbach) Outcome the nurse seeks to achieve.

Grand theory. Theory that covers broad areas of a discipline; may not be testable.

Growth and development. (King) The process in the lives of individuals that involves changes at the cellular, molecular, and behavioral levels and helps them move from potential to achievement.

Health problem.
> *Actual.* Client need that currently exists.
> *Potential.* Client need that may occur in the future and which may be averted with appropriate action.

Helicy. (Rogers) The nature and direction of human and environmental change; change that is continuously innovative, unpredictable, and characterized by increasing diversity of the human field and environmental field pattern emerging out of the continuous, mutual, simultaneous interaction between the human and environmental fields and manifesting nonrepeating rhythmicities.

Historicity. (Levine) Aspect of adaptation in which responses are based on past experiences.

Holism. A theory that the universe and especially living nature are correctly seen in terms of interacting wholes that are more than the mere sum of the individual parts.

Illness. (Levine) State of altered health.

Illness. (Neuman) State of insufficiency in which needs are yet to be satisfied.

Imaging. (Parse) The picturing or making real of events, ideas, and people, explicitly or tacitly.

Impoverishment. (Erickson, Tomlin, and Swain) A stress state in which the person needs external resources, including affliation.

Incompatibility. (Johnson) Two behavioral subsystems in the same situation being in conflict with each other.

Ineffective responses. (Roy) Behaviors that do not promote the integrity of the human system in terms of survival, growth, reproduction, mastery, and transformation of the system and environment.

Ingestive subsystem. (Johnson) The behavioral subsystem that relates to the meanings and structures of social events surrounding the occasions when food is eaten.

Innovator system. (Roy) A group control mechanism that involves change and growth.

Insufficiency. (Johnson) A behavioral subsystem that is not functioning adequately.

Integrality. (Rogers) The continuous, mutual, simultaneous process of human and environmental fields.

Interactions. (King) The observable, goal-directed, behaviors of two or more persons in mutual presence.

Interdependence mode. (Roy) The social context in which relationships occur; involves nurturing, respect, values, context, infrastructure, and resources.

Interpersonal stressors. (Neuman) Forces that occur between two or more individuals and evoke a reaction or response.

Intrapersonal stressors. (Neuman) Forces occurring within a person that result in a reaction or response.

Languaging. (Parse) Reflection of images and values through speaking and moving.

Lines of resistance. (Neuman) The internal set of factors (biological, psychological, sociocultural, developmental, and spiritual) that seek to stabilize the system when stressors break through the normal line of defense; the defense closest to the core.

Logical empiricism. Worldview in which truth must be confirmed by objective, sensory experiences that are to be relatively value free.

Means. (Wiedenbach) The activities and devices that enable the nurse to attain the desired goal.

Meeting. (Paterson and Zderad) The coming together of human beings characterized by the expectation that there will be a nurse and a nursed.

Metaparadigm. Core context of a discipline.

Metatheory. Theory about theory development.

Modeling. (Erickson, Tomlin, and Swain) Process used by the nurse to gain an understanding of the client's world as the client perceives it.

More-being. (Paterson and Zderad) The process of becoming all that is humanly possible.

Movement. (Newman) Change that occurs between two states of rest.

Need for help. (Orlando) A requirement for assistance in decreasing or eliminating immediate distress or in improving the sense of adequacy.

Normal line of defense. (Neuman) The biological-psychological-sociocultural-developmental-spiritual skills developed over a lifetime to achieve stability and deal with stressors.

Nurse reaction. (Orlando). Portion of the nursing process discipline in which the nurse responds to the patient's behavior through expressing the nurse's perception, thought, or feeling and seeking congruence between these and the patient's immediate need.

Nursing problem. (Abdellah) A condition faced by the client or client's family with which the nurse can assist through the performance of professional functions.

Nursing process. A deliberate, intellectual activity by which the practice of nursing is approached in an orderly, systematic manner. It includes the following components:

Assessment. The process of data collection and analysis that results in a conclusion or nursing diagnosis.

Diagnosis. A behavioral statement that identifies the client's actual or potential health problem, deficit, or concern that can be affected by nursing actions.

Outcomes identification. Establishing the desired results in terms that are culturally appropriate and realistic.

Planning. The determination of what can be done to assist the client, including setting goals, judging priorities, and designing methods to resolve problems.

Implementation. Action initiated to accomplish defined goals.

Evaluation. The appraisal of the client's behavioral changes that result from the action of the nurse.

Outcome evaluation. Evaluation based on behavioral changes.

Structure evaluation. Evaluation relating to the availability of appropriate equipment.

Process evaluation. Evaluation that focuses on the activities of the nurse.

Reassessment. The process of collecting additional data during the planning, implementing, and evaluation phases of the nursing process that may lead to immediate changes in those phases, or a change in the nursing diagnosis.

Nursing situation. (Boykin and Schoenhofer) Shared living experience in which personhood is enhanced through caring between nurse and nursed.

Nursing system. (Orem) Plan of care developed by the nurse to meet the person's self-care deficit.

Partly compensatory nursing system. A situation in which both nurse and patient perform care measures or other actions involving manipulative tasks or ambulation.

Supportive-educative nursing system. A situation in which the patient is able to, or can and should learn to, perform required therapeutic self-care measures but needs assistance to do so.

Wholly compensatory nursing system. A situation in which the patient has no active role in the performance of self-care.

Nurturer. (Hall) A fosterer of learning, growing, and healing.

Objective. A specific means by which one proposes to accomplish or attain the goal.

Ontology. A branch of metaphysics that studies the nature of being and of reality.

Organization. (King) An entity made up of individuals who have prescribed roles and positions and who use resources to achieve goals.

Orientation phase. (Peplau) The first phase of Peplau's nurse–patient relationship. Through assessment, the patient's health needs, expectations, and goals are explored and a care plan is devised. Concurrently, the roles of nurse and patient are being identified and clarified.

Originating. (Parse) A continuing process of creating personal uniqueness while in mutual energy exchange with the environment.

Outcome. The actual or desired result of actions taken.

Overt problem. Apparent or obvious condition of concern.

Paradigm. (Rogers) A way of viewing the world; a particular perspective of reality.

Pattern. (Newman) Movement, diversity, and rhythm that depict the whole.

Pattern. (Rogers) The distinguishing or identifying characteristic of an energy field.

Perceived view. Worldview that focuses on the person as a whole and values the lived experience of the person.

Perception. (King) An individual's view of reality that gives meaning to personal experience and involves the organization, interpretation, and transformation of information from sensory data and memory.

Phenomenology. The study of the meaning of phenomena to a particular individual; a way of understanding people from the way things appear to them.

Physiological-physical mode. (Roy) Involves the human system's physical response to and interaction with the environment.

Potential comforter. (Hall) The role of the nurse seen by the patient during the care aspect of nursing.

Potential painer. (Hall) The role of the nurse seen by the patient during the cure aspect of nursing.

Power. (King) A social force and ability to use resources to influence people to achieve goals.

Powering. (Parse) An energizing force the rhythm of which is the pushing–resisting interhuman encounters.

Prescription. (Wiedenbach) A directive for activity that specifies both the nature of the action and the necessary thought process.

Prescriptive theory. (Wiedenbach) A theory that conceptualizes both the desired situation and the activities to be used to bring about the desired situation.

Presence. (Paterson and Zderad) The quality of being open, receptive, ready, and available to another in a reciprocal manner.

Primary prevention. (Neuman) The application of general knowledge in a client situation to try to identify and protect against the potential effects of stressors before they occur.

Problem-solving process. Identifying the problem, selecting pertinent data, formulating hypotheses, testing hypotheses through the collection of data, and revising hypotheses.

Professional health system. (Leininger) Professional care or cure services offered by diverse health personnel who have been prepared through formal professional programs of study in special educational institutions.

Professional nursing action. (Orlando) What the nurse says or does for the benefit of the patient.

Proposition. A statement explaining relationships among concepts.

Qualitative research. Dynamic, organized investigations of the thoughts, feelings, and experiences of human beings.

Quantitative research. Systematic studies that involve empirical data analyzed through statistical methods.

Realities in the immediate situation. (Wiedenbach) At any given moment, all factors at play in the situation in which nursing actions occur; realities include the agent, the recipient, the goal, the means, and the framework.

Received view. *See* Logical empiricism.

Recipient. (Wiedenbach) The vulnerable and dependent patient who is characterized by personal attributes, problems, and capabilities, including the ability to cope.

Reconstitution. (Neuman) The increase in energy that occurs in relation to the degree of reaction to a stressor.

Redundancy. (Levine) Aspect of adaptation related to numerous levels of response available for a given challenge.

Reflective technique. (Hall) The process of helping the patient see who he or she is by mirroring what the person's behavior says, both verbally and nonverbally.

Regulator mechanism. (Roy) Coping mechanism subsystem that includes chemical, neural, and endocrine transmitters and autonomic and psychomotor responses.

Relating. (Paterson and Zderad) The process of nurse–nursed doing with each other, being with each other.

Residual stimuli. (Roy) Internal or external factors of the human system whose current effects are unclear.

Resonancy. (Rogers) The identification of the human field and the environmental field by wave pattern manifesting continuous change from lower-frequency longer waves to higher-frequency shorter waves.

Revealing–concealing. (Parse) Actions in interpersonal relationships that reveal one part of oneself and, as a result, conceal other parts.

Role. (King) The set of behaviors and rules that relate to an individual in a position in a social system.

Role function mode. (Roy) This mode involves knowing the relationship of the system to others so the system can behave appropriately.

Role Modeling. (Erickson, Tomlin, and Swain) Planning and implementing individualized care based on the client's model of the world to facilitate health.

Secondary prevention. (Neuman) Treatment of symptoms of stress reaction to lead to reconstitution.

Second-level assessment. (Roy) The collection of data about focal, contextual, and residual stimuli impinging on the person.

Self-care. (Orem) Practice of activities that individuals personally initiate and perform on their own behalf to maintain life, health, and well-being.

Self-care action. (Erickson, Tomlin, and Swain) Use of self-care knowledge and self-care resources.

Self-care agency. (Orem) The human ability to engage in self-care.

Self-care deficit. (Orem) The inability of an individual to carry out all necessary self-care activities; self-care demand exceeds self-care agency.

Self-care knowledge. (Erickson, Tomlin, and Swain) Knowledge about what has made one sick, lessened one's effectiveness, or interfered with one's growth; also includes knowledge of what will make one well, fulfilled, or effective.

Self-care requisites. (Orem) The impetus for self-care activities. Three types:

> ***Developmental self-care requisites.*** Maintaining conditions to support life and development or to provide preventive care for adverse conditions that affect development.

> ***Health deviation self-care requisites.*** Care needed by individuals who are ill or injured; may result from medical measures required to correct illness or injury.

Universal self-care requisites. Those requisites, common to all human beings throughout life, associated with life processes and the integrity of human structure and function.

Self-care resources. (Erickson, Tomlin, and Swain) An individual's strengths and supports that will help gain, maintain, and promote optimal health.

Self-concept-group identity mode. (Roy) Behaviors related to integrity; involves self-concept, body sensation, body image, self-consistency, self-ideal, moral-ethical-spiritual self, interpersonal relationships, and social milieu.

Set. (Johnson) An individual's predisposition to behave in a certain way.

Sexual subsystem. (Johnson) The behavioral subsystem that reflects socially acceptable behaviors related to procreation.

Simultaneity paradigm. (Parse) A view of humans as unitary beings who are in continuous interrelationship with the environment and whose health is a negentropic unfolding determined by the individual.

Social structure. (Leininger) The dynamic nature of interrelated structural and organizational factors of a particular culture (or society) and how those factors function to give meaning and structural order including educational, technological, and cultural factors.

Space. (King) A universal area, known also as territory, that is defined in part by the behavior of those who occupy it.

Specificity. (Levine) Aspect of adaptation in which responses are task specific and particular challenges lead to particular responses.

Stabilizer subsystem. (Roy) A group control mechanism that involves the structures, values, and daily activities that accomplish the work of the group.

Status. (King) The relationship of an individual to a group, or a group to other groups, including identified duties, obligations, and privileges.

Stress. (King) A positive or negative energy response to interactions with the environment in an effort to maintain balance in living.

Stressors. (Neuman) Stimuli that result in tensions and have the potential to create system instability.

Termination phase. (Peplau) The third and final phase of Peplau's nurse–patient relationship. This phase evolves from the successful completion of the previous phases. The patient and nurse terminate their therapeutic relationship as the patient's needs are met and movement is made toward new goals.

Tertiary prevention. (Neuman) Activities that seek to strengthen the lines of resistance after reconstitution has occurred.

Theory. Creative and systematic way of looking at the world or an aspect of it to describe, explain, predict, or control it.

Therapeutic interpersonal relationship. (Peplau) A relationship between patient and nurse in which their collaborative effort is directed toward identifying, exploring, and resolving the patient's need productively. The relationship progresses along a continuum as each experiences growth through an increasing understanding of one another's roles, attitudes, and perceptions.

Therapeutic self-care demand. (Orem) The sum or total of self-actions needed, during some period, to meet self-care requisites.

Time. (King) The relation of one event to another, uniquely experienced by each individual.

Totality paradigm. (Parse) View of man as a summative being, a combination of bio-psycho-social-spiritual aspects, surrounded by an environment of external and internal stimuli. Man interacts with the environment to maintain equilibrium and achieve goals. Health is a state of well-being measured against norms.

Transactions. (King) Observable behaviors between individuals and their environment that lead to the attainment of valued goals.

Transcultural nursing. (Leininger) A learned subfield or branch of nursing that focuses on the comparative study and analysis of cultures with respect to nursing and health–illness caring practices, beliefs, and values. The goal is to provide meaningful and efficacious nursing care services to people according to their cultural values and health–illness context.

Transformation. (Newman) Change occurring all-at-once.

Transforming. (Parse) The changing of change apparent in increasing diversity.

Transpersonal caring relationship. (Watson) A relationship that occurs with a caring consciousness in which the life space of another is entered, the other's state of being detected and experienced with a response that provides for the release of the other's feelings, thoughts, or tensions.

Unitary humans. (Rogers) Pandimensional, negentropic energy fields identified by pattern and manifesting characteristics and behaviors different from those of the parts, and which cannot be predicted from knowledge of the parts.

Valuing. (Parse) The process of living cherished beliefs while adding to one's worldview.

Veritivity. (Roy) The common purposefulness of human existence.

Well-being. (Paterson and Zderad) A steady state.

Working phase. (Peplau) The second phase of Peplau's nurse–patient relationship. The perceptions and expectations of the patient and nurse become more involved while building a working relationship of further identifying the problem and deciding on appropriate plans for improved health maintenance. The patient takes full advantage of all available services while feeling an integral part of the helping environment. Goals are met through a collaborative effort as the patient becomes independent during convalescence.

Worldview. (Leininger) The way in which people look at the world, or universe, and form a value stance about the world and their lives.

INDEX